Handbook of Oleoresins

Handbook of Oleoresins
Extraction, Characterization, and Applications

Edited by
Gulzar Ahmad Nayik, Amir Gull, and Tariq Ahmad Ganaie

CRC Press
Taylor & Francis Group
Boca Raton London New York

CRC Press is an imprint of the
Taylor & Francis Group, an **informa** business

First edition published 2022
by CRC Press
6000 Broken Sound Parkway NW, Suite 300, Boca Raton, FL 33487-2742

and by CRC Press
2 Park Square, Milton Park, Abingdon, Oxon, OX14 4RN

CRC Press is an imprint of Taylor & Francis Group, LLC

Library of Congress Cataloging-in-Publication Data
Names: Nayik, Gulzar Ahmad, editor. | Gull, Amir, editor. | Ganaie, Tariq Ahmad, editor.
Title: Handbook of oleoresins : extraction, characterization and applications / edited by Gulzar Ahmad Nayik, Amir Gull & Tariq Ahmad Ganaie.
Description: First edition. | Boca Raton : Taylor and Francis, 2022. | Includes bibliographical references and index.
Identifiers: LCCN 2021056707 (print) | LCCN 2021056708 (ebook) |
ISBN 9781032014005 (hardback) | ISBN 9781032030029 (paperback) | ISBN 9781003186205 (ebook)
Subjects: LCSH: Oleoresins. Classification: LCC RS201.O6 H36 2022 (print) | LCC RS201.O6 (ebook) |
DDC 583/.93—dc23/eng/20211124
LC record available at https://lccn.loc.gov/2021056707
LC ebook record available at https://lccn.loc.gov/2021056708

ISBN: 978-1-032-01400-5 (hbk)
ISBN: 978-1-032-03002-9 (pbk)
ISBN: 978-1-003-18620-5 (ebk)

DOI: 10.1201/9781003186205

Typeset in Minion
by codeMantra

Dedicated to my Late Grandparents
Ghulam Mohiuddin Naik & Raja Begam Binti Damsaaz

Contents

Preface

CONSUMER DEMAND FOR NATURAL AND HERBAL PRODUCTS CONTINUES TO RISE, and the desired focus for oleoresins is growing. Spices and condiments are known for their natural flavours. Similar to various plant extractives like essential oils, oleoresins form the largest category of flavourings available to the flavourists. Oleoresin represents the true essence of spices enriched with volatile and non-volatile essential oil and resinous fraction. India is the largest producer of spices (produces 683,000 tons per annum), which is around 31% of total world production. Oleoresin is a viscous liquid or semi-solid material obtained from spices, extracted with a hydrocarbon solvent such as acetone, ethanol, ethyl acetate, or ethylene dichloride, which contains the aroma and flavour of its source. A two-stage process is employed for their extraction, in which the oil is first recovered along with the resins by solvent extraction, and later the oil is recovered by steam distillation followed by solvent extraction for recovering the oleoresin. Oleoresins are 5–20 times stronger in flavour than their corresponding spices, whose pungency depends on the original powder's pungency, and the yield varies from 7% to 15% depending on varieties. The main components of an oleoresin include essential oils, fixed oils, pigments, pungent constituents, and natural antioxidants.

The oleoresin represents the wholesome flavour of the spice—a cumulative effect of the sensation of smell and taste. Therefore, it is designated as the "true essence" of the spice and can replace spice powders in food products without altering the flavour profile. The oleoresin may be rendered water-soluble using permitted emulsifiers or converted to powder form by dispersing on dry carriers. These plated products impart the strength of good-quality freshly ground spices and can be easily incorporated into food. Oleoresins have many advantages over whole or ground spices. Oleoresins are easy to store and transport because concentrated forms reduce space and bulk. They can be more heat-stable than raw spices and have a longer shelf life due to lower moisture content. Oleoresins have consistency in flavour, full release of flavour during cooking, and easy blendability to achieve the desired features. Oleoresins possess antioxidant, antibacterial, and antifungal properties. Oleoresins are extensively used in the treatment of anorexia, colic, cramp, flatulence, dyspepsia, heartburn, vomiting, indigestion, griping pains, and halitosis. These are also used in the treatment of fever, pulmonary diseases, and digestive problems.

The market for spice oleoresins is largely untapped, and Indian homes are still not familiar with the product. The world is moving towards natural products. Spices lend colour, taste, and flavour, and they are a good source of antioxidants and have preservative as well as therapeutic power. Therefore, it is important to understand and document the chemistry, characterization, properties, and applications of oleoresins. This book contains brief information on oleoresins—production, composition, properties, applications (medicinal and health properties), etc. It has been designed to be a practical tool for the many diverse professionals who develop and market spices and oleoresins.

Gulzar Ahmad Nayik
Amir Gull
Tariq Ahmad Ganaie

Editors

Dr. Gulzar Ahmad Nayik completed his Master's Degree in Food Technology at Islamic University of Science & Technology, Kashmir, India and PhD at Sant Longowal Institute of Engineering & Technology, Sangrur, Punjab, India. He has published over 55 peer-reviewed research and review papers and 31 book chapters, edited five books, published one textbook, and has delivered a number of presentations at various national and international conferences, seminars, workshops, and webinars. Dr Nayik was shortlisted twice for the prestigious Inspire-Faculty Award in 2017 and 2018 from Indian National Science Academy, New Delhi. He was nominated for India's prestigious National Award (Indian National Science Academy Medal for Young Scientists 2019–2020). Dr Nayik also fills the roles of editor, associate editor, assistant editor, and reviewer for many food science and technology journals. He has received many awards, appreciations, and recognitions and holds membership of various international societies and organizations. Dr Nayik is currently editing several book projects in Elsevier, Taylor & Francis, and Royal Society of Chemistry.

Dr. Amir Gull completed his Master's Degree in Food Technology at Islamic University of Science & Technology, Kashmir, India and PhD at Sant Longowal Institute of Engineering & Technology, Longowal, Sangrur, Punjab, India. Dr Gull has published 35+ peer-reviewed research and review papers in reputed journals. He has also published two edited books in Springer, 10+ book chapters and delivered many presentations in many national and international conferences. Dr Gull's main research activities include developing functional food products from millets. Dr. Gull is also serving as an editorial board member and reviewer of several journals. He is also an active member of the Association of Food Scientist & Technologist India. He is also the recipient of MANF from UGC India.

Dr. Tariq Ahmad Ganaie is working as Senior Assistant Professor and incharge Head in the Department of Food Technology, Islamic University of Science and Technology (IUST), Kashmir, India. He has worked as an Assistant Professor in the same from 2007 to 2013; after that, he was promoted as Senior Assistant Professor. He completed B.Sc. (Hons) in Chemistry in 1998, M.Sc. in Chemistry in 2001, and M.Tech (Agriculture Processing and Food Engineering) at Aligarh Muslim University, Aligarh, UP, India in

2005. In 2021, he completed his PhD (Food Science and Technology) at the University of Kashmir, India. He has published many papers in reputed national and international journals with high impact factors. He has organized many national and international conferences, workshops, and symposia. He has delivered many invited talks and is on the editorial board of many reputed national and international journals.

Contributors

Laura Natali Afanador-Barajas
Programa de Biología, Facultad de
    Ingeniería y Ciencias Básicas
Universidad Central
Bogotá D.C, Colombia

Tahmeena Ahad
University of Kashmir
Srinagar, India

Asif Ahmad
Institute of Food and
    Nutritional Sciences
PMAS-Arid Agriculture University
Rawalpindi, Pakistan

Sajid Ali
Institute of Agricultural Sciences
University of the Punjab
Lahore, Pakistan

Shinawar Waseem Ali
Institute of Agricultural Sciences
University of the Punjab
Lahore, Pakistan

Tahira Mohsin Ali
Department of Food Science and
    Technology
University of Karachi
Karachi, Pakistan

Aayeena Altaf
Department of Food Technology
Jamia Hamdard
New Delhi, India

Iqra Azam
Department of Food Science and
    Technology
University of Kashmir
Srinagar, India

Vikas Bansal
Department of Food Technology, School of
    Engineering & Technology
Jaipur National University
Jaipur, India

Cecilia Bañuelos
Programa Transdisciplinario en Desarrollo
    Científico y Tecnológico para la
    Sociedad
Centro de Investigación y de Estudios
    Avanzados del Instituto Politécnico
    Nacional
Ciudad de México, México

Barkha
Department of Agronomy, School of
    Agriculture
Lovely Professional University
Phagwara, India

Garima Bhardwaj
Department of Chemistry
Sant Longowal Institute of Engineering
    and Technology
Longowal, Sangrur, India

Suheela Bhat
Department of Food Engineering &
    Technology
Sant Longowal Institute of Engineering
    and Technology
Longowal, India

Tejasvi Bhatia
Department of Forensic Science,
    School of Bioengineering and
    Biosciences
Lovely Professional University
Phagwara, India

Hanuman Bobade
Department of Food Science and
    Technology
Punjab Agricultural University
Ludhiana, India

Tridip Boruah
PG Department of Botany
Madhab Choudhury College
Barpeta, India

Natasha Abbas Butt
Department of Food Science and
    Technology
University of Karachi
Karachi, Pakistan

Marycarmen Cortés-Hernández
Instituto de Ciencias Agropecuarias
Universidad Autónoma del Estado de
    Hidalgo
Hidalgo, México

Aamir Hussain Dar
Department of Food Technology
Islamic University of Science and
    Technology
Kashmir, India

Gargee Dey
PG Department of Botany
Madhab Choudhury College
Barpeta, India

Adriana Patricia Diaz-Morales
Programa de Biología, Facultad de
    Ingeniería y Ciencias Básicas
Universidad Central
Bogotá D.C, Colombia

Mujahid Farid
Department of Environmental Sciences
University of Gujrat
Gujrat, Pakistan

Apurba Gohain
Department of Chemistry
Assam University Silchar
Silchar, India

Adeel Hakim
Department of Food Science and
    Technology
MNS-University of Agriculture
Multan, Pakistan

Monika Hans
Govt. PG College for Women Gandhi
    Nagar
Jammu, India

Jashanpreet Kaur
Department of Chemistry
Mata Gujri College
Fatehgarh Sahib, India

Shaheen Khurshid
Department of Zoology
Govt. Degree College Tral
J&K, India

Muhammad Suhail Ibrahim
Institute of Food and Nutritional Sciences
PMAS-Arid Agriculture University
Rawalpindi, Pakistan

Shafeeqa Irfan
Institute of Food Science and Nutrition
University of Sargodha
Sargodha, Pakistan

Yash D. Jagdale
MIT School of Food Technology
MIT ADT University
Pune, India

Najeeb Jahan
Department of Ilmul Advia
   (Pharmacology)
National Institute of Unani Medicine
Bengaluru, India

Shweta Joshi
G.B. Pant University of Agriculture &
   Technology
Pantnagar, India

Rabia Kanwal
Institute of Food Science and Nutrition
University of Sargodha
Sargodha, Pakistan

Gurpreet Kaur
Department of Zoology
Mata Gujri College
Fatehgarh Sahib, India

Kamalpreet Kaur
Department of Chemistry
Mata Gujri College
Fatehgarh Sahib, India

Bababode Adesegun Kehinde
Department of Biosystems and
   Agricultural Engineering
University of Kentucky
Lexington, Kentucky

Ashwani Kumar Khajuria
Government Degree College
   for Women
Kathua, India

Jasmeet Kour
Govt. PG College for Women Gandhi
   Nagar
Jammu, India

Preeti Kukkar
Department of Chemistry
Mata Gujri College
Fatehgarh Sahib, India

Shailja Kumari
School of Applied Sciences and
   Biotechnology
Shoolini University of
   Biotechnology and Management
   Sciences
Solan, India

Tanu Malik
Department of Food Technology and
   Nutrition
Lovely Professional University
Phagwara, India

Lubna Masoodi
Department of Food Science and
    Technology
University of Kashmir
Srinagar, India

Gabriela Medina-Peréz
Instituto de Ciencias
    Agropecuarias
Universidad Autónoma del Estado de
    Hidalgo
Hidalgo, México

Sumera Mehfooz
Department of Ilmul Advia
    (Pharmacology)
National Institute of Unani Medicine
Bengaluru, India

Imtiyaz Ahmad Mir
AYUSH Department of
    Health & Medical Education
Government of Jammu & Kashmir
Srinagar, India

Mian Anjum Murtaza
Institute of Food Science
    and Nutrition
University of Sargodha
Sargodha, Pakistan

Vishal Mutreja
Department of Chemistry
University Institute of Science (UIS),
    Chandigarh University
Gharuan, India

Sabeera Muzzaffar
Department of Food Science and
    Technology
University of Kashmir
Srinagar, India

**Muhammad Modassar
Ali Nawaz Ranjha**
Institute of Food Science
    and Nutrition
University of Sargodha
Sargodha, Pakistan

Jassia Nisar
Department of Food Science and
    Technology
University of Kashmir
Hazratbal Srinagar, India

Gulzar Ahmad Nayik
Department of Food Science and
    Technology
Govt. Degree College
Shopian, India

Lisa F. M. Lee Nen That
School of Science
RMIT University
Bundoora, Australia

Navneet Kaur Panag
Department of Electrical
    Engineering
Baba Banda Singh Bahadur
    Engineering College
Fatehgarh Sahib, India

Vivek Pandey
Department of Nanomaterial
VET Centre for Nanoscience
Lucknow, India

Jessica Pandohee
Centre for Crop and Disease
    Management, School of
    Molecular and Life Sciences
Curtin University
Bentley, Australia

Sergio Rubén Peréz-Ríos
Instituto de Ciencias Agropecuarias
Universidad Autónoma del Estado de
    Hidalgo
Hidalgo, México

Shafiya Rafiq
Department of Food Technology and
    Nutrition
Lovely Professional University
Phagwara, India

Nighat Raza
Department of Food Science and
    Technology
MNS-University of Agriculture
Multan, Pakistan

Ume Roobab
School of Food Science and Engineering
South China University of Technology
Guangzhou, China

Sangeeta
Guru Nanak College
Budhlada, India

Muhamad Shafiq
Institute of Agricultural Sciences
University of the Punjab
Lahore, Pakistan

Bakhtawar Shafique
Institute of Food Science and Nutrition
University of Sargodha
Sargodha, Pakistan

Muhammad Shahbaz
Department of Food Science and
    Technology
MNS-University of Agriculture
Multan, Pakistan

Marium Shaikh
Department of Food Science and
    Technology
University of Karachi
Karachi, Pakistan

Ajay Sharma
Department of Chemistry
University Institute of Science (UIS),
    Chandigarh University
Gharuan, India

Renu Sharma
Department of Chemistry
Akal Degree College
Mastuana Sahib, India

Ruchi Sharma
School of Bioengineering & Food
    Technology
Shoolini University of Biotechnology and
    Management Sciences
Solan, India

Somesh Sharma
School of Bioengineering & Food
    Technology
Shoolini University of Biotechnology and
    Management Sciences
Solan, India

Arashdeep Singh
Department of Food Science and
    Technology
Punjab Agricultural University
Ludhiana, India

Baljit Singh
Department of Food Science and
    Technology
Punjab Agricultural University
Ludhiana, India

Vishakha Singh
Maharana Pratap University of
    Agriculture & Technology
Udaipur, India

Ghulamudin Sofi
Department of Ilmul Advia
    (Pharmacology)
National Institute of Unani Medicine
Bengaluru, India

Harvinder Singh Sohal
Department of Chemistry
University Institute of Science (UIS),
    Chandigarh University
Gharuan, India

Priyanka Suthar
Department of Food Science and
    Technology, Dr. Y. S. Parmar
    University of Horticulture and Forestry,
    Solan, India

Muhammad Rizwan Tariq
Institute of Agricultural Sciences
University of the Punjab
Lahore, Pakistan

Zakiya Usmani
Department of Pharmacy, School of
    Pharmaceutical Sciences
Lingayas Vidyapeeth
Faridabad, India

Edgar Vázquez-Núñez
Departamento de Ingenierías Química,
    Electrónica y Biomédica, División de
    Ciencias e Ingenierías
Universidad de Guanajuato
León, México

Syeda Mahvish Zahra
Institute of Food Science and Nutrition
University of Sargodha
Sargodha, Pakistan
Department of Environmental Design
    Health and Nutritional Sciences
Allama Iqbal Open University
Islamabad, Pakistan

Saadia Zainab
College of Food Science and Technology
Henan University of Technology
Zhengzhou, China

CHAPTER 1

Pepper Oleoresin

Properties and Economic Importance

Zakiya Usmani

Lingayas Vidyapeeth

Aamir Hussain Dar

Islamic University of Science and Technology Kashmir

Aayeena Altaf

Jamia Hamdard

Yash D. Jagdale

MIT ADT University

CONTENTS

DOI: 10.1201/9781003186205-1

1.1 INTRODUCTION

The discovery of bioactive compounds present in natural matrices has gained an increasing amount of attention during the past two decades. In addition to this fact, the awareness of the health benefits of eating healthy foods, as well as the development of analytical instruments, has contributed to the study of pepper fruits and their by-products as sources of bioactive compounds (Baenas, et al. 2019).

Pepper became so important in the Middle Ages that spice traders were dubbed "Pepperers" in England, "Poivriers" in France, and "Pfeffersacke" in Germany (Govindarajan and Stahl, 2009). Oleoresin can be obtained from different plants such as basil, capsicum (paprika), cardamom, celery seed, cinnamon bark and clove bud. Pepper (*Capsicum annuum* L.) is appreciated as a food additive, a pigment for its physiological and pharmaceutical uses due to its high level of antioxidants. Pepper spray has been widely used for decades by government agencies or military forces worldwide to combat interpersonal violence or civil unrest, law enforcement, criminal incapacitation, personal defence and sometimes even in controlling wild animals. Oleoresins are semi-solid extracts made up of resin and essential fatty oil that are obtained by evaporating the solvents used to make them (King, 2006). Naturally occurring oleoresins are referred to as Balsams. Oleoresin, often known as spice drops, includes all of the pungency and flavour components of pepper (Ravindran and Kallupurackal, 2012). The oleoresin, which is made up of volatile and non-volatile components, can be separated by squeezing the herb or using a solvent mixture to extract the volatile and non-volatile components (Peter, 2012).

1.2 ECONOMIC IMPORTANCE

In the Mexican culture, the wild chilli pepper that is also known as chile piquin (*C. annuum* var *glabriusculum*) plays a very significant role, serving as a staple food since prehistoric times. There are a variety of ways of preparing cilantro, whether fresh green, dried, used in dust, brine, sauces, salads, moles, stuffed chilli, sweet candies and other applications (Garcia et al., 2017). In Mexico, the chile is used for a variety of purposes, including Curanderos utilize it in various ceremonies, such as "cleansing," which refers to avoiding bad vibrations and is widely employed as an evil eye remedy. Prehispanic ethnic cultures, for example, were known to use medicinal plants (Martínez-Ávalos et al., 2018). The Aztecs employed them to treat toothaches, ear infections, constipation and labour pains, and the early Spaniards in America praised their use. It is used to treat dyspepsia in the digestive system, as well as toothaches, diarrhoea, ear pain, cough and fever because capsaicin promotes blood circulation. Some medicines have been made from oleoresins from *Capsicum* spp., and they act on the mucosa to relieve respiratory problems. Chilli with meals may be the most popular hangover treatment. Capsicum is an ornamental plant in Mexican culture, and it is used as an adornment in plates, altars, religious gatherings and amulets, among other things (Kunnumakkara et al., 2009). Chilli is also used in cosmetics, paintings, and meals, and it is used in industry to obtain oleoresins, from which capsaicin is made, and it is utilized in human and animal foods, such as birds, and even in personal defence (Baenas et al., 2019).

1.3 GEOGRAPHIC DISTRIBUTION AND ECOLOGY

C. annuum var *glabriusculum*'s distribution extends throughout Mexico, Central America, Colombia and down into several regions of Peru (Martínez-Ávalos et al., 2018). Mexico has registered this species in all 34 states, and it can be found in the coastal zone from Sonora to Chiapas on the Pacific, and from Tabasco to Yucatán and Quintana Roo on the Gulf of Mexico. Northeastern Mexico is typically found from sea level to approximately 1200 m and is particularly accessible to disturbed zones of small deciduous and thorny forest. However, a recent study on potential distribution modelling is being investigated. The temperature could be one of the key environmental variables affecting its spread from 18.3 Co, according to Martnez-valos and Venegas-Barrera (Martínez-Ávalos et al., 2018; Smith et al., 1957; kraft et al., 2014; Aguilar-Meléndez).

1.4 PRODUCTION

The production of chilli fruits in Mexico is one of the largest in the world, with the country growing 2.2 million tons of them each year from a surface area of 149,000 ha at a participation rate of 12,000 producers each year. Considering these facts, chilli is a significant commercial and social export product, with over 600,000 tonnes of green chilli produced each year, and its global consumption is growing every year. People from 9 cities in the states of Coahuila, Nuevo León and Tamaulipas favour the types jalapeno chilli (37.3%), piquin (29.6%) and serrano (24.0%), while the cities of Linares and Ciudad Victoria are the largest consumers of the variety "piquin." Harvesting wild chilli *Capsicum annum* var *glabriusculum* fruits by people living in rural areas is a popular activity in some Northern (Coahuila, Nuevo León, San Luis Potosi and Tamaulipas) and Northwestern (Baja California Sur, Sonora, Chihuahua and Sinaloa) Mexican states, as the price is always high and they are commercialized in both Mexico and the United States (Martínez-Ávalos et al., 2018; Govindrajan and Salzer, 1986).

1.5 EXTRACTION TECHNIQUES

1.5.1 Supercritical CO_2 Extraction

Extraction of supercritical CO_2 was either done in duplicate or using a dynamic extraction method consisting of an extracting column that is continuously supplied with solvent through a fixed solid bed (De Aguiar et al., 2013).

1.5.1.1 Global Yield (X0)

In order to determine X0, experiments were conducted in a dynamic extraction device (Applied Separations, Speed, Allentown, PA). In this experiment, 4.0 g of sample for the fixed bed was put in a stainless steel column with a volume of 5.6 mL. The effect of pressure and temperature on X0 was studied using a factorial design by repeating $2 \times 32 = 18$ experiments, each with three levels and two variables. The pressures and temperatures were 15, 25 and 35 MPa and 40°C, 50°C and 60°C, respectively. It was determined that pressure ranges below 15 MPa can reduce extraction rate and yield, while pressures over 35 MPa result in unfeasible costs compression. To avoid thermal degradation in the extract, levels of temperature were chosen over the critical temperature of CO_2 (31.1°C) and over 60°C, the upper limit. A flow rate of 1.98 10^{-4} kg/s was selected for the solvent flow. The extraction period was set at 320 minutes after initially testing. Using the chosen solvent flow rate showed that all of the immediately accessible solutes had been removed by convection. Glass flasks were used to collect the extracts, which were then weighed on an analytical balance (De Aguiar et al., 2013).

1.5.1.2 Kinetic Experiments

For kinetics, frozen and oven-dried pepper samples were used with the similar extraction unit used for global yield experiments, at pressures and temperatures that yielded the highest capsaicinoids yield and the conditions evaluated during the design of the experiment. The sample used for the assay constituted approximately 4.0 g, the quantity of which was fixed inside of a 5.6 mL column of stainless steel. Carbon dioxide (CO_2) was injected at a flow rate of 1.98 10^{-4} kg/s, and the average particle size of dry materials was 0.88 (*0.06) mm and 0.51 (*0.01) mm, respectively, for a freeze-dried and oven-dried sample. A curve showing the extraction flow was derived by measuring the mass of the extracted extract based on the time. According to the methodology presented, capsaicinoids were determined in the extract (De Aguiar et al., 2013).

1.5.2 Soxhlet Extraction

During the study, approximately 5 kg of fresh peppers were dried under the air circulation oven for 20 hours at approximately 70°C and lyophilized for 72 hours at approximately −40°C (highest capsaicinoids). As part of the extraction process, the samples were ground in a knife mill after drying; homogenization is important for them as it reduces resistance to mass transfer. An extraction technique suitable for Soxhlet extraction was selected, using hexane as a solvent. The extraction apparatus was packed with filter paper, and 5.0 g of freeze-dried sample was put in at a time. The system was heated to boiling (69°C) with hexane (0.15 L) added. The reflux was maintained for 6 hours, after which the solvent was evaporated under vacuum (at 25°C), and the recovered extract was weighed and stored for further analysis at −18°C (De Aguiar et al., 2013).

1.5.3 Microwave Reflux Extraction

Five grams of sieved samples were combined with solvents such as acetone and water hexane, and stirred with a magnetic stirrer. Soaking and stirring were performed to ensure that the sample and solvent were properly hydrated and homogeneous. In the microwave extractor, the sample was loaded and the orthogonal experimental design was used to irradiate it. To reduce the effects of superheating, a three-level microwave pulsed heating technique was used. For the pre-heating process, the sample was heated for 10 minutes at 100°C, irradiated as per the experimental design and cooled to 30°C for 5 minutes. In addition to the pre-heating irradiation cooling modes, pulsed heating modes are introduced to reduce the effects of temperature fluctuation on the system. A refrigerated centrifuge was then used to centrifuge the sample at 5000 rpm for 15 minutes after which it was removed from the extractor. An extraction yield was calculated from the final extract concentrate after concentrating the extract using a rotary evaporator. After storage at 4°C, the oleoresin extract concentrate was analysed and characterized by chemical techniques (Olalere et al. 2018; Mnadal, et al. 2007).

1.6 CHEMICAL CONSTITUENT

It contains approximately 0.5%–0.9% capsaicin, a volatile, colourless, crystalline and pungent compound. It also contains fixed oils, proteins and pigments, like capsanthin and carotene. Pigments are responsible for the red colour. Other ingredients of the drug include thiamine and ascorbic acid (Morais, et al. 2003). Because of the pungent taste associated with capsaicin present in pepper fruits, seeds and placenta, pepper fruits are consumed as spices in food preparations. When pepper fruits are consumed, they can create a burning sensation that can last for hours (Saleh, et al. 2018). The characteristic pungent flavour of pepper fruits can be attributed to capsaicinoids, which are a group of compounds. Associated with rheumatoid arthritis and gastric ulcers, capsaicinoids have also been shown to have therapeutic properties (Batiha, et al. 2020). There are 9–11 carbon chains, branched fatty acid vanillylamides in the capsicum, the most abundant of which are dihydrocapsaicin and capsaicin (Figure 1.1). They are accountable for 90% of the total pungency of pepper fruits. The major capsaicinoids reported in capsicum oleoresin are capsaicin (48.6%) followed by 6,7-dihydro capsaicin (36%), nordihydro-capsaicin (7.4%), homodihydrocapsaicin (2%), homocapsaicin (2%), pseudocapsaicine, capsanthin and capsorubin (Luo, et al. 2011).

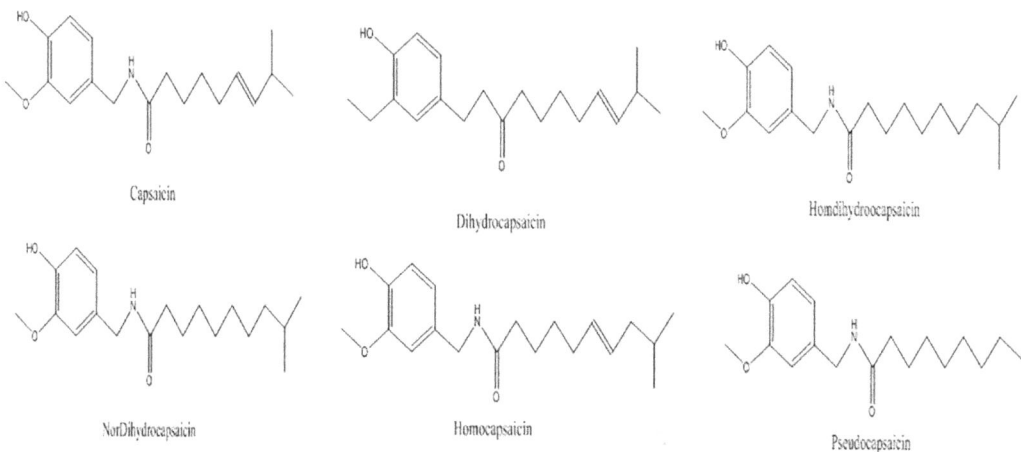

FIGURE 1.1   Structure of major capsaicinoids reported in capsicum.

1.7 APPLICATIONS

1.7.1 Antimicrobial Activity

The scientific community knows that bacteria are increasingly becoming resistant to antibiotics as time passes; therefore, the development of new treatments represents an important area of research. Pepper has been shown to have antimicrobial activity against a variety of bacteria, including *Proteus mirabilis, Pseudomonas aeruginosa, Staphylococcus aureus*, and *Escherichia coli* (Techawinyutham, et al. 2019; Dussault and Lacroix, 2014).

1.7.2 Antioxidant Activity

Leafy green vegetables with vibrant colours have high levels of antioxidants. Among these are pepper oleoresins, which were found to have antioxidant activity increased with the maturity stage of red, with nutrients like lycopene ascorbic acid and p-coumaryl alcohol ethoxyquin. It has been observed that isolated phytochemicals are efficacious against Fe(II)-induced lipid peroxidation. Methanolic extracts from *C. annuum* L. were found to prevent 4-hydroxy-2-nonenal-induced and H_2O_2-induced DNA damage in another investigation (Culafic, 2018; Maksimova, et al. 2014; oboh, et al. 2007).

1.7.3 Anti-Cancer

Capsaicin is responsible for the pungency of chilli. There has been evidence that capsaicin is effective at stopping, both in vitro and in vivo, the growth of prostate cancer cells. There is significant research demonstrating that capsaicinoid compounds, derived naturally from chilli, have antitumor properties, both in vitro and in vivo (Šaponjac, et al. 2014; Amruthraj, et al. 2014).

1.7.4 Other Application

- The capsicum fruit is used to create medication. Capsicum is used to treat a variety of digestive issues, including bloating, gas, stomach pain, diarrhoea and cramps (Pawar, et al. 2011).

- It's also used to treat heart and blood vessel problems like low circulation, excessive clotting of blood, high level of cholesterol and cardiac disease prevention (Sanati, et al. 2018).

- Toothaches, seasickness, drunkenness, malaria and fever are among the other uses. It's also used to aid those who have trouble swallowing. Capsicum is applied to the skin to treat shingles, osteoarthritis, rheumatoid arthritis and fibromyalgia discomfort (Gupta, et al. 2007; Madhumathy, et al. 2007).

The capsicum fruit is used to create medication. It is used to treat a variety of digestive issues, including bloating, gas, stomach pain, diarrhoea and cramps.

1.8 SAFETY, TOXICITY AND FUTURE SCOPE

The safety of capsaicin consumption or topical application has been a subject of controversy for centuries. Research studies suggest that capsaicin may either act as a carcinogen or act as a cancer-preventive agent, based on epidemiological evidence and basic research study findings. Despite limited safety studies, there is some evidence that pepper can be consumed in quantities several times the normal human intake without harming growth, organ weights, feed efficiency ratios, nitrogen balance, or chemistry of blood in Indian population. In comparison to other naturally occurring irritants, capsaicin is unique in that it provokes a short but refractory neuronal response, and there is a subsequent desensitization process (Srinivasan, 2016). It has therapeutic potential. For many years, creams containing capsaicin have been used to relieve a variety of painful conditions. Although some of their side effects are reported, they are highly debated as effective pain relievers. An increase in skin carcinogenesis was observed in mice treated with sunlight and capsaicin for a long period after chronic, long-term topical application (Bode and Dong, 2011).

1.9 CONCLUSION

A variety of pepper called *C. annuum* is an important crop in Northeastern Mexico, where its fruits are consumed and sold, generating much income for rural families. *C. annuum* contains varying amounts of capsaicinoids, explaining their high demand and the wide variability in capsaicinoids content. The chapter indicated that red pepper and its active constituent have antioxidant, anti-cancer, antimicrobial, and anti-hyperlipidemic effects. The antiobesity property of red pepper was partially similar to that of some antiobesity medications. The results of these studies suggest that red pepper could reduce the risk of mortality caused by cardiovascular disease and metabolic syndrome, but further clinical trials are needed to confirm its effectiveness in humans.

REFERENCES

Aguilar-Meléndez, A., Morrell, P. L., Roose, M. L. and Kim, S. C. (2009) Genetic diversity and structure in semiwild and domesticated chiles (*Capsicum Annuum*; Solanaceae) from Mexico, *American Journal of Botany*, 96(6), 1190–1202.

Amruthraj, N. J., Raj, P., Saravanan, S. and Lebel, L. A. (2014) In vitro studies on anticancer activity of capsaicinoids from Capsicum chinense against human hepatocellular carcinoma cells, *International Journal of Pharmacy and Pharmaceutical Sciences*, 6(4), 254–558.

Baenas, N., Belović, M., Ilic, N., Moreno, D. A. and García-Viguera, C. (2019) Industrial use of pepper (*Capsicum Annum* L.) derived products: Technological benefits and biological advantages, *Food Chemistry*, 274, 872–885.

Batiha, G. E. S., Alqahtani, A., Ojo, O. A., Shaheen, H. M., Wasef, L., Elzeiny, M., Ismail, M., Shalaby, M., Murata, T., Zaragoza-Bastida, A. and Rivero-Perez, N. (2020) Biological properties, bioactive constituents, and pharmacokinetics of some *Capsicum spp.* and capsaicinoids, *International Journal of Molecular Sciences*, 21(15), 5179.

Bode, A. M. and Dong, Z. (2011) The two faces of capsaicin, *Cancer Research*, 71(8), 2809–2814.

Culafic, D. M. (2018) Synergistic antioxidant activity of clove oleoresin with Capsicum oleoresin and Kalonji seeds extract in sunflower oil, *Biomedical Journal of Scientific & Technical Research*, 3(4), 3469–3474.

de Aguiar, A. C., Sales, L. P., Coutinho, J. P., Barbero, G. F., Godoy, H. T. and Martínez, J. (2013) Supercritical carbon dioxide extraction of Capsicum peppers: Global yield and capsaicinoid content, *The Journal of Supercritical Fluids*, 81, 210–216.

Dussault, D., Vu, K. D. and Lacroix, M. (2014) In vitro evaluation of antimicrobial activities of various commercial essential oils, oleoresin and pure compounds against food pathogens and application in ham, *Meat Science*, 96(1), 514–520.

García-Gaytán, V., Gómez-Merino, F. C., Trejo-Téllez, L. I., Baca-Castillo, G. A. and García-Morales, S. (2017) The chilhuacle chili (*Capsicum annuum* L.) in Mexico: Description of the variety, its cultivation, and uses, *International Journal of Agronomy*. https://doi.org/10.1155/2017/5641680

Govindarajan, V. S. and Salzer, U. J. (1986) Capsicum—Production, technology, chemistry, and quality—Part II. Processed products, standards, world production and trade, *Critical Reviews in Food Science & Nutrition*, 3(3), 207–288.

Govindarajan, V. S. and Stahl, W. H. (1977) Pepper—chemistry, technology, and quality evaluation, *Critical Reviews in Food Science & Nutrition*, 9(2), 115–225.

Gupta, R. S., Dixit, V. P. and Dobhal, M. P. (2002) Hypocholesterolaemic effect of the oleoresin of *Capsicum annum* L. in gerbils (*Meriones hurrianae Jerdon*), *Phytotherapy Research*, 16(3), 273–275.

King, K. (2006) Packaging and storage of herbs and spices. In *Handbook of Herbs and Spices*, pp. 86–102. Woodhead Publishing.

Kraft, K. H., Brown, C. H., Nabhan, G. P., Luedeling, E., Ruiz, J. D. J. L., d'Eeckenbrugge, G. C., Hijmans, R. J. and Gepts, P. (2014) Multiple lines of evidence for the origin of domesticated chili pepper, *Capsicum annuum*, in Mexico, *Proceedings of the National Academy of Sciences*, 111(17), 6165–6170.

Kunnumakkara, A. B., Koca, C., Dey, S., Gehlot, P., Yodkeeree, S., Danda, D., Sung, B. and Aggarwal, B. B. (2009) Traditional uses of spices: an overview, *Molecular Targets and Therapeutic Uses of Spices: Modern Uses for Ancient Medicine*, pp. 1–24.

Luo, X. J., Peng, J. and Li, Y. J. (2011) Recent advances in the study on capsaicinoids and capsinoids, *European Journal of Pharmacology*, 650(1), 1–7.

Madhumathy, A. P., Aivazi, A. A. and Vijayan, V. A. (2007) Larvicidal efficacy of *Capsicum annum* against Anopheles stephensi and Culex quinquefasciatus, *Journal of Vector Borne Diseases*, 44(3), 223–226.

Maksimova, V., Koleva Gudeva, L., Ruskovska, T., Gulaboski, R. and Cvetanovska, A. (2014) Antioxidative effect of Capsicum oleoresins compared with pure capsaicin, *IOSR Journal of Pharmacy*, 4(11), 44–48.

Mandal, V., Mohan, Y. and Hemalatha, S. (2007) Microwave assisted extraction—an innovative and promising extraction tool for medicinal plant research, *Pharmacognosy Reviews*, 1(1), 7–18.

Martínez-Ávalos, J. G., Venegas-Barrera, C. S., Martínez-Gallegos, R., Torres-Castillo, J. A., Santibáñez, F. E. O., Mora-Olivo, A., Guerra-Pérez, A., Arellano-Méndez, L. U. and Ocañas, F. G. (2018) A review on the geographical distribution, fruit production and concentration of capsaicinoids in *Capsicum annuum* var. glabriusculum in the northeastern region of Mexico, *Preprints* 2018110517, doi: 10.20944/preprints201811.0517.v1.

Morais, H., Rodrigues, P., Ramos, C., Forgács, E., Cserháti, T. and Oliveira, J. (2002) Effect of ascorbic acid on the stability of β-carotene and capsanthin in paprika (*Capsicum annuum*) powder, *Food/Nahrung*, 46(5), 308–310.

Olalere, O. A., Abdurahman, N. H., bin Mohd Yunus, R., Alara, O. R. and Kabbashi, N. A. (2018) Chemical fingerprinting of biologically active compounds and morphological transformation during microwave reflux extraction of black pepper, *Chemical Data Collections*, 17, 339–344.

Pawar, S. S., Bharude, N. V., Sonone, S. S., Deshmukh, R. S., Raut, A. K. and Umarkar, A. R. (2011) Chillies as food, spice and medicine: A perspective, *International Journal of Pharma and Bio Sciences*, 1(3), 311–318.

Peter, K. V. ed. (2012) *Handbook of Herbs and Spices*, Elsevier.

Ravindran, P. N. and Kallupurackal, J. A. (2012) Black pepper. In *Handbook of Herbs and Spices*, pp. 86–115. Woodhead Publishing.

Saleh, B. K., Omer, A. and Teweldemedhin, B. (2018) Medicinal uses and health benefits of chili pepper (*Capsicum spp.*): A review, *MOJ Food Processing & Technology*, 6(4), pp. 325–328.

Sanati, S., Razavi, B. M. and Hosseinzadeh, H. (2018) A review of the effects of *Capsicum annuum* L. and its constituent, capsaicin, in metabolic syndrome, *Iranian Journal of Basic Medical Sciences*, 21(5), 439–448

Šaponjac, V. T., Četojević-Simin, D., Ćetković, G., Čanadanović-Brunet, J., Djilas, S., Mandić, A. and Tepić, A. (2014) Effect of extraction conditions of paprika oleoresins on their free radical scavenging and anticancer activity, *Central European Journal of Chemistry*, 12(3), 377–385.

Smith, P. G. and Heiser Jr, C. B. (1957) Taxonomy of Capsicum sinense Jacq. and the geographic distribution of the cultivated Capsicum species, *Bulletin of the Torrey Botanical Club*, pp. 413–420.

Srinivasan, K. (2016) Biological activities of red pepper (*Capsicum annuum*) and its pungent principle capsaicin: a review, *Critical Reviews in Food Science and Nutrition*, 56(9), 1488–1500.

Techawinyutham, L., Siengchin, S., Dangtungee, R. and Parameswaranpillai, J. (2019) Influence of accelerated weathering on the thermo-mechanical, antibacterial, and rheological properties of polylactic acid incorporated with porous silica-containing varying amount of capsicum oleoresin, *Composites Part B: Engineering*, 175, 107108.

Uquiche, E., Millao, S. and del Valle, J. M. (2021) Extrusion affects supercritical CO_2 extraction of red pepper (*Capsicum annuum* L.) oleoresin, *Journal of Food Engineering*, 110829.

CHAPTER 2

Chemistry and Properties of Coriander Oleoresin

Hanuman Bobade, Arashdeep Singh, and Baljit Singh

Punjab Agricultural University

CONTENTS

2.1 INTRODUCTION

Coriander (*Coriandrum sativum* L.) included in the family of Apiaceae (Umbelliferae) is an annual herbaceous crop. The taxonomical details of the coriander herb are presented in Table 2.1. Coriander plant usually grows to the average height of about 50 cm

DOI: 10.1201/9781003186205-2

TABLE 2.1   Taxonomical Classification of the
Coriander Plant

Kingdom	Plantae
Subkingdom	Tracheobionta
Division	Magnoliophyta
Class	Magnoliopsida
Sub-class	Rosidae
Order	Apiales (Umbellales)
Family	Apiaceae (Umbelliferae)
Genus	*Coriandrum* L.
Species	*Coriandrum sativum* L.

with upright branched pattern and green stem and leaves which become dark violet or red at the time of flowering of coriander. Coriander plant generally matures between 90 and 120 days from its cultivation. The flowers of this plant are arranged in umbels and are whitish to pinkish in color. The flowers, on the maturity of the herb, bear small fruits of about 1.5–3.0 mm diameter. The immature and young coriander herb has a peculiar odor that resembles the aroma of essential oil. The particular look of the coriander herb differs with ecotype and location (Rajeshwari and Andallu 2011; Small 2006).

The origin of coriander herb is not precisely known due to a lack of authentic historical data about this herb. This herb grows well in the fertile areas of the tropical regions and therefore Southern Europe, the Mediterranean, Western Australia, and the Middle East are suitable for coriander cultivation (Seidemann 2005). It is considered that coriander has its origin nearby the Mediterranean.

The coriander plant is mainly cultivated for the production of seeds and green leaves which are depicted in Figure 2.1. The seeds and foliage of coriander are extensively regarded for their wide-ranging applications not only in food but also in the medicinal and pharma industry (Bhat, et al. 2014). Besides, seeds and foliage, nearly all parts of the coriander herb find applications, specifically in food, and have distinct dwellings in a traditional as well as a modern kitchen. For instance, the leaves of this coriander have considerable use as a flavor enhancer in many food preparations (Carrubba 2009). The addition of coriander leaves improves aroma, taste, appearance of many dishes prepared from vegetables, pulses, and meats and of products like pickle, soup, salads, and other cooked foods. Recently, coriander is also used for flavoring bakery products like bread, biscuits, cakes, pastry, and buns. Some liquors, particularly gin, are also being flavored with this herb (Sharma and Sharma 2012). Apart from this primary function as a flavor enhancer, powdered seeds of the coriander herb are also utilized to improve the thickness of curries, soups, and other cuisines (Maroufi, et al. 2010).

Coriander varies widely in its chemical composition. The chemical composition of coriander green leaves and mature dry seeds is presented in Table 2.2. Carbohydrate is the major constituent of green leaves, whereas mature seeds contain a substantial amount of ether extract. The oil content in seeds of coriander differs broadly with geographical

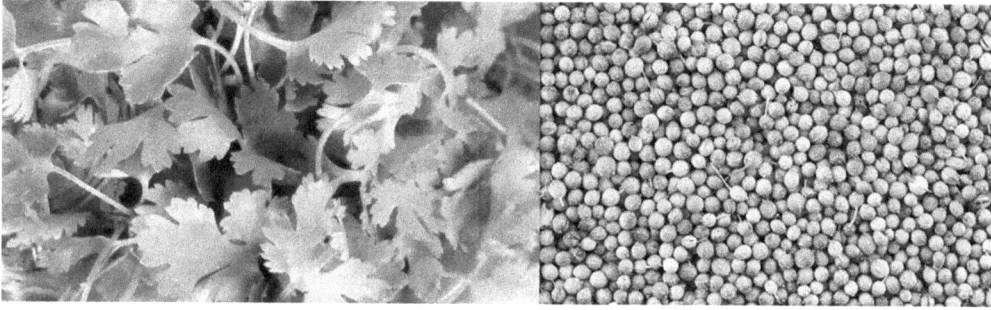

FIGURE 2.1   Leaves and seeds of coriander.

TABLE 2.2   Chemical Composition of Green Leaves and Mature Seeds of Coriander

Sr. No.	Parameter	Green Leaves	Mature Seed
1	Moisture (%)	87.90	6.3–8.0
2	Carbohydrates (%)	6.50	24.0
3	Proteins (%)	3.30	1.3
4	Fats (ether extract) (%)	0.60	31.5
5	Mineral matter (%)	1.70	5.3

Source: Adapted from Sharma & Sharma, 2012.

location. Indian coriander is known to have less oil content compared to Norwegian coriander and Bulgarian coriander except for CS-4 and CS-6 Indian coriander varieties (Sharma and Sharma 2012).

The essential oil and extracts of coriander are regarded for containing high-value compounds like linalool, pinene, terpinene, camphor, and geraniol. Coriander offers many health benefits and possesses several medicinal properties. This is because of the existence of the aforementioned bioactive molecules. Coriander is considered diuretic, carminative, aphrodisiac, and stomachic antibilious (Sharma and Sharma 2012). The coriander offers considerable antimicrobial (Zare-Shehneh, et al. 2014), antioxidative (Wangensteen, et al. 2004), and anti-inflammatory properties (Sabogal-Guáqueta, et al. 2016).

2.2 DISTRIBUTION, PRODUCTION, AND ECONOMIC IMPORTANCE

Historically, the coriander has been in use for a long time; it has been in use since 1000 BC. However, the corianders were said to be cultivated long back even before their reported history of use. The coriander is reported to be the first spice ever used by human beings (Small 1997). Its reference is found in Sanskrit literature long back in 5000 BC and is also mentioned in Greek Eber Papyrus in about 1550 BC (Uhl 2000). The coriander herb is claimed to be cultivated in the Hanging Gardens of Babylon for the first time in 2000 BC. The Egyptians then brought coriander seeds to Europe, for preserving their meat, and later to other parts of the globe. The Egyptians termed this herb as 'spice of happiness' which might be because of coriander's consideration as an aphrodisiac. It is also believed that Romans introduced coriander in Great Britain (Livarda and van der Veen 2008). The coriander is considered to have its origin in the Mediterranean and Middle Eastern parts of the world. The coriander etymology is thought to be derived from the *korannon* (Greek word), an amalgamation of two Greek words *koris* and *annon* meaning aromatic anise (Uchibayashi 2001). The dried seeds of the coriander have experienced their utilization for more than 700 years (Kiple and Ornelas 2000). The coriander is known in Indian from the Vedic period; however, in the ancient history, the use of coriander was limited to fresh leaves. The seeds were not used in India as a spice until the arrival of Muslims. This elucidates the bulk consumption of coriander seeds in Mughlai preparations, which is undoubtedly of Muslim origin (Sharma and Sharma 2012). Coriander is now widespread and is grown in almost every part of the world.

The coriander is extensively cultivated in China, India, Iran, Indonesia, Russia, Bulgaria, Turkey, and Tanzania for their varied uses (Ashraf, et al. 2020). India is one of the major countries for farming and producing coriander in considerable quantity. The farming of coriander in India is done on an area of about 0.52 million hectares and has an annual production of about 0.31 million tons (Sharma and Sharma 2012).

The essential oil extracted from coriander ranks second-most in annual world production followed by essential oil extracted from orange pointing that this herb is the most prominent commercial herb of the globe (Lawrence 1993). India is also a leading exporter of coriander seeds in the global market. India accounts for 35.9% of total global export trade followed by Bulgaria. India, Bulgaria, Morocco, and Canada account for over 75% of the global export trade of coriander seed (Sharma and Sharma 2012).

2.3 EXTRACTION TECHNIQUES

Extraction has a critical part in determining the quality and composition of the extract. Many techniques of extraction exist for the recovery of the constituent of notice from the food matrix. These extraction techniques can be categorically classified into two broad types: a. conventional extraction techniques and b. non-conventional or advanced techniques of extraction as illustrated in Figure 2.1. Each of these techniques has its advantages and limitations. Therefore, it necessitates the careful selection of extraction technique/method and a comprehensive understanding of its process parameters (Figure 2.2).

2.3.1 Non-Conventional Extraction Techniques

2.3.1.1 Ultrasound-Assisted Extraction Technique

This technique uses ultrasound waves for extracting the compound of interest from the food matrix. Ultrasound waves are kind of sound waves with a frequency of more than 16 kHz. Based on frequency, intensity, and power, there are two types of ultrasound waves: (a) low-intensity low power ultrasounds having a frequency range of 1–10 MHZ and power intensity below 1 W/cm^2 and (b) high-intensity high power ultrasounds having a frequency less than 100 kHz and power above 10 W/cm^2. The later type of ultrasounds is used for extraction purposes. The principle of ultrasound is founded on cavitation and de-cavitation that lead to compression and rarefaction effects on material subjected to ultrasound. This

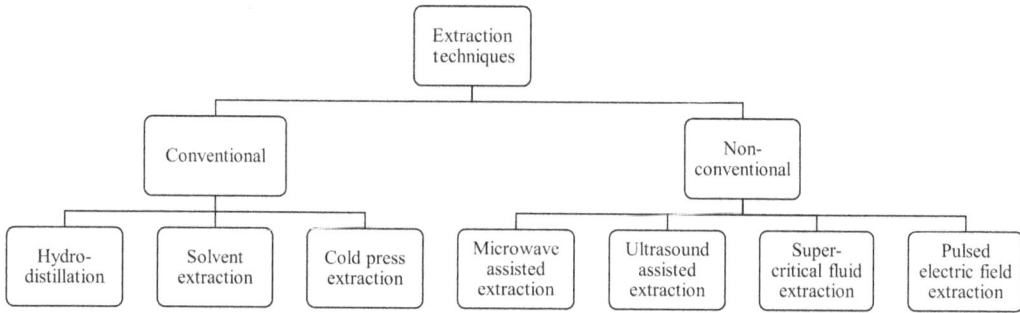

FIGURE 2.2 Types of extraction techniques.

results in altering the permeability of the cell wall and thus enhanced mass transfer rates (Bermúdez-Aguirre, et al. 2011).

Rahmani et al. (2015) found that yield of the coriander oil extracted with ultrasound is comparable with microwave-assisted extraction; however, the former technique results in the loss of some essential compounds from the extracted coriander oil. The coriander seed oil extracted with ultrasound extraction technique consists of polar compounds in large amounts (Zeković, et al. 2015). It has been found that ultrasound-assisted extraction is more suitable for the extraction of constituents with a higher proportion of polar compounds. The ultrasound-assisted extraction technique, specifically when used at relatively higher frequencies, is likely to give a low yield with more risk of degrading valuable compounds in food matrices in comparison to different non-conventional methods (Ashraf, et al. 2020).

2.3.1.2 Supercritical Fluid Extraction

Extraction using supercritical fluid is carried out by a fluid that has desirable properties of both liquid (density and solubility) and gas (viscosity and diffusivity). The fluid at its critical temperature and critical pressure is mixed with the food matrix from which the constituent of interest has to be extracted. The fluid solubilizes the constituent and the mixture of fluid-constituent is allowed to separate from the food matrix. The constituent is then separated from the fluid by regulating the temperature–pressure conditions of the fluid. The solubility of extracting components is higher in supercritical fluids and also enhances the mass transfer rate. Moreover, it permits extraction of a particular component of interest by easily manipulating the process parameters like temperature and pressure (Illés, et al. 2000; Mendiola, et al. 2007). Many fluids are used for extraction using supercritical technology; however, the utmost regular choice is CO_2 for its easy availability, non-toxicity, stability, and non-inflammability. Contrary to ultrasound extraction, supercritical fluid extraction is more preferred and highly viable for constituents with more non-polar molecules. This technique, nevertheless, can also be used to extract polar analytes by modifying the polarity of CO_2 with co-solvents (Mhemdi, et al. 2011).

Supercritical fluid extraction technology gives a comparatively higher yield of coriander seed oil than conventional extraction techniques. Moreover, the coriander seed oil received by supercritical fluid extraction has an improved fragrance than obtained by the hydro-distillation method (Shrirame, et al. 2018). Grosso et al. (2008) have performed the extraction of coriander seed oil with supercritical fluid extraction and found that the best conditions of supercritical fluid extraction are 90 bar pressure, 40°C temperature, 1.10 kg/h flow rate, and 0.6 mm particle size. Further, the composition of oil obtained by extracting at a pressure between 90 and 100 bar was found close to that obtained by hydro-distillation. Zeković et al. (2017) extracted the coriander seed oil by use of supercritical fluid through CO_2 as a medium. The optimized processing conditions achieved by artificial neural network included 200 bar pressure, 40°C temperature, and 0.4 kg/hour flow rate. Yield and the composition of coriander seed oil were adversely affected by replacing CO_2 with propane as a supercritical fluid (Illés, et al. 2000). This outlines that CO_2 is better than other fluids to be used in supercritical fluid extraction.

2.3.2 Conventional Techniques

2.3.2.1 Hydro-Distillation

Water is used as a medium in this technique for the extraction of polar components from the food matrix. Hydro-distillation is usually performed using a Clevenger apparatus or steam distillation unit. Material, from which the constituent of interest is to be extracted, is mixed with water and boiled for evaporation of the volatile components in the Clevenger apparatus, whereas steam is allowed to diffuse through the bed of material in steam distillation (Ashraf, et al. 2020). Zeković et al. (2015) reported that hydro-distillation produces a lower yield of extract of coriander seed as compared to the Soxhlet extraction technique. Hydro-distillation and steam distillation are considered contemporary techniques of isolating the desired oil from the plant sources and present the problem of hydrolysis and thermal degradation of the product. Heat-induced degradation of some compounds and large energy consumptions are certain limitations of this method as pointed out by Balbino et al. (2021). These limitations of the distillation technique can be overcome with the use of modern methods of extractions like supercritical fluid extraction (Grosso et al. 2008).

Many studies (Eikani, et al. 2007; Sovová and Aleksovski 2006; Zeković, et al. 2015) involving the extraction using hydro-distillation methods have reported issues in the yield of essential oil compared to different methods of extraction.

2.3.2.2 Solvent Extraction

The solvent extraction technique is widely used for extraction and is considered the standard reference technique to compare and determine the efficacy of other methods (Balbino, et al. 2012). In this technique, a suitable solvent is used as an extraction medium instead of water and is usually performed in the Soxhlet apparatus. Solid material after size reduction is kept above the flask in which the medium of extraction (solvent) is boiled. The vapors of the solvent then diffuse through this material and solubilize the compatible material from the food matrix. The solvent vaporizes with solubilized material after condensation are dropped back in the solvent reservoir. The solvent is then separated from the mix by other suitable techniques like evaporation (Ashraf, et al. 2020).

Balbino, et al. (2021) have carried out the solvent extraction of oil from coriander seed and observed that the yield of coriander seed oil with solvent extraction is 20.46%. Pavlić, et al. (2015) compared the traditional techniques with modern methods for extraction of oil from coriander seed and observed that the recovery of coriander seed oil obtained with Soxhlet extraction (14.45%) is more than the supercritical fluid (8.88%) and subcritical fluid extraction (0.36%) methods. Further, Zeković, et al. (2015) also found that the yield of extract obtained from coriander seed is more in Soxhlet extraction compared to the supercritical fluid extraction technique. This outlines that the traditional methods like Soxhlet extraction are better for the yield of coriander seed oil than the modern methods like supercritical fluid extraction techniques. Solvent extraction is reported to yield about 19.4% oil from the coriander seed (Eikani, et al. 2007; Ramadan, et al. 2003); however, the implementation of this technique is restricted to fixed oils. Further, complete separation of solvent from the oil is difficult and traces of solvent remain in the extracted oil. Heat-induced degradation of essential and thermolabile components of the extract is the principal disadvantage of this technique (Zeković, et al. 2015). Balbino, et al. (2012) mentioned some serious limitations of this method with organic solvents. This method necessitates many exchanges of solvents, is laborious and relatively unfeasible to apply on a commercial scale.

2.3.2.3 Cold Pressing

In this technique, pressure is applied on the ground plant material and the liquid matter is squeezed off. Pressure application results in mechanical rupture of oil-bearing organelles and initiates the flow of oil from the cells, irrespective of the polarity of oil. The cold pressing technique is simple, eco-friendly, and viable for the extraction of oils from dried and size-reduced plant materials. However, this method suffers yield and leads to adulteration of oil as other liquid material along with the oil is also extracted with the application of pressure. For the same reason, this method is unsuitable for the extraction of essential oil (Ashraf, et al. 2020).

The oil extracted by cold pressing technique from coriander seeds is found to have good quality (Sriti, et al. 2010). This may be due to fact that the oils extracted by cold pressing are reported to have more oxidative stability (Ramadan, et al. 2003) and less detrimental effect on components of extracted coriander seed oil (Ashraf, et al. 2020). The recovery of oil extracted by cold pressing of coriander seed varies from 0.03% to 2.6% (Eidi and Eidi 2011).

2.4 CHARACTERIZATION, CHEMISTRY, AND PROPERTIES

The coriander oleoresins are generally obtained by the process of steam distillation of dried material. The coriander oleoresins can also be extracted with solvent extraction technique. The seeds are subjected to size reduction to reduce particle size in order to increase surface area and improve oil yield. The coriander oleoresins contain fatty oil, volatile oil, and some other extractive matter; the amount of these fractions is governed by the type of source material, the processing methodology adopted and its parameters, and the choice of medium. The oleoresins extracted from coriander are usually reported to comprise on an average 90% fatty oil and 5% steam-volatile oil. The oleoresin obtained from the seeds of coriander is affluent in lipid fraction but miserable in essential oil content (Salzer 1977). The coriander seeds, on average, contain about 18% fat and 0.84% essential oil. The oil content of coriander extract is affected by many factors including geographical location, stage of maturity, and size of the seed. The microcarpum varieties (mainly Russian and European types) have higher oil content than the tropical or sub-tropical varieties. Further, the small-sized seeds of coriander yield more oil than the bold seeded type and for this reason, the small-sized seeds are favored for distillation purposes, whereas the bigger seeds with good semblance are seeming fit for their application as a spice (Sharma and Sharma 2012).

Linalool constitutes the principal component of the oleoresins extracted from the coriander seed. More than two-third portion of coriander oleoresins constitutes linalool. The principal constituents of oil removed from coriander seeds besides linalool are presented in Table 2.3. The minor components of the coriander seed essential oil include β-pinene, myrcene, dipentene, limonene, camphene, p-cymol, borneol, α-terpinene, and esters of acetic acid (Sharma and Sharma 2012). The chemical structures of elements of coriander oil are depicted in Figure 2.3. It is reported that coriander seed contains about 122 different constituents (BACIS 1999); however, the actual number of constituents may be more than 200. Further, about 97% proportion of coriander oil is constituted by 18 major compounds. It is also believed that not these major compounds but the compounds present in trace amounts constituting about 0.01% or less are principally responsible for contributing to the primary sensory properties of coriander oil (Burdock and Carabin 2009).

TABLE 2.3 Composition of Coriander Seed Essential Oil

Sr. No.	Constituent	Amount (%)
1	Linalool	67.7
2	A-pinene	10.5
3	Γ-terpinene	9.0
4	Geranyl acetate	4.0
5	Camphor	3.0
6	Geraniol	1.9

Source: Adapted from Sharma and Sharma, 2012.

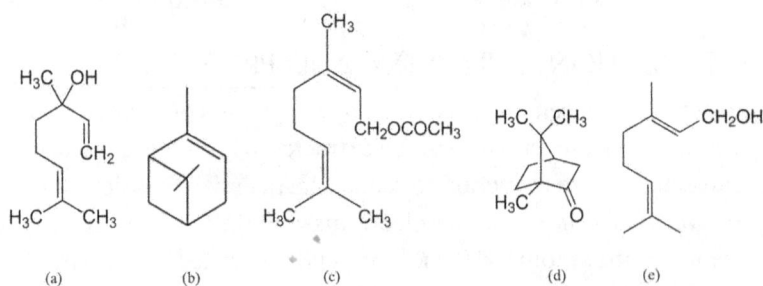

FIGURE 2.3 Chemical structures of chief constituents of coriander seed oil: (a) linalool, (b) α-pinene, (c) geranyl acetate (d) camphor, and (e) Geraniol.

The coriander extract is known to comprise a large quantity of monounsaturated fatty acids, predominantly petroselinic acid (Pavlić, et al. 2015; Uitterhaegen, et al. 2016). Petroselinic acid (C-18) is a kind of monounsaturated ω-12 fatty acid and is a positional isomeric compound of octadecenoic acid. The concentration of petroselinic acid in coriander oil varies from 68% to 83% (Laribi, et al. 2015; Kiralan, et al. 2009). Besides petroselinic acid, other key fatty acids that are contained in coriander oil include linoleic acid, oleic acid, palmitic acid, and stearic acid. Many bioactive compounds are available in coriander oleoresins, these compounds include essential oils, lipids, and polyphenols, among others (Laribi, et al. 2015; Msaada, et al. 2017). The oil drawn out from the seeds of coriander using supercritical fluid extraction technology at optimum conditions of 40°C temperature and 90 bar pressure contained 65%–79% linalool, 4%–7% γ-terpinene, 3% camphor, 2%–4% geranyl acetate, 1%–3% α-pinene, 1%–3% geraniol, and 1%–2% limonene as analyzed by GC and GC/MS (Grosso, et al. 2008). Further, it has been observed that the chief elements of coriander oil extracted by Soxhlet as well as subcritical water extraction are similar (Pavlić, et al. 2015). Micić, et al. (2019) isolated the oil from seeds of the coriander by water-distillation method and characterized it with GC/MS. The study discovered the occurrence of 38 different compounds in the essential oil extracted from coriander. The linalool was present as the chief compound constituting 64.04% along with the presence of other compounds including α-pinene (7.31%), geranyl acetate (5.76%), γ-terpinene (5.59%), camphor (4.24%), p-cymene (3.83%), and limonene (1.6%).

The coriander seed oil is reported to contain different compounds in varying quantities. The thin layer chromatography analysis of coriander oil seed reported the existence of such molecules as linalool, α-pinene, geranyl acetate, limonene, geraniol, linalyl acetate, limonene, and other compounds (Rastogi and Mehrotra 1993). Telci, et al. (2006) mentioned that the oil primarily consisted of 50%–60% linalool and 20% terpenes (limonene, pinene, camphene, γ-terpinene, myrcene, cymene, and α-terpinene). The study of Bhuiyan, et al. (2009) found that the coriander seeds essential oil had about 53 molecules. From these molecules, the principal compounds identified were linalool (37.65%), geranyl acetate (17.57%), and γ-terpinene (14.42%). Besides these principal compounds, the other minor compounds identified were α-cedrene (3.87%) citronellal (1.96%), geraniol (1.87%), β-pinene (1.82%), β-sesquiphellandrene (1.56%), citral (1.36%), citronellyl acetate (1.36%), citronellol (1.31%), m-cymene (1.27%), and α-farnesene (1.22%). Although many of these and other studies (Leung and Foster 1996; Pino, et al. 1996) reported variation in the composition of oil, most of these studies found no variation concerning the presence/absence of the particular constituent. The variation in the make-up of coriander seed oil maybe because of the agronomical practices adopted during the cultivation and growth of coriander (Gil, et al. 2002; Zheljazkov, et al. 2008) and the harvesting or maturity stage of the coriander (Msaada, et al. 2007).

The seeds of coriander are reported to contain some antinutritional factors like glucosinolate (27.5 μmol/g), condensed tannins (1.1 mg/g), and inositol phosphate at the level of 17.4 mg/g (Matthäus and Angelini 2005).

The coriander oil is characterized by unique specifications. The oil or oleoresin extract of coriander seed is colorless to pale yellow with peculiar taste and aroma of coriander. It has a pleasant, sweet, warm, and aromatic flavor (Telci, et al. 2006). The coriander oil is identified for its infrared absorption spectrum. The refractive index of coriander oil varies between 1.462 and 1.472 at 20°C, whereas its specific gravity ranges from 0.863 to 0.875. The maximum and minimum angular rotations of coriander oil are 15° and 8°, respectively. Coriander oil is fairly soluble in alcohol. The solubilization of 1 ml coriander oil requires about 3 ml (70%) alcohol (FCC 2003).

2.5 APPLICATIONS

Coriander is regarded for many health benefits and medicinal properties including anti-inflammatory, antimicrobial, antioxidant, antihypertensive, and diuretic activities (Zeb 2016). The health benefits and medicinal properties of coriander seed oil are illustrated in Figure 2.4. Coriander has diverse food applications and at least one part of coriander is used in food preparations, primarily to enhance the flavor and appearance. Coriander seed oil when incorporated in food increases their storage stability and act as a preservative through its antioxidant and antimicrobial activity (Ashraf, et al. 2020). Some of the applications of coriander extract are presented in Table 2.4.

2.5.1 Antioxidant Activity

The antioxidant activity of coriander oil varies widely as reported by earlier researchers (Samojlik, et al. 2010; Teixeira, et al. 2013; Wangensteen, et al. 2004). Wangensteel, et al. (2004) observed that coriander oil had weak antioxidant activity, whereas Teixeira, et al. (2013) reported that oils extracted from coriander have nearly no antioxidant potential. The coriander oil is believed to possess moderate antioxidant activity (Samojlik, et al. 2010) with IC_{50} value of 5.35%. The oil extracted from coriander is used as an antioxidant to inhibit browning in fruits and vegetables as it has the potential to significantly reduce the peroxidase activity (Mousavizadeh and Sedaghathoor 2011a; 2011b). The coriander oil is also used to inhibit the peroxidation of lipids in meat and meat products (Marangoni and de Moura 2011a, 2011b). Coriander essential oil addition at the level of 0.05%–0.15% results in inhibiting the generation of oxidation products in baked products like cake. The cake prepared with the addition of coriander essential oil at 0.05% level has sensory characteristics of cake prepared without the addition of oil from coriander (Darughe, et al. 2012). The extract or essential oil obtained from coriander prolongs the lipid oxidation in food and food products. The biofilms developed with the use of coriander extract also display similar activity against the oxidation of lipids (Silva, et al. 2020). The oil extracted from coriander contains many antioxidant compounds including phenolics, flavonoids, linalool, and phytosterols. The extract obtained by cold pressing of seeds of coriander contains these antioxidants in substantial amounts (Wangensteen et al., 2004).

The monoterpenes contained in coriander seed oil possess hypoglycemic activity and aid in the metabolization of carbohydrates. These monoterpenes inhibit the enzymes in the gastrointestinal tract and thereby hinder glucose assimilation in the gastro-intestine (Ramadan, et al. 2008). Coriander oil is diuretic and has hypotensive potential (Jasbeen, et al. 2009).

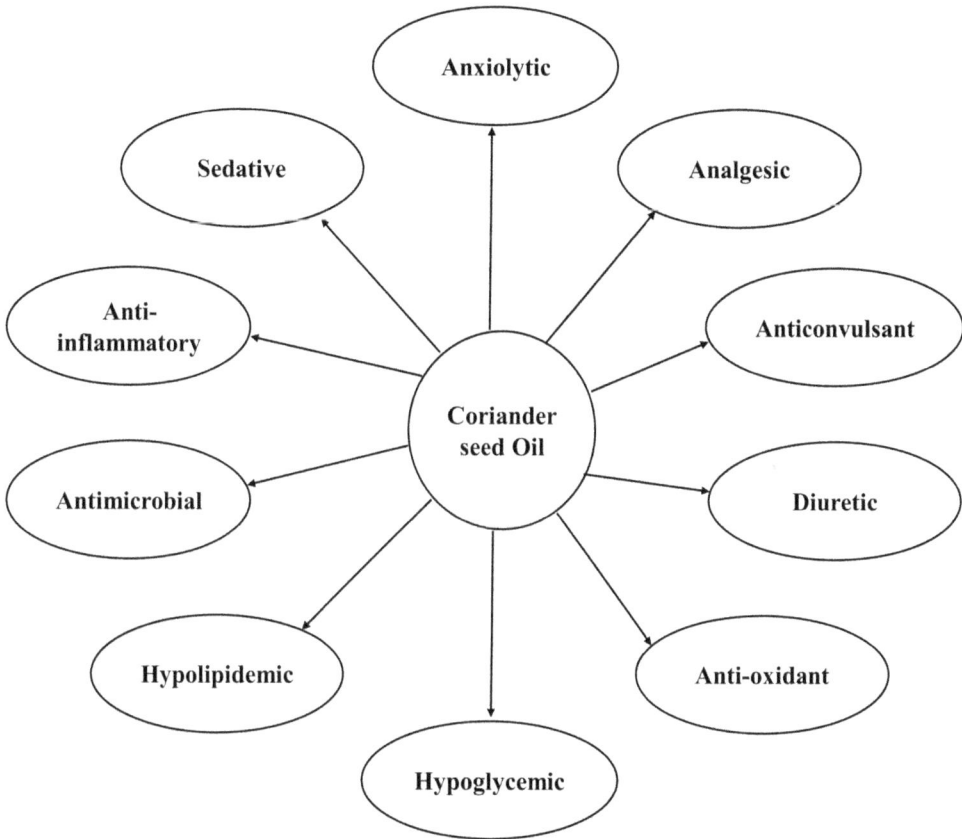

FIGURE 2.4 Health benefits and medicinal properties of coriander seed oil.

TABLE 2.4 Applications of Coriander Extract in Food and Food Products

Type of Coriander Extract	Food/Food Product	Effect	Reference
Essential oil	Apple and quince	Prevented activity of peroxidase enzyme, decreased enzymatic browning	Mousavizadeh and Sedaghathoor (2011a)
Essential oil	Celery, spinach, lettuce	Reduced peroxidase activity	Mousavizadeh and Sedaghathoor (2011b)
Essential oil	Minced beef meat	Inhibited the growth of Enterobacteriaceae and lactic acid bacteria	Michalczyk, et al. (2012)
Seed essential oil	Tomato sauce	Inhibited the growth of *Byssochlamys fulva* with an MIC value of 2700 ppm	Zamindar, et al. (2016)
Seed essential oil	Minced chicken and beef meat	Inhibited the growth of *C. jejuni* with an MIC value of 0.03%–0.06%	Rattanachaikunsopon and Phumkhachorn (2010)
Leaf powder	White bread	Improved crumb moisture content, sensory characteristics, and increased antioxidant content	Das, et al., (2012)
Seed extract	Turkey meatballs	Delayed lipid oxidation and inhibited growth of aerobic microorganisms	Gantner, et al., (2016)

2.5.2 Antimicrobial Activity

The essential oil extracted from coriander displays significant antimicrobial potential against almost all kinds of microorganisms including bacteria, yeast, fungi, and viruses. The antimicrobial action of essential oil extracted from the coriander is because of the existence of long-chain alcohols and aldehydes (Zeb 2016). Coriander oil is reported to reduce the *Campylobacter jejuni* bacteria count in beef and chicken meat stored at 4°C and 32°C. The antimicrobial activity of essential oil obtained from coriander is not affected by the type of meat and its storage temperature. The inhibition zone of oil of coriander against *C. jejuni* ranges from about 23 to 27 mm in diameter (Rattanachaikunsopon and Phumkhachorn 2010). Coriander oil depicts considerable antibacterial potential inhibiting the multiplication of Gram-positive as well as Gram-negative bacteria because of the occurrence of bioactive molecules (Laribi, et al. 2015). The extract or oil collected from coriander when utilized in food preparation reduces the growth and count of Gram-positive (*L. monocytogenes, S. aureus*) as well as Gram-negative bacteria (Enterobacteriaceae, *Aeromonas hydrophila*) and fungi (*Byssochlamys fulva*). The biofilms incorporated with coriander extract also exhibit similar activity against microorganisms (Silva, et al. 2020). Plantaricin CS, an antimicrobial peptide found in coriander, is reported to exhibit antibacterial activity (Zare-Shehneh, et al. 2014). Further, the silver nanoparticles constituting coriander extract function as a capable antimicrobial agent through their interaction with the bacterial external membrane, collapsing bacterial DNA, and inhibiting the mechanism responsible for the reproduction of bacteria (Ashraf, et al. 2019). Secondary metabolites like polyphenols and flavonoids in coriander oil also confer microbial activity (Bhat, et al. 2014).

2.5.3 Analgesic Activity

The aqueous extract of coriander seed is reported to have an analgesic effect, the mechanism of which may be facilitated by the inhibition of pain receptors (Pathan, et al. 2011). The chief element of the oil of coriander seed, linalool, is thought to be majorly accountable for the analgesic potential of coriander oil (Guimares, et al. 2013). In this respect, researchers (Peana, et al. 2003) have documented that the linalool possesses antinociceptive activity. Linalool elicited antinociceptive activity in mice is supported by the glutamatergic system (Batista, et al. 2008). Further, it is also found in experimental pain protocols that linalool complexed with β-cyclodextrin have better antinociceptive activity compared to free linalool (Quintans-Junior, et al. 2013).

2.5.4 Anti-Inflammatory Activity

Many studies have found the anti-inflammatory potential of coriander extract and essential oil of coriander seeds (Gupta, et al. 2010; Reuter, et al. 2008; Wu, et al. 2010). The ethanolic extract of coriander seeds showed inhibition of edema in rats. The application of this coriander seed extract at a concentration of 200 mg/kg yields 40.81% edema inhibition in rats after 3 hours (Gupta, et al. 2010). The anti-inflammatory effect of coriander oil is because of the existence of rutin, β-sitosterol, β-sitosterolene, and other bioactive compounds. Besides, these compounds also inhibit aggregation, macrophage inactivation, and infiltration (Sabogal-Guáqueta, et al. 2016).

2.5.5 Hypoglycemic Activity

Several research reports have indicated the efficacy of coriander extract for lowering the glycemic effect in biological systems (Aissaoui, et al. 2011; Rajeshwari, et al. 2011; Naquvi, et al. 2012; Waheed, et al. 2006). However, modest data is available depicting the anti-diabetic and hypoglycemic potential of essential oil extracted from coriander in experimental animals. It is suggested that the combined impact of various bioactive molecules, namely, linalool, γ-terpinene, and geranyl acetate, is responsible for the hypoglycemic potential of coriander essential oil (Abou El-Soud, et al. 2012). Many researchers (Gallagher, et al. 2003; Pandeya, et al. 2013) have opined that the hypoglycemic activity of coriander is related to stimulation of insulin excretion and improved uptake of glucose and its subsequent metabolization by muscles, which reflects the influence of several bioactive compounds simultaneously. These researchers found coriander as a prospective resource of valuable dietary supplements for enhanced regulation of blood glucose level and prevention of enduring impediments in such ailments as type 2 diabetes mellitus.

2.5.6 Hypolipidemic Activity

The hypolipidemic potential of coriander is documented by many research studies (Dhanapakiam, et al. 2008; Lal, et al. 2004) conducted to assess the influence of coriander seed extract administration in several characteristics of metabolization of lipid in experimental animals. Similar to hypoglycemic activity, the lipid-lowering ability of coriander seed is also attributed to the interactive action of several bioactive molecules existing in the coriander seed extract (Rajeshwari et al., 2011). Moreover, it has been found that certain fatty acids (palmitic acid, stearic acid, oleic acid, linoleic acid) and ascorbic acid available in the extract of coriander are responsible for reducing cholesterol. These compounds are also effective in reducing the accumulation of cholesterol in arteries and veins (Ertas, et al. 2005). This reduction in blood and tissue cholesterol level as a result of coriander seed extract administration is considered to be facilitated by enhanced degradation of biles and sterols (Dhanapakiam, et al. 2008; Lal, et al. 2004). Hence it is believed that the coriander can get promoted as a household herbal preparation having preclusive and healing potential for anti-hyperlipidemic activity (Lal, et al. 2004).

Besides, aforementioned health benefits and medicinal properties, coriander is also considered effective for bettering memory power, and therefore it is aspiring to investigate this prospective of coriander in the control and regulation of Alzheimer's disease (Cioanca, et al. 2013; Mani and Parle 2009). Further, the extract of coriander seeds also has sedative-hypnotic potential. However, the principal components responsible for this effect are reported to exist in the aqueous extract of coriander (Emamghoreishi and Heidari-Hamedani 2006). The crude extracts of coriander are useful in the stimulation of the gut and have inhibitory and hypotensive potential. The coriander extract can also be used for treating hypertension as it has diuretic properties (Jabeen, et al. 2009). Coriander extract also exhibits protective potential in renal tissue for toxicity caused by lead (Kansal, et al. 2011).

2.6 SAFETY, TOXICITY, AND FUTURE SCOPE

The coriander has been in use in many food preparations as a flavor enhancer for a long time. The applications of coriander also extend beyond food like in cosmetics without any reports of intense adverse side effects. The oil obtained from coriander has gained a GRAS status for utilization in food products by food and drug administration as well as by flavor and extracts manufacturers' Association. The coriander oil is also authorized for its food applications by the European Council. Therefore, oleoresin extract can be safely used in food preparations for its varied functions. The average level of its incorporation in food varies from 0.1 to 100 ppm. Very few scientific reports are available depicting the comprehensive toxicity effect of coriander oil. The coriander oil has no observed adverse effect level (NOAEL) of about 250 mg/kg/day and the developmental NOAEL was found to be 500 mg/kg/day. The reported NOAEL value of linalool, the principal component of oil extracted from coriander is 50 mg/kg/day (Burdock and Carabin 2009). Coriander is classified as a class I herb, that is the group of substances usually utilized for human consumption without harm in an appropriate amount (McGuffin, et al. 1997). The oil extracted from coriander has been regarded as a novel food ingredient and its utilization as a food supplement by a normal human being at the highest dosage level of 600 mg/day is considered safe (Uitterhaegen, et al. 2016).

The acute toxicity of coriander oil is well reported with its LD_{50} value of 2.48–6.14 g/kg of body weight in rats upon oral administration, whereas the coriander oil produces acute dermal toxicity in rabbits with LD_{50} value of more than 5 g/kg. Treating rabbit skin with coriander oil for 24 hours was found to result in skin irritation (Hart 1971). However, coriander oil, as well as linalool in petrolatum at a concentration of 6% and 20%, did not prove irritant in human beings (Kligman 1971; Kligman 1970). The toxicity at the acute level (LD_{50}) of the principal component of coriander oil, linalool, is more than 2.79 g/kg body weight in rats (Jenner, et al. 1964). In one of the other sub-chronic toxicity studies, it was found that the coriander oil administered at a concentration of 1% in methylcellulose and concentrations of 160, 400, and 1000 mg/kg/day produced no effect on survival rates, clinical symptoms, body weight, food consumption (Letizia, et al. 2003). However, it seems that this concentration is too low to cause any visible toxicity effects in experimental animals.

The coriander oil was observed to not produce any effect on the immune function when administered at a concentration of 313, 625, and 1250 mg/kg/day for 5 days in rats (Gaworski, et al. 1994).

2.7 CONCLUSION

Oil and oleoresins obtained from coriander seed find wide application in the food processing industry, particularly as a flavor enhancer. Coriander oil and oleoresin are mainly attained with steam distilling the dried seeds of coriander. The coriander extract and oleoresins offer tremendous health benefits and medicinal properties. The protective properties of this herb need to be emphasized as an encouraging ingredient for fostering the welfare of the impending generation of senescent society with lifestyle-adjudicated ailments. The majority of purported issues of coriander oil are ascribed to the existence of linalool as later is the chief constituent of coriander oil and forms more than two-third of its proportion. However, the information available on the toxicity of coriander oleoresins is ambiguous though despite the long history of coriander use in various food preparations for human consumption, has not recorded any lethal effect indicating it is safe to use in foods. It is, therefore, resolutely suggested that coriander extract is remarkably harmless for human consumption at the appropriate dosage and it would be beneficial to consider coriander oil and oleoresins to use in daily diet.

REFERENCES

Aissaoui, A., Zizi, S., Israili, Z. H. and Lyoussi, B. 2011 Hypoglycemic and hypolipidemic effects of *Coriandrum sativum* L. in Meriones shawi rats, *Journal of Ethnopharmacology*, 137: 652–61.

Ashraf, A., Zafar, S., Zahid, K., Shah, M. S., Al-Ghanim, K. A., Al-Misned, F. and Mahboob, S. 2019 Synthesis, characterization, and antibacterial potential of silver nanoparticles synthesized from *Coriandrum sativum* L, *Journal of Infection and Public Health*, 12: 275–81.

Ashraf, R., Ghufran, S., Akram, S., Mushtaq, M. and Sultana, B. 2020 Cold pressed coriander (*Coriandrum sativum* L.) seed oil, In *Cold Pressed Oils: Green Technology, Bioactive Compounds, Functionality, and Applications*, ed. M. F. Ramadan, 345–356. London: Academic Press.

BACIS 1999 *Coriander Seed*. Database of Volatile Compounds in Food, *TNO Nutrition and Food Research*, Boelens Aroma Chemical Information Service, The Netherlands.

Balbino, S., Repajić, M., Obranović, M., Medved, A. M., Tonković, P. and Dragović-Uzelac, V. 2021 Characterization of lipid fraction of Apiaceae family seed spices: Impact of species and extraction method, *Journal of Applied Research on Medical and Aromatic Plants*, 25. (December) 100326. Doi: 10.1016/j.jarmap.2021.100326.

Batista, P. A., de Paula Werner, M. F., Oliveira, E. C., Burgos, L., Pereira, P., da Silva Brum, L. F. and Dos Santos, A. R. S. 2008 Evidence for the involvement of ionotropic glutamatergic receptors on the antinociceptive effect of (–)-linalool in mice, *Neuroscience Letters*, 440: 299–303.

Bermúdez-Aguirre, D., Mobbs, T., and Barbosa-Cánovas, G. V. 2011 Ultrasound applications in food processing. In *Ultrasound Technologies for Food and Bioprocessing*, ed. H. Feng, G. V. Barbosa-Cánovas and J. Weiss, 65–105. New York: Springer.

Bhat, S., Kaushal, P., Kaur, M. and Sharma, H. K. 2014 Coriander (*Coriandrum sativum* L.): Processing, nutritional and functional aspects, *African Journal of Plant Science*, 8: 25–33.

Bhuiyan, M. N. I., Begum, J. and Sultana, M. 2009 Chemical composition of leaf and seed essential oil of *Coriandrum sativum* L. from Bangladesh, *Bangladesh Journal of Pharmacology*, 4: 150–53.

Burdock, G. A. and Carabin, I. G. 2009 Safety assessment of coriander (*Coriandrum sativum* L.) essential oil as a food ingredient, *Food and Chemical Toxicology*, 47: 22–34.

Carrubba, A. 2009 Nitrogen fertilisation in coriander (*Coriandrum sativum* L.): A review and meta-analysis, *Journal of the Science of Food and Agriculture*, 89: 921–26.

Cioanca, O., Hritcu, L., Mihasan, M. and Hancianu, M. 2013 Cognitive-enhancing and antioxidant activities of inhaled coriander volatile oil in amyloid β (1–42) rat model of Alzheimer's disease, *Physiology and Behavior*, 120: 193–202.

Darughe, F., Barzegar, M. and Sahari, M. A. 2012 Antioxidant and antifungal activity of Coriander (*Coriandrum sativum* L.) essential oil in cake, *International Food Research Journal*, 19: 1253–60.

Das, L., Raychaudhuri, U. and Chakraborty, R. 2012 Supplementation of common white bread by coriander leaf powder, *Food Science and Biotechnology*, 21: 425–33.

Dhanapakiam, P., Joseph, J. M., Ramaswamy, V. K., Moorthi, M. and Kumar, A. S. 2007 The cholesterol lowering property of coriander seeds (*Coriandrum sativum*): Mechanism of action, *Journal of Environmental Biology*, 29: 53–56.

Eidi, M. and Eidi, A. 2011 Effect of Coriander (*Coriandrum sativum L.*) seed ethanol extract in experimental diabetes. *In Nuts and Seeds in Health and Disease Prevention*, ed. V. R. Preedy and R. R. Watson, 395–400. Academic Press.

Eikani, M. H., Golmohammad, F. and Rowshanzamir, S. 2007 Subcritical water extraction of essential oils from coriander seeds (*Coriandrum sativum L.*), *Journal of Food Engineering*, 80: 735–40.

El-Soud, N. H. A., El-Lithy, N. A., El-Saeed, G. S. M., et al. 2012 Efficacy of *Coriandrum sativum* L. essential oil as antidiabetic, *Journal of Applied Sciences Research*, 8: 3646–55.

Emamghoreishi, M., Heidari-Hamedani, G., Emam, G. M. and Heydari, H. G. 2006 Sedative-hypnotic activity of extracts and essential oil of coriander seeds, *Iranian Journal of Medical Sciences*, 31: 22–27.

Ertas, O. N., Guler, T., Ciftci, M., Dalkilic, B. and Yilmaz, O. 2005 The effect of a dietary supplement coriander seeds on the fatty acid composition of breast muscle in Japanese quail, *Revue de médecine vétérinaire*, 156: 514–18.

FCC 2003 Coriander Oil. *Food Chemicals Codex*, Washington, DC: National Academy Press.

Gallagher, A. M., Flatt, P. R., Duffy, G. A. W. Y. and Abdel-Wahab, Y. H. A. 2003 The effects of traditional antidiabetic plants on in vitro glucose diffusion, *Nutrition Research*, 23: 413–24.

Gantner, M., Guzek, D., Najda, A., et al. 2017 Oxidative and microbial stability of poultry meatballs added with coriander extracts and packed in cold modified atmosphere, *International Journal of Food Properties*, 20: 2527–37.

Gaworski, C. L., Vollmuth, T. A., Dozier, et al. 1994 An immunotoxicity assessment of food flavouring ingredients, *Food and Chemical Toxicology*, 32: 409–15.

Gil, A., De La Fuente, E. B., Lenardis, A. E., et al. 2002 Coriander essential oil composition from two genotypes grown in different environmental conditions, *Journal of Agricultural and Food Chemistry*, 50: 2870–77.

Grosso, C., Ferraro, V., Figueiredo, A. C., Barroso, J. G., Coelho, J. A. and Palavra, A. M. 2008 Supercritical carbon dioxide extraction of volatile oil from Italian coriander seeds, *Food Chemistry*, 111: 197–203.

Guimarães, A. G., Quintans, J. S. and Quintans-Júnior, L. J. 2013 Monoterpenes with analgesic activity—A systematic review, *Phytotherapy Research*, 27: 1–15.

Hart, E.P. 1971 Report to the Research Institute for Fragrance Materials (RIFM), (cited in Opdyke 1973).

Illés, V., Daood, H. G., Perneczki, S., Szokonya, L. and Then, M. 2000 Extraction of coriander seed oil by CO_2 and propane at super-and subcritical conditions, *The Journal of Supercritical Fluids*, 17: 177–86.

Jabeen, Q., Bashir, S., Lyoussi, B. and Gilani, A. H. 2009 Coriander fruit exhibits gut modulatory, blood pressure lowering and diuretic activities, *Journal of Ethnopharmacology*, 122: 123–30

Jenner, P. M., Hagan, E. C., Taylor, J. M., Cook, E. L. and Fitzhugh, O. G. 1964 Food flavourings and compounds of related structure I. Acute oral toxicity, *Food and Chemical Toxicology*, 2: 327–43.

Kansal, L., Sharma, V., Sharma, A., Lodi, S. and Sharma, H. 2011 Protective role of *Coriandrum sativum* (coriander) extracts against lead nitrate induced oxidative stress and tissue damage in the liver and kidney in male mice, *International Journal of Pharmaceutical Sciences and Research*, 2: 65–83.

Kiple, K. F. and Ornelas, K. C. 2000 Coriander. The Cambridge World History of Food. New York: Cambridge University Press.

Kiralan, M., Calikoglu, E., Ipek, A., Bayrak, A. and Gurbuz, B. 2009 Fatty acid and volatile oil composition of different coriander (*Coriandrum sativum*) registered varieties cultivated in Turkey, *Chemistry of Natural Compounds*, 45: 100–02.

Kligman, A. M. 1970 Report to the Research Institute for Fragrance Materials (RIFM), (cited in Opdyke 1975).

Kligman, A.M., 1971 Report to the Research Institute for Fragrance Materials (RIFM), (cited in Opdyke 1973).

Lal, A., Kumar, T., Murthy, P. B. and Pillai, K. S. 2004 Hypolipidemic effect of *Coriandrum sativum* L. in triton-induced hyperlipidemic rats, *Indian Journal of Experimental Biology*, 42: 909–12.

Laribi, B., Kouki, K., M'Hamdi, M. and Bettaieb, T. 2015 Coriander (*Coriandrum sativum* L.) and its bioactive constituents, *Fitoterapia*, 103:9–26.

Lawrence, B. M. 1993 A planning scheme to evaluate new aromatic plants for the flavor and fragrance industries. In *New crops*, ed. J. Janick and J. E. Simon, 620–627. New York:Wiley.

Letizia, C. S., Cocchiara, J., Lalko, J. and Api, A. M. 2003 Fragrance material review on linalool, *Food and Chemical Toxicology*, 41: 943–64.

Leung, A. Y. and Foster, S. 1996. *Encyclopaedia of common natural ingredients used in food, drugs and cosmetics*. New York: John Wiley & Sons, Inc.

Livarda, A. and Van der Veen, M. 2008 Social access and dispersal of condiments in North-West Europe from the Roman to the medieval period, *Vegetation History and Archaeobotany*, 17: 201–09.

Mani, V. and Parle, M. 2009 Memory-enhancing activity of *Coriandrum sativum* in rats, *Pharmacologyonline*, 2: 827–39.

Marangoni, C. and Moura, N. F. D. 2011a Antioxidant activity of essential oil from *Coriandrum Sativum* L. in Italian salami, *Food Science and Technology*, 31: 124–28.

Marangoni, C. and Moura, N. F. D. 2011b Sensory profile of Italian salami with coriander (*Coriandrum sativum* L.) essential oil, *Food Science and Technology*, 31: 119–23.

Maroufi, K., Farahani, H. A. and Darvishi, H. H. 2010 Importance of coriander (*Coriandrum sativum* L.) between the medicinal and aromatic plants, *Advances in Environmental Biology*, 4: 433–36.

Matthäus, B. and Angelini, L. G. 2005 Anti-nutritive constituents in oilseed crops from Italy, *Industrial Crops and Products*, 21: 89–99.

McGuffin, M., Hobbs, C., Upton, R. and Goldberg, A. 1997 *Botanical Safety Handbook*. Boca Raton, Florida: CRC Press LLC36.

Mendiola, J. A., Herrero, H., Alejandro Cifuentes, A. and Elena Ibañez, E. 2007 Use of compressed fluids for sample preparation: Food applications, *Journal of Chromatography A* 1152: 234–246.

Mhemdi, H., Rodier, E., Kechaou, N. and Fages, J. 2011 A supercritical tuneable process for the selective extraction of fats and essential oil from coriander seeds, *Journal of Food Engineering*, 105: 609–16.

Michalczyk, M., Macura, R., Tesarowicz, I. and Banaś, J. 2012 Effect of adding essential oils of coriander (*Coriandrum sativum* L.) and hyssop (*Hyssopus officinalis* L.) on the shelf life of ground beef, *Meat Science*, 90: 842–50.

Micić, D., Ostojić, S., Pezo, L., Blagojević, S., Pavlić, B., Zeković, Z. and Đurović, S. 2019 Essential oils of coriander and sage: Investigation of chemical profile, thermal properties and QSRR analysis, *Industrial Crops and Products*, 138: 111438.

Mousavizadeh, S. J. and Sedaghathoor, S. 2011a Apple and quince peroxidase activity in response to essential oils application, *African Journal of Biotechnology*, 10: 12319–25.

Mousavizadeh, S. J. and Sedaghathoor, S. 2011b Peroxidase activity in response to applying natural antioxidant of essential oils in some leafy vegetables, *African Journal of Biotechnology*, 5: 494–99.

Msaada, K., Hosni, K., Taarit, M. B., Chahed, T., Kchouk, M. E. and Marzouk, B. 2007 Changes on essential oil composition of coriander (*Coriandrum sativum* L.) fruits during three stages of maturity, *Food Chemistry*, 102: 1131–34.

Msaada, K., Jemia, M. B., Salem, N., Bachrouch, O., Sriti, J., Tammar, S. and Marzouk, B. 2017 Antioxidant activity of methanolic extracts from three coriander (*Coriandrum sativum* L.) fruit varieties, *Arabian Journal of Chemistry*, 10: S3176–83.

Naquvi, K. J., Ali, M. O. H. D. and Ahmad, J. 2004 Antidiabetic activity of aqueous extract of Coriandrum sativum L. fruits in streptozotocin induced rats. *Indian Journal of Experimental Biology* 42: 909–12.

Pandeya, K. B., Tripathi, I. P., Mishra, et al. 2013 A critical review on traditional herbal drugs: An emerging alternative drug for diabetes, *International Journal of Organic Chemistry*, 3: 1–22.

Pathan, A. R., Kothawade, K. A. and Logade, M. N. 2011 Anxiolytic and analgesic effect of seeds of *Coriandrum sativum* Linn, *International Journal of Research in Pharmacy and Chemistry*, 1: 1087–99.

Pavlić, B., Vidović, S., Vladić, J., Radosavljević, R. and Zeković, Z. 2015 Isolation of coriander (*Coriandrum sativum* L.) essential oil by green extractions versus traditional techniques, *The Journal of Supercritical Fluids*, 99: 23–28.

Peana, A. T., Paolo, S. D., Chessa, M. L., Moretti, M. D., Serra, G. and Pippia, P. 2003 (–)-Linalool produces antinociception in two experimental models of pain, *European Journal of Pharmacology*, 460: 37–41.

Pino, J. A., Rosado, A. and Fuentes, V. 1996 Chemical composition of the seed oil of *Coriandrum sativum* L. from Cuba, *Journal of Essential Oil Research*, 8: 97–98.

Quintans-Júnior, L. J., Barreto, R. S., Menezes, P. P., et al. 2013 β–Cyclodextrin-complexed (–)-linalool produces antinociceptive effect superior to that of (–)-linalool in experimental pain protocols, *Basic & Clinical Pharmacology & Toxicology*, 113(3): 167–72.

Rahmani, S., Khorrami, A. R. and Mizani, F. 2015 A survey of the effects of coriander seed essential oil by solvent-free microwave extraction and ultrasonic waves on control of the growth of Salmonella typhimurium bacteria, *Journal of Applied Environmental and Biological Sciences*, 5: 65–71.

Rajeshwari, U. and Andallu, B. 2011 Medicinal benefits of coriander (*Coriandrum sativum* L), *Spatula DD*, 1: 51–58.

Rajeshwari, U., Shobha, I. and Andallu, B. 2011 Comparison of aniseeds and coriander seeds for antidiabetic, hypolipidemic and antioxidant activities, *Spatula DD*, 1: 9–16.

Ramadan, M. F., Amer, M. M. A. and Awad, A. E. S. 2008 Coriander (*Coriandrum sativum* L.) seed oil improves plasma lipid profile in rats fed a diet containing cholesterol, *European Food Research Technology*, 227: 1173–82.

Ramadan, M. F., Kroh, L. W. and Mörsel, J. T. 2003 Radical scavenging activity of black cumin (*Nigella sativa* L.), coriander (*Coriandrum sativum* L.), and niger (*Guizotia abyssinica* Cass.) crude seed oils and oil fractions, *Journal of Agricultural and Food Chemistry*, 51: 6961–69.

Rastogi, R. P. and Mehrotra, B. N. 1990 *Compendium of Indian Medicinal Plants*. Lucknow: Central Drug Research Institute.

Rattanachaikunsopon, P. and Phumkhachorn, P. 2010 Potential of coriander (*Coriandrum sativum*) oil as a natural antimicrobial compound in controlling *Campylobacter jejuni* in raw meat, *Bioscience Biotechnology and Biochemistry*, 74: 31–35.

Reuter, J., Huyke, C., Casetti, F., et al. 2008 Anti–inflammatory potential of a lipolotion containing coriander oil in the ultraviolet erythema test, *Journal der Deutschen Dermatologischen Gesellschaft*, 6: 847–51.

Sabogal-Guáqueta, A. M., Osorio, E. and Cardona-Gómez, G. P. 2016 Linalool reverses neuropathological and behavioral impairments in old triple transgenic Alzheimer's mice, *Neuropharmacology*, 102: 111–20.

Salzer, U. J. and Furia, T. E. 1977 The analysis of essential oils and extracts (oleoresins) from seasonings-A critical review, *Critical Reviews in Food Science and Nutrition*, 9: 345–73.

Samojlik, I., Lakic, N., Mimica-Dukic, N., Đaković-Švajcer, K. and Bozin, B. 2010 Antioxidant and hepatoprotective potential of essential oils of coriander (*Coriandrum sativum L.*) and caraway (Carum carvi L.) (Apiaceae), *Journal of Agricultural and Food Chemistry*, 58: 8848–53.

Seidemann, J. 2005 *World Spice Plants: Economic Usage, Botany, Taxonomy*. Berlin: Springer Science & Business Media.

Sharma, M. M. and Sharma, R. K. 2012 Coriander. In *Handbook of Herbs and Spices*, ed. K. V. Peter, 216–249. Cambridge: Woodhead Publishing.

Shrirame, B. S., Geed, S. R., Raj, A., et al. 2018 Optimization of supercritical extraction of coriander (*Coriandrum sativum* L.) seed and characterization of essential ingredients, *Journal of Essential Oil Bearing Plants*, 21: 330–44.

Silva, F., Domeño, C. and Domingues, F. C. 2020 Coriandrum Sativum L.: Characterization, biological activities, and applications. In *Nuts and Seeds in Health and Disease Prevention* ed. V. R. Preedy and R. R. Watson, 497–519. Cambridge: Academic Press.

Small, E. 2006 *Culinary Herbs*. Ottawa: NRC Research Press.

Sonika, G., Manubala, R. and Deepak, J. 2010 Comparative studies on anti-inflammatory activity of Coriandrum sativum, Datura stramonium and Azadirachta indica, *Asian Journal of Experimental Biological Sciences*, 1: 151–54.

Sovová, H. and Aleksovski, S. A. 2006 Mathematical model for hydrodistillation of essential oils, *Flavour and Fragrance Journal*, 21: 881–89.

Sriti, J., Wannes, W. A., Talou, T., Mhamdi, B., Cerny, M. and Marzouk, B. 2010 Lipid profiles of Tunisian coriander (*Coriandrum sativum*) seed, *Journal of The American Oil Chemists' Society*, 87: 395–400.

Teixeira, B., Marques, A., Ramos, C., et al. 2013 Chemical composition and antibacterial and antioxidant properties of commercial essential oils, *Indian Crops and Products*, 43: 587–95.

Telci, I., Toncer, O. G. and Sahbaz, N. 2006 Yield, essential oil content and composition of *Coriandrum sativum* varieties (var. vulgare Alef and var. microcarpum DC.) grown in two different locations, *Journal of Essential Oil Research*, 18: 189–93.

Uchibayashi, M. 2001 The coriander story, *Yakushigaku zasshi*, 36: 56–57.

Uhl, S.R. 2000 *Handbook of Spices, Seasonings, and Flavorings*. Boca Raton: CRC Press.

Uitterhaegen, E., Sampaio, K. A., Delbeke, E. I., et al. 2016 Characterization of French coriander oil as source of petroselinic acid, *Molecules*, 21: 1202–2014.

Waheed, A., Miana, G. A., Ahmad, S. I. and Khan, M. A. 2006 Clinical investigation of hypoglycemic effect of *Coriandrum sativum* in type-2 (NIDDM) diabetic patients, *Pakistan Journal of Pharmacology*, 23: 7–11.

Wangensteen, H., Samuelsen, A. B. and Malterud, K. E. 2004 Antioxidant activity in extracts from coriander, *Food Chemistry*, 88: 293–97

Wu, T. T., Tsai, C. W., Yao, et al. 2010 Suppressive effects of extracts from the aerial part of *Coriandrum sativum* L. on LPS-induced inflammatory responses in murine RAW 264.7 macrophages, *Journal of the Science of Food and Agriculture*, 90: 1846–54.

Zamindar, N., Sadrarhami, M. and Doudi, M. 2016 Antifungal activity of coriander (*Coriandrum sativum* L.) essential oil in tomato sauce, *Journal Food Measurement and Characterization*, 10: 589–94.

Zare-Shehneh, M., Askarfarashah, M., Ebrahimi, L., et al. 2014 Biological activities of a new antimicrobial peptide from Coriandrum sativum, *International Journal of Biosciences*, 4: 89–99.

Zeb, A. 2016 Coriander (*Coriandrum sativum*) oils. In *Essential Oils in Food Preservation, Flavor and Safety*, ed. V. R. Preedy, 359–364. London: Academic Press.

Zeković, Z., Bera, O., Đurović, S. and Pavlić, B. 2017 Supercritical fluid extraction of coriander seeds: Kinetics modelling and ANN optimization, *The Journal of Supercritical Fluids*, 125: 88–95.

Zeković, Z., Bušić, A., Komes, D., Vladić, J., Adamović, D. and Pavlić, B. 2015 Coriander seeds processing: Sequential extraction of non-polar and polar fractions using supercritical carbon dioxide extraction and ultrasound-assisted extraction, *Food and Bioproducts Processing*, 95: 218–27.

Zheljazkov, V. D., Pickett, K. M., Caldwell, C. D., Pincock, J. A., Roberts, J. C. and Mapplebeck, L. 2008 Cultivar and sowing date effects on seed yield and oil composition of coriander in Atlantic Canada, *Industrial Crops and Products*, 28: 88–94.

CHAPTER 3

Characterization of Capsicum Oleoresin

Asif Ahmad and Muhammad Suhail Ibrahim

PMAS-Arid Agriculture University Rawalpindi

CONTENTS

DOI: 10.1201/9781003186205-3

3.1 INTRODUCTION

Capsicum is a flowering plant that belongs to the family Solanaceae and has about 55,000 cultivars. Among these, six cultivars, including *C. annuum*, *C. baccatum*, *C. chinese*, *C. frutescens*, and *C. pubescen*, are predominately cultivated globally. Although these can be cultivated in a diversified environment, they prefer to grow in a damp hot environment, thus cultivated largely in tropical and subtropical regions. The fruit of capsicum is available in a wide range of colors and varieties ranging from shades of green, yellow, red, orange, purple, white, and brown. The color differences are attributed to the existence of carotenoid and anthocyanin pigments, which add antioxidant characteristics and are good for providing health benefits that can be capitalized on to develop nutraceutical foods (Akhtar, et al. 2019).

Moisture is the predominant component in *Capsicum* fruits; good amounts of carbohydrates including fibers are also present. Minor amounts of protein, ash, and lipid also exist that may vary from cultivar to cultivar. An appreciable amount of volatile and nonvolatile oils exist in the whole fruit, but the major part concentrates on seeds. Capsicum fruit also contains important minerals including K, Na, Ca, P, Fe, Cu, and Mn. CO is among these plant-based derivatives. Regulatory restriction of using synthetic chemicals as food additives has made plant-based derivatives a safe, economical, and nutritious alternative. Capsicum flowering plant species were predominately cultivated in America. It was brought by Columbus to the rest of the world. *Capsicum* spp. are cultivated for their various potential uses in food and pharmaceuticals (Perry, et al. 2007). Several cuisines around the globe require *Capsicum* for its unique sensory attributes that make the food delicious (Giuffrida, et al. 2013; Ozdemir, et al. 2008). The therapeutic effect of capsicum is attributed to the presence of ant diabetic and antioxidants substances that make it ideal as a nutraceutical vegetable. Some of the functional characteristics that can be derived from capsicum are shown in Figure 3.1.

Based on functional properties in plant resources, these materials and their derivatives have gained the attention of researchers, processors, nutritionists, and consumers. These compounds are being used as food additives in various cuisines (Fernández-Ronco, et al. 2010). Among these, capsicum-based varieties are gaining the attention of producers, processors, and consumers due to the high production potential of oleoresins. Some of these members having the potential of oleoresins formation are depicted in Figure 3.2, hence widely used in various food products as coloring and flavoring agents (Pino, et al. 2007). Oleoresins belong to terpenoids synthesized by epithelial cells localized in the stem and

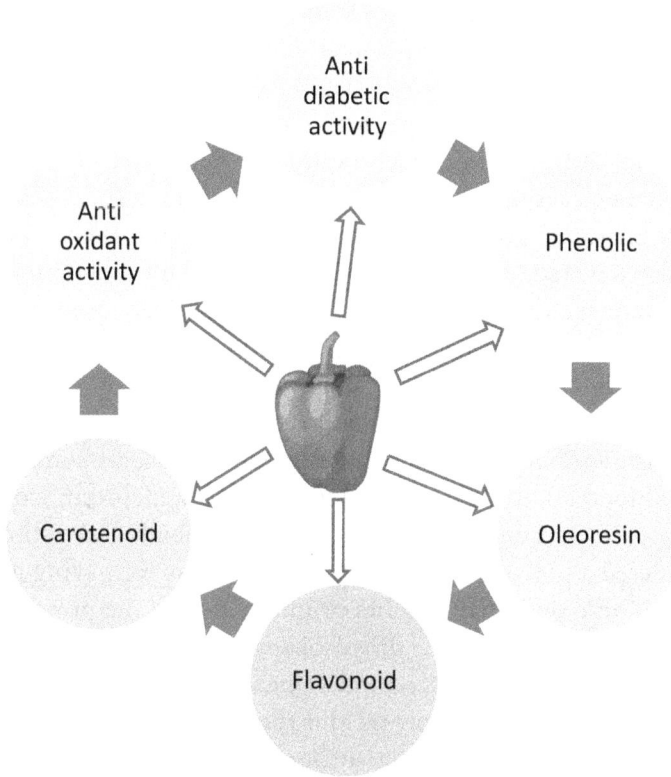

FIGURE 3.1   Functional importance of capsicum.

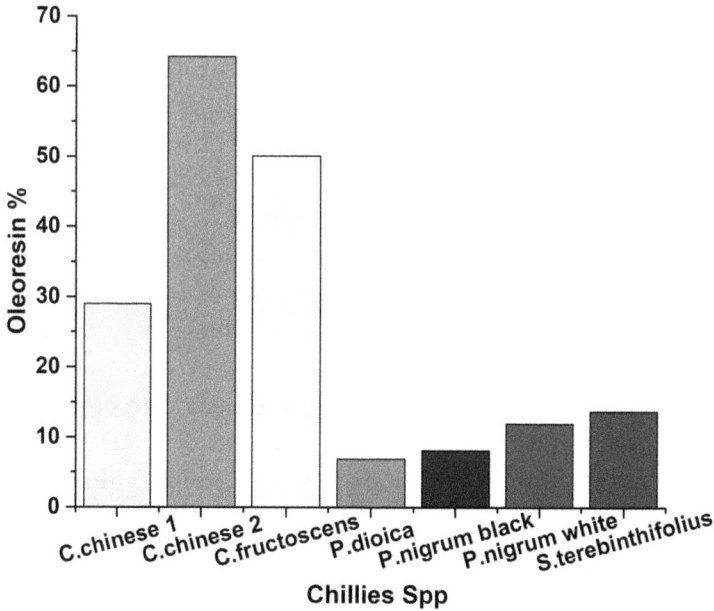

FIGURE 3.2   Oleoresin percentage in various capsicum cultivars.

roots (Keeling, et al. 2006). These oleoresins from capsicum not only bear unique taste and flavor but are also equipped with the potential bioactive moieties, hence preferred over traditional spices.

Different extraction techniques are being used for the extraction of oleoresin from the capsicum. Among these techniques, solvent extraction, sonication, and microwave-assisted extraction are the preferred ones and are considered environmental friendly. Pure capsaicin got the attention of pharmaceutical chemists for its broad biological activity. Reversed HPLC is being used for its ultimate purity and analysis (Riquelme and Matiacevich, 2017). Hexane is predominately used in solvent extraction for its better efficacy and low extraction time. It is also recommended by the FDA (Alós et al., 2008). *C. frutescens* is a commercial source of oleoresin. *C. annuum* is an economic alternative of *C. frutescens* for its unique reddish color, antioxidant potential, and antimicrobial properties that further increase its commercial potential as a nutraceutical food additive. In some Asian markets, oleoresin from various capsicum varieties possesses anti-inflammatory, antimicrobial, and antioxidant properties and is considered a potential source of a food additive for having its unique color, taste, and flavor. These potential benefits originate due to the presence of capsaicin, norhydrocapsaicin, homocapsaicin, dihydrocapsaicin, and homodihydrocapsaicin (Korkutata and Kavaz, 2015). Capsaicin has pharmacological application as analgesic properties and is used in osteoporosis and rheumatoid arthritis for pain management. Capsaicin is exploited for its anti-inflammatory, antimicrobial, antibacterial, antioxidant, and anticancer potential. Being volatile, the macroporous resin is used for its absorption and maximum recovery. Sophisticated analytical techniques can have a potential role in the quantification and identification of these components in oleoresins and other products. Among these analytical techniques, FTIR and TGA have a great future potential to be adopted at an industrial scale and is of great interest for researchers working in this field (Gourava, 2019; Pérez-Alonso et al., 2008; Haiyee, et al. 2009). For these bioactive substances, FTIR spectroscopy observed peaks at 1050–1055, 2900–2905, and 3350 cm^{-1} corresponding to vibrations NH, OH, and CH bonds. Spectroscopy of CO observed peaks at 1378, 1627, and 1650 cm^{-1} and capsaicin at 1347 cm^{-1}. TGA and DSC are used to define its stability when subjected to various industrial processes and its ultimate use. The presence of carbonyl groups in these substances provides redox properties and acts as a reducing agent. Other components that reinforce these properties are β-carotene, capsanthin, capsorubin, cryptoxanthin, protocatechuic, chlorogenic, cinnamic, ferulic, coumaric, and caffeic acid. Capsaicin showed the inhibitory effect against *Escherichia coli* and *Listeria monocytogenes*, when used in a concentration of 200–300 µg/mL. Capsaicin inhibited the growth of *Aspergillus flavus*, *Aspergillus niger*, and *Rhizopus* sp. up to 60% (Bacon, et al. 2015; Omolo, et al. 2014).

3.1.1 Economic Importance of Capsicum Oleoresin

Oleoresins are widely used as a flavoring agent and have tremendous economic value due to the variation of substances they may contain. Commercial products may contain both volatile and nonvolatile constituents. Oleoresin can be used as a substitute for traditionally used spice without masking the flavor and taste of the finished product; this will enable the processor to use lesser amounts, but in the purified form usually, solvent extraction is practiced for extraction of oleoresin and solvent can be recovered through the vacuum evaporation process. To achieve economic benefits and improved commercial activity, certain factors may drive the market of oleoresins. These factors include unique flavor and aroma to the finished product, ultimately increasing its overall acceptability. Evaporation intends to reduce the volume of finished product ultimately increase its heat stability, storage and transport convenience. Focusing on these factors may boost oleoresin markets across the globe. The global oleoresin market is estimated at USD 1.44 billion in 2017 (Kumareswaran, et al. 2018). The major part of these oleoresins products is being consumed in processed meat, confectionery, and baked products. Global market trends are based on its application, sale, and region. On an application basis, the oleoresin market is segmented into food and beverages, cosmetic, and pharmaceutical industries. The food and beverage segment is further subsegmented into confectionery, bakery, seasoning, sauces, dairy industry, convenience foods, desserts, ice cream, meat products, juices, etc. The cosmetic industry is subsegmented into skincare and hair care products. Oleoresin has wide application in the food and beverage industry as a coloring agent and oil soluble form is used in beverages. On the sale basis, it is further categorized into a direct and indirect sale (trader, wholesaler, and trader retailer). Europe, North America, and India are the major contributors to the global oleoresin market. There is a lot of attraction in the oleoresin market for the rest of the world (Weber, et al. 2020).

3.2 PHYSICOCHEMICAL CHARACTERIZATION OF *CAPSICUM ANNUUM*

3.2.1 Proximate and Bioactives Profile

The composition of raw material, i.e., capsicum fruit, is important in determining the composition of oleoresins. As the capsicum fruit is dried to a low moisture level, the average carbohydrates percentage tends to increase on a dried weight percentage basis. The proximate composition of capsicum is shown in Figure 3.3. The average values for moisture, crude protein, ash, crude fiber, crude fat, and carbohydrate contents were observed 14, 12, 11.1, 13.2, 21.1, and 61.8 g/100 g (DWB), respectively. Chemical characterization of capsicum showed that it contains piperine, dihydrocapsiconiate, quercetin, dihydrocapsaicin, rutin, capsiate, dihydrocapsiate, capsaicin, nordihydrocapsiate, capsiconiate, and beta-carotene. These components influence the composition of oleoresins from capsicum and have an impact on the cuisines and pharmaceuticals' characteristics. The phytochemistry is quite variable in the plant material from this family, thus affecting the physicochemical properties of the end product.

3.2.2 Mineral Profile of *Capsicum Annuum*

The mineral composition shown to calcium, magnesium, phosphorous, potassium, sulfate, copper, iron, manganese, sodium, and zinc is up to 131, 162.4, 280.1, 3504, 228.4, 1.1,7.7,1.1, 24, and 2.2 mg/100g, respectively (Zou, et al. 2015; Kim, et al. 2019), and the data is depicted in Figure 3.4.

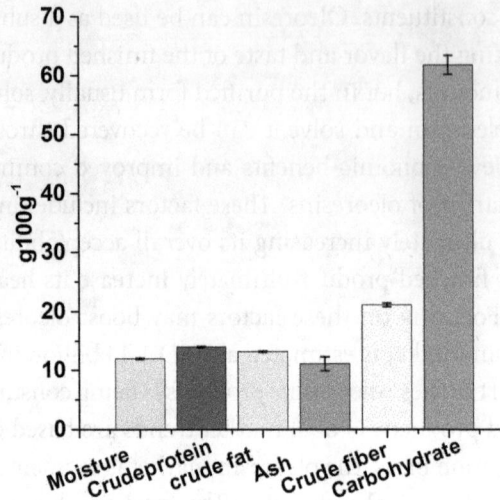

FIGURE 3.3   Mineral profile of *Capsicum annuum*.

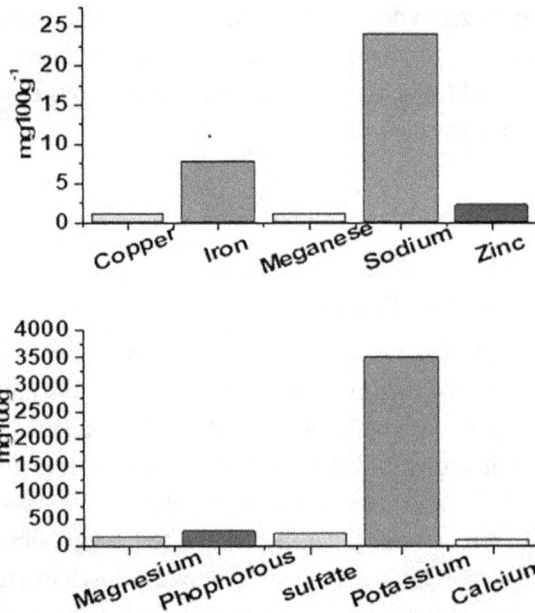

FIGURE 3.4   Mineral profile of capsicum.

3.2.3 Fatty Acid Profile of Capsicum

The fatty acid profile of capsicum on a dry weight basis is shown in Figure 3.5: Myristic 5.09, Palmitic 17.6, Stearic 4.4, Oleic 9.5, Linoleic 40.2, Linolenic 18.1, Lauric 22.1, Stearic 4.4, Arachidic 0.76, and Behenic acid 0.55% (Kim, et al. 2019). Capsicum is rich in polyunsaturated fatty acids, having health-beneficial effects. Capsicum is the richest source of PUFA and SFA, both are predominant due to elevated levels of linolenic acid. Food has

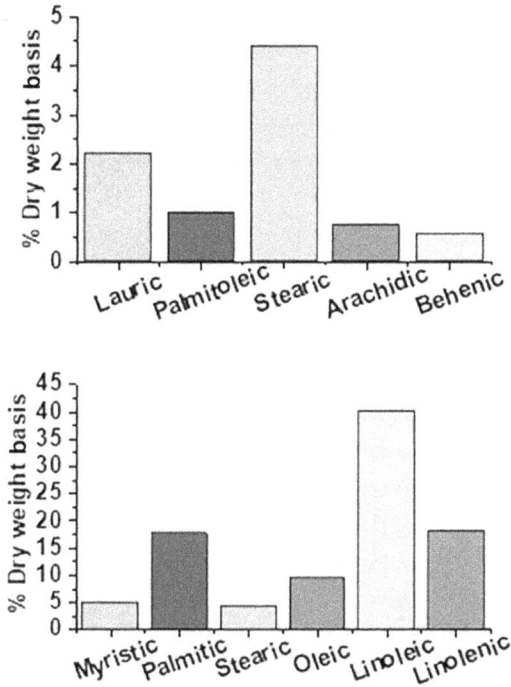

FIGURE 3.5   Fatty acid composition of capsicum.

the highest fraction of polyunsaturated fatty acids particularly PUFA/SFA tends to reduce body fat deposition and total cholesterol (Simopoulos, 2002). The most predominant fatty acid in CO was reported to include oleic (18:1), linoleic (18:2), and palmitic acid (16:0). It is studied that C18 is a major fraction of CO fatty acid (~87%), and linolenic (18:2) is the most predominant fatty acid in CO (Tepić, et al. 2009).

3.2.4 Amino Acid Profile of Capsicum

The amino acid profile of the capsicums is shown in Figure 3.6: Arginine (3.6), Cysteine (1.33), Glutamic acid (10.2), Glycine (3.23), Histidine (1.21), Isoleucine (1.97), Lysine (2.69), Methionine (0.69), Phenylalanine (2.5), Leucine (3.67), Alanine (3.8), Proline (5.2), Serine (3.7), Threonine (3.2), Aspartic Acid (23), Tryptophan (0.5), Tyrosine (1.4), and Valine (3%) of protein. The amino acid profile indicates that these are potential sources of amino acids as well. It also contains lysine—an essential amino acid necessary to be included in the food. The inclusion of capsicum in the food basket not only will impart unique taste and flavor to the foodstuff but also be a potential source of essential nutrients ((Kim, et al. 019; Simopoulos, 2002; Tepić, et al. 2009).

3.3 BIOSYNTHESIS OF OLEORESIN

Oleoresins are terpenoids and are resultant of plant defensive system, resulting in insect damage and fungal infection (Franceschi, et al. 2005). Oleoresin accumulates at the injury site of the plant and provides a natural barrier at the site of injury and is synthesized by the

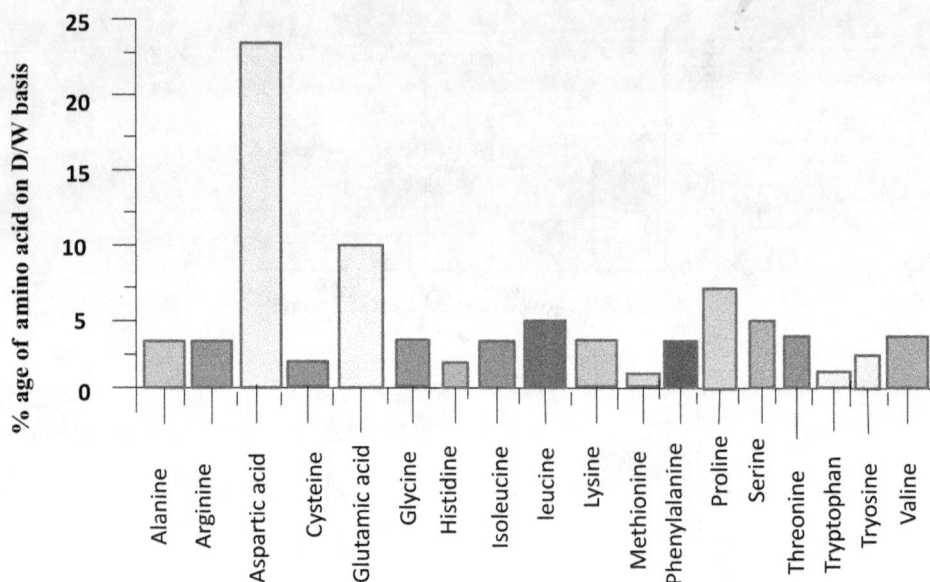

FIGURE 3.6   amino acid profile of capsicum.

epithelial cell of parenchyma tissue (Martin, et al. 2002). Defense response is an important factor that triggers the flow of oleoresin from the specialized duct system. Phenolic acid and oleoresin both prevent fungal infection. Oleoresin is a monoterpene retard of fungal mycelia by having a growth inhibitory effect. Various biotic factors determine the concentration of synthesized oleoresin (Martin et al., 2002; Kaleem, and Ahmad, 2018).

Biosynthetic pathways of oleoresin constituents are currently unknown. Synthesis of isopentenyl diphosphate in mevalonic acid or methylerythritol phosphate pathway eventuates synthesis of oleoresin. The five-carbon building blocks of terpenoids dimethylallyl diphosphate are gone through consecutive condensation to produce the intermediates including farnesyl diphosphate, geranyl diphosphate, and geranylgeranyl diphosphate. These largest molecules are terpenes, forerunners of monoterpenes, sesquiterpenes, and diterpenes. Terpenoids production in plants is a complex process, occurring in different stages (Rodrigues and Fett-Neto 2009). The initial phase of terpenoids biosynthesis proceeds in the cytosol, endoplasmic reticulum, and plastids, respectively. This process is followed by the synthesis of mono- and di-terpenoids with the support of the MEP pathway in plastids, some of the sesquiterpenoids are also formed during this process but their location of synthesis is cytosol. The support of P450 is essentially required during the whole mechanism for modification of mono, sesqui, and di-terpenoids in the endoplasmic reticulum. Oleoresin synthesis and major compounds in oleoresins with molecular formulae are shown in Figures 3.7 and 3.8 and Table 3.1, respectively.

3.4 EXTRACTION TECHNIQUES

Various extraction processes are designed to extract botanical essential oils and resin constituents. These provide aromatic and flavoring resins and can be extracted by various solvents. Their volatile and nonvolatile constituents impart characteristics of spicy flavor to the savory dishes. Being carrying antimicrobial characteristics, these extracted materials

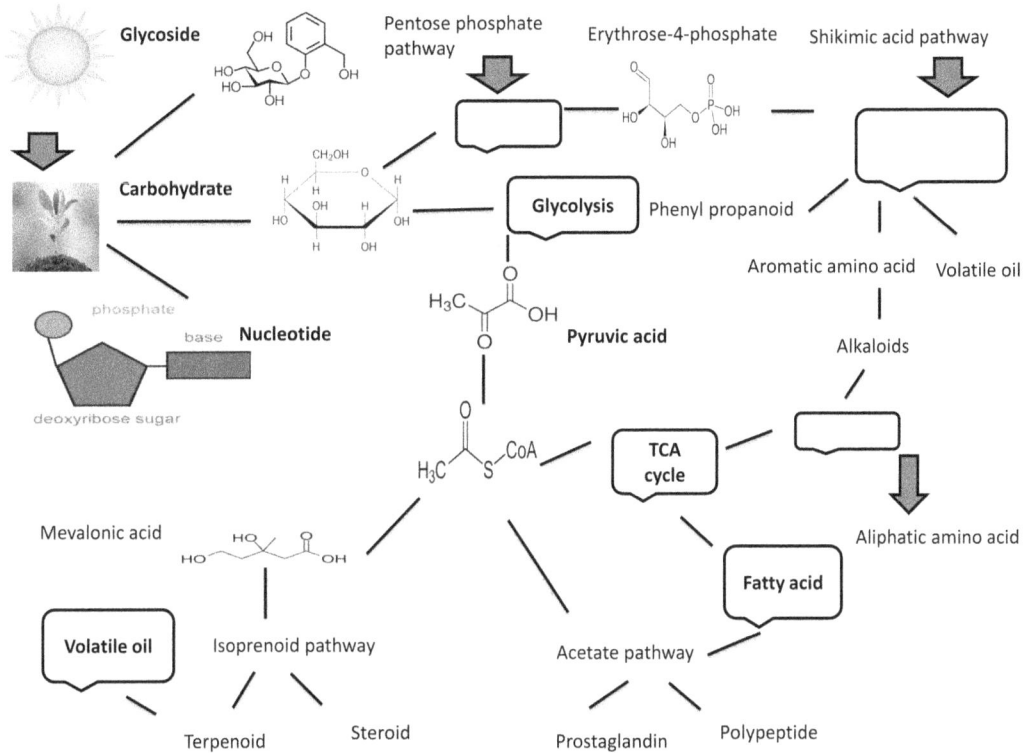

FIGURE 3.7   biosynthesis of Capsicum oleoresin.

also improve the shelf stability of food products. Before processing for actual extraction, some pretreatments may improve the recovery of active constituents and may improve the efficiency of the extraction process.

3.4.1 Preextraction Treatment of Capsicum Fruit

Quality characteristics of dehydrated capsicum fruit depend upon various chemical pre-treatments. Chemical used before dehydration includes NaOH, KOH, $K_2S_2O_{5,}$ $K_2CO_3 \cdot nH_2O$, $C_6H_8O_6$, $C_6H_8O_7$, and methyl and ethyl ester emulsions. Pretreatment with $C_6H_8O_7$ and $C_{20}H_{38}O_2$ increases dehydration efficacy including time and mass-transfer resistance (Doymaz and Kocayigit, 2012). Pretreatment with an aqueous solution of $CaCl_2$, NaCl, and $Na_2S_2O_3$ at 70°C exhibited better color tonality and firmness (Vega-Gálvez, et al. 2008). Pretreatment of fruit with ethyl oleate $C_6H_8O_7$ and citric acid ($C_{20}H_{38}O_2$) preserves the red color of fruit and its slices (Doymaz and Kocayigit, 2012). Soaking capsicum in sodium metabisulfite with $CaCl_2$ and putting it in boiling water before chemical treatment resulted in better color stability (Sharma, et al. 2015). Some of the pretreatment techniques are summarized in Table 3.2.

3.4.2 Osmotic/Hot Air/Sun Drying

Osmotic dehydration is an innovative dehydration technique that maintains the equilibrium of moisture among concentrated solute matrix and cellular matrix through a semi-permeable membrane. It reduces the moisture contents of foodstuff from 30% to 70% and

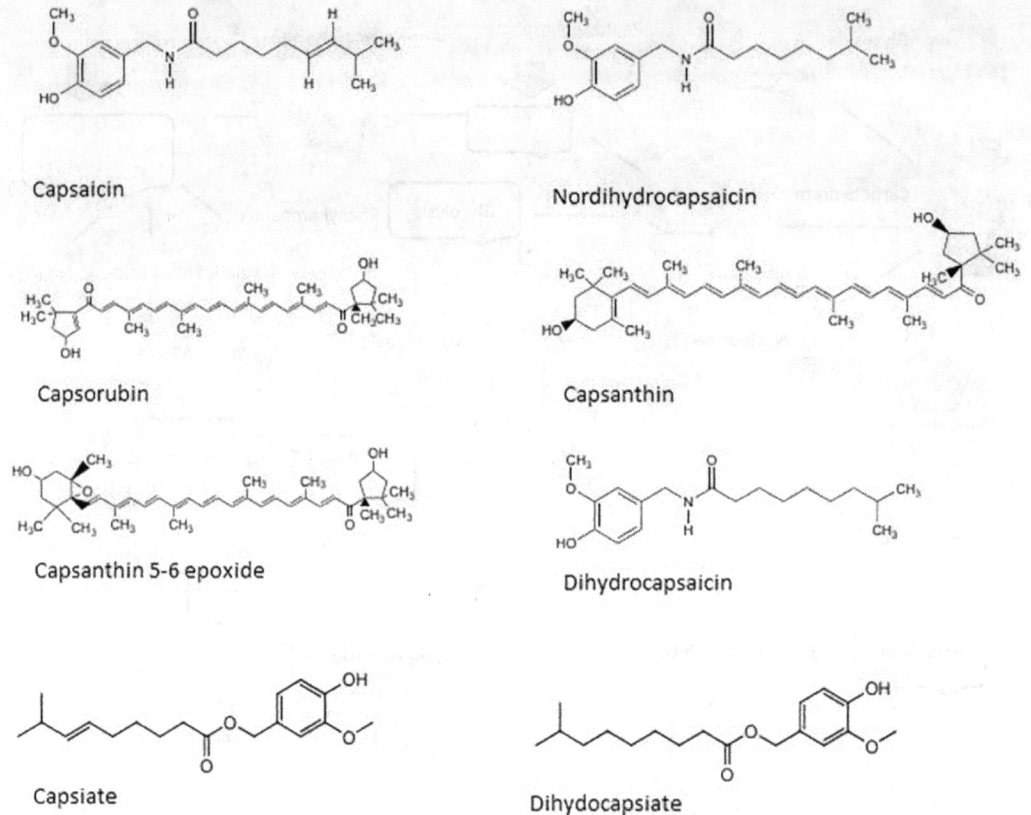

FIGURE 3.8 Chemical constituents of Capsicum oleoresin.

enhances the efficacy of further processing operations to which foodstuff is exposed (Levent and Ferit, 2012). It also sustained various quantitative and qualitative properties of food. Osmotic agents, including sodium chloride, corn syrup, sucrose, fructose, and fructose, are used individually or in combination. In combination, these ingredients exhibit synergistic and positive effects on their quality and color (Falade and Oyedele, 2010; Quintero-Chávez, et al. 2012). Osmotic dehydration cannot remove all moisture contents from food, thus final product is not shelf-stable. Osmotic agents, such as sorbitol and salt, increase weight loss, TSS, and Brix and decrease water activity (Ozdemir, et al. 2018). Sucrose and salt when used in combination make the processing more economical and reduce processing time and energy. Salt and sucrose are abundantly used in combination with enhanced efficacy (Zhao, et al. 2013). Drying reduces water activity, and hence enhances the shelf life of food and retards biochemical and microbial deterioration. Removals of moisture from food decrease its volume weight, ultimately reducing its storage, packaging, and logistic cost (Doymaz and Kocayigit, 2012). Drying in a hot air medium is a widely used drying technique for *Capsicum* spp. due to short time, uniform heating, and hygiene. The hot air drying temperature is usually between 45°C and 70°C and reduces drying time and ensures maximum color retention and less volatile deterioration (Arslan and Özcan, 2011). Sun drying is another traditional and oldest drying technique, in which material absorbs

TABLE 3.1   Biochemical Profile of Bioactive Moieties Extracted from *Capsicum annuum*

Compound	Synonyms	Chemical Formula	Plant Source	References
Piperine	1-Piperoylpiperidine	$C_{17}H_{19}NO_3$	Constituent of pepper spp	Haynes and Herring (1981)
Dihydrocapsiconiate	Coniferyl 8-methylnonanoate	$C_{20}H_{30}O_4$	Capsicum genus of plants	Kobata, et al. (2008)
Quercetin	Xanthaurine	$C_{15}H_{10}O_7$	Pepper fruit	Buczkowska, et al. (2016)
Dihydrocapsaicin	6,7-Dihydrocapsaicin	$C_{18}H_{29}NO_3$	pepper (*C. annuum*)	Andrews (1995)
Rutin	Quercetin 3-rutinoside	$C_{27}H_{30}O_{16}$	Fruits	Materska and Perucka (2005)
Capsiate	(4-hydroxy-3-methoxyphenyl)methyl (E)-8-methylnon-6-enoate	$C_{18}H_{26}O_4$	Capsicum genus of plants	Fayos, et al. (2008)
Dihydrocapsiate	4-Hydroxy-3-methoxybenzyl 8-methylnonanoate	$C_{18}H_{28}O_4$	Capsicum genus of plants	Fayos, et al. (2008)
Capsaicin	Capsaicin	$C_{18}H_{27}NO_3$	Capsicum fruits	Fayos, et al. (2008)
Nordihydrocapsiate	4-hydroxy-3-methoxybenzyl 7-methyloctanoate	$C_{17}H_{26}O_4$	Capsicum genus of plants	Fayos, et al. (2008)
Capsiconiate	Coniferyl (E)-8-methyl-6-nonenoate	$C_{20}H_{28}O_4$	Capsicum genus of plants	Perucka and Materska (2007)
Nordihydrocapsaicin	N-(4-hydroxy-3-methoxybenzyl)-7-methyloctanamide	$C_{17}H_{27}NO_3$	Eed pepper (*C. annuum*)	
beta-Carotene	Provitamin A	$C_{40}H_{56}$	*Capsicum* genus of plants	Perucka and Materska (2007); Kawaguchi, et al. (2004)

TABLE 3.2   Pretreatments of Capsicum Before Drying

Species	Common Name	Treatment Conditions	Pre Treatments	References
C. annuum L.	Charliston	Ambient Temperature for 1 minute	Ethyl oleate+K_2CO_3(2:3)+0.5% Citric acid	Doymaz and Kocayigit (2012)
C. annuum L.	Kahramanmaras	Ambient Temperature for 1 minute	Ethyl oleate+K_2CO_3(2:4) ethyl oleate+K_2CO_3(2:5) ethyl oleate+K_2CO_3(2:6)	Doymaz and Kocayigit (2012)
C. annuum L.	Paprika	23 °C/1 minute 60 °C/1 minute	2% Ethyl oleate (33°C), ethyl oleate+NaOH (23°C) 2% each, ethyl oleate, NaOH, K_2CO_3 (23°C) (2:2:4), 2% Ethyl oleate (60°C), ethyl oleate NaOH (60°C)[2:2].ethyl oleate, NaOH, K_2CO_3 (60°C) ()2:2:4	Vega-Gálvez, et al. (2008)
C. annuum L.	Lamuyo variety	25°C/ 10 min	20% NaCl +1.0% $CaCl_2$+0.3% NaS_2O_5	Sharma, et al. (2015)

sunlight to remove its free water contents. This technique needs more space and time for complete drying (ELkhadraoui, et al. 2015). Foodstuff subjected to sun drying is more amiable to physical, chemical, and microbial damage due to its exposure to the external environment. It has a detrimental effect on the quality and quantity of the final product (Fudholi, et al. 2013).

3.4.3 Water-Assisted Extraction

Water is the most economical solvent used for the extraction of hydrophilic compounds, and being solvent, it ensures the nutritional quality of the extract. Extraction with water can be carried out with hot, cold, or boiling water depending upon the final matrix ultimately centrifuged and dried for further characterization (Ergüneş and Tarhan, 2006). Hydrodistillation and infusion are the most traditionally used extraction techniques. This technique is now in a process of replacement with modern techniques. The latest innovative techniques reported in the literature are ultrasound-assisted extraction, pressurized hot water extraction, negative pressure-assisted extraction, and pulsed electric field extraction. These techniques can be used alone or in combination with conventional techniques. Using these modern techniques along with conventional techniques often improves the efficiency of the extraction process (Vega-Gálvez, et al. 2008). Water being a polar solvent has a low affinity with nonpolar or less polar compounds that intends to be extracted including capsaicinoids such as homocapsaicin, dihydrocapsaicin, and homodihydrocapsaicin (Vega-Gálvez, et al. 2008; Arvanitoyannis, et al. 2012). Steam distillation followed by condensation and decantation is an easy process of removing essential oil from plant material. Temperature and time of extraction are the most important factors determining extracted oils. Prolonged temperature leads to hydrolysis, polymerization, and decomposition, ultimately retarding the quality of the final product. Reduced-pressure steam distillation ensures retention of flavoring compounds (Aliakbarlu, et al. 2014).

3.4.4 Pressurized Water Extraction

This is a green and environment-friendly extraction technique. Elevated temperature attenuates water viscosity and surface tension, hence increasing capsaicinoids solubility and diffusivity. Pressurized hot water extraction has an advantage over traditional Soxhlet extraction. PHWE is the most convenient green extraction technology, where pressurized water is used as a solvent for the extraction of bioactive. It is reported that temperature and pressure variation alters the polarity of water and it acts like alcohol; hence, it can dissolve a wide range of medium and low polarity analytes (Meng and Lozano, 2014; Barbero, et al. 2006). PHWE (pressurized hot water extraction) has reduced organic solvent consumption and has made extraction more economical and easy as compared to solvent extraction. Disposal of solvent used for extraction may cause adverse effect on human health and environment.

3.4.5 Maceration

Maceration is mixing solid matrix to a solvent bulk at room temperature for a long period of light protected with daily agitation. It could also be carried out under a vacuum. The solvent used for maceration may be methanol, ethanol, or their mixture (Jang, et al. 2008).

Homogenization with nitrogen (expensive technique) and carbon maceration are being used at an experimental level. Filtration or centrifugation is done to separate solid matrix from liquid after maceration.

3.4.5.1 Olive Oil Maceration

Maceration by using olive oil enhances sensorial characteristics of the extracted oil but should be used in low quantity to prevent over-aromatization (Kim, et al. 2009). Mixing capsicum fruit with olive oil before cold pressing yields oleoresin with low functional properties and yield (Deng, et al. 2005). Second, seeds are cold-pressed that results pungent extracted oil and retard its consumer acceptability. Maceration for 3 months in darkness at ambient temperature conserves the functional and nutritional quality of oil (de Aguiar, et al. 2013). Traditional extraction techniques yield maximum capsaicinoids fraction, while in olive oil flavored extraction using a microwave, ultrasound results in superior quality oil with reduced time extraction (Sousa, et al. 2015).

3.4.5.2 Vegetable Oil Maceration

Medicinal oil and vegetable oil are being used for maceration of dehydrated capsicum to extract capsaicin and capsaicinoids, and different time and temperature combinations are being used to enhance extraction efficacy followed by filtration and centrifugation to get solid matrix (Baiano, et al. 2009). Vegetable and medicinal oil extracts ensured higher antioxidant activity with good sensorial characteristics, especially when macerated with corn oil. Ozonated oil is an industrial-used technique but has some hazards. Cold press is the most recent extraction technique that involves mechanical shear without heating. This yields good quality oil that doesn't need further refining (Caporaso, et al. 2013). The watery emulsion is obtained as a result of cold pressing, but it's concentrated by centrifugation. Soxhlet extraction with any organic solvent gives more yield but impart toxicological and environmental effects, which has less consumer acceptability.

3.4.6 Organic Solvent Extraction

Conventional techniques make use of solvent extraction, mechanical presses, or a combination of both for the extraction of oils from plant sources. These conventional techniques are being widely used for capsicum oil and bioactive extraction. Organic solvent dissolves reactant solvate molecules that eventually separate oil from the insoluble plant material. Unfortunately, these organic solvent has serious health impact as a residual effect in the extracted product, also imparting pungency of that particular organic solvent in the finished product. The efficiency of extraction solvent is based on various factors; among them, the occurrence of polar substances in the raw material and extraction conditions plays a vital role for high efficiencies (Paduano, et al. 2014). A lot of organic solvents are being used for the extraction of bioactive moieties from plant material. The most traditionally used organic solvents include methanol, ethanol, hexane, acetonitrile, isopropanol, acetone, propane, and dimethyl ether under low or atmospheric pressure. Capsaicin and capsaicinoids contents vary among different cultivars, are lipophilic, and are effectively extracted in lipophilic solvents. The solvent extraction technique is being used by researchers for the characterization of bioactive substances of capsicum for major antioxidants, phenolic substances, carotenoids, and flavonoids. The antioxidants extracted in this way can be analyzed further for DPPH, ABTS, and hydrogen peroxide radical scavenging activities (Amruthraj, et al. 2014; Khalid, et al. 2016; Khalid, et al. 2017).

The toxicological effects of these solvents may not be overlooked. Inhalation of n-hexane, used as an organic solvent for extraction of oleoresin, causes a serious effect on the CNS and prolonged exposure may lead to polyneuropathy. The solvent-extracted CO is predominately used as an additive (color and flavor). ERC (European Regulation Commission) allows a maximum of 50 mg/kg residue of organic solvent in finished products. During the extraction process, the polarity of organic solvents may induce a significant increase in the extraction rate. Hexane and methanol are widely used organic solvents used for the extraction of CO. Other solvents were used for the extraction of oleoresin acetonitrile, acetone, ethanol, and isopropanol (Amruthraj, et al. 2014). Use of nonpolluting and nontoxic solvents is now being preferred, especially ethanol, which imparts less toxic effect to human health (Vian, et al. 2014). The organic solvent, having a narrow boiling point of 63°C –65°C, has better oil solubility, recovery, and recycling. Acetone, a polar aprotic solvent, has better capsaicinoid extraction efficacy, especially for pharmacological purposes. Acetonitrile is another solvent which is not allowed in food due to its toxicity. Finally it was concluded that ethanol is the best option among all the organic solvents (Chinn, et al. 2011).

3.4.7 Innovative and Green Extraction Technologies

Technologies amenable to automation, especially time-efficient, low use of solvent, energy-efficient, and environment-friendly, are being preferred by the processors and researchers. Among these innovative extraction techniques, UAE (ultrasound-assisted extraction), MAE (microwave-assisted extraction), and SFE (supercritical fluid extraction) are emerging environment-friendly green extraction technologies.

3.4.7.1 UAE (Ultrasound-Assisted Extraction)

Sound waves above the audible range are being applied for the extraction of various plants' bioactive. Sonication enhances the extraction by mass transfer between liquid and solid phase by creating an acoustic effect. A brief mechanism is shown in Figure 3.9.

The acoustic effect produces bubbles that disrupt near-solid surfaces, cause disruption, and increase the surface area of the solid matrix. Solvents penetrate most effectively, ultimately enhancing the extraction of bioactive (Dong, et al. 2014). Sonication is a widely used extraction technique for capsaicin and capsaicinoids from capsicum species using methanol as solvent. Extraction is usually carried out at low temperatures for a shorter time. Sonication is also being used for the extraction of coloring compounds from capsicum species by using ethanol as a solvent. Sonication is carried out at a low temperature and for a shorter time, ultimately ensures the quality and quantity of extract (Kaleem, et al. 2019).

3.4.7.2 MAE (Microwave-Assisted Extraction)

MAE is also a recent and emerging extraction technique to extract water from the material for enhancing the drying rate and quality of the finished product (Singh, et al. 2014).

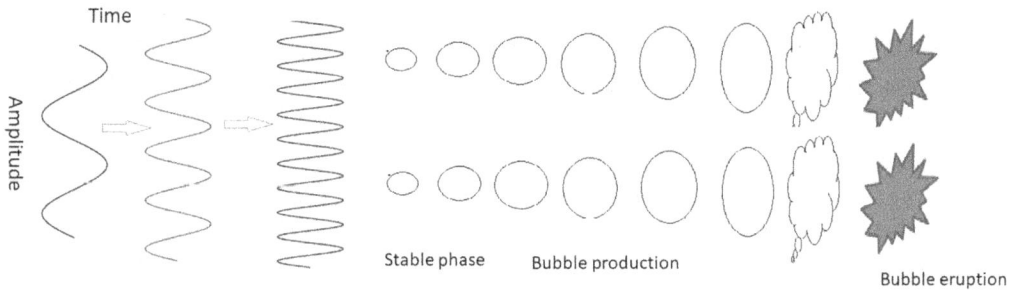

FIGURE 3.9   Acoustic effect of ultrasound in solid-liquid matrix.

MAE, efficacy and selectivity, depends on the polarity and dielectric constant of the solvent. MAE results in a higher recovery rate as compared to conventional techniques. It is also a cost-effective extraction technique.

MAE includes different variants, the most important are microwave hydrodiffusion, vacuum microwave hydrodistillation, solvent-free microwave extraction, and compressed air microwave distillation. MAE with hexane is widely used for the extraction of oleoresin from capsicum. Fruit is immersed in nonabsorptive hexane, which is finally evaporated by microwave energy and has better extraction efficacy as compared with traditional extraction techniques. MAE produces thermal stress that ruptures cells and causes releases of volatile from the matrix. Usually, 1–10 g of sample is immersed in approximately 40 mL of the solvents for up to 30 minutes, and then microwaves are applied. It is reported that MAE causes no degradation to capsaicin and capsaicinoids up to 150°C. Osmotic dehydration is an efficacious pretreatment of capsicum before MAE for prompt drying, thereby sustaining product quality (Mason, et al. 2011).

3.4.7.3 SFE (Supercritical Fluid Extraction)

Carbon dioxide is used for the fractional separation of bioactive substances; during this process, lipid-based fractions are separated containing a bunch of bioactive substances. It has the advantage over traditional extraction solvent for inertness, low cost, nonflammability, nontoxicity, and good extraction efficacy. Extraction of oleoresin from capsicums was carried out in two phases using CO_2. In the first phase, pungent oleoresin is obtained that may also be turned into essential oils. If a viscous paste-like extract is obtained during this process, it creates issues of bioactive recovery from separation vessels. High pressure is needed to recover it. The pressure applied determines the quality of extract (Swain, et al. 2012). Capsaicin, an orange-yellow pungent extract along with carotenoids, was extracted at low pressure in the first phase of extraction. A crude dark color suspension was obtained, which was a typical mixture of carotenoids, anthocyanins, fatty acid, and some other substances (Gogus, et al. 2015). Further separation and fractionation of carotenoids can be obtained in the second phase using high pressure and selective solvents along with carbon dioxide (Quintero-Chávez, et al. 2012; Fernández-Ronco, et al. 2011; Santos, et al. 2015; Araus, et al. 2012).

3.5 OLEORESIN CHARACTERIZATION

3.5.1 Color Analysis

The color tonality of CO was measured (Figure 3.10) by using a computer vision system (previously calibrated). This system makes use of a complex system comprising various shades of natural lights (D65) and a black box, and the system was equipped with a digital camera. The camera and sample were maintained at a suitable distance. The camera lens was set to have light at a 45° angle. The whole system allows the development of photographs for reference color shades. CO photographs were taken in triplicate by using a white background, so for that purpose, 2 mL of CO was uniformly spread in a Petri dish having a diameter of 5 cm (Matiacevich, et al. 2012; Pedreschi, et al. 2006).

To have standardized color parameters with digitized parameters (RGB space), software like Adobe Photoshop or Adobe Illustrator can be used to interpret and save these parameters into machine language and transform it into CIE $L*a*b*$, where $a*$ is the red–green axis, $L*$ indicates lightness, and $b*$ is the blue–yellow axis.

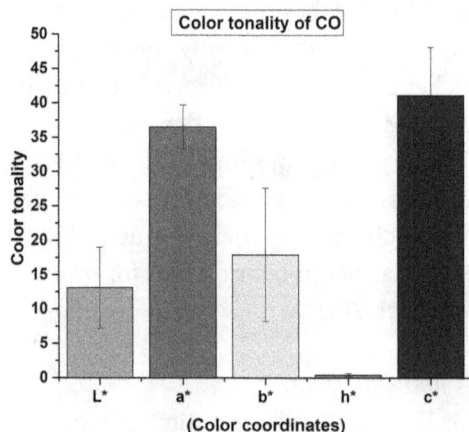

FIGURE 3.10   Color tonality of Capsicum oleoresin.

3.5.2 Use of FTIR Spectroscopy for Oleoresin Characterization

The oleoresin and capsaicin can be well characterized using FTIR spectroscopic technique. This technique is valuable in providing information about the chemical nature of bioactive substances and may validate the chemical composition obtained through the chemical analysis process. Based on this technique, differences or similarities among the bioactive substances may be explored. The authenticity of results can be improved when it is used with ATR (attenuated total reflectance) unit in the range of 450–4000 cm^{-1}; using 16 scans to develop spectra neglecting the effects of noise, the authenticity can be further improved by increasing the number of replications.

The Capsicum oleoresin (CO) was characterized by FTIR. The peaks observed at wavenumbers 1050, 2900, and 3350 cm^{-1} correspond to vibrations of bonds C-O-C, CH, and OH, respectively (Riquelme and Matiacevich, 2017). The same peaks in microcapsules of capsaicin were also observed. Peaks at wavenumber 1600 and 1630 cm^{-1}, which correlates with amides and peaks groups at 1300 cm^{-1}, corresponding to C–N groups. Peaks such as 1378, 1627, and 1650 cm^{-1} for CO and 1347 cm^{-1} for capsaicin were also observed. Peaks at wavenumbers 1036, 1517, and 2857 cm^{-1} were observed in both capsaicin in the CO. It is evident from FTIR spectra that capsaicinoid is found in a larger proportion in CO and is about 90% of the capsaicinoids (Riquelme and Matiacevich, 2017; Simonovska et al., 2016).

3.5.3 Antioxidant Properties

SRA of the oleoresin and capsaicin was determined using two DPPH (2-diphenyl-1-picrylhydrazyl) methods. A standard curve from a Trolox (6-hydroxy-2,5,7,8-tetramethylchroman-2-carboxylic acid) solution was prepared at an initial concentration of 1×10^{-3} g/mL. Aliquots of 3 mL of different dilutions of Trolox solution or sample reacted with 0.3 mL of DPPH solution at 7.9×10^{-4} g/mL, for 30 minutes in darkness, and then its absorbance was taken at 517 nm by using a spectrophotometer (UVmini-1240, Shimadzu, Japan). Similarly, capsaicin and OCc reacted with DPPH solution, and its absorbance was taken at 517 nm, after 30 min in the dark. The results were expressed in the g Trolox/g sample. Phenol group molecular structure determines antioxidant properties of capsaicinoids and capsicin in oleoresin. Apart from capsaicinoids and capsicin, different flavonoids and phenolics also contribute to the antioxidant properties of CO (Maksimova, et al. 2014; Ahmad, et al. 2020) and can be analyzed through HPLC techniques (Kaleem, et al. 2016; Kaleem and Ahmad, 2018). Oleoresin compounds, including capsanthin, β-carotene, capsorubin, and cryptoxanthin, exhibit antioxidant characteristics due to their redox ability (Deepa, et al. 2007). It is reported that the antioxidant properties of oleoresins from capsicum are contributed by the concentration of capsaicin, deducing that capsaicin is mainly responsible for the antioxidant ability of oleoresins. Oleoresin is composed of constituents, which have phenolic nature, and having the same oil concentration of capsaicin, it is directly proportional to the antioxidant activity of oleoresin (Zimmer, et al. 2012).

3.5.4 Antibacterial Properties of Capsicum Oleoresin

CO has a potential inhibitory effect on both Gram +ve (*Staphylococcus epidermidis* and *Staphylococcus aureus*) and Gram −ve (*Escherichia coli* and *Pseudomonas aeruginosa*) strains. It is reported that CO has inhibited the Gram-positive bacteria more effectively as compared to Gram-negative. This may be attributed because of structural differences (Diao, et al. 2014) among both strains, especially peptidoglycan, which is the structural component of Gram-positive bacteria. Two capsicum cultivar red chilies and curly red chilies oleoresin were compared for their efficacy against bacterial strains. The results revealed that oleoresin from curly red chilies has more efficacious against the Gram-positive bacteria as compared to red chilies oleoresin. Both the cultivars have compositional differences and capsaicin is the potential compound that exhibited antimicrobial activity (Liu, et al. 2012). It was reported that curly red chili oleoresin for *S. epidermis*, *S. aureus*, *P. aeruginosa*, and *E coli* was 17, 18.25, 2.9, and 24 mm, respectively (Nurjanah, et al. 2014), while oleoresin from red chilies for the same bacteria were 2.02, 2.86, 1.65, and 1.06 mm, respectively. Oleoresin from *C. annuum* L. has more potential as an antibacterial agent. It was studied that CO exhibited antibacterial properties when used in the concentration of 200–300 μg/mL, while the dose of 50–150 μg/mL is less effective. Capsaicin and capsaicinoids have no significant effect on *L. monocytogenes* (Dorantes, et al. 2000). A brief activity of oleoresins against bacteria is depicted in Figure 3.11.

Capsicum is the predominant component in CO and amounts to 51.06 mg/. It was reported that nanoemulsion of the CO reduced *S. aureus* and *E. coli* populations significantly ($p \leq 0.05$) [82]. In lecithin nanoemulsion, it ranged from 2.84 to 3.40 log for *E. coli*. It was reported that capsaicin is used in a concentration of 25 μg/mL, retarding the growth

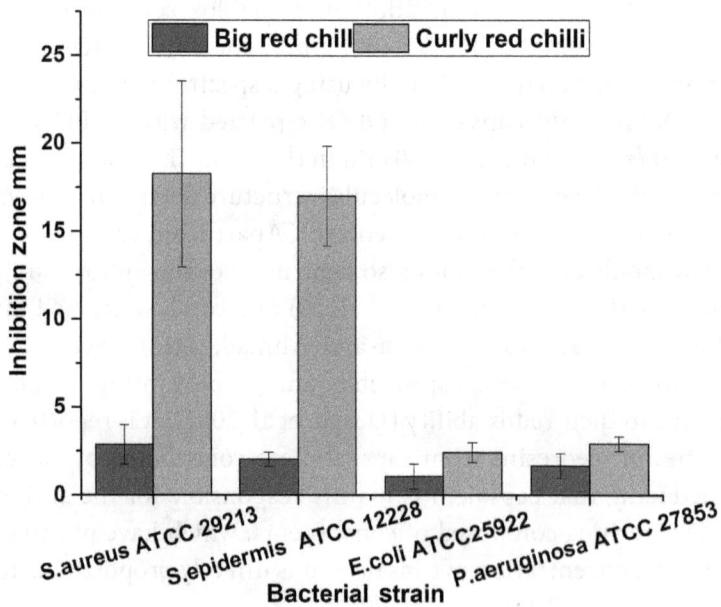

FIGURE 3.11 Oleoresin against bacterial strains.

of *Bacillus subtilis* (El Abed, et al. 2014), and a dose of 200 or 300 μg/mL retarded *E. coli* growth significantly. It was reported that a capsicin dose of 1.5 mL/100 g of meat showed a lethal impact on *L. monocytogenes* count (Molina-Torres, et al. 1999). *C. annum* and NaCl were used in combination to explore their efficacy. It was reported that salmonella is salt tolerant, and hence the proposed less salt and more pepper extract can retard the *L. monocytogenes* growth more effectively. The effect of capsicum extract on *P. aeruginosa* was studied. A dose of 0.5–1.5 mL/100 g has a bacteriostatic effect. The extract from 4 to 5 mL/100 g of meat drastically decreased the *L. monocytogenes* count and *S. aureus* (Careaga, et al. 2003). It was evaluated that capsaicin decreased MIC of ciprofloxacin 2–4 times against *S. aureus* (Kalia, et al. 2012). It was reported that the extract from sweet fennel, red chili, and white pepper inhibited virulence expression of *Vibrio cholerae* (Chatterjee, et al. 2010). It was studied that 10 μg/mL of capsicum extract and some other plant-based bioactives significantly reduced the *Helicobacter pylori* count (Jones, et al. 1997; Ahmed, et al. 2019).

3.5.5 Characterization of Capsicum Oleoresin and Pungency Level

Sonication is the innovative and adopted technique of extraction of bioactive. Capsicum extract after sonication was quantified for capsaicin and dihydrocapsaicin and total capsaicinoids by RP-HPLC-PDA. Capsaicin and capsaicinoids eluted at a retention time of 5.70 and 6.87 min, respectively. Quantification of capsaicin, dihydrocapsaicin, and total capsaicinoids is shown in Figure 3.12. Both the capsaicin and capsaicinoids showed linearity in the range of 50–10,000 ng/mL. Fourteen cultivars of capsaicin were evaluated for capsaicin, dihydrocapsaicin, and total capsaicinoids and their pungency. Different physiological factors including light intensity, temperature, fruit age, and fruit position determine capsaicinoid contents of different cultivars. Capsaicinoids contents in all cultivars varied from 614 to 25,976 mg/kg for capsaicin and 609–22,130 mg/kg for dihydrocapsaicin (Sricharoen et al., 2017). Pungency is calculated in SHU calculated by multiplying the capsaicinoid fraction (ppm) by the coefficient of the heat value for each compound which is for nonivamide (9.2), nordihydrocapsaicin (9.3), and for both capsaicin and dihydrocapsaicin (16.1) (Bajer, et al., 2015).

$$SHU = 16.1 \times \left[CAP(ppm) + DHC(ppm) \right]$$

There are five levels of the pungency classified using SHU: nonpungent (0700), mildly pungent (700–3000), moderately pungent (3000–25,000), highly pungent (25,000–70,000), and very highly pungent (>80,000 SHU) (Othman et al., 2011).

3.5.6 Antidiabetic Activity of Capsicum Oleoresins

Reducing sugar exists in capsicum that may be extracted (from selected capsicum cultivars) in oleoresins, these sugars may be analyzed by optical absorbance (Perla, et al. 2016). It was quantified as dinitro salicylic acid which reacts with sugar-free carbonyl group in the alkaline condition and forms 3-amino-5-nitrosalicylate, an aromatic compound having absorption at 540 nm. The antidiabetic effect of these compounds can be quantified by inhibition%. α-Amylase catabolism carbohydrate is responsible for

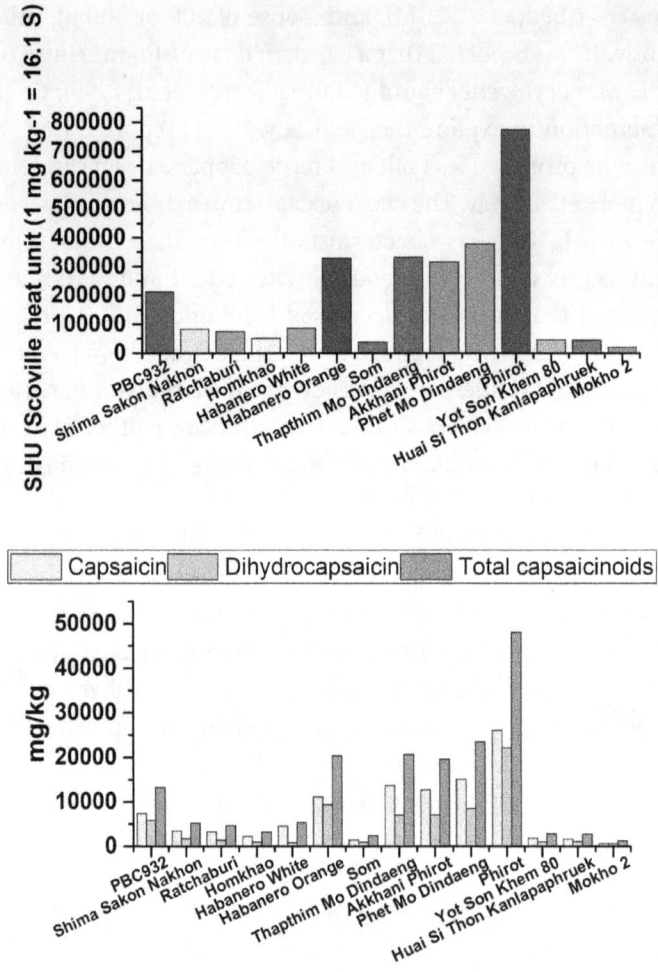

FIGURE 3.12   Characterization of capsicum extract for scoville heat value.

the release of glucose by its digestion. If its activity is inhibited, it retards its catabolic activity and releases glucose, ultimately reducing the glycemic index. Oleoresin from capsicum annum has the best inhibition%; therefore, oleoresin from this cultivar can be used as a therapeutic agent in attenuating glycemic index (Gupta et al., 2021). The results of reducing sugar contents, α-amylase, and inhibition percentage age are shown in Figure 3.13.

3.5.7 Capsicum Oleoresin, Phenolics, Carotenoid, and Flavonoid Contents

Phytochemical and oleoresin quantification of capsicum variety is shown in Figure 3.14. The results showed that oleoresin in selected cultivars ranged from 19.23 to 45.13 g/100 g DW. Total phenolic contents varied from 6392 to 12,115 mg CE/kg DW. Carotenoid contents varied from 99.47 to 350.12 mg βCE/kg DW. Flavonoid contents varied from 6,541 to 23,110 mg CE/kg DW. The details of selective therapeutic bioactive are shown in Table 3.3.

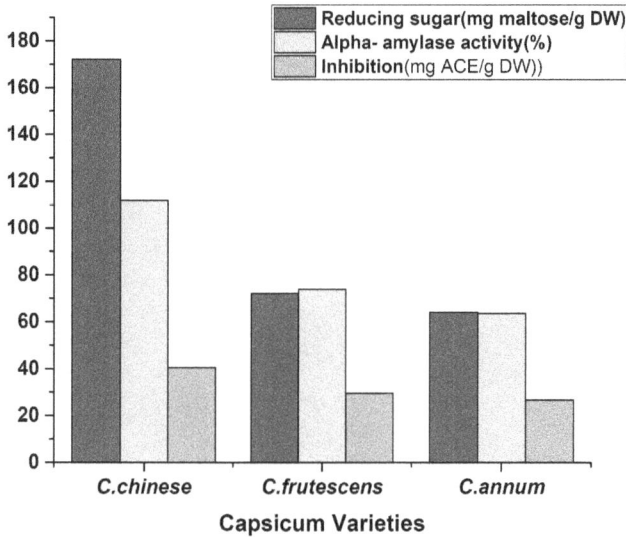

FIGURE 3.13   Reducing sugar, α-amylase, and % inhibition.

3.6 SAFETY/TOXICITY AND FUTURE SCOPE

Oleoresin causes immediate changes in the chemical and mechanical sensitivities of corneal tissues. This change is associated with damage of the corneal nerve which is usually unmyelinated nerve fibers (Chularojmontri, et al. 2011). Capsicum spray can cause chemical injury to the conjunctiva and cornea (Vesaluoma, et al. 2000). The toxicological effect of capsaicin as existing in oleoresins or somewhere else is shown in Table 3.4.

Incredible growth for oleoresins was observed in the last decade that likely to further grow in the future. In the year 2019, the worldwide market for oleoresins stood at 1.2 billion USD, and it is anticipated to attain a figure of 1.7 billion USD by 2025 with an expected cumulated annual growth rate of 6%. There is a rising trend in the use of natural flavors and botanical resins in the processed food and pharmaceutical industry that increases the demand for oleoresins. Industry and people are migrating from synthetic flavors toward health-promoting natural substances with phytomedicine characteristics that are extracted from botanical sources. Based on that, there is a great potential for these products to be used in sauces, soups, salad dressings, snacks, seafood, meat products, processed foods, nutraceuticals, and pharma foods.

3.7 CONCLUSION

Plant-based nutraceuticals and related substances have gained consumer attention due to these potential health benefits. CO is being used as a flavoring agent due to its sharp taste, while paprika oleoresin is widely used as a colorant in different food products. Various solvents could be potentially used to prepare the commercial products through various available techniques. Besides, conventional chemical analysis, advanced machine analysis such as FTIR, TGA, and DSC are valuable techniques for characterization and analysis of oleoresins. COs are also renowned for their antioxidant, antifungal, and antimicrobial

TABLE 3.3 Therapeutic Effect of Bioactive Extracted from *Capsicum annuum*

Therapeutic Effect	Models	Extract	Bioactive Compound/Mechanism	References
Antimicrobial effects	*Micrococcus sp., Bacillus, E. Coli, Pseudomonas sp.,* and *Citrobacter sp.* (*Salmonella typhimurium* and *Pseudomonas aeruginosa, Staphylococcus aureus* UFPEDA02, *Enterococcus faecalis* ATCC6057, *Bacillus subtilis* UFPEDA 86), and Gram negative (*Escherichia coli* ATCC25922, *Klebsiella pneumonia* ATCC29665, *Pseudomonas aeruginosa* UFPEDA416) bacteria and one yeast strain (*Candida albicans* UFPEDA 1007) *Saccharomyces cerevisiae, Candida albicans, Candida parapsilosis, Candida tropicalis, Pichia membranifaciens, Kluyveromyces marxiannus* and *Candida guilliermondii, Aspergillus flavus, Aspergillus niger*	Butanol extract of *Capsicum annuum* fruit The ethanol extract *C. frutescens* extract. *C. frutescens* extracts	Capsaicin CAY-1, a novel saponin obtained from *C. frutescens*, peptides obtained from chili pepper seeds	Abdou Bouba, et al. (2012); Kappel, et al. (2008)
Antiviral	Guinea pigs against cutaneous herpes simplex virus	Capsicum extract	Capsaicin	Bourne, et al. (1999)
Insecticidal, anthelmintic and Larvicidal effects	*A. aegypti* mosquitoes Cercaria of *Schistosoma mansoni*	*Capsicum frutescens* extracts	Water-soluble unsaturated compounds with repellent properties	Kollmannsberger, et al. (2011)
Antioxidant properties	Adult men and women	*Capsicum annuum* leaves extracts	Antioxidant properties of capsaicinoids	Popovich, et al. (2014)
Anti-inflammatory properties	Rat hind paw inflammation induced by subplantar injections of fresh egg albumin (0.5 mL/kg)	*Capsicum annuum* extract	Carotenoids	Jolayemi (2012)
Cardiovascular effect	Anesthetized dogs iv injections	Ethyl acetate *C. frutescens* extract	Capsaicin	Chularojmontri, et al. (2011)
Antithrombotic and vasodilatory properties	Gerbil males Feed rabbits for 12 weeks with a diet rich in cholesterol (1%) and chili pepper (1%),	Capsaicin (10–300 µg/kg). Pepper oleoresin. Chili pepper (1%).	Decreasing exogenous absorption of cholesterol Antiatherosclerotic effects	Dos Santos, et al. (2021)

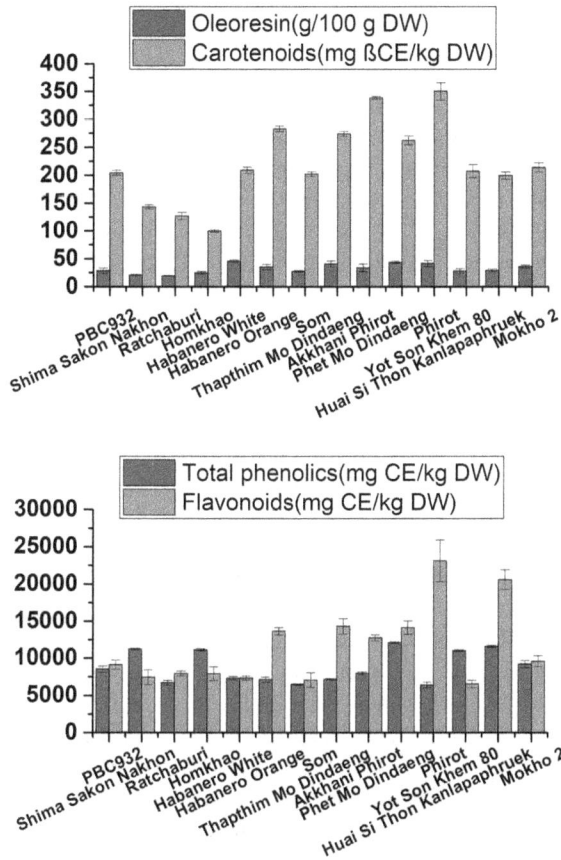

FIGURE 3.14 Flavonoid, total phenolics, and carotenoids contents.

TABLE 3.4 Toxicological Effect of Capsaicin

Toxic Activities	Bioactive Compound/Type of Extract	Mechanism of Action of Toxicity	References
Hemorrhage of the gastric fundus	Capsaicin 161.2 mg/kg (rats) and 118.8 mg/kg (mice)	Triggers painful irritation of the mucous membrane	Das, et al. (2005)
Myocardial infarction	40-year-old man admitted to emergency division with complaints of chest discomfort and dyspnea after exposure to pepper gas	Irritation of the mucous membrane	Cil, et al. (2012)
Tenacious dermatitis	Capsaicin	Irritation of the skin	Batiha, et al. (2020)

activities and have several documented health benefits, thus widely used in medication to treat minor aches, muscular, and joint pain. Capsaicin, an active compound in oleoresin, is beneficial for liver health as it reduces activation of hepatic stellate cells. Based on these characteristics, these oleoresins may contribute to future pharmaceuticals, food, and nutraceutical industry.

REFERENCES

Abdou Bouba, A., Njintang Yanou, N., Foyet, H., Scher, J., Montet, D. and Mbofung, C.M. 2012 Proximate composition, mineral, and vitamin content of some wild plants used as spices in Cameroon, *Food and Nutrition Sciences*, 3(4): 423–432.

Ahmad, A., Zulfiqar, S. and Chatha, Z.A. 2020 Development of roasted flaxseed cookies and characterization for chemical and organoleptic parameters, *Pakistan Journal of Agricultural Sciences*, 57(1): 229–235.

Ahmed, M., Masud, T., Ahmad, A., Ismail, A., Ibrahim M.T., and M.S. Ibrahim 2019 Isolation and antimicrobial susceptibility testing of Helicobacter Pylori strain from gastric biopsies from Pakistani patients, *Pakistan Journal of Pharmaceutical Sciences*, 32(5): 2279–2285.

Akhtar, M., Ahmad, A., Masud, T. and Wattoo, F.H. 2019 Phenolic, carotenoid, ascorbic acid contents and their antioxidant activities in bell pepper, *Acta Scientiarum Polonorum Hortorum Cultus*, 18(1): 13–21. DOI: 10.24326/asphc.2019.1.2.

Aliakbarlu, J., Mohammadi, S., and Khalili, S. 2014 A study on antioxidant potency and antibacterial activity of water extracts of some spices widely consumed in I Iranian diet, *Journal of Food Biochemistry*, 38(2): 159–166.

Alós, E., Roca, M., Iglesias, D. J., et al. 2008 An evaluation of the basis and consequences of a stay-green mutation in the navel Negra citrus mutant using transcriptomic and proteomic profiling and metabolite analysis, *Plant Physiology*, 147(3): 1300–1315.

Amruthraj, N. J., Preetam Raj, J. P., and Antoine Lebel, L. 2014 Effect of vegetable oil in the solubility of capsaicinoids extracted from Capsicum chinense Bhut Jolokia, *Asian Journal of Pharmaceutical and Clinical Research*, 7(1): 48–51.

Andrews, J. 1995 *Peppers: The Domesticated Capsicums*. University of Texas Press.

Araus, K. A., del Valle, J. M., Robert, P. S., and Juan, C. 2012 Effect of triolein addition on the solubility of capsanthin in supercritical carbon dioxide, *The Journal of Chemical Thermodynamics*, 51: 190–194.

Arslan, D. and Özcan, M.M. 2011 Dehydration of red bell pepper (*Capsicum annuum* L.): Change in drying behavior, color, and antioxidant content, *Food and Bioproducts Processing*, 89(4): 504–513.

Arvanitoyannis, I. S., Veikou, A., and Panagiotaki, P. 2012 Osmotic dehydration: Theory, methodologies, and applications in fish, seafood, and meat products, *Progress in food preservation*, 161–189.

Bacon, K., Boyer, R., Denbow, C., O'Keefe, S., Neilson, A. and Williams, R. 2017 Antibacterial activity of jalapeño pepper (*Capsicum annuum var. annuum*) extract fractions against select foodborne pathogens, *Food Science & Nutrition*, 5(3): 730–738.

Baiano, A., Terracone, C., Gambacorta, G. and La Notte, E. 2009 Changes in quality indices, phenolic content, and antioxidant activity of flavored olive oils during storage, *Journal of the American Oil Chemists' Society*, 86(11): 1083–1092.

Bajer, T., Bajerová, P., Kremr, D., Eisner, A., and Ventura, K. 2015 Central composite design of pressurised hot water extraction process for extracting capsaicinoids from chili peppers, *Journal of Food Composition and Analysis*, 40: 32–38.

Barbero, G. F., Palma, M., and Barroso, C.G. 2006 Pressurized liquid extraction of capsaicinoids from peppers, *Journal of Agricultural and Food Chemistry*, 54(9): 3231–3236.

Batiha, G. E. S., Alqahtani, A., Ojo, O. A. et al. 2020 Biological properties, bioactive constituents, and pharmacokinetics of some *Capsicum spp.* and capsaicinoids, *International Journal of Molecular Sciences* 21(15): 5179.

Bourne, N., Bernstein, D. I., and L.R. Stanberry. 1999 Civamide (cis-capsaicin) for treatment of primary or recurrent experimental genital herpes, *Antimicrobial Agents and Chemotherapy* 43(11): 2685–2688.

Buczkowska, H., Michalojc, Z., and R. Nurzynska-Wierdak 2016 Yield and fruit quality of sweet pepper depending on foliar application of calcium, *Turkish Journal of Agriculture and Forestry*, 40(2): 222–228.

Caporaso, N., Paduano, A., Nicoletti, G., and R. Sacchi 2013 Capsaicinoids, antioxidant activity, and volatile compounds in olive oil flavored with dried chili pepper (*Capsicum annuum*), *European Journal of Lipid Science and Technology*, 115(12): 1434–1442.

Careaga, M., Fernández, E., Dorantes, L., Mota, L., and M. E. Jaramillo 2003 Antibacterial activity of capsicum extract against salmonella typhimurium and pseudomonas aeruginosa inoculated in raw beef meat, *International Journal* of *Food Microbiology*, 83: 331–335

Chatterjee, S., Asakura, M., Chowdhury, N., Neogi, S.B., and Sugimoto, N. 2010 Capsaicin, a potential inhibitor of cholera toxin production in Vibrio cholera, *FEMS Microbiology Letters*, 306: 54–60.

Chinn, M. S., Sharma-Shivappa, R. R., and Cotter, J. L. 2011 Solvent extraction and quantification of capsaicinoids from Capsicum Chinense, *Food and Bioproducts Processing* 89(4): 340–345.

Chularojmontri, L., Suwatronnakorn, M., and Wattanapitayakul, S. K. 2011 Influence of capsicum extract and capsaicin on endothelial health, *Journal of the Medical Association of Thailand*, 93(2): 92–100.

Cil, H., Atilgan, Z. A., Islamoglu, Y., Tekbas, E. O. and Dostbil, Z. 2012 Is the pepper spray a triggering factor in myocardial infarction? A case report, *European Review for Medical and Pharmacological Sciences*, 16(Suppl 1): 73–74.

Das, S., Chohan, A., Snibson, G. R., and Taylor, H. R. 2005 Capsicum spray injury of the eye. *International Ophthalmology*, 26(4): 171–173.

de Aguiar, A. C., Sales, L. P., Coutinho, J. P., Barbero, G. F., Godoy, H. T., and Martínez, J. 2013 Supercritical carbon dioxide extraction of Capsicum peppers: Global yield and capsaicinoid content, *The Journal of Supercritical Fluids*, 81: 210–216.

Deepa, N., Kaur, C., George, B., Singh, B., and H.C. Kapoor 2007 Antioxidant constituents in some sweet pepper (*Capsicum annuum L.*) genotypes during maturity, *LWT-Food Science and Technology*, 40(1): 121–129.

Deng, C., Ji, J., Wang, X., and Zhang, X. 2005 Development of pressurized hot water extraction followed by headspace solid-phase microextraction and gas chromatography-mass spectrometry for determination of ligustilides in Ligusticum chuanxiong and Angelica sinensis, *Journal of Separation Science*, 28(11): 1237–1243.

Diao, W.R., Zhang, L.L., Feng, S.S., and J.G. Xu. 2014 Chemical composition, antibacterial activity, and mechanism of action of the essential oil from *Amomum kravanh*, *Journal Food Protection*, 77(10): 1740–1746.

Dong, X., Li, X., Ding, L., Cui, F., Tang, Z., and Liu, Z. 2014 Stage extraction of capsaicinoids and red pigments from fresh red pepper (Capsicum) fruits with ethanol as solvent. *LWT-Food Science and Technology*, 59(1): 396–402.

Dorantes, L., Colmenero, R., Hernandez, H., Mota, L. and Jaramillo, M. E. 2000 Inhibition of growth of some foodborne pathogenic bacteria by *Capsicum annum* extracts, *International Journal of Food Microbiology*, 57: 125–128.

Dos Santos, L., de Oliveira Maciel, L., Gracia, E. K. I. et al. 2021 Ethereal extract of pepper: Preventing atherosclerosis and left ventricle remodeling in LDL receptor knockout mice. *Preventive Nutrition and Food Science*, 26(1): 51–57.

Doymaz, İ., and Kocayigit, F. 2012 Effect of pre-treatments on drying, rehydration, and color characteristics of red pepper ('Charliston'variety), *Food Science and Biotechnology*, 21(4), 1013–1022.

El Abed, N., Kaabi, B., Smaali, M. I. et al. 2014 Chemical composition, antioxidant and antimicrobial activities of Thymus capitata essential oil with its preservative effect against Listeria monocytogenes inoculated in minced beef meat, *Evidence-Based Complementary and Alternative Medicine*. https://doi.org/10.1155/2014/152487

ELkhadraoui, A., Kooli, S., Hamdi, I., and Farhat, A. 2015 Experimental investigation and economic evaluation of a new mixed-mode solar greenhouse dryer for drying of red pepper and grape, *Renewable Energy*, 77: 1–8.

Ergüneş, G. and Tarhan, S. (2006) Color retention of red peppers by chemical pretreatments during greenhouse and open sun drying, *Journal of Food Engineering*, 76(3), 446–452.

Falade, K. O., and Oyedele, O. O. 2010 Effect of osmotic pretreatment on air drying characteristics and colour of pepper (*Capsicum spp*) cultivars, *Journal of Food Science and Technology*, 47(5): 488–495.

Fayos, O., Barbero, G. F., Savirón, M., et al. 2018 Synthesis of (±)-3, 4-dimethoxybenzyl-4-methyloctanoate as a novel internal standard for capsinoid determination by HPLC-ESI-MS/MS (QTOF), *Open Chemistry*, 16(1): 87–94.

Fernández-Ronco, M. P., Gracia, I., De Lucas, A. and Rodríguez, J. F. 2011 Measurement and modeling of the high-pressure phase equilibria of CO_2-Oleoresin Capsicum, *The Journal of Supercritical Fluids*, 57(2): 112–119.

Fernández-Ronco, M. P., Ortega-Noblejas, C., Gracia, I., De Lucas, A., García, M. T., and Rodríguez, J. F. 2010 Supercritical fluid fractionation of liquid oleoresin capsicum: Statistical analysis and solubility parameters, *The Journal of Supercritical Fluids*, 54(1): 22–29.

Franceschi, V. R., Krokene, P., Christiansen, E., and Krekling, T. 2005 Anatomical and chemical defenses of conifer bark against bark beetles and other pests, *New Phytologist*, 167(2): 353–376.

Fudholi, A., Othman, M. Y., Ruslan, M. H., and Sopian, K. 2013 Drying of Malaysian Capsicum annuum L.(red chili) dried by open and solar drying, *International Journal of Photoenergy*, 13: 1–9.

Giuffrida, D., Dugo, P., Torre, et al. 2013 Characterization of 12 Capsicum varieties by evaluation of their carotenoid profile and pungency determination, *Food Chemistry*, 140(4): 794–802.

Gogus, F., Ozel, M. Z., Keskin, H., Yanık, D. K., and Lewis, A.C. 2015 Volatiles of fresh and commercial sweet red pepper pastes: processing methods and microwave assisted extraction, *International Journal of Food Properties*, 18(8): 1625–1634.

Gourava, J. 2019 Characterization of indian pine oleoresin and evidence for the existence of silicon compounds, *Journal for Foundations and Applications of Physics*, 6(1): 95–102.

Gupta, R., Kapoor, B., Gulati, M., Singh, S. K., and Saxena, D. 2021 The two faces of capsiate: Nutraceutical and therapeutic potential, *Trends in Food Science & Technology*, 110: 332–348.

Haiyee, Z. A., Saim, N., Said, M., Illias, R. M., Mustapha, W. A. W., and Hassan, O. (2009) Characterization of cyclodextrin complexes with turmeric oleoresin, *Food Chemistry* 114(2), 459–465.

Haynes, R., and Herring, S. 1981 Performance of drip-irrigated bell peppers, *Arkansas Farm Research*.

Jang, H. W., Ka, M. H., and Lee, K. G. 2008 Antioxidant activity and characterization of volatile extracts of *Capsicum annuum L.* and *Allium spp*, *Flavour and Fragrance Journal*, 23(3): 178–184.

Jolayemi, A. T. E. 2012 Studies on some pharmacological properties of Capsicum frutescens-driven capsaicin in experimental animal models (Doctoral dissertation).

Jones, N.L., Shabib, S., and P.M. 1997 Capsaicin as an inhibitor of the growth of the gastric pathogen Helicobacter pylori, *FEMS Microbiology Letters*, 146: 223–227.

Kaleem, M., Ahmad, A., Amir, R. M., and Kaukab, R.G. 2019 Ultrasound-assisted phytochemical extraction condition optimization using response surface methodology from perlette grapes (*Vitis vinifera*), *Processes* 7(10): 749–759.

Kaleem, M., Ahmad, A., Khalid, S., and Azam, M.T. 2016 HPLC condition optimization for identification of flavonoids from Carissa opaca, *Science International (Lahore)*, 28(1), 343–348.

Kaleem, M., and Ahmad, A. 2018 Flavonoids as nutraceuticals, In: *Therapeutic, Probiotic and Unconventional Foods*, ed A. M., Grumezescu and A.M., Holban, 137–155, Elsevier Academic Press. USA.

Kalia, N.P., Mahajan, P., Mehra, R., Nargotra, A., and Sharma, J.P. 2012 Capsaicin, a novel inhibitor of the NorA efflux pump, reduces the intracellular invasion of Staphylococcus aureus, *Journal of Antimicrobial Chemotherapy*, 67: 2401–2408

Kappel, V. D., Costa, G. M., Scola, G. et al. 2008 Phenolic content and antioxidant and antimicrobial properties of fruits of Capsicum baccatum L. var. pendulum at different maturity stages, *Journal of Medicinal Food*, 11(2): 267–274.

Kawaguchi, Y., Moriya, T., Yanae, K., Setoguchi, Y., and Kato, M. 2004 Method of acid value determination for oils containing alkali-labile esters, *Journal of Oleo Science*, 53(7): 329–336.

Keeling, C. I., and Bohlmann, J. 2006 Diterpene resin acids in conifers, *Phytochemistry*, 67(22): 2415–2423.

Khalid, S., Ahmad, A, Kaleem, M. 2017 Antioxidant activity and phenolic contents of Ajwa date and their effect on lipo-protein profile, *Functional Foods in Health and Disease*, 7(6): 396–410.

Khalid, S., Ahmad, A., Masud, T., Asad, M.J., Sandhu, M. 2016 Nutritional assessment of ajwa date flesh and pits in comparison to local varieties, *Journal of Animal and Plant Sciences*, 26(4): 1072–1080.

Kim, E. H., Lee, S. Y., Baek, D. Y., et al. 2019 A comparison of the nutrient composition and statistical profile in red pepper fruits (*Capsicums annuum L.*) based on genetic and environmental factors, *Applied Biological Chemistry*, 62(1): 1–13.

Kim, W. J., Kim, J., Veriansyah, B., et al. 2009 Extraction of bioactive components from Centella asiatica using subcritical water, *The Journal of Supercritical Fluids*, 48(3): 211–216.

Kobata, K., Tate, H., Iwasaki, Y., et al. 2008 Isolation of coniferyl esters from Capsicum baccatum L., and their enzymatic preparation and agonist activity for TRPV1, *Phytochemistry*, 69(5): 1179–1184.

Kollmannsberger, H., Rodríguez-Burruezo, A., Nitz, S., and Nuez, F. 2011 Volatile and capsaicinoid composition of ají (*Capsicum baccatum*) and rocoto (*Capsicum pubescens),* two Andean species of chile peppers, *Journal of the Science of Food and Agriculture*, 91(9): 1598–1611.

Korkutata, N. F., and Kavaz, A. 2015 A comparative study of ascorbic acid and capsaicinoid contents in red hot peppers (*Capsicum annum L.*) grown in southeastern Anatolia region. *International Journal of Food Properties*, 18(4): 725–734.

Kumareswaran, T., Jolia, P., Maurya, M., Maurya, A., Abbasmandri, S., and Kamalvanshi, V. 2018 Export scenario of Indian agriculture: A review, *Journal of Pharmacognosy and Phytochemistry*, 7(6): 2733–2736.

Kwon, Y. I., Apostolidis, E., and Shetty, K. 2007 Evaluation of pepper (Capsicum annuum) for management of diabetes and hypertension, *Journal of Food Biochemistry*, 31(3): 370–385.

Levent, İ. A., and Ferit, A.K. 2012 Partial removal of water from red pepper by immersion in an osmotic solution before drying, *African Journal of Biotechnology*, 11(6): 1449–1459.

Liu, X., Lin, T., Peng, B., and Wang, X. 2012 Antibacterial activity of capsaicin-coated wool fabric, *Texture Research Journal*, 82(6):584–590.

Maksimova, V., Koleva Gudeva, L., Ruskovska, T., Gulaboski, R., and Cvetanovska, A. 2014 Antioxidative effect of Capsicum oleoresins compared with pure capsaicin, *IOSR Journal of Pharmacy*, 4(11): 44–48.

Martin, D., Tholl, D., Gershenzon, J., and Bohlmann, J. 2002 Methyl jasmonate induces traumatic resin ducts, terpenoid resin biosynthesis, and terpenoid accumulation in developing xylem of Norway spruce stems, *Plant Physiology*, 129(3): 1003–1018.

Mason, T., Chemat, F., and Vinatoru, M. 2011 The extraction of natural products using ultrasound or microwaves, *Current Organic Chemistry*, 15(2): 237–247.

Materska, M. and Perucka, I. 2005 Antioxidant activity of the main phenolic compounds isolated from hot pepper fruit (*Capsicum annuum L.*), *Journal of Agricultural and Food Chemistry*, 53(5), 1750–1756.

Matiacevich, S., Silva, P., Osorio, F., and Enrione, J. 2012 Color in food: Technological and psychophysical aspects, *Evaluation of Blueberry Color during Storage Using Image Analysis*, 211–218.

Meng, L., and Lozano, Y. 2014 Innovative technologies used at pilot plant and industrial scales in water-extraction processes. In *Alternative Solvents for Natural Products Extraction*, pp. 269–315. Springer, Berlin, Heidelberg.

Molina-Torres, J., García-Chávez, A., and Ramírez-Chávez, E. 1999 Antimicrobial properties of alkamides present in flavouring plants traditionally used in Mesoamerica: affinin and capsaicin, *Journal of Ethnopharmacology*, 64: 241–248.

Nurjanah, S., Sudaryanto, Z., Widyasanti, A., and Pratiwi, H. 2014 Antibacterial activity of Capsicum annuum L. oleoresin. In *XXIX International Horticultural Congress on Horticulture: Sustaining Lives, Livelihoods and Landscapes (IHC2014): V World 1125*, pp. 189–194.

Omolo, M. A., Wong, Z. Z., Mergen, K., Hastings, J. C., Le, N. C., Reil, H. A., and Baumler, D.J. 2014 Antimicrobial properties of chili peppers. *Journal of Infectious Diseases and Therapy*, 2(4):2–14.

Othman, Z. A. A., Ahmed, Y. B. H., Habila, M. A. and Ghafar, A. A. (2011) Determination of capsaicin and dihydrocapsaicin in Capsicum fruit samples using high performance liquid chromatography, *Molecules*, 16(10): 8919–8929.

Ozdemir, M., Ozen, B. F., Dock, L. L., and Floros, J. D. 2008 Optimization of osmotic dehydration of diced green peppers by response surface methodology, *LWT-Food Science and Technology*, 41(10): 2044–2050.

Ozdemir, N., Pola, C. C., Teixeira, B. N., Hill, L. E., Bayrak, A., and Gomes, C.L. 2018 Preparation of black pepper oleoresin inclusion complexes based on beta-cyclodextrin for antioxidant and antimicrobial delivery applications using kneading and freeze drying methods: A comparative study, *LWT Food Science & Technology*, 91: 439–445.

Paduano, A., Caporaso, N., Santini, A., and Sacchi, R. 2014 Microwave and ultrasound-assisted extraction of capsaicinoids from chili peppers (*Capsicum annuum L.*) in flavored olive oil, *Journal of Food Research*, 3(4): 51–59.

Pedreschi, F., León, J., Mery, D. and Moyano, P. 2006 Development of a computer vision system to measure the color of potato chips, *Food Research International*, 39(10): 1092–1098.

Pérez-Alonso, C., Cruz-Olivares, J., Barrera-Pichardo, J. F., Rodríguez-Huezo, M. E., Báez-González, J. G., and Vernon-Carter, E.J. 2008 DSC thermo-oxidative stability of red chili oleoresin microencapsulated in blended biopolymers matrices, *Journal of Food Engineering*, 85(4): 613–624.

Perla, V., Nimmakayala, P., Nadimi, M. et al. 2016 Vitamin C and reducing sugars in the world collection of Capsicum baccatum L. genotypes, *Food Chemistry*, 202: 189–198.

Perry, G. H., Dominy, N. J., Claw, K.G. et al. 2007 Diet and the evolution of human amylase gene copy number variation, *Nature Genetics*, 39(10): 1256–1260.

Perucka, I. and Materska, M. (2007) Antioxidant vitamin contents of Capsicum annuum fruit extracts as affected by processing and varietal factors, *ACTA Scientiarum Polonorum Technologia Alimentaria*, 6(4), 67–73.

Pino, J., González, M., Ceballos, et al. 2007 Characterization of total capsaicinoids, colour and volatile compounds of Habanero chilli pepper (*Capsicum chinense Jack.*) cultivars grown in Yucatan, *Food Chemistry*, 104(4): 1682–1686.

Popovich, D. G., Sia, S. Y., Zhang, W., and Lim, M. L. 2014 The color and size of chili peppers (Capsicum annuum) influence Hep-G2 cell growth, *International Journal of Food Sciences and Nutrition*, 65(7): 881–885.

Quintero-Chávez, R., Quintero-Ramos, A., Jiménez-Castro, J. et al. 2012 Modeling of total soluble solid and NaCl uptake during osmotic treatment of bell peppers under different infusion pressures, *Food and Bioprocess Technology*, 5(1): 184–192.

Riquelme, N., and Matiacevich, S. 2017 Characterization and evaluation of some properties of oleoresin from C apsicum annuum var. cacho de cabra, *CyTA-Journal of Food*, 15(3): 344–351.

Rodrigues, K. C., and Fett-Neto, A.G. 2009 Oleoresin yield of Pinus elliottii in a subtropical climate: Seasonal variation and effect of auxin and salicylic acid-based stimulant paste. *Industrial Crops and Products*, 30(2): 316–320.

Santos, P., Aguiar, A. C., Barbero, G. F., Rezende, C. A., and Martínez, J. 2015 Supercritical carbon dioxide extraction of capsaicinoids from malagueta pepper (*Capsicum frutescens L.*) assisted by ultrasound, *Ultrasonics sonochemistry*, 22: 78–88.

Sharma, R., Joshi, V. K., and Kaushal, M. 2015 Effect of pre-treatments and drying methods on quality attributes of sweet bell-pepper (*Capsicum annum*) powder, *Journal of Food Science and Technology*, 52(6): 3433–3439.

Simonovska, J., Yancheva, D., Mikhova, B. et al. 2016 Spectral analysis of extracts from red hot pepper (*Capsicum annuum L.*). Your hosts Macedonian Pharmaceutical Association and Faculty of Pharmacy, Ss Cyril and Methodius University in Skopje, *Macedonian Pharmaceutical Bulletin*, 62: 491–492.

Simopoulos, A. P. 2002 The importance of the ratio of omega-6/omega-3 essential fatty acids, *Biomedicine & Pharmacotherapy*, 56(8): 365–379.

Singh, S., Das, S. S., Singh, G., Schuff, C., de Lampasona, M. P., and Catalan, C.A. 2014 Composition, in vitro antioxidant and antimicrobial activities of essential oil and oleoresins obtained from black cumin seeds (*Nigella sativa L.*), *BioMed Research International*, 2014.

Sousa, A., Casal, S., Malheiro, R., Lamas, H., Bento, A., and Pereira, J. 2015 Aromatized olive oils: Influence of flavouring in quality, composition, stability, antioxidants, and antiradical potential, *LWT-Food Science and Technology*, 60(1): 22–28.

Sricharoen, P., Lamaiphan, N., Patthawaro, P., Limchoowong, N., Techawongstien, S., and Chanthai, S. 2017 Phytochemicals in Capsicum oleoresin from different varieties of hot chilli peppers with their antidiabetic and antioxidant activities due to some phenolic compounds, *Ultrasonics Sonochemistry*, 38: 629–639.

Swain, S., Samuel, D. V. K., Bal, L. M., Kar, A., and Sahoo, G.P. 2012 Modeling of microwave assisted drying of osmotically pretreated red sweet pepper (*Capsicum annum L.*), *Food Science and Biotechnology*, 21(4): 969–978.

Tepić, A., Zeković, Z., Kravić, S., and Mandić, A. 2009 Pigment content and fatty acid composition of paprika oleoresins obtained by conventional and supercritical carbon dioxide extraction, *CyTA–Journal of Food*, 7(2): 95–102.

Vega-Gálvez, A. L. M. S., Lemus-Mondaca, R., Bilbao-Sáinz, C., Fito, P., and Andrés, A. 2008. Effect of air drying temperature on the quality of rehydrated dried red bell pepper (var. Lamuyo), *Journal of Food Engineering*, 85(1): 42–50.

Vesaluoma, M., Müller, L., Gallar, J. et al. 2000 Effects of oleoresin capsicum pepper spray on human corneal morphology and sensitivity, *Investigative Aphthalmology and Visual Science*, 41(8): 2138–2147.

Vian, M. A., Allaf, T., Vorobiev, E., and Chemat, F. 2014 Solvent-Free Extraction: Myth or Reality?. In *Alternative Solvents for Natural Products Extraction*, pp. 25–38. Springer, Berlin, Heidelberg.

Wang, J., Dong, X., Chen, S., and Lou, J. 2013 Microencapsulation of capsaicin by solvent evaporation method and thermal stability study of microcapsules, *Colloid Journal*, 75(1): 26–33.

Weber, M., Salhab, J., Sanchez-Quintela, S., and Tsatsimpe, K. 2020 *Medicinal and Aromatic Plants in the North-West of Tunisia: Findings from a Value Chain and Jobs Survey*. World Bank.

Zhao, D., Zhao, C., Tao, H., An, K., Ding, S., and Wang, Z. 2013 The effect of osmosis pretreatment on hot-air drying and microwave drying characteristics of chili (C apsicum annuum L.) flesh, *International Journal of Food Science & Technology*, 48(8): 1589–1595.

Zimmer, A. R., Leonardi, B., Miron, D., et al. 2012 Antioxidant and anti-inflammatory properties of Capsicum baccatum: from traditional use to scientific approach, *Journal of Ethnopharmacology*, 139(1): 228–233.

Zou, Y., Ma, K., and Tian, M. 2015 Chemical composition and nutritive value of hot pepper seed (Capsicum annuum) grown in Northeast Region of China, *Food Science and Technology*, 35(4): 659–663.

ABBREVIATIONS

HPLC	High-performance liquid chromatography
DPPH	2,2-Diphenyl-1-picrylhydrazyl
FTIR	Fourier transform infrared
CO	Capsicum oleoresin
NH	Amino group
μg	Microgram
OH	Hydroxy group
mL	Milliliter
Cu	Copper
Na	Sodium
K	Potassium
Ca	Calcium
P	Phosphorous
Fe	Ferric
Mn	Manganese
FDA	Federal drug authority
TGA	Thermogravimetric analysis
DSC	Diffraction scanning calorimetry
PUFA	Polyunsaturated fatty acid
SFA	Shortchain fatty acid
MEP	Mevalonic acid pathway
HD	Hydro distillation
NPAE	Negative pressure-assisted extraction
PHWE	Pressurized hot water extraction
MIC	Minimum inhibitory concentration
PEFE	Pulsed electric field extraction)
DPPH	2,2-Diphenyl-1-picrylhydrazyl
ABTS	2, 2′-Azino-bis-3-ethylbenzothiazoline-6-sulfonic acid
ERC	European Regulation Commission
CNS	Central nervous system
MAE	Microwave-assisted extraction
SFE	Supercritical fluid extraction
UAE	Ultrasound-assisted extraction
VMH	Vacuum microwave hydrodistillation
CAMD	Compressed air microwave distillation
MHD	Microwave hydro diffusion
SFME	Solvent-free microwave extraction
SHU	Scoville heat units

DHC   Dihydrocapsaicin
RP-HPLC-PDA   Reverse phase high performance liquid chromatography photodiode
                            array
ATR   Attenuated total reflectance
SRA   Scavenging radical activity

CHAPTER 4

Health and Medicinal Properties of Saffron

Sabeera Muzzaffar and Iqra Azam

University of Kashmir

CONTENTS

DOI: 10.1201/9781003186205-4

4.1 INTRODUCTION

Saffron (*Crocus sativus* Linn.), a small perennial, triploid sterile plant is considered the king of the spice world. It belongs to the family Iridaceae and is also known as red gold. The crocus genus comprises approximately 90 species, out of which some are grown for flowers only. It is planted between June and mid-September, and it flowers during the months of November and December (Dar et al., 2017). This spice has been around for over 4000 years and is one of the main ingredients in folk medicine, where it is used to cure around 90 different medical conditions (Shokrpour, 2019; Mousavi and Bathaie, 2011). It has six tepals, three stamens and a solitary pistil with three red filaments defining the stigma. Saffron is used as a spice and a colourant because of this solitary pistil, which is the most valuable portion of the flower. Its flowers are usually purple in colour, and one to seven flowers are usually produced by each bulb (Muzaffar, et al. 2019). Each flower has generally up to three stigmas extended over the petals and is usually 25–30 mm long (Gohari et al., 2013). For producing 1 kg of saffron, almost 1,50,000 flowers are needed (Pandita, 2021).

4.2 DISTRIBUTION, PRODUCTION AND ECONOMIC IMPORTANCE

This spice has adapted to different environmental conditions and is widely distributed in areas ranging from southern Europe to the Mediterranean basin and the Middle East to

Asia Minor (Giaccio, 2004). It thrives in arid and semi-arid climates with chilly winters and hot, dry summers. Calcium-rich and well-drained sandy soil is best suited for saffron cultivation, making the Mediterranean countries and west of Asia the preferred areas for its cultivation. Saffron is grown in Iran, India, Spain, Italy and Greece, as well as Morocco, France, Switzerland, Turkey, Israel, Azerbaijan, Pakistan, China, Egypt, the United Arab Emirates, Japan, Afghanistan, Iraq, Tasmania, Australia and Mexico (Dar, et al. 2017). The annual production of saffron is about 418 tonnes with 90% of global production contributed by Iran. In Iran, Khorasan province accounts for almost 46,000 ha of area followed by Fars Province. From 2007 to 2017, Iran has witnessed an increase in saffron production from 59,000 ha and 230 tonnes to 108,000 ha and 376 tonnes (Koocheki, et al. 2019). Saffron is farmed exclusively on the Karewas of Kashmir and Kishtwar in Jammu and Kashmir, with a total area of 3674 ha (Ganaie and Singh, 2019; Pandita, 2021). In Jammu and Kashmir, around 3715 hectares of land is under saffron cultivation with a production of 16 MT and a productivity of 4 kg/ha. In Afghanistan, it is grown on an area of about 7557 ha, with Herat Province contributing more than 90% to it. In Greece, 1000 ha of land is under saffron cultivation, while Morocco and Spain have 850 and 150 ha, respectively (FAO, 2018). Most of the saffron-growing countries have witnessed a sharp decline in production, which might be attributed to different factors like unavailability of a good quality corm, declining soil fertility, disease infestations, poor infrastructure, and absence of postharvest management and marketing (Ganaie and Singh, 2019).

According to 2019 trade data, saffron is the 3550th most traded commodity in the world, with a total trade value of 229 million dollars. Exports of saffron fell by 41% from 388 million dollars in 2018 to 229 million dollars in 2019. Saffron commerce accounts for 0.0013% of global trade. Iran was the top saffron exporter in 2019 ($102 million), followed by Spain ($49.8 million), Afghanistan ($28.9 million), China ($5.73 million) and Hong Kong ($5.48 million). However, Spain ($34.1M) was the top most importer of saffron in 2019, followed by Hong Kong, Saudi Arabia, the United Arab Emirates and India importing about $33.6 M, $19.8 M, $18.6 M and $18.3 M worth of saffron, respectively. Iran was held at first and Spain at the second place in saffron exports between 2012 and 2016. Greece occupied third place in most years with Afghanistan ranking ahead of Greece in the year 2016. Afghanistan and Hong Kong have recently become the largest saffron exporters and thus are relatively competitive with other major exporters (Shahnoushi, et al. 2020).

4.3 CHEMISTRY AND PROPERTIES OF SAFFRON

Over the past two decades, numerous researchers have been intrigued by the chemical composition of saffron stigmas (Bathaie and Mousavi, 2010). More than 150 volatile terpenes, terpene alcohols, aldehydes, esters and nonvolatile compounds including proteins, amino acids, minerals, carbohydrates, vitamins (especially B_1 and B_2) and pigments were indicated to be primarily present in its stigmas (Bukhari, et al. 2018). The beneficial compounds like Vitamin B2, hexadecanoic acid, lauric acid, 4-hydroxydihydro-2(3H)-furanone and stigmasterol are abundantly present in its perianth, stamen and corm (Charles, 2012). However, what makes saffron the most sought-after spice is the presence of specific carotenoids in it. Carotenoids (both water-soluble and fat-soluble) are by far the most important

TABLE 4.1 Proximate Analysis of Dried Stigmas of Saffron

Component	Mass Percentage
Water-soluble compounds	53.0
Gums	10.0
Pentosans	8.0
Pectins	6.0
Starch	6.0
α-Crocin	2.0
Other carotenoids	1.0
Fibre (crude)	5.0
Lipids	12.0
Nonvolatile oils	6.0
Volatile oils	1.0
Proteins	12.0
Inorganic matter (ash)	6.0
HCl-soluble ash	0.5
Water	10.0

constituents of saffron because they are responsible for its colour and flavour (Muzaffar, et al. 2019). The principal bioactive constituents of saffron are water-soluble carotenoids such as apocarotenoid crocetin ($C_{20}H_{24}O_4$), crocin, safranal and picrocrocin (Bagur, et al. 2019; Maggi, et al. 2020). The stigmas of *C. sativus* contain phytosterols such as stigmasterol and b-sitosterol, while the petals contain fucosterol, stigmasterol and β-sitosterol.

Furthermore, chemical analysis has shown that the most important compounds in saffron petals are Quercetin and Kaempferol glycoside derivatives. Quercetin ($C_{15}H_{10}O_7$) having a molecular weight of 302.236 g/mol is the aglycone form of flavonoid glycoside having the potential of pharmacological activities. Kaempferol ($C_{15}H_{10}O_6$) is a flavonoid, an antioxidant and anti-inflammatory compound present in its petals and has a molecular weight of 286.23 g/mol. The principal flavonoids in these types of flowers are kaempferol glycosides forming 70%–90% of the total amount and are found in the perianth and the leaves. Seven kaempferol glycosides as well as a corresponding aglycone have been found in saffron floral bio residues. Kaempferol glycoside is the main flavonoid found in stigmas, whereas methylated flavonoids, kaempferide and isorhamnetin glycosides are found in pollen (Bagur, et al. 2019; Boskabady and Farkhondeh, 2016). The proximate analysis of dried stigmas of saffron is shown in Table 4.1.

4.4 COMPOUNDS RESPONSIBLE FOR COLOUR

Saffron is valued for both its prominent colour and odour (Gohari, et al. 2013). Carotenoids are believed to be responsible for saffron's distinct hue and are thus used as natural colourants in the food processing sector (Abu-Izneid, et al. 2020). The presence of glycosylated esters (mono- and di-) of crocetin's dicarboxylic acid stimulates crocetin to turn orange in water, making it more adaptable for food colouring. These crocins account for around 3.5% of the total weight of saffron stigmas, with crocin 1 being the most prominent one. Further, the sugar moieties are responsible for their high solubility. Upon being hydrolysed, crocin, which is a conjugated polyene dicarboxylic acid, produces crocetin and gentiobiose. Both of these hydrolysis products are oil soluble and hydrophobic. Further, crocetin, on being esterified with two water-soluble gentiobioses (sugars), produces a water-soluble carotenoid product, α-Crocin (Rahimi, 2015). Crocin, just like its precursor, is available in both 13-cis and all-trans isomeric forms. Crocin owes its presence for being available in different varieties to the fact that its carbohydrates have the capability of esterifying one or both carboxyl groups (Maggi, et al. 2020). Except for crocin 1, most crocin derivatives are thought to exist in cis–trans isomeric forms (Bukhari, et al. 2018). The principal crocins present in saffron are trans-crocin-2 (TC2), trans-crocin-3 (TC3), trans-crocin-4 (TC4), cis-crocin-2 (CC2), cis-crocin-3 (CC3), cis-crocin-4 (CC4) and trans-crocin-5. However, the most common crocin studied was trans-crocin-4 (TC4), followed by trans-crocin-3 (TC3) and cis-crocin-4 (CC4). Although synthesised in lower concentrations, trans-crocin-2 and cis-crocin-2 were found in all farmed samples (Karkoula, et al. 2018). Moreover, the substituents and configurations of these crocins differ; however, other properties like polarity are very similar (Maggi, et al. 2020). Oral ingestion of crocins present in saffron is not bio-available in the cellular system. In the presence of intestinal epithelium enzymes, crocins are rapidly hydrolysed to trans-crocetin. This hydrolysed product of crocins is absorbed via the intestinal mucosal layer through passive diffusion (Abu-Izneid, et al. 2020). Crocin structure is elucidated in Figure 4.1.

Crocetin (Figure 4.2), the second most bioactive component of saffron, is a natural carotenoid dicarboxylic acid that does not dissolve in water or most organic solvents. Approximately 94% of total crocetin present in saffron is available in the form of glycoside molecules, while the remaining (6%) is free crocetin (Abu-Izneid, et al. 2020). On the side chain of crocetin's glucosyl ester, there are seven conjugated double bonds and four methyl groups. Only six crocetin glycosides were previously reported to exist in saffron (Bukhari, et al. 2018).

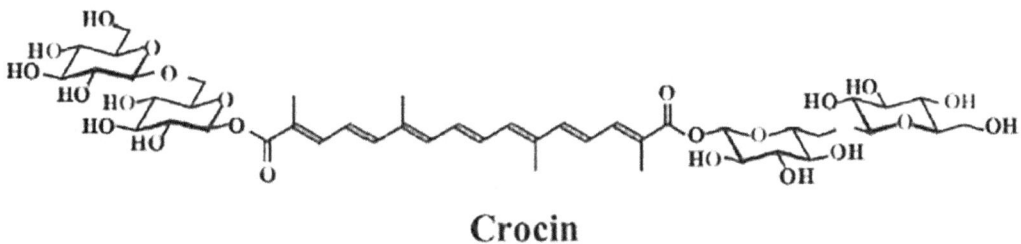

Crocin

FIGURE 4.1   Structure of crocin.

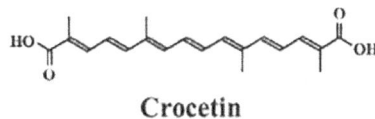

Crocetin

FIGURE 4.2   Structure of crocetin.

High-performance liquid chromatography, medium-pressure liquid chromatography, preparative thin-layer chromatography, molecularly imprinted polymer solid-phase extraction, macroporous resin, crystallisation method and reversed-phase chromatography and extraction with various solvents have been used to isolate TC4 and other crocins (water, methanol, ethyl acetate). The compound crocetin is difficult to get using the aforementioned methods, and it is mostly produced through crocin hydrolysis (acidic and/or alkaline) (Karkoula, et al. 2018). When HPLC was paired with a UV/vis photodiode array and spectrometry, the number of crocetin esters along with their cis–trans isomers increased significantly (Bukhari, et al. 2018).

4.5 PROPERTIES OF CROCIN AND CROCETIN

Crocin: Crocin (MW: 976.96 g/mol) is a unique hydrophilic carotenoid present in saffron, easily dissolves in water and gives an orange-red solution, with a melting point of 186°C (Abu-Izneid, et al. 2020). Crocetin and glucose are produced by acid hydrolysis in an airless environment, whereas crocetin and gentiobiose are produced by alcoholic ammonia hydrolysis of crocin. Crocin is highly responsive to dilute aqueous potassium hydroxide, resulting in an increase in the yield of crocetin (potassium salt). Crocetin mono- and dimethyl esters are produced after treating these with aqueous methyl alcoholic potash. When crocin is dissolved in strong sulphuric acid, it forms a blue solution with a deep colour. Similar to carotene, it turns to violet, red and finally brown when let to stand, and turns green when exposed to nitric acid (Sampathu, et al. 1984).

Crocetin: Crocetin (MW: 328.4 g/mol) is an apocarotenoid produced from cleavage of zeaxanthin (carotenoid) by carotenoid cleavage oxygenase (CCD) (Abu-Izneid, et al. 2020). There are the three forms of crocetin: α-Crocetin is the stable trans-isomer of the dicarboxylic acid crocetin commonly known as crocetin I.

Crocetin II, a labile cis-isomer, is the second version. The monomethyl and dimethyl esters of crocetin I are β-Crocetin and γ-Crocetin, respectively. Other than the xanthone-carotenoid glycosidic compound known as mangicrocin, saffron contains trans-crocetin isomers and 13-cis-crocetin isomers. Crocetin is a crocin breakdown product that is not soluble in water and most organic solvents. However, it is exceptionally soluble in pyridine which is used to isolate it from red-coloured leaves. Moreover, the potassium and sodium salts of crocetin are yellowish in colour. β-Crocetin which is its monomethyl ester has a melting point of 218°C and gets separated from the combination of chloroform and methyl alcohol as reddish-yellow plates. The unstable cis-isomer is converted to the stable trans-form by light exposure. The latter separates as orange-red plates in a combination of chloroform and methyl alcohol, with optical maxima in chloroform at 463 and 434.5 nm. This compound turns bright blue in colour, followed by violet, then by brown after being rubbed with a drop of concentrated H_2SO_4 (Sampathu, et al. 1984). The stable trans forms of crocetin I have a high melting point, while the labile cis forms of crocetin II have a low melting point.

4.6 COMPOUNDS RESPONSIBLE FOR BITTERNESS

Picrocrocin (4-(-D-glucopyranosyloxy)-2,6,6-trimethyl-1-cyclohexene-1-carboxaldehyde) has a molecular weight of 330.37 g and is regarded as the main contributor to saffron's bitter

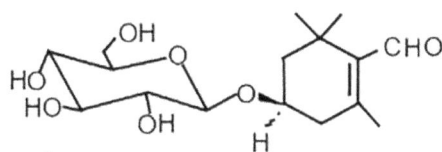

Picrocrocin

FIGURE 4.3 Structure of picrocrocin.

flavour (Bagur, et al. 2019). Saffron essential oil contains picrocrocin, a monoterpene glycoside that is a precursor to safranal. Picrocrocin (Figure 4.3) is made up of a carbohydrate and a safranal (systematic name:2,6,6-trimethylcyclohexa-1,3-diene-1-carboxaldehyde) aldehyde sub-element (Mir et al., 2013). Picrocrocin ($C_{16}H_{26}O_7$) is the second most common constituent (in terms of weight), contributing 3.7% of the stigma's total weight. It gives saffron its distinct flavour and forms up to 1%–13% of the total dry matter (Muzaffar et al., 2019). Picrocrocin, the molecular marker for saffron, whose flavour cannot be duplicated by any other seasoning or spice can be used to recognise its genuineness (Bagur, et al. 2019). It is found to have insecticidal and pesticidal properties, and upon thermal treatment from 5°C to 70°C, picrocrocin has been found to have more stability than the esters of crocetin (Bagur, et al. 2019; Rahimi, 2015). Khun and Winterstein established the structure of picrocrocin in 1934 (José Bagur, et al. 2017).

Picrocrocin is a colourless glycoside that melts at 156°C (Sampathu, et al. 1984). Picrocrocin degrades into safranal, the most abundant component of saffron's volatile fractions, and D-glucose through thermal degradation or a dual-step enzyme/dehydration process that includes the intermediate compound, viz. HTCC (4-hydroxy-2,6,6-trimethyl -1-cyclohexen-1-carboxaldehyde, $C_{10}H_{16}O_2$). It has a maximum absorbance wavelength of 257 nm (Bagur, et al. 2019).

4.7 COMPOUNDS RESPONSIBLE FOR THE AROMA

Around 40 chemicals have been identified as being associated with saffron's distinct aroma, with safranal being the most prominent and essential. The hydrolysis and dehydration of picrocrocin and bio-oxidative cleavage of zeaxanthin yield safranal. Safranal is a monoterpene aldehyde found in the essential oil of saffron and is basically an aglycon of picrocrocin (Abu-Izneid, et al. 2020).

Safranal and 2,6,6-trimethyl-1,4-cyclohexadiene-1-carboxaldehyde are the primary volatile chemicals identified in it (Muzaffar, et al. 2019). Safranal ($C_{10}H_{14}O_7$) is the primary segment that gives saffron its aroma and records for 60%–70% of the unpredictable parts of saffron (Bukhari, et al. 2018). Fresh stigmas lack safranal content and are produced by the action of β-glucosidase on its precursor i.e., picrocrocin during postharvest dehydration and storage conditions. The perfume of 2-hydroxy-4,4,6-trimethyl-2,5-cyclohexa-dien-1-one (saffron, dry hay-like) is the second component of saffron's aroma (Rahimi, 2015). The structures of safranal and zeaxanthin are shown in Figures 4.4 and 4.5, respectively.

The molecular weight of safranal ($C_{10}H_{10}O$), a monoterpene aldehyde, is 150.21. Saffron typically has a safranal concentration of 0.1%–0.6% (José Bagur, et al. 2017). At 330 nm,

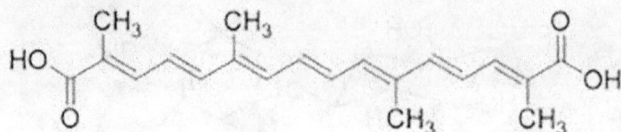

FIGURE 4.4 Structure of safranal.

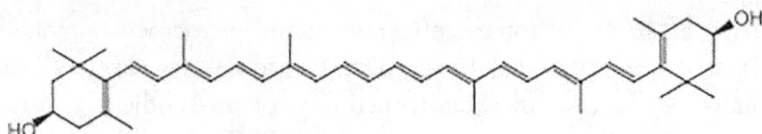

FIGURE 4.5 Structure of zeaxanthin.

it has the highest absorbance; however, other chemicals also adsorb at this wavelength. Several analytical procedures have been developed to determine and characterise the volatile fraction of saffron, including gas chromatography/mass spectrometry (GC-MS), olfactometry, ultrasound-assisted extraction by UV-Vis or HPLC–MS/MS and HPLC-DAD (Diode-Array Detection). Only the HPLC-DAD method can be used to identify and quantify safranal. Safranal has been proven to have a significant antioxidant capacity and cytotoxicity against specific oncogenic cells in vitro, as well as its typical spicy aromatic note (Bagur et al., 2019).

When exposed to light, heat and oxygen, or when the enzyme-glucosidase is active, nonvolatile precursors like carotenoids generate some volatile compounds although in small quantities (Muzaffar, et al. 2019). On the treatment of cyclocitral with selenious acid, Kuhn and Wendt were able to synthesise safranal. In Germany, they were also granted a safranal patent (Sampathu, et al. 1984).

4.8 MISCELLANEOUS

Aspartic acid, glutamic acid (GA), cystine, serine, glycine, threonine, tyrosine, arginine, histidine, lysine, proline, phenylalanine, leucine, valine and methionine, as well as the sugar glucose, are all found in saffron bulbs. The additional compounds include two saponins, viz. oleanolic acid glycoside and steroid saponin (Sampathu, et al. 1984). In addition to safranal, saffron contains roughly 30% crocins, 5%–15% picrocrocin and approximately 2.5% volatile chemicals (Schmidt, et al. 2007).

4.9 HEALTH AND MEDICINAL PROPERTIES OF SAFFRON

Saffron is farmed for its stigmas, which besides being a valued spice, have a variety of therapeutic applications (Jan, et al. 2014). Traditionally, saffron extracts have been used since ages to treat a number of syndromes and disorders (José Bagur et al., 2017). Saffron has long been used as an anti-asthma, sedative, emmenagogue, expectorant, adaptogenic agent and anti-spasmodic in folk and Ayurvedic medicine. It is also utilised for lumbar discomfort, bronchial spasms, heart illness, small pox, eupeptic, menstrual cramps, scarlet fever and common cold. During the 16th and 19th centuries, it was used in various opioid formulations for managing pain (Bukhari et al., 2018; Gohari et al., 2013). Saffron is used by administering orally, through injections and topically in the treatment of various diseases (Bathaie and Mousavi, 2010). Active components of saffron have pharmacological properties because of their distinct chemical structure (Razak et al., 2017). Due to its anti-tumour, anti-inflammatory, antioxidant, anticonvulsant, neuron protection and anti-neurodegenerative disease capabilities, degradative derivatives of carotenoids have become extremely important in modern pharmacological research. These carotenoids have also been linked to anticancer, anti-nociceptive, antidepressant, relaxing and anxiolytic activities. There has also been evidence of an inhibitory influence on platelet aggregation, radical scavenging property, anti-tyrosinase activity, apoptotic effect, enzymatic activity, catalase activity, effect on uterine and oestrus cycle, glutathione S-transferase (GST) activity and immunomodulating action (Bukhari et al., 2018; Muzaffar et al., 2019). Figure 4.6 shows different medicinal uses of saffron and its components.

4.9.1 Saffron and Brain Conditions

Saffron with its constituents is being experimented for therapeutic benefits for treatment of several brain conditions which include Alzheimer's disease, Parkinson's disease, depression, cerebral ischaemia, vascular dementia, posttraumatic stress disorder, mood and anxiety disorders, aging, seizure, insomnia and sleep disorder, brain tumour, multiple sclerosis

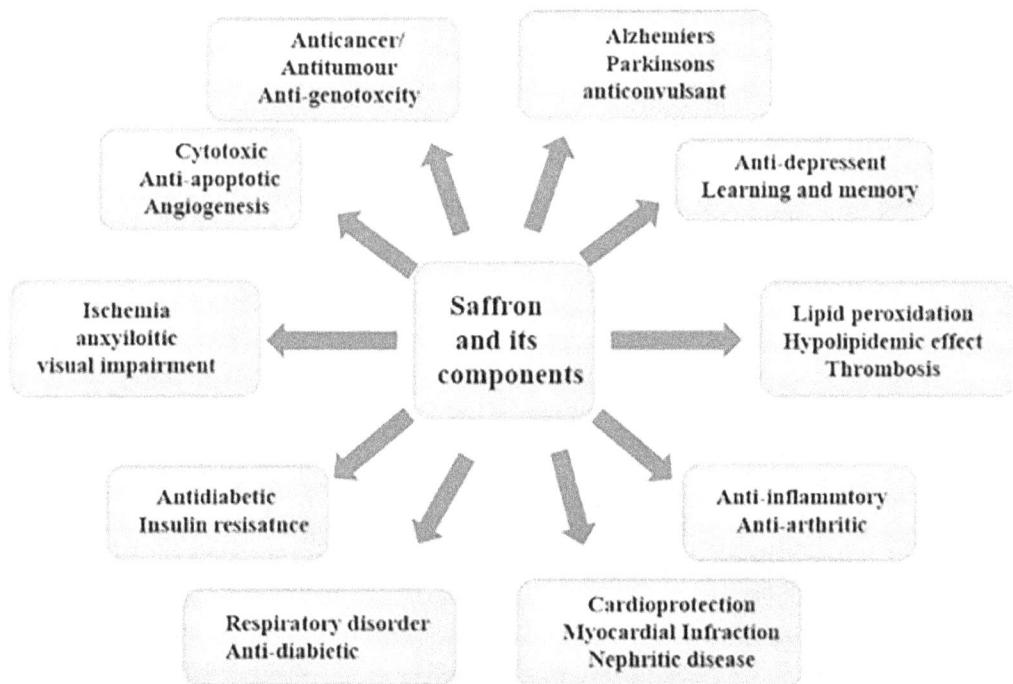

FIGURE 4.6 Different medicinal uses of saffron and its components.

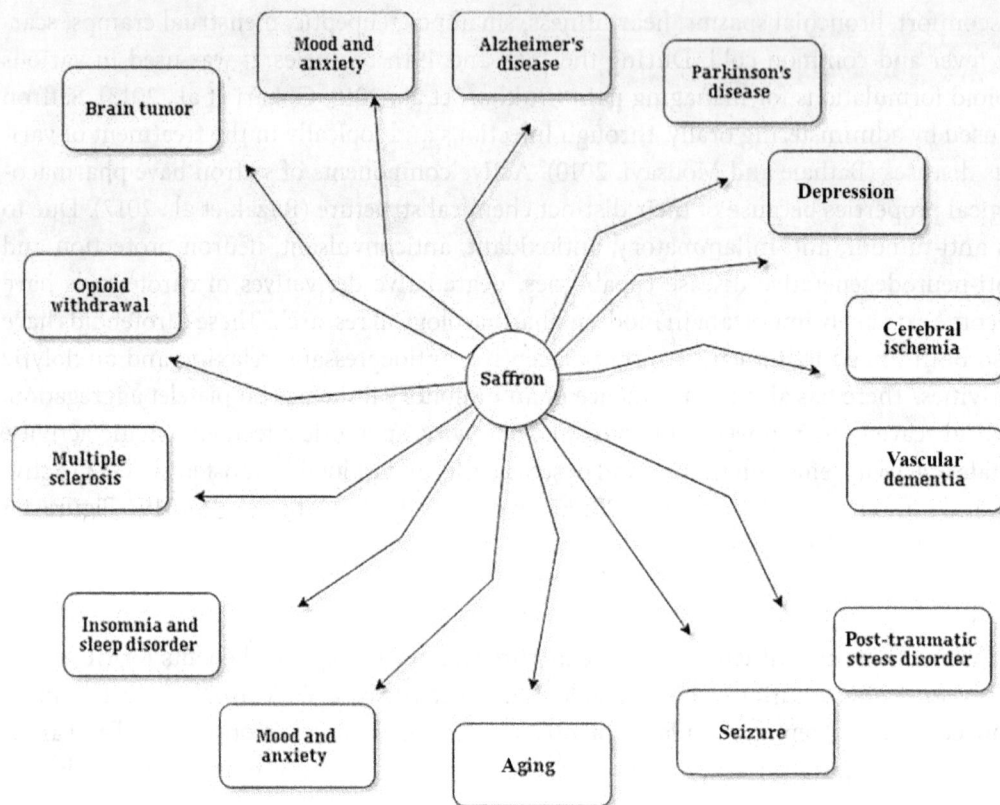

FIGURE 4.7 Saffron and different brain-related diseases.

(MS) and opioid withdrawal (Sharma et al., 2020). A diagram showing saffron and different brain-related diseases is shown in Figure 4.7.

4.9.2 Saffron: An Antidepressant/Anxiolytic Herb

Anxiety and sadness are among the psychiatric diseases that have been demonstrated to react to the treatment of saffron and its metabolites. Saffron is reported to raise oxidative stress levels through raising oxidative stress markers such as malondialdehyde, which causes depression, as well as a decrease in antioxidant defences due to decreased antioxidant enzymes including superoxide dismutase (SOD), catalase and glutathione peroxidase. The boost in CAT activity in liver tissue is credited to safranal and crocin and increased SOD levels and glutathione availability is because of all three active saffron constituents (Razak, et al. 2017). The use of 50 mg quantity of saffron twice daily for 12 weeks has been shown to benefit elderly people with anxiety and sadness. In most patients suffering from depression, while a quantity of 40 mg/day for 6 weeks has been proven effective in the treatment of depression, other research has discovered that taking 30 mg/day of saffron for 9 weeks lowers anxiety and sleep problems in mild to moderate co-morbid depression-anxiety patients (Samarghandian and Farkhondeh, 2020). The intake of 30 mg of saffron per day, according to several clinical trials, maybe more helpful than fluoxetine or imipramine in treating depression (José Bagur et al., 2017).

4.9.3 Alzheimer's Disease

Alzheimer's is counted amongst the most common and dreaded age-related neurode-generative diseases that cause a considerable decline in cognitive functions (José Bagur, et al. 2017). The presence of polypeptide-amyloid-loaded brain plates on blood vessels and the outer surface of neurons in the brain, as well as intracellular aggregation of significant tau protein tangles, distinguishes the molecular mechanism of Alzheimer's disease. Saffron's inhibitory effect on acetylcholinesterase activity is another mechanism involved in its anti-Alzheimer impact (José Bagur, et al. 2017). Crocetin an important constituent of saffron carries significant positive effects in treating Alzheimer's disease. It helps in the inhibition of Ab fibrillisation as well as stabilisation of Ab oligomers in the hippocampus, cerebellum and cerebral cortex while also decreasing total insoluble amyloid, insoluble Ab42 and soluble Ab40 levels which enhances learning and memory. Both crocin-1 and crocetin have been demonstrated to reduce Ab aggregation, while crocin-1 inhibits tau protein aggregation. Crocin components have also been discovered to suppress amyloid aggregation in vitro (Sharma, et al. 2020). Patients with mild to severe Alzheimer's disease found that taking 30 mg of saffron per day (15 mg twice per day) for 16 weeks had a considerably better cognitive performance than placebo, with no evident side effects (Saeedi and Rashidy-Pour, 2021).

4.9.4 Parkinson's Disease

The aggregation of alpha-synuclein (αS) in the brain causes damage to the neurons of the substantia nigra (dopaminergic neurons) (Venda et al. 2010). The main causes of this condition are inflammation and oxidative stress. Furthermore, amyloidogenesis plays a key part in aetiology of Parkinson's disease. Crocin was discovered to have a stronger inhibitory impact on fibrillation in amyloidogenesis than safranal. Crocin administration has also been successful in preventing behaviours like organophosphate OP-induced Parkinson in rats by inhibiting not only the lipid peroxidation but also the inflammation caused by the disease (Samarghandian and Farkhondeh, 2020). Crocetin, like crocin and safranal, has been shown to lessen the risk of Parkinson's disease. The level of thiobarbituric acid, a chemical component found in the substantia nigra, was protected by many doses of crocetin given over a 7-day period, suggesting that crocetin protects against lipidic peroxidation-induced damage (José Bagur, et al. 2017).

4.9.5 Cerebral Ischaemia

Ischaemia is a disease affecting the neuronal cells by way of delaying and selective death of these cells. The mechanisms used in pathogenesis of the disease include inflammation, oxidative stress and apoptosis. Crocin protects against cerebral ischaemia by slowing the activation of the matrix metalloproteinase pathway in old rats, preserving the integrity of the blood–brain barrier (BBB). In this disorder, safranal is an effective drug for protecting the brain. With the creation of an ischaemia-reperfusion injury, safranal was found to maintain a balance between the oxidant and antioxidant systems, which helped to alleviate behavioural changes. Safranal reduces total sulfhydryl in the brain while raising thiobarbituric acid reactive compounds (TBARS) in the hippocampus in doses ranging from 145 to 72.5

mg/kg. The positive effects of the bioactive compound safranal on ischaemia-reperfusion injury are basically due to a reduction in the production of free radicals (Samarghandian and Farkhondeh, 2020).

4.9.6 Epilepsy

It is basically a neurodegenerative disease, which manifests through the loss of consciousness, sensations and also unusual behaviour with pathogenesis involving mainly oxidative stress. The utilisation of saffron as an anti-convulsant in the dosage of 800 and 400 mg/kg for animal models has effectively demonstrated an anti-epileptic effect in a model for pentylenetetrazol-induced seizures. Pentylenetetrazol-induced seizures were reduced not only in frequency but also in duration by safranal (0.35 and 0.15 mL/kg). It also slowed down the onset of convulsions and protected death in the mice (Rahmani, et al. 2017; Samarghandian and Farkhondeh, 2020). It was found that crocin when administered to an animal model exposed to penicillin showed a considerable anticonvulsant impact. Crocin's anticonvulsant mechanism is mostly based on the alteration of GABA (A)-benzo-diazepine receptors. Crocin (20 mg/kg) reduces the likelihood of a generalised seizure (Samarghandian and Farkhondeh, 2020).

4.9.7 Multiple Sclerosis

It is considered an autoimmune disease wherein the body's immune system attacks its own tissues. This immune system malfunction actually destroys the fatty substance that forms the coating and thereby protecting the nerve fibres in the brain and spinal cord (myelin). Antioxidant protection has been proposed as one of the potential therapies for MS, as reactive oxygen species (ROS) play a crucial role in the disease's early and late stages. The aetiology of illnesses is intimately linked to the imbalance between the generation of ROS and levels of antioxidant. Endoplasmic reticulum (ER) stress is a well-known inflammatory mechanism. GA and quinolinic acid (QA) cause inflammation and demyelination in neurological diseases like MS. They primarily work by activating oligodendrocytes and producing too many free radicals (Samarghandian and Farkhondeh, 2020). Numerous studies have found that MS plates are subjected to a wide range of oxidative injury and that the damage induced because of ROS begins at the earliest stages of neuroinflammation. Saffron has been found effective in improving MS symptoms. In a type of experimental autoimmune encephalomyelitis, clinical symptoms and leukocyte infiltration reduced after an ethanol extract of saffron were administered, suggesting that demyelination and neurodegeneration might be prevented by the glycosidic esters of crocetin. Crocin (100 mg/kg) has also been shown to help in demyelination. Safranal (0.1, 1, 10, 50, 100, and 200 µM) protects OLN-93 oligodendrocytes from GA or QA-induced damage by reducing oxidative stress. This data suggests that saffron can be effective in treating MS by reducing oxidative stress and preventing leukocyte infiltration into the CNS (José Bagur, et al. 2017; Samarghandian and Farkhondeh, 2020).

4.9.8 Learning Behaviour and Memory

Majority of neurodegenerative disorders are linked to changes in memory and learning. MS is also characterised by memory loss, albeit the risk factors for this have yet to be established.

Literature review suggests that the saffron extract, i.e., crocin and crocetin have a favourable effect on memory and learning skills in mice and rats with ethanol-induced learning behaviour deficits (Bukhari et al. 2018). Saffron reportedly increases learning and memory, has a genoprotective impact and protects against genotoxin-induced oxidative stress because of the varied spectrum of bioactives present in it. Crocin was also found to help older mice avoid learning impairment, reduce oxidative stress and improve memory according to a study. The benefits of saffron and its constituents have been linked to their antioxidant properties which help to scavenge free radicals that cause memory loss (Abu-Izneid, et al. 2020).

4.9.9 Cardiovascular Diseases

Cardiovascular diseases are generally considered "the world's first killer" and include diseases like heart failure and myocardial infarction (MI), mostly affecting middle-aged and elderly people. High blood pressure and cholesterol, diabetes mellitus (DM), smoking, obesity, lack of physical activity, ethnicity and family history are all variables that contribute to cardiovascular diseases (Razak, et al. 2017).

Heart failure, MI, reperfusion injury, ischaemic heart disease, cardiomyopathy and other cardiovascular illnesses are associated with apoptosis, also known as programmed cell death. Several factors have been found to activate this highly controlled cell death pathway in cardiac myocytes, which include inflammatory cytokines and oxidative stress. By blocking apoptotic signalling pathways and decreasing cardiac cell death, antioxidants may prove to be a viable medicinal intervention in preventing and treating cardiovascular diseases. Crocin was found to prevent the down-regulation of Bcl-2 gene expression as well as the up-regulation of Bax mRNA expression, lowering apoptosis in a dose-dependent manner in several animal and in vitro investigations (Ghaffari and Roshanravan, 2019).

The two key members of the Bcl-2 family that play a role in the intrinsic signalling system are Bax, a pro-apoptotic protein, and Bcl-2, an anti-apoptotic protein (mitochondrial apoptosis). During apoptosis, the balance of these two proteins is crucial. The Bax/Bcl-2 ratio was lowered by saffron extracts, particularly crocin and cardiac myocytes and other cells were protected from apoptosis.

A severe form of myocardial necrosis produced by an imbalance in coronary blood flow and myocardial demand is known as MI. It affects lipid peroxidation, free radical damage, hyperlipidemia and hyperglycemia, among other biochemical parameters. The role of saffron in the electrophysiological remodelling of the atrioventricular (AV) node when the zone of concealment and AV nodal refractoriness develops in atrial fibrillation has been acknowledged and well accepted (Bukhari, et al. 2018). Saffron has been found cardioprotective at all doses, prevents hemodynamic and left ventricular activities, maintains structural integrity and increases antioxidants. Tea with saffron contains lycopene which is actually a flavonoid antioxidant may lower the risk of cardiovascular disease. The administration of crocin intravenously decreased myocardial injury, LDH and creatine kinase (CK) levels, though it was not positive when crocin was given orally, presumably due to its poor absorption in GI tract (Razak, et al. 2017).

The development of atherosclerosis, the major cause of cardiovascular disease, is aided by inflammation. In the early phases of atherogenesis, there is the release of cytokines, chemokines and adhesion molecules which are all proinflammatory in nature. Furthermore, oxidative stress has a role in a wide range of CVD symptoms. Moreover, because cardiac tissue has greater oxidative metabolism and a low antioxidant defence when compared to other organs, it is vulnerable to oxidative damage (José Bagur, et al. 2017).

The antioxidant and anti-inflammatory impact of saffron is well-known, with carotenoids, flavonoids and anthocyanins being regarded as the main antioxidant and anti-inflammatory components of its extract. Saffron's carotenoid compounds, crocin and crocetin, were found to be the most effective at radical scavenging in experiments, followed by safranal. These components have a high radical scavenging activity due to their proclivity for donating a single hydrogen atom to free radicals. Saffron extracts (particularly crocetin and crocin) have been shown to reduce plasma malondialdehyde formed by ROS (Razak, et al. 2017).

The antioxidant, anti-inflammatory and anti-apoptotic characteristics in saffron extract make it a valuable cardioprotective agent. Its anti-inflammatory properties are aided by its radical scavenging properties. The anti-inflammatory characteristics of saffron components are believed to considerably inhibit the effects of enzymes cyclooxygenase 1 and 2, as well as the synthesis of prostaglandin E2. Crocetin reduces inflammation and vascular injury by inhibiting immune cell adhesion and infiltration into inflamed endothelium (Ghaffari and Roshanravan, 2019).

The anti-atherosclerotic advantages of saffron are credited to crocetin, which reduces the levels of cardiac indicators such as lactate dehydrogenase (LDH/p), CK and MDA. It also enhances the mitochondrion capacity in noradrenaline-treated cardiac myocytes. Crocetin plays a potential role as an anti-atherosclerotic agent (Bukhari, et al. 2018). Crocetin-fed rats had lower cholesterol deposits in the aorta, atheroma, foam cells and atherosclerotic lesions. Crocetin improves oxygen transport in blood plasma, counteracting the reduction caused by increased cholesterol levels and lowering blood cholesterol levels in people with atherosclerosis (José Bagur, et al. 2017).

4.9.10 Hypotensive and Hypolipidemic Properties

The prevalence of hyperlipidemia and hypertension are both well-established factors in the development of cardiovascular disease. Crocetin, in atherosclerosis increases O_2 absorption in blood plasma, negating the reduction caused by the increase in cholesterol. It also lowers cholesterol levels in the blood. Saffron contains antioxidant qualities as well as calcium antagonistic (calcium channel blocking) capabilities, making it a potential smooth muscle relaxant. Furthermore, the components of saffron, especially crocin, block the transfer of extracellular Ca^{2+} into the ER and the release of intracellular Ca^{2+}. These proposed mechanisms may relax blood vessels and reduce blood pressure (Ghaffari and Roshanravan, 2019). Crocin and crocetin, on the other hand, were proposed to initiate different mechanisms in the vasoconstriction pathway, specifically improving aortic contraction problems, better known as the hypotensive effect (Razak, et al. 2017). In saffron extract, the main ingredients crocins and safranal have been found to be hypotensive, though some credit it to the anti-oxidative properties of the same plant. Experiments have also shown safranal to be of critical importance in lowering blood pressure in rats. In the previous study, an aqueous saffron extract (safranal and crocin) had a dose-dependent effect on lowering the mean pressure of the arteries (Imenshahidi, et al. 2010). It was discovered that saffron (400 mg) reduced not only the systolic blood pressure but the mean arterial pressure as well. The use of the same quantity of saffron reduced the mean arterial pressure in healthy subjects also (Modaghegh, et al. 2008).

Hyperlipidemia is considered one of the important risk factors for the development and progression of atherosclerotic lesions and cardiovascular disorders. Elevated serum cholesterol, very low-density lipoproteins, low-density lipoproteins, fatty acids, TGs and disruption of other biochemical markers are also linked to it (Bukhari, et al. 2018). CETP (cholesteryl ester transfer protein), a serum protein implicated in the control of plasma lipid profiles and lipoprotein levels, can be considered as a novel technique for lowering the risk of cardiovascular diseases when it is suppressed (Ghaffari and Roshanravan, 2019).

According to one study, crocin supplements given to patients with this metabolic syndrome lowered CETP and increased HDL levels after treatment. Pancreatic lipase inhibitory characteristics, fat and cholesterol malabsorption, a decrease in lipoprotein oxidation and oxidative stress regulation are all possible reasons for saffron's lipid-lowering properties (Sheng, et al. 2006). Crocin, when administered at 25–100 mg/kg body weight, is demonstrated to have a hypolipidemic impact in diet-induced hyperlipidemic rats by blocking pancreatic lipase and inducing fat and cholesterol malabsorption, culminating in a hypolipidemic effect (Razak, et al. 2017).

4.9.11 Treatment of Cancers

Cancer is considered as one of the dreaded diseases in the world with its frequency rising continuously in emerging as well as the developed nations. It is one of the most serious non-communicable illnesses that endanger global health (Bhandari, 2015). Cancer is defined by uncontrolled cell development that results from an intricate interplay between inherited genetic composition and different environmental variables (Pharaoh, et al. 2004). Cancer can be caused by a variety of factors including genetics, immune system, carcinogens, and age (Tseng, et al. 2008). Crocin, crocetin and safranal were discovered to have effective anticancer properties against a variety of tumours including prostate cancer (CaP), leukaemia, lung cancer, colorectal cancer (CRC), breast cancer, pancreatic cancer (PC) and ovarian cancer (Samarghandian, et al. 2013). The antitumor activity is mainly caused by one of the many factors like inhibition of DNA and RNA synthesis, suppression of cancer cell proliferation, apoptosis, inhibition of metastasis and angiogenesis and changes in the expression pattern of oncogenes or tumour-suppressive genes (Lambrianidou, et al. 2021). Crocin has been seen to inhibit the growth of cancerous cells; however, it does not affect the normal/or noncancerous cells. It was also found that the invasion, migration and adhesion activity of cancer cells were severely affected by the use of saffron and its derivatives (Arzi, et al. 2018).

Saffron was found to be more beneficial when taken orally, while its chemopreventive efficacy could be improved by encapsulating it in liposomes (Lambrianidou, et al. 2021). Crocetin caused death in human gastric cancer cells by many possible mechanisms, like disrupting mitochondrial membrane potential, enhancing caspase 3 activation and cytochrome c translocation (Bhandari, 2015). Further, crocin also demonstrated cytotoxicity against an adenocarcinoma AGS cell line in a dose and time-dependent manner and caspase activity and flow were used to confirm crocin-induced apoptosis (Hoshyar, et al. 2013).

CRC is the most common cancer and its incidence increases as people get older. Crocin, a major constituent of saffron extract, although found to have an adverse effect on the growth of CRC cells had no such impact on the normal cells (Aung, et al. 2007).

Hepatocellular carcinoma is the third leading cause of cancer-related deaths and its incidence is increasing. The majority of its cases are linked to chronic viral hepatitis. Due to the reduction of cell growth and promotion of apoptosis, saffron has a significant chemo-preventive impact against liver cancer. According to one study, saffron appears to protect rat livers from cancer by regulating oxidative damage and decreasing the response caused by inflammation (Amin, et al. 2011).

PC is the fourth biggest cause of cancer-related deaths in the world. PC has a dismal prognosis and a low incidence of radical resection. Crocetin was discovered to have a substantial anticancer impact on pancreatic cells both in vitro and in vivo via activation of apoptosis in a number of researches conducted to comprehensively determine if it significantly influences PC growth (Bakshi, et al. 2010).

Prostate cancer is a disease that progresses slowly and frequently with higher prevalence in older age. In all malignant cell lines, saffron extract and its primary ingredient crocin, suppressed cell growth in a manner that was time and dosage-dependent but not in non-malignant cells. These potential components also stop cell cycle progression, inhibit cell proliferation and induce apoptosis in prostate cancer (D'Alessandro, et al. 2013).

Lung cancer results in the highest cancer-related fatalities worldwide, owing to the fact that the vast majority of patients are detected after the disease has progressed to an advanced stage. Crocetin has been linked to cancer prevention and its effect on lung cancer-bearing mice was studied in both the pre- and post-initiation phases. Crocetin therapy significantly reduced the elevated values of lipid peroxidation marker enzymes, glutathione metabolising enzymes and enzymic antioxidant activity in carcinogen-treated mice. The pathological changes visible in cancerous animals were considerably normalised by crocetin administration (Magesh, et al. 2006). Crocetin from saffron has anticancer properties because it not only inhibits cell proliferation but also promotes apoptosis in cancer cells by activating caspase-dependent pathways (Samarghandian, et al. 2013).

Breast cancer has been the reason for the largest number of cancer-related deaths among females worldwide. Its present treatment which includes surgery, radiotherapy and adjuvant chemotherapy or hormone therapy has not been successful enough to decrease its morbidity or mortality rate (Khorasanchi, et al. 2018). The use of saffron extracts along with its constituents, trans-crocin-4, safranal and crocetin inhibited the proliferation of breast cancer cell tumour lines (MDAMB-231 and MCF-7) considerably. Saffron inhibits the proliferation of MCF-7 cells and induces apoptosis in these cells in the doses of 10–50 ug/mL, through many mitochondrial signalling pathways which involved caspase-8 activation, up-regulation of Bax, disruption of the potential of mitochondrial membrane and release of cytochrome c. Thus, saffron is considered a promising chemotherapeutic agent in the treatment of this type of cancer (Bhandari, 2015).

4.10 OTHER MISCELLANEOUS ROLES

4.10.1 Saffron as an Anti-diabetic Agent

Diabetes which is characterised by high blood sugar levels is one of the most prevalent non-communicative diseases in the world (Siddique, et al. 2020). Diabetes-related complications are initiated and progressed as a result of an increase in oxidative stress and faulty antioxidant defence systems. Encephalopathy is one of the most serious complications of DM (Bukhari, et al. 2018). Saffron has been experimented with as a potent drug for diabetes due to the fact that the main active constituents of saffron viz., crocin, crocetin and safranal provide an anti-diabetic response. They increase insulin signalling and prevent diabetes by increasing insulin sensitivity while being ineffective on blood serum glutamic oxaloacetic transaminase, serum glutamic-pyruvic transaminase or creatinine levels (Razak, et al. 2017; Yaribeygi, et al. 2019).

4.10.2 Saffron as a Relaxant on Smooth Muscles

Saffron and its constituents have a relaxing effect on the smooth muscles of organs, including blood vessels, trachea, GI and urogenital tract. This effect has been credited to the mechanisms which include stimulatory effect on b2-adrenoreceptors, inhibitory effect on muscarinic receptor, inhibitory effect on histaminic (H1) receptors, inhibitory effect on calcium channel, endothelium-dependent relaxation (EDR) effect and the impact of the use of saffron and its constituents on intracellular cyclic adenosine monophosphate (cAMP) and besides the effect on intracellular cAMP (Boskabady, et al. 2020).

4.10.3 Saffron in Ocular Diseases

The presence of polar carotenoids, crocin and crocetin in saffron makes it a strong antioxidant and has been effective in treating age-related macular degeneration (AMD) and glaucoma. These polar carotenoids when taken at daily doses of 20–50 mg for 3 months protect retinal cells from oxidation and helps in treatment. Clinical studies statistically revealed a significant improvement compared with the control group in performing their functions when used in the treatment of age-related maculopathy (Koşar and Hüsnü Can Başer, 2020).

4.10.4 Saffron as Immunomodulatory Agent

The immune system is a complex biological system comprising innate and adaptive immunity. Moreover, the innate immune system is responsible for an efficient first line of host defence and is necessary for triggering the adaptive immune response. The immunomodulatory effects of saffron have been observed in vivo and in vitro and in a few clinical studies as well. These studies have shown that the use of saffron and crocin, which is one of saffron's main constituents, augmented not only the production of hormonal immune responses but also modulated the total and differential leukocyte counts. Saffron has been found to improve the immune system, the main components of which are the T and B cells.

In saffron-treated groups, IgG levels saw an increase, while there was a decrease in the IgM levels. Besides, it was also found to regulate immune reactivity by inhibiting histamine (H1) and muscarine receptors (Zeinali, et al. 2019).

4.10.5 Saffron as an Antimicrobial Agent

Antimicrobial properties have been reported in various parts of the saffron plant. The antimicrobial property of saffron against bacteria (*Micrococcus luteus, Staphylococcus epidermitis, Staphylococcus aureus* and *Escherichia coli*) and fungi (*Candida albicans, Aspergillus niger*, and *Cladosporium* sp.) has been reported when the ethyl acetate extracts of stigma, stamen, leaves and corolla were used (Razak, et al. 2017; Siddique, et al. 2020).

4.10.6 Saffron as Anti-Inflammatory Agent

Neutrophil cells are central cells in acute inflammatory processes and the use of saffron has been recommended as a curative herbal agent to prevent afflictions caused by these cells. It has been found that in the inflammatory processes, mobility, the number, lifespan, tissue influx ability and phagocytic activity of neutrophil cells increases. Saffron's anti-inflammatory properties are undoubtedly linked to its powerful antioxidant and radical scavenging abilities, which are primarily attributed to the presence of crocetin and crocin in saffron (Mokhtari-Zaer, et al. 2020; Zeinali, et al. 2019).

4.11 BIOACTIVE COMPOUNDS OF SAFFRON AND THEIR EXTRACTION

Saffron contains crocin, crocetin, safranal, picrocrocin, minerals, essential oils and traces of B1 and B2 vitamins. Extraction and purification techniques are required to obtain many important substances, such as bioactive chemicals found naturally in plants. Green chemistry needs like safety, environmental friendliness, low or no contaminants, efficiency and economies should all be addressed by a highly effective bioactive extraction process (Garavand, et al. 2019). The compounds of saffron have been found to be of great significance in the treatment of various health issues and their extraction is of paramount importance. However, a wide range of extraction processes are currently available and it is the end product that is the deciding factor as to which one of these extraction processes ought to be used. Saffron compounds are typically extracted for medicinal purposes, so the safety of the end product is the primary concern. As a result, numerous alternative extraction procedures have been tried to extract the high-value bioactives from the saffron portion, either alone or in combination. Previous work on the extraction of saffron volatile compounds reveals that it was mostly done the old-fashioned way, with chemicals or water as a solvent, and that it was more suitable for lab-scale extraction. However, in recent years, technology-assisted extraction has gained immense importance as the use of these extraction methods prevents cell disruption of essential compounds present in saffron (Suali, 2020).

Traditional extraction processes, like Soxhlet, maceration or solvent extraction, vapour or hydro-distillation, need high volumes of organic toxic solvents, are non-selective, necessitate extensive extraction durations and in some cases destroy thermoactive substances like bioactives (Heydari and Haghayegh, 2014). In order to remove the difficulties in these types of extraction processes, novel extraction methods are invented and suggested as replacements for such processes. These modern and latest extraction techniques, known as "green methods", are more efficient, safer, environmentally friendly, faster and more accurate. Green extraction techniques for saffron include emulsion liquid membranes (ELMs), supercritical fluid extraction (SFE), microwave-assisted extraction (MAE), enzyme-assisted extraction (EAE), ultrasound-assisted extraction (UAE) or sonication and pulsed electric field (PEF) extraction. In general, the effectiveness of extraction processes is largely determined by the choice of appropriate solvents, use of complementary or co-extraction methods and consideration of solvent-solute affinity (Azmir, et al. 2013).

4.11.1 Conventional Techniques

The category of these types of extraction methods is typically relying on the strength of the various solvents that are used, as well as the use of high temperature and/or mixing. This category includes Soxhlet extraction, solvent extraction or maceration/soaking and hydro- or steam distillation (Jafari, et al. 2020).

4.11.2 Soxhlet Extraction

The Soxhlet extraction process, developed by Soxhlet, a German chemist, in 1879 is considered the gold standard for extracting bioactive substances, fats, oils and essential oils. For extraction, the dried saffron is put in a porous cellulose thimble and then a flask containing the solvent is heated, upon which the solvent is evaporated and then condensed to a liquid that trickles into the extraction chamber containing the saffron. Picrocrocin is extracted using a Soxhlet method with different solvents like diethyl ether, light petroleum and methanol. Methanol is the best solvent for extracting picrocrocin, primarily to understand its anticancer and therapeutic properties (Garavand, et al. 2019; Jafari, et al. 2020). Long extraction durations, considerable solvent and energy usage, impure extracts, low safety and lesser extraction efficiency are the main disadvantages of this approach (Gupta, et al. 2012).

4.11.3 Solvent Extraction

Solvent extraction also known as maceration/soaking is counted as the best and most common extraction process for extracting whole saffron. This extraction process begins with the mixing of a predetermined quantity of saffron with the solvent, accompanied by a time and speed-dependent stirring, filtering and measuring the absorbance of the resultant product with a UV-Vis spectrophotometer. The dried saffron is kept in a closed vessel and menstruum, a solvent is added to it. After some time, the liquid is strained out and the solid component called marc is thereafter compressed to recover high amounts of the inhibited solution. Saffron bioactive components are typically extracted using solvents such as methanol, ethanol, water and petroleum ether. According to reports, methanol (50% v/v) is the best solvent for extracting the largest amounts of saffron active compounds, seconded by ethanol (50% v/v) and water (Garavand, et al. 2019).

4.11.4 Hydro- or Steam Distillation

It is a process that uses water, steam or a combination of the two without the use of organic solvents and is done before drying the plant material. The hydro-/steam-distillation technique recovers both bioactives and essential oils from plant tissues. Saffron stigmas are kept either in water or in a mixture comprising of both water and alcohol for a while, before being heated to boiling point in this process. Volatile substances are ferried by the steam to a condenser, where they are liquefied for collection and cooled down by a jet stream of water. The reason that water is used in three different states, viz. liquid, vapour or steam is because it has no chemical effect on bioactive compounds (Jafari, et al. 2020). As a result, bioactives can be vigorously separated from water by simple decantation after extraction. The method is suitable for extracting bioactive substances from different parts of the plant, including blooms, petals, stems and roots (Yang, et al. 2011). In any case, the technique has several drawbacks, which include a lengthy extraction time, a few chemical changes including cyclisation and hydrolysis, contact of terpenic atom with bubbling water, besides the loss of polar molecules because of overheating (Garavand et al., 2019).

4.12 NOVEL EXTRACTION TECHNIQUES

4.12.1 Emulsion Liquid Membrane (ELM)

This process comprises a membrane phase, dispersed phase and a feed. ELM systems are double emulsions (W1/O/W2), wherein W1 represents the internal aqueous phase which contains the stripping agents, "O" represents the organic membrane phase which has the diluent, surfactant, carrier and in some cases co-surfactant, and W2 represents the external aqueous phase (feed phase) enriched with the target ingredients in ELM systems. Using a recently developed ELM system, saffron bioactive compounds were extracted from dried saffron stigmas in an aqueous solution. The following conditions were observed when using the one-factor-at-a-time method to optimise extraction: Span 80 was prepared as a surfactant at a concentration of 2.5%, n-decane as a membrane diluent, a phase ratio of 0.8 (internal aqueous phase – membrane phase), a treat ratio of 0.3 (emulsion – external aqueous phase) and an agitating speed of 300 rpm. In optimal conditions, nearly 90% of saffron and its bioactives including picrocrocin, safranal and crocins were accumulated into the aqueous phase of the emulsion globules (Mokhtari and Pourabdollah, 2013).

4.12.2 Microwave-Assisted Extraction (MAE)

Microwave heating involves dispersion of electromagnetic waves in magnetrons in laboratories at frequencies ranging from 0.915 to 2.45 GHz for food, medical, nutraceutical and pharmaceutical purposes. Heat and mass transfer occur from the inside of the plant material in the same direction to the solvent medium in MAE (Garavand, et al. 2019). In novel extraction practices like MAE, there is no degradation of saffron metabolites, the extraction time is reduced and there is also a considerable reduction in undesired by-product thereby, saving energy, time and use of solvents (Sarfarazi, et al. 2020). The best solvent to extract safranal and picrocrocin is ethanol and water used in equal proportions and for crocin 1 the best one is a mixture of methanol and water in equal proportions (Sobolev, et al. 2014).

4.12.3 Ultrasound-Assisted Extraction (UAE)

This method of extraction is known as sonication and actually involves sound waves in 20 kHz–100 MH range, which are simultaneously expanded and compressed. Because of the cavitation phenomenon, sonication entails the generation, amplification and collapse of microbubbles. Ultrasound wave extraction is used to release bounded organic and inorganic compounds by increasing solvent contact with the target compounds and exacerbating mass transfer. The UAE technique has several advantages over traditional extraction methods including faster extraction, higher selectivity, high purity finish product, improved mass and energy transfer and economical in nature. Crocetin esters, volatile compounds of saffron (safranal and isophorone), crocin derivatives, picrocrocin and bioactives such as quercetin, myricetin and kaempferol in saffron have all been studied in the UAE using various organic and aqueous solvents or both at a frequency ranging between 20 and 60 kHz like ethanol:water (50:50), distilled water, methanol:acetonitrile (38:62) diethyl ether, water:methanol, petroleum ether and diethyl ether. The most remarkable benefits of UAE-assisted extraction of saffron bioactives are smaller extraction durations, higher yield and optimum results at ambient temperatures (Ferrara, et al. 2014; Garavand, et al. 2019).

4.12.4 High Hydrostatic Pressure (HHP)

High hydrostatic pressure extraction is a non-thermal way of extraction that has shown effectiveness in increasing the quality, yield and accelerated transfer of bioactive compounds by mass transfer generated by the ultra-high hydraulic pressures ranging between 1000 and 8000 bars. This extraction method affects noncovalent associations (ionic, hydrogen and hydrophobic bonds), as contrasted to thermal extractions, which affect covalent bonds. Plant compartments with high molecular weight (proteins, carbohydrates, etc.) have noncovalent bonds that gets deformed or denatured by using ultra-high pressure, preventing them from releasing into the solvent and resulting in formation of a pure solute. If compared to conventional extraction procedures, HPP extraction results in increased permeability of solutes and faster extraction times by deprotonating the charged groups. This disrupts salt bridges and hydrophobic connections in cell membranes, resulting in enhanced solute permeability. The benefits of the HHP extraction method include energy and time savings, environmental friendliness, high purity extraction, minimal use of solvents, and the ability to obtain a large number of useful compounds (Garavand, et al. 2019).

The HPLC analysis revealed that increasing the applied pressure in the range of 1000–6000 bars resulted in an increase in the extract quality to the extent of 52–63% of crocin, 54%–85% of picrocrocin and 55–62% of safranal. However, extraction temperatures ranging from 30°C to 70°C resulted in a significant drop in crocin content (25–36%). The best operation settings for HHP extraction of saffron bioactive components were reported to be 5800 bars at 50°C for 5 minutes (Shinwari and Rao, 2018).

4.12.5 Enzyme-Assisted Extraction (EAE)

Different enzymes can be used as pre-treatments to speed up the extraction of bioactive material from the matrix of a plant. However, the cell walls of the plants not only get damaged but bioactive substances bound to carbohydrate and lipid chains can also be degraded while using the enzyme-assisted extraction. In solvent and pressurised hot water extraction, the use of naturally occurring enzymes such as cellobiase, cellulase, pectin-esterase, hemi-cellulase, fructosyltransferase, pectinase, α-amylase and protease have been demonstrated to boost the yield of premium quality extract. Traditional extraction methods as well as their subsequent filtration and purification processes consume a lot of time and energy (Garavand, et al. 2019). The EAE approach can save both time and energy and is preceded by the use of a cold press or solvents (water). EAE is categorised as a "green extraction technology" since it uses natural enzymes and water instead of harmful organic and toxic solvents and co-extractors.

The quality of enzyme-assisted extraction depends on the water content, particle size, chemical characteristics of the plant matrix, dosage, type, solvent to solid ratio and the required conditions for enzyme and time-temperature configuration of the extraction procedure (Azmir, et al. 2013).

As per Lotfi, et al. (2015), Pectinex, a commercial enzyme mixture, containing cellulase, pectinase and hemicellulose in various concentrations, dissolved in distilled water was used to isolate anthocyanins from saffron at 40°C with different extraction durations. The optimised EAE was found to recover 40% more anthocyanins from saffron tepals than solvent extraction with ethanol (reference method). The extract obtained by enzyme-assisted had a distinct colour and more consistent quality, whereas the solvent-extracted compound was pale and susceptible to degradation.

4.12.6 Pulsed Electric Field (PEF) Extraction

PEF can be used as a non-thermal method of extraction that leaves the minimum quantity of bioactive compounds, product appearance and nutritional components unaltered. The tissue membrane of the plant is ruptured by electric fields, especially in low power ranging between 20 and 80 kV/cm. There is also a temporary or permanent loss of semi-permeability of membrane at the plant interface which encourages the release of embedded bioactive components (Barba, et al. 2015). The obtaining of plant-derived materials using PEF is such a promising method for recovering vitamins, phenolic and other value-added components. The newly found advantages of PEF extraction include extraction efficiency, increased mass transfer, reduced processing temperature and extraction time, support for sensitive bioactives, minimal environmental risks and energy savings. The target compounds are not degraded, hydrolysed or polymerised as a result of such non-thermal extraction. In comparison to solvent extraction, PEF treatment at 1–5 kV/cm to extract major saffron bioactive ingredients resulted in a 14% increase in crocin, 15.5 in safranal and 10.2 in picrocrocin content of stigma (Garavand, et al. 2019).

4.12.7 Supercritical Fluid Extraction (SFE)

The role of supercritical CO_2 in chemical extraction has attracted more attention recently. SFE as an extraction method uses supercritical fluids as solvents for extraction. Carbon dioxide (CO_2), without any toxic and negative effects, known as a green solvent, is a common supercritical solvent for SFE. CO_2 is, in fact, the most used supercritical fluid because of the interesting properties of fluidic density, low viscosity, non-toxicity, high diffusiveness and selective extraction capacities. In the instance of safranal, SFE using carbon dioxide (SFE-CO_2) does better with components having less polarity. Aqueous or organic solvents like ethanol are used as entrainers to broaden the use of this procedure towards polar component extraction and to separate polar constituents (crocin, crocetin etc.) from saffron. Significant variables for saffron extraction with supercritical CO_2 within the extraction vessel are temperature and pressure. To optimise extraction conditions of saffron bioactives, operational parameters such as carbon dioxide volume velocity, temperature, extraction time and gas pressure are used (Garavand, et al. 2019; Jafari, et al., 2020; Suali, 2020).

Nerome et al. (2016) combined CO_2-mediated SFE with methanol and aqueous solutions to use these as entrainers as opposed to the conventional extraction methods which used methanol and water solutions to extract the phytochemicals present in saffron. HPLC studies revealed increased production of several saffron bioactives especially safranal, picrocrocin and certain derivatives of crocin when SFE was used in comparison to methods using traditional solvent extraction. It was found that crocin derivatives and picrocrocin produced their highest yields at 30 MPa and 80°C, while safranal and HTCC produced their highest yields at 40 MPa and 80°C. The best entrainer for recovering crocin derivatives was aqueous solvent, while methanol entrainer maximised extraction yield and was more effective in extracting HTCC, safranal, and picrocrocin (Garavand, et al. 2019).

Apart from the above extraction techniques, other new extraction techniques for the bioactive extraction of saffron are solid-phase microextraction, stir-bar sorptive extraction and dispersive liquid–liquid microextraction which have the advantages of ease of running and development, simplicity and low cost (Jafari, et al. 2020).

4.13 CHARACTERISATION OF SAFFRON AND ITS BIOACTIVE COMPOUNDS

4.13.1 UV-Vis Spectrophotometry

UV-Vis spectrophotometry has been almost solely employed to identify and assess the concentration of crocins, picrocrocin, and safranal in the samples of saffron till now. This technique is a part of ISO 3632-2 (2010) standard, which is concerned with determining the main saffron constituent (Rajabi, et al. 2019). An aqueous saffron extract is prepared, a spectrum in the range of 200–700 nm is observed. Thereafter, absorbance values at specific wavelengths of 440, 250 and 330 nm are used to quantify the concentration of crocins, picrocrocin and safranal in a saffron sample (Jafari et al., 2020) as measurements of colour, flavour and scent strength, respectively.

$$E^{1\%}_{\lambda max} = \frac{D \times 10,000}{m(100-H)}$$

where D represents the absorbance value at 440 nm (the colouring strength), 330 nm (the aroma strength) and 250 nm (the flavour strength); m represents the mass of the test portion (g); and H represents the moisture and volatile content of the sample (%, w/w).

Zalacain, et al. (2005) used derivative UV-Vis spectrophotometry to detect various artificial colourants in saffron including quinoline yellow, naphthol yellow, tartrazine, allura red, azorubine, amaranth, red 2G and ponceau 4R. In another study, Ordoudi, et al. (2017) discovered that adding 2% w/w carminic acid, a naturally occurring colourant when added to saffron to increase colouring strength, resulted in the significant alteration of the second derivative spectrum of authentic saffron. The authors hypothesised that even modest levels of the second derivative could confirm the availability of carminic acid in saffron. Many researchers have questioned whether absorbance at 257 nm is connected to crocin glycosidic linkages and not to picrocrocin and whether absorbance at 330 nm is connected to cis-crocins and not safranal. Furthermore, because crocins, picrocrocin and safranal have different polarities, only the first two should be included in an aqueous saffron extract made in accordance to ISO 3632-2. Nonpolar safranal, on the other hand, is unlikely to be fully extracted by the use of water. Despite this, researchers continue using the ISO 3632-2 extraction protocol, which is followed by UV-Vis analysis to determine crocins, picrocrocin and safranal. Maggi et al. (2011), for example, used UAE to prepare saffron extracts using chloroform or diethyl ether as extraction solvents. The researchers found a good correlation between the amount of safranal measured by UV-Vis spectrometry at 330 nm and the amount measured by GC-MS (Jafari, et al. 2020).

4.13.2 High-Performance Liquid Chromatography (HPLC)

It is a new method for determining crocetin and thus total crocins in saffron raw material; thus, this approach has the potential to be used as a saffron quality check. This is the first saffron analysis protocol to include the ability to determine total crocin content and is based on the alkaline hydrolysis of crocins to yield crocetin, which is then quantified using an HPLC method. The segregation of apocarotenoids from saffron takes place on reversed-phase C18 chromatographic columns having lengths between 100 and 250 mm, internal diameters ranging between 2.1 and 4.9 mm, with particle sizes ranging from 4 to 10 m. Despite reports of temperatures as high as 30°C, majority of the research is done at room temperature. Saffron apocarotenoids are almost exclusively separated using gradient elution. Polar organic solvents such as methanol or acetonitrile are commonly used in the mobile phase. It has also been proposed that acids including acetic and phosphoric/formic acids (0.25–1%) can be used as pH regulators to enhance peak resolution as their use limits the ionisation of substances while analysis is being done. Whether or not connected to a mass detector, UV-Vis and DADs are often employed to detect crocins, picrocrocin and safranal (Jafari, et al. 2020). A total of 42 samples of saffron with different drying conditions, origins and ages were taken to separate the two isomers of crocins (trans- and cis-isomers) by Rocchi, et al. (2018) who used a UHPLC-MS/MS system with a reversed-phase Kinetex C18 column. Moras, et al. (2018) put forth the UHPLC-DAD/MS process in order to analyse saffron quality and detect adulteration using *Gardenia jasminoides Ellis*. Thirty-five compounds were found, including picrocrocin, kaempferol derivatives and trans- and cis-crocins. The use of UHPLC methodology instead of an HPLC technique should be examined in the future revision of the ISO 3632-2 for the analysis of saffron apocarotenoids. Since there is no commercial standard available in the market and the ones available come with a high cost, the quantification of saffron apocarotenoids is really difficult. Column chromatography and a C18 adsorbent were used by Saenchez, et al. (2009) to isolate picrocrocin of which the purity was found to be 96% by calculating it as a percentage of the total peak area at 250 nm. Cossignani, et al. (2014) reported the isolation of picrocrocin using thin-layer chromatography. The development of HPLC-DAD technique in order to quantify the trans-4-GG and trans-3-Gg crocetin esters, including their cis-isomers and trans-2-gg crocetin ester, was reported by Koulakiotis, et al. (2015). These constituents were isolated and identified and had a purity of 98%. Commercially available standards are typically used to quantify safranal using HPLC (Jafari, et al. 2020).

4.13.3 Gas Chromatography-Mass Spectrometry (GC-MS)

Given the volatile nature of safranal, other methods such as GC combined with MS were used to determine its content over the years. In order to study safranal and its volatiles, capillary chromatographic columns ranging between 30 and 60 m in lengths and internal diameters ranging between 0.22 to 0.32 mm, with particle sizes ranging between 0.25 and 0.5 m are utilised. In order to analyse safranal and rest of the saffron volatiles, capillary chromatographic columns with lengths ranging from 30 to 60 m, internal diameters ranging from 0.22 to 0.32 mm and particle sizes ranging from 0.25 to 0.5 m are used. In the case of safranal, as with HPLC, quantification is usually done by using the relevant calibration curves of high purity standards which are available commercially (Jafari, et al. 2020).

4.13.4 Electronic Nose Technique

This technique doesn't need a particular sample preparation, is fast and powerful and is used to determine a product's overall volatile profile. E-noses, in particular, are devices that are made up of a variety of sensors that can simulate the olfactory nerves. The sensors are subjected to a range of chemical compounds, which are odour-responsive. These odour-responsive compounds leave a distinct smell print on the sensors. It has already been claimed that e-nose can be used to assess the quality or authenticity of a variety of products, including coffee, milk, olive oil, honey and tea, although the use of this technique has its own limitations when used for saffron. In order to detect adulteration in saffron, Heidarbeigi, et al. (2015) used the e-nose metal oxide semiconductor (MOS) gas sensors connected to the principal component analysis (PCA). The writers looked at the volatile fingerprints of not only pure whole saffron and yellow stamens but safflower as well. At levels of adulteration greater than 10%, this e-nose system was able to distinguish between pure and adulterated saffron samples. The discrimination of saffron samples from different regions of Iran was done by Kiani, et al. (2016) by using a portable e-nose having 10 MOS gas sensors connected to a multilayer perceptron artificial neural network. According to the authors, this system is low-cost, non-destructive and has been found to achieve 100% success rate. Safranal content can be determined without prior extraction by non-destructive method using the e-nose technique.

4.14 SAFETY, TOXICITY AND FUTURE SCOPE

Saffron and its main bioactive components have been used as a spice and medicinal herb for centuries. It contains a variety of constituents that have both health-promoting and toxic effects. According to the latest reports of studies on human toxicity, the human body can tolerate a maximum dose of 1.5 g/d of saffron when taken orally. However, oral use of saffron in a quantity of 5 g/kg body weight was found to be toxic and a dose of 20 g/kg body weight was found to a have lethal effect on the human body. There were no significant clinical changes associated with biochemical, haematological and hormonal or urinary parameters in short-term human safety trials (7–30 days), when saffron and crocin intakes of (30–400 mg/day) and (20 mg/day) were administered, respectively. Induction of abortion has been seen if doses above 10 g have been used per day. At this dose, some side effects that have been reported include vomiting, uterine bleeding, haematuria, gastrointestinal mucosa bleeding, vertigo and dizziness. Saffron and crocin (15 mg twice daily) did not show any toxic effects on thyroid, liver, kidneys or haematologic systems. Furthermore, in term pregnancies having a gestational age between 39 and 41 weeks, the consumption of three saffron pills of 250 mg each, within 24 hours increased the cervix readiness without any negative effects. Another clinical study that involved persons with anxiety and depression showed that a 50 mg saffron capsule taken two times daily for 12 weeks manifested a substantial improvement in the condition of these patients. The researchers also investigated the long-term effects of crocetin usage in adult volunteers without any underlying health conditions and found that taking a 7.5 mg per capsule for 3 months or 37.5 mg per day for 4 weeks had no side effects and was equally effective. Another clinical study proved the safety and efficacy of saffron (30 mg/day, BID) for 10 weeks in the treatment of mild to moderate obsessive-compulsive disorder. One saffron tablet (100 mg) was given to healthy men every day for 6 weeks in order to study its impact on the human immune system. After 3 weeks, saffron increased IgG levels while decreasing IgM levels, basophil percentage and platelet count, but increased monocyte percentage and no adverse reports were reported. In short, in clinical practice, the common effective doses of saffron (30–50 mg/day) were considerably less than those of toxicity (>5 g/day) (Mehri, et al. 2020). It has also been found that less than 400 mg/day of saffron is likely safe for human consumption. As such, pure saffron extracts, or as a part of bioactive mixtures, is commercially available in the market in a dozen odd forms. These commercially available extracts supply saffron constituents in between 30 and 88 mg/capsule, to a daily dose of up to 180 mg, where dosing is recommended as such. Affron, which is a proprietary product, is being used in some studies, is available in the market and sold as a high-pressure liquid chromatography standardised extract, representing 0.3% of a crocin, picrocrocin and safranal mixture with a daily recommended dosage of 28 mg. Similarly, a stigma extract containing 88 mg/capsule, Satiereal is another product used in the trial, which is standardised to 0.3% safranal. Another one, SaffroMood of which 2 capsules have been recommended on a daily basis has 15 mg extract/capsule present in it (Singletary, 2020). To improve the characterisation of safety, it should be examined to determine the dose-related safety of gender, age and health status of the consumers by considering longer oral intake of saffron. Existing scientific data indicate that *C. sativus* extract and its bioactive components are a potent medicinal plant for neurodegenerative disorders, cardioprotective disorders, diabetes, immune-related disorders, inflammation, cancer/tumour and other related complications based on in vivo and in vitro models as well as clinical trials. In order to authenticate its toxicological profiles, more studies should also be done to determine the bio-accessibility and bioavailability of various components of *C. sativus*. This plant and its essential compounds could, therefore, be vital for the development of medicinal products used in disease management (Bostan, et al. 2017).

4.15 CONCLUSION

Saffron has been a part of the human diet for ages now and thereafter found its importance in traditional medicines, therapeutic use and even as an important compound of Ayurvedic medicines. Because of the wide range of elements that contribute to saffron quality, thorough quality and inspection of the input/raw material is of primal importance and requirement, particularly when it comes to the utilisation and reproduction of saffron in the laboratory for clinical use. Despite the increase in production from a few tonnes to around 450 tonnes, it is still the most sought-after spice in the world owing to its colour and taste. The discovery and the identification of the crocetins in saffron have increased its importance as these crocetins are promising in the treatment of a wide range of diseases, and in time with more scientific experiments, its medicinal and health benefits seem to be an increasing manifold with each passing day.

The list of diseases that can be treated by saffron and its bioactives is very long and usually, the ones which are extremely expensive to treat with the methods available presently. The research to explore the health and medicinal benefits of saffron and its constituents is of immense importance now than ever before to find cost-effective and efficient treatments for these diseases which are among the leading life-threatening diseases around the world.

REFERENCES

Abu-Izneid, T., Rauf, A., Khalil, A.A., Olatunde, A., Khalid, A., Alhumaydhi, F.A., Aljohani, A.S., Sahab Uddin, M., Heydari, M., Khayrullin, M. and Shariati, M.A. 2020 Nutritional and health beneficial properties of saffron (*Crocus sativus L*): A comprehensive review, *Critical Reviews in Food Science and Nutrition*, 17: 1–24.

Amin, A., Hamza, A.A., Bajbouj, K., Ashraf, S.S. and Daoud, S. 2011 Saffron: a potential candidate for a novel anticancer drug against hepatocellular carcinoma, *Hepatology*, 54: 857–867.

Arzi, L., Riazi, G., Sadeghizadeh, M., Hoshyar, R. and Jafarzadeh, N. 2018 A comparative study on anti-invasion, antimigration, and antiadhesion effects of the bioactive carotenoids of saffron on 4T1 breast cancer cells through their effects on Wnt/β-catenin pathway genes, *DNA and Cell Biology*, 37: 697–707.

Aung, H.H., Wang, C.Z., Ni, M., Fishbein, A., Mehendale, S.R., Xie, J.T., Shoyama, A.Y. and Yuan, C.S. 2007 Crocin from *Crocus sativus* possesses significant anti-proliferation effects on human colorectal cancer cells, *Experimental Oncology*, 29: 175.

Azmir, J., Zaidul, I.S.M., Rahman, M.M., Sharif, K.M., Mohamed, A., Sahena, F., Jahurul, M.H.A., Ghafoor, K., Norulaini, N.A.N. and Omar, A.K.M. 2013 Techniques for extraction of bioactive compounds from plant materials: A review, *Journal of Food Engineering*, 117: 426–436.

Bakshi, H., Sam, S., Rozati, R., Sultan, P., Islam, T., Rathore, B., Lone, Z., Sharma, M., Triphati, J. and Saxena, R.C. 2010 DNA fragmentation and cell cycle arrest: A hallmark of apoptosis induced by crocin from Kashmiri saffron in a human pancreatic cancer cell line, *Asian Pacific Journal of Cancer Prevention*, 11(3): 675–679.

Barba, F.J., Parniakov, O., Pereira, S.A., Wiktor, A., Grimi, N., Boussetta, N., Saraiva, J.A., Raso, J., Martin-Belloso, O., Witrowa-Rajchert, D. and Lebovka, N. 2015 Current applications and new opportunities for the use of pulsed electric fields in food science and industry, *Food Research International*, 77: 773–798.

Bathaie, S.Z. and Mousavi, S.Z. 2010 New applications and mechanisms of action of saffron and its important ingredients, *Critical Reviews in Food Science and Nutrition*, 50(8): 761–786.

Bhandari, P.R. 2015 *Crocus sativus L.* (Saffron) for cancer chemoprevention: A mini review, *Journal of Traditional and Complementary Medicine*, 5(2): 81–87.

Boskabady, M.H. and Farkhondeh, T. 2016 Antiinflammatory, antioxidant, and immunomodulatory effects of *Crocus sativus L.* and its main constituents, *Phytotherapy Research*, 30(7): 1072–1094.

Boskabady, M.H., Mokhtari-Zaer, A., Khazdair, M.R., Memarzia, A. and Gholamnezhad, Z. 2020 *Crocus sativus L.* (Saffron) and its components relaxant effect on smooth muscles and clinical applications of this effect, In *Saffron* 219–231. Academic Press.

Bostan, H.B., Mehri, S. and Hosseinzadeh, H. 2017 Toxicology effects of saffron and its constituents: A review, *Iranian Journal of Basic Medical Sciences*, 20(2): 110.

Bukhari, S.I., Manzoor, M. and Dhar, M.K. 2018 A comprehensive review of the pharmacological potential of *Crocus sativus* and its bioactive apocarotenoids, *Biomedicine & Pharmacotherapy*, 98: 733–745.

Charles, D.J. 2012 Saffron, In: *Antioxidant Properties of Spices, Herbs and Other Sources*, Springer, New York, NY. https://doi.org/10.1007/978-1-4614-4310-0_49

Cossignani, L., Urbani, E., Simonetti, M.S., Maurizi, A., Chiesi, C. and Blasi, F. 2014 Characterisation of secondary metabolites in saffron from central Italy (*Cascia, Umbria*), *Food Chemistry*, 143: 446–451.

D'Alessandro, A. M., Mancini, A., Lizzi, A. R., De Simone, A., Marroccella, C. E., Gravina, G. L., Tatone, C. and Festuccia, C. 2013 *Crocus sativus* stigma extract and its major constituent crocin possess significant antiproliferative properties against human prostate cancer, *Nutrition and Cancer*, 65(6): 930–942.

Dar, R.A., Shahnawaz, M., Malik, S.B., Sangale, M.K., Ade, A.B. and Qazi, P.H. 2017 Cultivation, distribution, taxonomy, chemical composition and medical importance of *Crocus sativus*, *Journal of Phytopharmacology*, 6(6): 356–358.

FAOSTAT [INTERNET]. Fao.org.2021 [cited 2 May 2021]. Available from: http://www.fao.org/faostat/en/

Ferrara, L., Naviglio, D. and Gallo, M. 2014 Extraction of bioactive compounds of saffron (*Crocus sativus L.*) by ultrasound assisted extraction (UAE) and by rapid solid-liquid dynamic extraction (RSLDE), *European Scientific Journal*, 10(3).

Ganaie, D.B. and Singh, Y. 2019 Saffron in Jammu & Kashmir, *International Journal of Research in Geography*, 5: 1–12.

Garavand, F., Rahaee, S., Vahedikia, N. and Jafari, S.M. 2019 Different techniques for extraction and micro/nanoencapsulation of saffron bioactive ingredients, *Trends in Food Science & Technology*, 89: 26–44.

Ghaffari, S. and Roshanravan, N. 2019 Saffron; An updated review on biological properties with special focus on cardiovascular effects, *Biomedicine & Pharmacotherapy*, 109: 21–27.

Giaccio, M. 2004 Crocetin from saffron: An active component of an ancient spice, *Critical Reviews in Food Science and Nutrition*, 44(3): 155–172.

Gohari, A.R., Saeidnia, S. and Mahmoodabadi, M.K. 2013 An overview on saffron, phytochemicals, and medicinal properties, *Pharmacognosy Reviews*, 7(13): 61.

Gupta, A., Naraniwal, M. and Kothari, V. 2012 Modern extraction methods for preparation of bioactive plant extracts, *International Journal of Applied and Natural Sciences*, 1(1): 8–26.

Heidarbeigi, K., Mohtasebi, S.S., Foroughirad, A., Ghasemi-Varnamkhasti, M., Rafiee, S. and Rezaei, K. 2015 Detection of adulteration in saffron samples using electronic nose, *International Journal of Food Properties*, 18(7): 1391–1401.

Heydari, S. and Haghayegh, G.H. 2014 Extraction and microextraction techniques for the determination of compounds from saffron, *Canadian Chemical Transactions*, 2: 221–247.

Hoshyar, R., Bathaie, S.Z. and Sadeghizadeh, M. 2013 Crocin triggers the apoptosis through increasing the Bax/Bcl-2 ratio and caspase activation in human gastric adenocarcinoma, AGS, cells, *DNA and Cell Biology*, 32(2): 50–57.

Imenshahidi, M., Hosseinzadeh, H. and Javadpour, Y. 2010 Hypotensive effect of aqueous saffron extract (*Crocus sativus L.*) and its constituents, safranal and crocin, in normotensive and hypertensive rats, *Phytotherapy Research*, 24(7): 990–994.

Jafari, S.M., Tsimidou, M.Z., Rajabi, H. and Kyriakoudi, A. 2020 Bioactive ingredients of saffron: Extraction, analysis, applications. In *Saffron*, pp. 261–290. Woodhead Publishing.

Jan, S., Wani, A.A., Kamili, A.N. and Kashtwari, M. 2014 Distribution, chemical composition and medicinal importance of saffron (*Crocus sativus L.*), *African Journal of Plant Science*, 8(12): 537–545.

José Bagur, M., Alonso Salinas, G.L., Jiménez-Monreal, A.M., Chaouqi, S., Llorens, S., Martínez-Tomé, M. and Alonso, G.L. 2018 Saffron: An old medicinal plant and a potential novel functional food, *Molecules*, 23(1): 30.

Karkoula, E., Angelis, A., Koulakiotis, N.S., Gikas, E., Halabalaki, M., Tsarbopoulos, A. and Skaltsounis, A.L. 2018 Rapid isolation and characterization of crocins, picrocrocin, and crocetin from saffron using centrifugal partition chromatography and LC–MS, *Journal of Separation Science*, 41(22): 4105–4114.

Khorasanchi, Z., Shafiee, M., Kermanshahi, F., Khazaei, M., Ryzhikov, M., Parizadeh, M.R., Kermanshahi, B., Ferns, G.A., Avan, A. and Hassanian, S.M. 2018 *Crocus sativus* a natural food coloring and flavoring has potent anti-tumor properties, *Phytomedicine*, 43: 21–27.

Kiani, S. and Minaei, S. 2016 Potential application of machine vision technology to saffron (*Crocus sativus L.*) quality characterization, *Food Chemistry*, 212: 392–394.

Koocheki, A., Moghaddam, P.R. and Seyyedi, S.M. 2019 Depending on mother corm size, the removal of extra lateral buds regulates sprouting mechanism and improves phosphorus acquisition efficiency in saffron (*Crocus sativus L.*), *Industrial Crops and Products*, 141: 111–779.

Koşar, M. and Başer, K.H.C., 2020. Beneficial effects of saffron (*Crocus sativus L.*) in ocular diseases, In *Saffron*, pp. 155–161. Academic Press.

Koulakiotis, N.S., Gikas, E., Iatrou, G., Lamari, F.N. and Tsarbopoulos, A. 2015 Quantitation of crocins and picrocrocin in saffron by hplc: Application to quality control and phytochemical differentiation from other crocus taxa, *Planta Medica*, 81(07): 606–612.

Lambrianidou, A., Koutsougianni, F., Papapostolou, I. and Dimas, K. 2021 Recent advances on the anticancer properties of saffron (*Crocus sativus L.*) and its major constituents, *Molecules*, 26(1): 86.

Lotfi, L., Kalbasi-Ashtari, A., Hamedi, M. and Ghorbani, F. 2015 Effects of enzymatic extraction on anthocyanins yield of saffron tepals (*Crocos sativus*) along with its color properties and structural stability, *Journal of Food and Drug Analysis*, 23(2): 210–218.

Maggi, L., Sánchez, A.M., Carmona, M., Kanakis, C.D., Anastasaki, E., Tarantilis, P.A., Polissiou, M.G. and Alonso, G.L. 2011 Rapid determination of safranal in the quality control of saffron spice (*Crocus sativus L.*), *Food Chemistry*, 127(1): 369–373.

Maggi, M.A., Bisti, S. and Picco, C. 2020 Saffron: Chemical composition and neuroprotective activity, *Molecules*, 25(23): 5618.

Magesh, V., Singh, J.P.V., Selvendiran, K., Ekambaram, G. and Sakthisekaran, D. 2006 Antitumour activity of crocetin in accordance to tumor incidence, antioxidant status, drug metabolizing enzymes and histopathological studies, *Molecular and Cellular Biochemistry*, 287(1): 127–135.

Mehri, S., Razavi, B.M. and Hosseinzadeh, H. 2020 Safety and toxicity of saffron. In *Saffron*, pp. 517–530. Woodhead Publishing.

Mir, J.I., Qadri, R.A. and Ahmed, N., 2013 *Clonal Identification and Molecular Characterization of Saffron (Crocus sativus L.) Clones (Doctoral dissertation, University of Kashmir.*

Modaghegh, M.H., Shahabian, M., Esmaeili, H.A., Rajbai, O. and Hosseinzadeh, H. 2008 Safety evaluation of saffron (*Crocus sativus*) tablets in healthy volunteers, *Phytomedicine* 15(12): 1032–1037.

Mokhtari, B. and Pourabdollah, K. 2013 Extraction of saffron ingredients and its fingerprinting by nano-emulsion membranes.

Mokhtari-Zaer, A., Saadat, S., Ghorani, V., Memarzia, A. and Boskabady, M.H. 2020 The effects of saffron (*crocus sativus*) and its constituents on immune system: experimental and clinical evidence. In *Saffron* 193–217. Academic Press.

Moras, B., Loffredo, L. and Rey, S. 2018 Quality assessment of saffron (*Crocus sativus L.*) extracts via UHPLC-DAD-MS analysis and detection of adulteration using gardenia fruit extract (*Gardenia jasminoides Ellis*), *Food Chemistry*, 257: 325–332.

Moratalla-López, N., Bagur, M.J., Lorenzo, C., Martínez-Navarro, M.E., Salinas, M.R. and Alonso, G.L. 2019 Bioactivity and bioavailability of the major metabolites of *Crocus sativus L.* Flower, *Molecules*, 24(15): 2827.

Mousavi, S.Z. and Bathaie, S.Z. 2011 Historical uses of saffron: Identifying potential new avenues for modern research, *Avicenna Journal of Phytomedicine*, 1(2): 57–66.

Muzaffar, S., Sofi, T.A. and Khan, K.Z. 2019 Chemical composition of saffron: A review. *International Journal of Biological and Medical Research*, 10(4): 6910–6919.

Pandita, D. 2021 Saffron (*Crocus sativus L.*): Phytochemistry, therapeutic significance and omics-based biology. In *Medicinal and Aromatic Plants*, 325–396. Academic Press.

Pharoah, P.D., Dunning, A.M., Ponder, B.A. and Easton, D.F. 2004 Association studies for finding cancer-susceptibility genetic variants, *Nature Reviews Cancer*, 4(11): 850–860.

Rahimi, M. 2015 Chemical and medicinal properties of saffron, *Bulletin of Environment, Pharmacology and Life Sciences*, 4: 69–81.

Rahmani, A.H., Khan, A.A. and Aldebasi, Y.H. 2017 Saffron (*Crocus sativus*) and its active ingredients: Role in the prevention and treatment of disease, *Pharmacognosy Journal*, 9(6).

Rajabi, H., Jafari, S.M., Rajabzadeh, G., Sarfarazi, M. and Sedaghati, S. 2019 Chitosan-gum Arabic complex nanocarriers for encapsulation of saffron bioactive components, *Colloids and Surfaces A: Physicochemical and Engineering Aspects*, 578: 123–644.

Razak, S.I.A., Anwar Hamzah, M.S., Yee, F.C., Kadir, M.R.A. and Nayan, N.H.M. 2017 A review on medicinal properties of saffron toward major diseases, *Journal of Herbs, Spices & Medicinal Plants*, 23(2): 98–116.

Rocchi, R., Mascini, M., Sergi, M., Compagnone, D., Mastrocola, D. and Pittia, P. 2018 Crocins pattern in saffron detected by UHPLC-MS/MS as marker of quality, process and traceability, *Food Chemistry*, 264: 241–249.

Saeedi, M. and Rashidy-Pour, A. 2021. Association between chronic stress and Alzheimer's disease: Therapeutic effects of Saffron. *Biomedicine & Pharmacotherapy*, 133: 110–995.

Samarghandian, S., Borji, A., Farahmand, S.K., Afshari, R. and Davoodi, S. 2013 *Crocus sativus L.* (saffron) stigma aqueous extract induces apoptosis in alveolar human lung cancer cells through caspase-dependent pathways activation, *BioMed Research International*, 2013.

Samarghandian, S. and Farkhondeh, T. 2020 Saffron and Neurological Disorders. In *Saffron* 103–116. Academic Press.

Sampathu, S.R., Shivashankar, S., Lewis, Y.S. and Wood, A.B. 1984 Saffron (Crocus sativus Linn.)—Cultivation, processing, chemistry and standardization, *Critical Reviews in Food Science & Nutrition*, 20(2): 123–157.

Sánchez, A.M., Carmona, M., del Campo, C.P. and Alonso, G.L. 2009 Solid-phase extraction for picrocrocin determination in the quality control of saffron spice (*Crocus sativus L.*), *Food Chemistry*, 116(3): 792–798.

Sarfarazi, M., Jafari, S.M., Rajabzadeh, G. and Galanakis, C.M. 2020 Evaluation of microwave-assisted extraction technology for separation of bioactive components of saffron (*Crocus sativus L.*), *Industrial Crops and Products*, 145: 111978.

Schmidt, M., Betti, G. and Hensel, A. 2007 Saffron in phytotherapy: Pharmacology and clinical uses, *Wiener Medizinische Wochenschrift*, 157(13): 315–319.

Shahnoushi, N., Abolhassani, L., Kavakebi, V., Reed, M. and Saghaian, S. 2020 Economic analysis of saffron production, In *Saffron*, 337–356. Woodhead Publishing.

Sharma, B., Kumar, H., Kaushik, P., Mirza, R., Awasthi, R. and Kulkarni, G.T. 2020 Therapeutic benefits of Saffron in brain diseases: New lights on possible pharmacological mechanisms, In *Saffron*, 117–130. Academic Press.

Sheng, L., Qian, Z., Zheng, S. and Xi, L. 2006 Mechanism of hypolipidemic effect of crocin in rats: crocin inhibits pancreatic lipase, *European Journal of Pharmacology*, 543(1–3): 116–122.

Shinwari, K.J. and Rao, P.S. 2018 Thermal-assisted high hydrostatic pressure extraction of nutraceuticals from saffron (*Crocus sativus*): Process optimization and cytotoxicity evaluation against cancer cells, *Innovative Food Science & Emerging Technologies*, 48: 296–303.

Shokrpour M. 2019 Saffron (*Crocus sativus L.*) breeding: Opportunities and challenges. In: Al-Khayri J., Jain S., Johnson D. (eds) *Advances in Plant Breeding Strategies: Industrial and Food Crops*. Springer, Cham. https://doi.org/10.1007/978-3-030-23265-8_17

Siddique, H.R., Fatma, H. and Khan, M.A. 2020 Medicinal properties of saffron with special reference to cancer—A review of preclinical studies, *Saffron*, 233–244.

Singletary, K. 2020 Saffron: Potential health benefits, *Nutrition Today*, 55(6): 294–303.

Sobolev, A.P., Carradori, S., Capitani, D., Vista, S., Trella, A., Marini, F. and Mannina, L. 2014 Saffron samples of different origin: An NMR study of microwave-assisted extracts, *Foods*, 3(3): 403–419.

Suali, E. 2020 Extraction of phytochemicals from saffron by supercritical carbon dioxide. In *Green Sustainable Process for Chemical and Environmental Engineering and Science*, 133–148. Elsevier.

Tseng, C.W., Hung, C.F., Alvarez, R.D., Trimble, C., Huh, W.K., Kim, D., Chuang, C.M., Lin, C.T., Tsai, Y.C., He, L. and Monie, A. 2008 Pretreatment with cisplatin enhances E7-specific CD8+ T-cell–mediated antitumor immunity induced by DNA vaccination, *Clinical Cancer Research*, 14(10): 3185–3192.

Venda, L.L., Cragg, S.J., Buchman, V.L. and Wade-Martins, R. 2010 α-Synuclein and dopamine at the crossroads of Parkinson's disease, *Trends in neurosciences*, 33(12): 559–568.

Yang, B., Jiang, Y., Shi, J., Chen, F. and Ashraf, M. 2011 Extraction and pharmacological properties of bioactive compounds from longan (*Dimocarpus longan Lour.*) fruit—A review, *Food Research International*, 44(7): 1837–1842.

Yaribeygi, H., Zare, V., Butler, A.E., Barreto, G.E. and Sahebkar, A. 2019 Antidiabetic potential of saffron and its active constituents, *Journal of Cellular Physiology*, 234(6): 8610–8617.

Zeinali, M., Zirak, M.R., Rezaee, S.A., Karimi, G. and Hosseinzadeh, H. 2019 Immunoregulatory and anti-inflammatory properties of *Crocus sativus* (Saffron) and its main active constituents: A review, *Iranian Journal of Basic Medical Sciences*, 22(4): 334.

CHAPTER 5

Ajwain Oleoresin

Characterization and Properties

Lubna Masoodi, Tahmeena Ahad, and Jassia Nisar
University of Kashmir

Shaheen Khurshid
Govt. Degree College Tral

CONTENTS

5.1 INTRODUCTION

- Kingdom: Plantae

- Division: Magnoliophyta

- Order: Apiales

- Class: Magnoliopsida

- Family: Apiaceae

- Genus: Trachyspermum

- Species: Ammi

DOI: 10.1201/9781003186205-5

Ajwain or *Trachyspermu ammi* is often known as bishop's weed, thymol seeds, ajowan caraway, or carom. It is an aromatic seed spice, coumarin-rich, highly nutritious and medicinally significant herb and is commonly grown in dry and semi-arid regions where the soil contain high amount of salts. Ajwain's small, oval-shaped, seed-like fruits are pale brown schizocarps that look like the seeds of other Apiaceae plants like cumin, fennel and parsley. Its fruit shucks appear like seeds and are grey in colour. They have a bitter, pungent flavour that is reminiscent of anise and oregano. As they contain thymol, they smell almost identical to thyme but are more aromatic and less delicate in flavour.

5.2 DISTRIBUTION AND PRODUCTION

It belongs to the Apiaceae family with a diploid chromosome number of $2n = 18$, making it a significant rabi season seed spice. Ajwain is indigenous of Egypt and is grown primarily in Egypt, Persia, Pakistan, Afghanistan, Iran and India. The main ajwain exporting countries to India are Yemen, Dubai, Malaysia, Pakistan, Saudi Arabia, Indonesia, Singapore, the United Arab Emirates. In India, Rajasthan, Gujarat, Madhya Pradesh, Uttar Pradesh, Maharashtra, West Bengal, Bihar, Telangana, and Andhra Pradesh are the main states where ajwain is grown. The production of ajwain seed during 2018–2019 was 25,000 tons. The present productivity of ajwain is 0.71 t/ha. Rajasthan is the largest producer of ajwain, with an area of 15,430 hectares and a yield of 10,540 t per year. Rajasthan accounts for 73% of India's entire ajwain production. Telangana leads the way in output in south India, with 5,720 tons in 1380 hectares. Ajwain farming has exploded in the Karnataka towns of Gulbarga, Raichur, Vijayapur, and Bagalkote in recent years.

5.3 CHEMICAL COMPOSITION/CHARACTERISTICS

The seeds and oil of ajwain are high in nutrients. Protein, minerals, fats, fibre, and carbohydrate make up 17.1%, 21.8%, 7.8%, 21.2% and 24.6%, respectively. Moreover, calcium, potassium, sodium, phosphorus, thiamine, iron, and niacin are also found in it. Ajwain seeds contain nearly 50% of thymol along with 3.83% of γ-terpinene and 3.37% cymene. It has a strong germicidal, fungicidal, and antispasmodic effect. The most important use of ajwain is the home remedy for indigestion. Its seeds and oils are largely used for its stimulant, antioxidants, preservatives, aromatic and carminative properties. Table 5.1 displays the chemical composition of Ajwain seed oil.

5.4 AJWAIN OLEORESIN

The oleoresin of ajwain represents the spice's overall flavour profile. It's made up of essential oil and a viscous fraction with flavourings. Ajwain oleoresin is a pastel green greasy liquid with a distinct scent and a strong flavour. It is good for therapeutic usage due to its high thymol concentration. It is soluble in oil but insoluble in water and inhibit development of harmful microorganisms. Hence, it is used in treatment of intestinal symbiosis and is useful in curing gastrointestinal symptoms.

Ajwain can be used in a variety of ways in food, including powder, whole spices, essential oils, and oleoresins. Spice extracts are a more modern alternative. The natural ingredients

TABLE 5.1 Chemical Composition of Ajwain Seed Oil

S. No.	Components	Concentrations (%)							
		India		Iran		Pakistan		Egypt	Turkey
		Delhi	Gorukhpur	Kehsan	Tehran	Jaipur	Peshawar	Cairo	Şanlıurfa
1	Thymol	15.56	39.1	45.9	64.51	16.77	–	42.0	24.1
2	α-Terpinene	1.32	0.2	–	–	2.62	0.36	–	–
3	4-Terpineol	0.65	0.8	0.1	–	–	–	–	–
4	γ-Terpinolene	–	0.2	–	–	55.63	–	–	–
5	cis-β-Terpineol	0.42	–	–	–	0.39	–	–	–
6	α-Thujene	–	0.2	0.4	0.17	–	–	–	–
7	α-Pinene	2.29	0.2	0.3	0.06	2.91	0.20	–	–
8	β-Pinene	8.12	1.7	1.9	0.39	8.95	1.42		
9	p-Cymene	12.30	30.8	–	16.16	13.50	–	24.00	33.1
10	o-Cymene	–	–	19.0	–	–	37.44	–	–
11	β-Myrcene	1.67	0.4	0.7	0.33	1.11	0.60	–	–
12	β-Phellendrene	0.97	0.6	0.4	–	0.91	–	–	–
13	α-Phellendrene	–	–	–	–	–	0.52	–	–
14	cis-Limonene oxide	0.7	–	–	–	–	–	–	–
15	Limonene	0.44	–	0.2	–	0.57	–	–	–
16	Sabinene	0.29	–	–	0.02	–	0.44	–	–
17	cis-β-Terpineol	0.42	–	–	–	–	0.39	–	–
18	p-Cymene-3-ol	–	–	–	–	–	–	38.0	–
18	γ-Terpinene	55.75	23.2	20.6	17.52	–	21.07	24.00	28.6

Source: Hassan, 2016.

that are used in flavour creations are often separated from essential oils. A variety of methods are used to extract oils and oleoresins, including

- Supercritical carbon dioxide extraction

- Enzymatic treatment and fermentation

- Chlorinated solvent extraction

- Steam distillation

- Hydrocarbon extraction

These extraction methods have a significant impact on the concentration of essential oil. Supercritical carbon dioxide extraction from herbs is now being done on a commercial scale. It results in solvent residue-free essential oils, fewer terpenes, and enhanced black notes. Increased yields and quality of essential oil are also a result of enzymatic treatment and fermentation of raw botanicals. Ketones, natural esters and other flavouring materials can now be made by the use of recombinant DNA and genetic engineering on the bacteria and fungi used in fermentation. Flavourists benefit from cloning and single-cell culture techniques, which can be used to cultivate flavour cells from black pepper, cardamom, or thyme instead of growing the entire plant. In vitro synthesis of secondary metabolites may lower market prices of traditionally grown spices in the future.

The oil extracted from the seeds of ajwain using the supercritical CO_2 extraction process smells like dill but has a light thyme aroma. It has long been used in Ayurvedic medicine. Steam distillation of ajwain seeds produces a dark-brown liquid with a distinct odour and a pleasant warm taste. It is primarily used in the preparation of essential oils for the treatment of various ailments and has a wide range of applications in Indian cuisine. Ajwain is a spice used in Indian curry. Ajwain essential oil has almost 26 recognized components, accounting for 96.3% of the total amount. Thymol (39.1%), p-cymene (30.8%), terpinene (23.2%), pinene (1.7%) and terpinene-4-ol (0.8%) were found to be main components. Furthermore, oil showed a broad spectrum of fungitoxic behaviour against all tested fungi like *Aspergillus flavus*, *Aspergillus niger*, *Aspergillus ochraceus*, *Aspergillus oryzae*, *Fusarium graminearum*, *Fusarium moniliforme*, *Penicillium viridicatum*, *Penicillium citrinum*, and *Penicillium madriti*.

5.5 FUNCTIONAL PROPERTIES

Phenolic, flavonoids, protein, minerals, and essential oil are all abundant in *T. ammi*. It also exhibited a variety of pharmaceutical properties, such as analgesic, anxiolytic, anticonvulsant, and anti-inflammatory properties. Its seeds are also usually used as a seasoning agent. Furthermore, the seeds have shown many beneficial effects and have been traditionally used to combat dyspepsia, gas, stomach pain, diarrhoea, and indigestion. Ajwain seed oil showed significant antiviral, antifungal, and antibacterial effects. Moreover, it showed good antioxidant, bronchodilator, and antitumor properties. It has a strong antispasmodic, fungicidal and germicidal effect. The most important use of ajwain is the home remedy for indigestion. Its seeds and oils are largely used for its stimulant, antioxidants, preservatives, aromatic, and carminative properties. The other major use of ajwain in flavouring of foods.

Like other classes in the Apiaceae family, ajwain is famous for its brown-coloured oleoresin, which is responsible for its smell and taste. Thymol is the core component of ajwain essential oil, and it can be found in concentrations ranging from 35% to 60%. Gamma-terpinene, para cymene alpha-pinene, beta pinene, -terpinene, styrene, terpinene-4-ol, beta phyllanderene, delta-3-carene, and carvacrol are all found in the non-thymol fraction (Thymene).

Some studies reported the concentration of carvone, limonene, and dillapiole was 46.2%, 38.1%, and 8.9% respectively, which were found to be important oil components. The fatty acids present in ajwain are oleic, linoleic, palmitic, petroselinic, and resinic. Some glycosyl constituents are recently reported from fruits of Ajwain, i.e. 6-hydroxycarvacrol, 2-O-β-D-glucopyranoside, 3, 5-dihydroxytoluene, and 3-O-β-D-galactopyranoside. A steroid-like chemical and a compound known as 6-O-glucopyranosyloxythymol have also been discovered in the fruits.

Hyperlipidaemia is a well-known risk factor for cardiovascular disease, particularly coronary artery disease (CAD). A definite link between cardiovascular events and excessive cholesterol levels has been demonstrated in numerous researches. According to a report by the World Health Organization, cardiovascular diseases are the leading cause of death worldwide, accounting for almost 16.7 million deaths each year. Phytochemical studies revealed that *T. ammi* contains a significant amount of polyunsaturated fatty acids as well as a good source of dietary fibres. It can act as anti-hyperlipidemic agent by sharing the mechanism of action of statins along with ameliorating the oxidative stress in vital organs.

Carom seed powder was found to lower total cholesterol, LDL (bad) cholesterol, and triglyceride levels in rabbits. Similarly, carom seed extract was found to help lower total cholesterol, triglyceride, and LDL (bad) cholesterol levels while increasing heart-protective HDL (good) cholesterol levels in rats.

Hypertension, or high blood pressure, is a common condition that raises your risk of heart disease and stroke. Medications such as calcium-channel blockers are used in traditional treatment. These blockers stop calcium from entering your heart's cells and relax and stretch blood arteries, lowering blood pressure. According to certain studies, thymol (a key component of carom seeds) may have calcium-channel-blocking properties, which could help decrease blood pressure. However, there is still a lack of evidence on the efficiency of carom seeds in decreasing blood pressure. More research is needed to determine how the seeds may affect human blood pressure.

5.6 CONCLUSIONS

Ajwain has been used as a traditional medicinal plant to treat indigestion, dyspepsia, and a variety of other gastric problems. It is enriched with micro and macrocompounds like antioxidants, vitamins and essential minerals. The plant is also rich in essential oils which makes it responsible for a wide range of therapeutic properties.

REFERENCES

Anonymous. Department of Agriculture and Cooperation, Hand book on Horticulture Statistics, New Delhi 2018, 135–143.

Bhatt, V., Kumar, M.M., and Selvam, P.S. 2018 Antimicrobial effect of ajwain seed ethanolic extract against food borne pathogenic bacteria, *International Food Research Journal*, 25(3): 908–912.

Chahal, K. K., Dhaiwal, K., Kumar, A., Kataria, D., and Singla, N. 2017 Chemical composition of Trachyspermum ammi L. and its biological properties: A review, *Journal of Pharmacognosy and Phytochemistry*, 6(3): 131–140.

Choudhury, S., Ahmed, R., Kanjilal, P.B., and Leclercq, P.A. 1998 Composition of the seed oil of *Trachyspermum ammi* (L.) Sprague from Northeast India, *Journal of Essential Oil Research*, 10(5): 588–90.

Gurdip, S., Sumitra, M.C., Catalan, M.P., and Lampasona 2004 Chemical constituents, antifungal and antioxidative effects of ajwain essential oil and its acetone extract, *Journal of Agriculture and Food Chemistry*, 52(11): 3292–3296.

Hassan, W., Gul, S., Rehman, S., Noreen, H., Shah, Z., Mohammadzai, I., and Zaman, B. 2016 Chemical composition, essential oil characterization and antimicrobial activity of *Carum copticum*, *Vitamin Minerals*, 5: 1–5.

Ijaz, J., Zia-ur-Rehman, Khan, M.Z., Mohammad, F., Aslam, B.M., Zahid, I., Sultan, J.I., and Ijaz, A. 2009 Antihyperlipidaemic efficacy of *Trachyspermum ammi* in albino rats, *ACTA Veterinaria Brno*, 78: 229–236.

Meena, S.S., Kakani, R.K., Singh, B., Meena, R.S., Mehta, R.S., Kant, K. et al. 2014 AA 93: An early maturing variety of ajwain developed at NRCSS for all ajwain growing areas, *International Journal of Seed and Spices*, 4(2): 91–93.

Minija, J., and Thoppil, J.E. 2002 Essential oil composition of Trachyspermum ammi (l.) sprague from South India, *Indian Journal of Pharmaceutical Sciences*, 64(3): 250–51.

Mohsenzadeh, S., Zaboli, J., Jaime, A., Silva, T. D. 2012. Allelopathic potential of ajwain (*Trachyspermum copticum*), *Medical Aromatic Plant Science Biotechnology*, 6(1): 72–74.

Muvel, R., Naruka, I.S., Chundawat, R.S., Shaktawat, R.P.S., Rathore, S.S., and Verma, K.S. 2015 Production, productivity and quality of ajwain (*Trachyspermum ammi L.*) as affected by plant geometry and fertilizer levels, *International Journal of Seed Spices*, 5(2): 32–37.

Ravindrababu, Y., Prajapati, D.B., and Patel, M. 2012 Characterization and evaluation of indigenous ajwain (*Trachyspemum ammi*) germplasms under North Gujarat condition, *International Journal of Seed Spices*, 22(1): 59–62.

Sadgrove, N.J., and Jones, G.L. 2015 A contemporary introduction to essential oils: Chemistry, bioactivity and prospects for Australian agriculture, *Agriculture*, 5(1): 48–102.

Uzma, S., Saba, R., Bashir, A., and Mohammad S. 2017 Pharmacological screening of *Trachyspermum ammi* for antihyperlipidemic activity in triton X-100 induced hyperlipidemia rat model, *Pharmacognosy Research*, 9(1): 34–40.

Zarshenas, M.M., Petramfar, P., Semani, S.M., and Moein, M. 2014 Analysis of the essential oil components from different Carum copticum L. samples from Iran, *Pharmacognosy Research*, 6: 62–66.

CHAPTER 6

Extraction Techniques, Production and Economic Importance of Asafoetida Oleoresin

Garima Bhardwaj

Sant Longowal Institute of Engineering and Technology

Ajay Sharma

Chandigarh University

Apurba Gohain

Assam University Silchar

Harvinder Singh Sohal

Chandigarh University

Tejasvi Bhatia

Lovely Professional University

Vishal Mutreja

Chandigarh University

DOI: 10.1201/9781003186205-6

CONTENTS

6.1 INTRODUCTION

Herbal medicines are a priceless gift from nature to humanity, as they facilitate the treatment of several ailments and have several uses in the realms of cosmetics, colours, drinks, food flavouring, preservatives and many others. The assurance of safety, relatively low cost and eco-friendliness of herbal medicines make them a valuable asset around the world (Singh 2015). For over 5000 years, evidence of the use of medicinal herbs has been documented in traditional literature such as ancient Indian scriptures (Rig Veda, Atharva Veda, Charaka Samhita and Sushruta Samhita), Chinese, Egyptian, Greek, Roman, and Syrian literary works, and many others. According to a survey conducted by the World Health Organization (WHO), around 80% of the world's population relies on plant-based herbal remedies to cure a variety of disorders (Srivastava, et al. 1996). Additionally, the WHO acknowledged the presence of herbal plant-based approaches hundreds of years prior to the emergence of contemporary medicines. According to the WHO's fundamental concerns, three important features of any herbal medication are authenticity, identity and nontoxicity. According to those recommendations, traditional medicines that lack a botanical identity are considered controversial drugs. Plant-based biologically active drugs have the potential to be an effective source of treatment in the recent era, owing to their fewer side effects and superior integration with biological processes in several conditions (Gurav and Gurav 2014).

Plants have long been a source of medicines, and finding new therapeutic agents from medicinal plants has recently received a lot of attention. Most people nowadays tend to use herbal medicines rather than chemical medications. The usage of herbal plants to cure diseases goes all the way back to the beginning of time and has been prevalent ever since. About 25%–30% of all current drugs are estimated to be derived directly or indirectly from natural sources. Although medicinal plants are present throughout the world, they are more prevalent in tropical areas due to the favourable environmental conditions (Cragg and Newman 2013; Newman and Cragg 2014). Plants or historically utilized combinations of plants contain a diverse range of biological compounds of varying physicochemical properties and, as a consequence, exhibit a variety of biological modes of action. As a result, plants or traditionally used plant combinations hold tremendous expectations for the development of new drugs to fight the myriad diseases that mankind faces. Medicinal plants synthesize biologically active secondary metabolites (SMs) such as alkaloids, quinines, flavonoids, sterols, terpenes, anthraquinones, glycosides, tannins, saponins, resins and lactones. Injections, syrups, concoctions, decoctions, essential oils, ointments, enriched oil and creams are only a handful of the ways that important biological chemicals are processed and used in daily life. Due to their prolonged biogenic action in biological systems, the SMs s found in plants are mostly utilized in on-going clinical trials for haemorrhoids, osteoporosis, memory loss, tumours, AIDS and malaria, along with other ailments (Cragg and Newman 2013; Newman and Cragg 2014; Joshi et al. 2016).

Numerous plant genera in the eastern Himalayas are well known for their large bioactive SMs s (SMs) and therapeutic properties. The genus *Ferula* is one among them. The genus *Ferula* is the third largest genus of family Apiaceae (Yaqoob 2016), which comprises 180–185 species found in Central and Southwest Asia (India, Pakistan, China, Turkey, Iran and Saudi Arabia) and throughout the Mediterranean basin (Pimenov and Leonov 1993). Totally 19 species of *Ferula* have been reported from the western Himalayas (*F. baluchistanica, F. collina, F. costata, F. foetid, F. heuffelii, F. hindukushensis, F. jaeschkeana Vatke* (Figure 6.1), *F. karelini, F. kokanica, F. lehmanni, F. lycocarpum, F. macrocolea, F. microloba Boiss, F. narthex, F. oopoda, F. ovina, F. propinqua, F. reppiae* and *F. stewartiana*) and 3 from India (*F. narthex, F. thomsonii* and *F. jaeschkeana Vatke*) (Yaqoob et al. 2016).

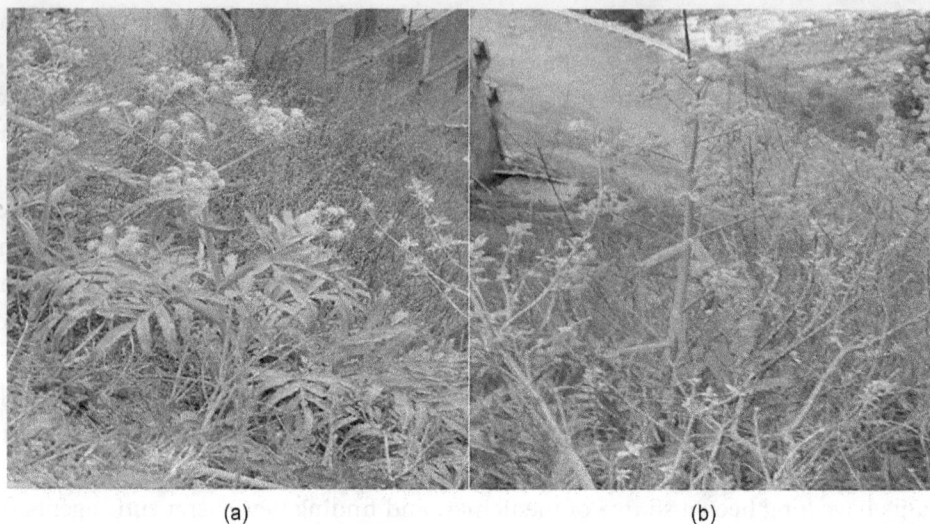

FIGURE 6.1 (a) *F. jaeschkeana* plant and (b) Inflorescence of *F. jaeschkeana* (*Ferula* species commonly found in western Himalayas of India).

6.2 THE GENUS *FERULA*

The botanical classification of the genus *Ferula* is as follow:

Kingdom: Plantae
Class: Angiosperms
Order: Apiales
Family: Apiaceae (Umbelliferae)
Genus: *Ferula*
Category: Perennial
Flower colour: Yellow
Flowering: April–June

Most of the species of *Ferula* have been used as spices. Being a rich source of aromatic gum resin (asafoetida), which possesses anthelmintic, antispasmodic, antiseptic, digestive, carminative, expectorant, analgesic, laxative, diuretic and sedative properties, it has also been used in folklore medicine (Yaqoob 2016). Sesquiterpenes and sesquiterpene coumarins are the major classes of SMs s isolated from the genus *Ferula* (Kojima et al. 2000). The plants of this genus also possess various sulphur-containing compounds and their derivatives along with other classes of SMs (phenolic acids, glycosides, steroids, tannins, etc.) (Iranshahi 2013).

Generally, the different species of genus *Ferula* are similar in morphology, which makes the genus *Ferula* monophyletic. Recent research on genus *Ferula* unveiled that besides traditional uses, the species has also exhibited innumerous pharmacological properties such as antifungal, antibacterial, antioxidant, antinociceptive, anti-inflammatory, anti-convulsant, anticancer, antispasmodic, anti-mycobacterial and hypotensive (Iranshahi 2013; Iranshahi et al. 2007; Maggi et al. 2009; Sayyah et al. 2002) (Table 6.1). Many species have also been used in various foods as flavouring agents. The species have also been used

TABLE 6.1   Biological Activity of Different Species of Genus *Ferula*

Activity	*Ferula* Species	References
Antimicrobial	*F. badrakema*	Asili et al. (2009)
–	*F. glauca*	Maggi et al. (2009)
–	*F. latisecta*	Iranshahi (2013)
–	*F. gummosa*	Ghasemi et al. (2005)
Antibacterial	*F. kuhistanica*	Tamemoto et al. (2001)
–	*F. gummosa*	Eftekhar et al. (2004)
–	*F. pseudalliacea*	Dastan et al. (2016)
Effect on sexual behaviour	*F. hermonis*	El-Thaher et al. (2001)
Antifungal	*F. latisecta*	Sahebkar and Iranshahi (2010)
Antioxidant	*F. orientalis*	Kartal et al. (2007)
–	*F. szovitsiana*	Dehghan et al. (2007)
Anticonvulsant and anti-inflammatory	*F. gummosa*	Mandegary et al. (2004)
Hypotensive effect	*F. asafoetida*	Iranshahi (2013)
Cancer chemopreventive	*F. diversivittata*	Iranshahi et al. (2007)
–	*F. vesceritensis*	Gamal-Eldeen and Hegazy (2010)
Antileishmanial	*F. szovitsiana*	Iranshahi et al. (2007)
Cytotoxic	*F. lutea*	Znati et al. (2014)
–	*F. hezarlalehzarica*	Hajimehdipoor et al. (2012)
–	*F. oopoda*	Kasaian et al. (2014)

as a condiment and can be mixed with almost all dishes. The hot-water extract of different parts of *Ferula asafoetida* has been used as an analgesic, antispasmodic, vermifuge, diuretic, aphrodisiac and anthelmintic (Elisabetsky, et al. 1992). *Ferula communis* has been used in curing many diseases both externally and orally. Externally with olive oil, it has been used in the treatment of a variety of skin diseases and to heal the cracks in the feet, and orally, it has been used as a powerful analgesic, antihelmintic, diuretic, rheumatism, vermifuge and female sterility agent. The essential oil isolated from *F. gummosa* has been known to decrease the impact of caffeine (Rashidi, et al. 2013). Therefore, it has been prescribed against the injurious effects of caffeine on foetuses. *Ferula persica* has been used for the treatment of rheumatism, diabetes and backache. In addition to this, it has also been used as anti-hysteric, laxative and carminative (Sahebkar and Iranshahi 2010). The roots and seeds of *F. persica* have been prescribed for the curing of infertility, sexual weakness and asthma (Fulder et al. 2003), and the resin has been used to improve male sexual potency (Lev and Amar 2002).

6.3 ASAFOETIDA – *FERULA* OLEORESIN

Asafoetida, a gum resin often used as a condiment, is obtained from *F. asafoetida* – a native plant of central Asia. Ferula in Latin means a vehicle or a carrier, while, asafoetida is a combination of "asa" and "foetida" which means "resin" and "smelling unpleasant," respectively. This magical herb is known by various names in different languages *like* asafoetida in Spanish; anghuzeh in Farsi; aza in Greek; asafoetida or awei in Chinese; haltit or tyib in Arabic; stinkasant or teufelsdreck in German; devil's dung, férulepersique or merdedudiable in French and hing in Hindi and Sanskrit. Different common/vernacular names of asafoetida are presented in Table 6.2 (Mahendra and Bisht 2012).

Likewise, asafoetida has been used for ages in all possible ways, especially from a tempting spice to a trusted medicine for its ability as an appetizer and a restorer of consciousness respectively (Eigner and Scholz 1999). Asafoetida is such a highly esteemed condiment that it is called "food of the Gods" in Persia (Eigner and Scholz 1999). Although it is bitter in taste, unctuous and hot in effect, it is a vital constituent of several spice mixtures and is often used to flavour pickles, curries and meatballs in many parts of the world. It stands high on the list of Indian medicines and cookery; however, it is not native to India.

TABLE 6.2   Common/Vernacular Name of Asafoetida

Name of Country	Common/Vernacular Name
India	Hing, Kayam, Perungayam, HinguInguva, Raamathan, Hengu, Perunkaya, Ingu
Bangladesh	Hing
Pakistan	Anjadana, Kama I anguza
United States, France, England, Germany, Russia, Croatia, Finland, Poland, Spain, Netherlands, Guyana, Estonia, Sweden, Iceland and Lithuania	Asafoetida
France	AssaFoetida, Merde du diable
United States	Devil's dung
Italy	Assafetida
China	A-wei
Greece	Aza
Denmark, Netherlands, Norway, Sweden, Latvia	Dyvelsdrak
Iceland	Djoflatao
Netherlands	Godenvoedsel
Afghanistan	Kama I anguza
Hungary	Ordoggyoker
Finland	Pirunpaska, Pirunpihka
Netherlands	Sagapeen
Germany	Stinkasant
Mozambique	Mvuje
Myanmar	Sheingho
United States	Stinking gum
Latvia	Velna suds
Poland	Zapaliczkacuchnaca
Turkey	Setanbokosu, Seytantersi
Germany	Teufelsdreck
Iran	Rechinafena, Zaz
France	Ferule persique
Finland	Hajupihka
Laos	Ma ha hing
Sri Lanka	Perunkayan
Tibet	Shing-kun
Iran	Zaz

It is chiefly grown in Afghanistan and Iran to export to the rest of the world (Eigner and Scholz 1999).

6.3.1 Distribution of Oleoresin

Apiaceae (Umbelliferae) family has 455 genera and about 3600–3750 species. This family is further sub-divided into three sub-families, in which Hydrocotyloideae sub-family (320 species) is distributed in the southern hemisphere, while Saniculoideae and Apioideae are distributed in the northern hemisphere having 250 and 1950 species, respectively. Apiaceae family is widely distributed in countries like China (677 species in 108 genera), Turkey (450 species in 109 genera), Iran (350 species in 111 genera), Georgia (185 species in 77 genera), Syria (173 species in 68 genera), Azerbaijan (169 species in 73 genera), Iraq (148 species in 62 genera), Armenia (138 species in 70 genera), Lebanon (120 species in 56 genera), Israel (90 species in 44 genera), Jordan (79 species in 46 genera), Cyprus (73 species in 37 genera) and India (43 genera and 180 species) (Yaqoob 2016).

The genus *Ferula* mostly grows in mountains or in arid climate regions. It is chiefly grown in Afghanistan and Iran, and some species are reported in Pakistan, India and western Himalayas. In India, it is grown in Kashmir and a few regions of Punjab. The two main variants of asafoetida are Hing Lal (red asafoetida) and Hing Kabuli Sufaid (milky white asafoetida). Because of sulphur compounds in the asafoetida, it has a strong pungent smell and is acrid and bitter in taste. The white or pale variant is soluble in water, while the dark or black variant is soluble in oil. Due to its strong flavour, instead of selling it pure, it is generally mixed with starch and gum to sell it in bricket form. It can be bought in tablet or free-flowing form also (Yaqoob 2016; Sood 2020).

6.3.2 Economic Importance of Asafoetida

India is the largest consumer of asafoetida in the world with a total consumption of 40% of the world's total production. The elementary raw material is mainly imported from Afghanistan and Iran, which is finally processed into tablet and powder form for the national and export markets. It is estimated that in 2015–16, India imported about 1199 MT of asafoetida that cost Rs. 527.42 crores. Out of this, around 885 MT that cost around Rs. 46.27 crores was exported after processing (Sood 2020). The demand for superior-quality asafoetida is very high both in the national as well as in international markets. The United Kingdom, Switzerland, Belgium, Yemen, Kenya, Oman, the United Arab Emirates and Malaysia are the foremost importing countries of asafoetida. The value of superior-quality asafoetida in the national market may vary between Rs. 10,000 and 15,000/Kg, and it may fetch up to $469–$536 (Rs. 35,000–40,000/Kg) in the international market (Sood 2020).

As asafoetida is not cultivated in India, the government data states that during the financial years 2007–2016, imports hiked by 84.26%, worth from $16.52 million to $80.16 million. This is about 1,200 tonnes and about $89 million in the financial year 2017. This import is chiefly from Afghanistan, Iran and Uzbekistan. Here alone, Afghanistan's share is 92% (Marar 2020; Kumar 2017). It is exported to other parts of the world for its diversified utilities in the different regions; it is mainly used in food as a condiment, as a spice to aid digestion and in pickles (Saleem et al. 2001). Apart from these, it has many traditional uses (Table 6.3) as well as pharmacological uses also.

6.3.3 Traditional Uses of Asafoetida

Traditionally, asafoetida is used to treat a variety of ailments such as asthma, intestinal parasites, gastrointestinal disorders, intestinal parasites, dyspepsia, earache, wound healing, epilepsy, microbial infections and nervous disorders (Farhadi et al. 2019). In Afghanistan, it is believed that the hot-water extract of dried oleoresin gum administrated orally can treat ulcers, hysteria and whooping cough (Iranshahy and Iranshahi 2011). While Brazilians like to take the hot-water extract of the dried stem and leaves orally as an aphrodisiac for males (Iranshahy and Iranshahi 2011; Bayrami et al. 2013), Chinese take the decoction of the plant orally as a vermifuge (Iranshahy and Iranshahi 2011; Bayrami et al. 2013). In Egypt, it is considered contraceptive, when its dried gum is applied to vagina (Shweta et al. 2021). While oral administration of hot-water extract of the dried root can act as an antispasmodic and an analgesic. In Fiji; whooping cough is treated by applying a paste to the chest made from dry resin. Fried *Ferula* with sugar and *Allium sativum* is taken to cleanse the new mother, while with hot-water extract, it treats upset stomach (Bayrami et al. 2013). Malaysian females chew the gum for amenorrhea (Mahendra and Bisht 2012). In Saudi Arabia, dried gum is used to treat asthma, bronchitis and whooping cough. In the United States also, fluid extract of the resin is used as is taken orally as an aphrodisiac, a stimulating expectorant, an anthelmintic, a powerful antispasmodic and a stimulant to the brain and nerves when administrated orally (Mahendra and Bisht 2012). In India, dried gum hot-water extract is consumed orally as an antispasmodic, expectorant and carminative in chronic bronchitis. Extract of dried *F. asafoetida* combined with rock salt and *Brassica alba* is administrated orally after diluted with vinegar as an abortifacient. It is used to treat cholera in combination with sweet flag and cayenne pepper. It is used for the prevention of guinea worm disease, exudate of the dried gum resin is eaten as such. A paste of gum resin with bark juice of *Moringa pterygosperma* and salt is applied externally to get relief from stomach aches. It is a good remedy for gallstones and kidney stones, when 200–300 mg of *Ferula* is mixed with dry *Lampyris noctiluca* (without head) is taken in the mornings and evenings (Zimmerman and Yarnell 2018). Hyperglycemia and diabetes can be regulated by ethanolic *Ferula* extract. It is found to be effective in relieving menstrual cramps and increases anti-apoptotic factor Bcl-2 expression that produces a rejuvenating effect (Asma et al. 2017). The various traditional uses of asafoetida are presented in Table 6.3.

6.3.4 Pharmacological *Ferula* Oleoresin

Other than the traditional utilities *Ferula asafoetida*, clinical trials have shown great potencies of pharmacological activities.

6.3.4.1 Allergenic Activity

Oleoresin powder applied externally was found active against dermatitis on fingertip (Christensen and Brandt 2006).

TABLE 6.3   Traditional Uses of Asafoetida

Region/Country	Traditional Uses	Reference
Afghanistan	It is believed that the hot-water extract of dried oleoresin gum administrated orally can treat ulcers, hysteria and whooping cough	Iranshahy and Iranshahi (2011)
Brazil	Hot-water extract from the dried leaf and stem is consumed as an aphrodisiac by males orally. The extract is administered as a nerve and general tonic orally. Oleoresin powder is used as a condiment and crushed with a fingertip.	Elisabetsky et al. (1992); Seetharam (2021)
China	Decoction of the plant is taken orally as a vermifuge.	James and Edward (2021)
Egypt	Dried gum is used vaginally before or after coitus as a contraceptive. This strategy was used by 52% of the women interviewed and 48% of them relied on indigenous practices and/or extended breastfeeding. The warm water extract from the dried root is administered orally as diuretic, vermifuge and analgesic.	Buddrus et al. (1985)
Fiji	The paste formed of dried resin is used for whipping cough on the chest. Fried *Ferula* is used to clean the new mother with *Allium sativum* and sugar. Orally, fried *Ferula*, *Cinnamomum camphora* and *Piper nigrum* are used to treat headaches and toothaches. Oral administration of the dried resin hot-water extract is used to treat digestive problems.	Singh (1986)
India	Dried *F. asafoetida* extract along with rock salt and *Brassica alba* is given orally as an abortifacient. In chronic bronchitis, the dried gum hot-water extract is given orally as an expectorant, carminative and antispasmodic. It is used in combination with cayenne pepper and sweet flag as a cholera remedy. The dried gum resin exudate is consumed to prevent guinea worm illness. Externally, gum resin combined with salt and *Moringa pterygosperma* bark juice is used to treat stomach aches. For gallstones and kidney stones, a dry *Lampyris noctiluca* without the head is combined with 200–300 mg of *Ferula* and eaten in the mornings and nights. Potassium nitrate is added to the mixture to dissolve older stones. As an emmenagogue, a hot-water extract of the dried resin is administered orally.	Venkataraghavan and Sundareesan (1981); Joshi (1991); John (1984); Tiwari et al. (1979); Kamboj (2021)
Malaysia	Females chew gum to treat amenorrhea.	Gimlette (1939)
Morocco	Oleoresin gum is chewed as an antiepileptic.	Bellakhdar et al. (1991)
Nepal	As an anthelmintic, the resin water extract is given orally.	Bhattarai (1992)
Saudi Arabia	Whooping cough, asthma and bronchitis can all be treated with dried gum.	Mahendra and Bisht (2012)
United States	The resin fluid extract is taken orally as an emmenagogue, anthelmintic, stimulating expectorant, aphrodisiac and stimulant to the nerves and brain. It is also used as a powerful antispasmodic.	Mahendra and Bisht (2012)

6.3.4.2 Antibacterial Activity
Dried gum resin was found potent against *Clostridium perfringens* and *Clostridium sporogenes* (Bhatnager et al. 2021).

6.3.4.3 Anticarcinogenic Activity
Oral administration of dried resin at doses of 1.25% and 2.5% w/w of the diet to Sprague–Dawley rats not only resulted in a significant reduction of tumour growth but also increased the percentage of life span by 52.9% (Amalraj and Gopi 2017).

6.3.4.4 Anti-Coagulant Activity
Oral administration of hot-water extract of the gum was found active in dogs and rats (Fatehi et al. 2004).

6.3.4.5 Antifungal Activity
Dried gum ethanol extract exhibited significant results at various concentrations against many fungal agents like *Microsporum gypseum*, *Trichophyton rubrum*, *Trichophyton equinum* and *Aspergillus parasiticus* (Amalraj and Gopi 2017).

6.3.4.6 Anti-Hypertensive Effect
Intravenously administrated with dried gum resin hot-water extract was found to be active in the dogs (Kazemi et al. 2020).

6.3.4.7 Anti-Inflammatory Effect
The dried resin ethanol extract produced significant results against irritable colon in a group of 50 patients (Vijayasteltar et al. 2017).

6.3.4.8 Apoptosis Effect
Sodium ferulate induced apoptosis on the administration to human lymphocytes cell culture (Devanesan et al. 2020).

6.3.4.9 Cytotoxic Activity
Water extract of the dried gum at 500 μg/mL concentration on CA-mammary-microalveolar cells produced a weak activity (Devanesan et al. 2020). The list of activities and clinical trials is long with significantly potent results; however, proper study and investigation can be done before the conversion into commercial drugs.

6.4 EXTRACTION TECHNIQUES

6.4.1 Collection and Harvesting
In 5 years span, the crop grows up to 2 m tall trees. The resin gum material is mainly secluded from the rhizomes and roots of the plants. The elder plants are extra productive than the younger ones. The best time to start the harvesting of oleoresin gum from the rhizome, roots and succulent stem is just earlier than flowering. The time of March and April months is the suitable time for harvesting (Golmohammadi 2016). The cut is

given vertically on the stem close to the roots of a tree. The roots having a diameter near 6–10 cm are mainly recommended for the isolation of asafoetida. A white milky liquid is discharged from the bare surface. This white milky liquid gets hardened when comes in contact with air. This process is repeated at the interval of 4–5 days on the stems of plant, till resin gum stops discharging (Eigner and Scholz, 1999; Shah and Zare 2014; Ali 2019).

The effects of various cutting approaches (crown cutting, conventional method, surface and concave cutting) and the number of cuts (13, 10 and 5 times) on the amount of asafoetida produced in its usual habitation in Iran was evaluated by Barat and Faravani (2014). The amount of gum produced was determined by the counts of cuts. The study revealed that the highest yield and the best tree rejuvenation were attained via the concave technique with 10 cuts. The study also revealed that the traditional technique of cutting abolishes the buds and causes the death of the plant. It was also reported by Damanch and Sharafatmandrad (2017) that the conventional incision approaches were fatal to the plant. The study revealed that the 45° cutting technique and concave method were the finest incision practices. The pure and fresh resin gum seems to be greyish-white and gets darkened to a profound yellow or amber colour upon drying. Lumps of asafoetida resin gum are cut off to be sold commercially. The resin gum is rarely sold in its pure state. It is frequently combined with Arabic gum, rice or wheat flour, and turmeric and sold commercially as compounded asafoetida (Damanch and Sharafatmandrad 2017; Sood 2020; NIFTEM 2021). The structure of different parts of the asafoetida plant, crude asafoetida and powder form is presented in Figure 6.2.

6.4.2 Yield

Usually, a single plant produces about 40 to 900 g of fresh resin gum (Moghaddam and Farhadi 2015; Sood 2020). The price of 1 kg dried resin gum in the international bazaar is about 130–170$ USD (Golmohammadi 2016). The amount of essential oil produced may vary between 2.53% and 20.85%. This large variation in yield of essential oil may

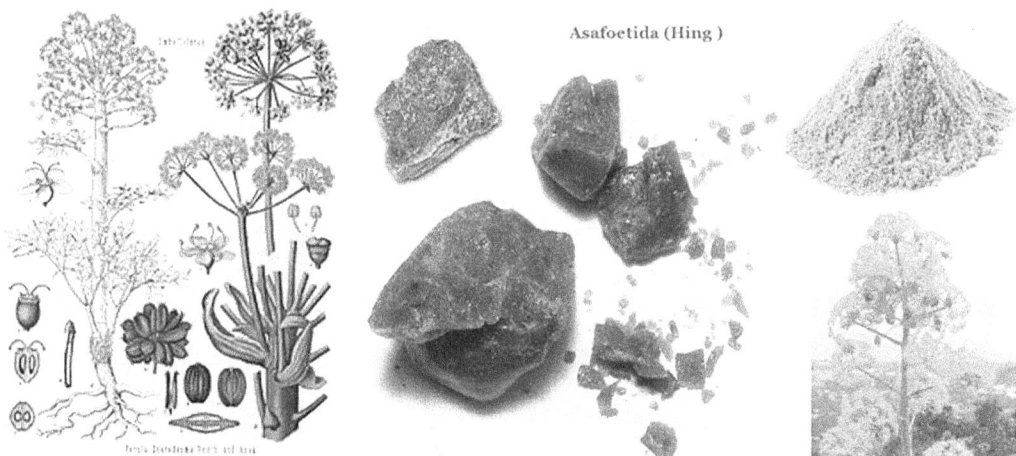

FIGURE 6.2   Different parts of *F. asafoetida* and its oleoresin (Mahendra and Bisht 2012).

be attributed to the different climatic conditions at the place of cultivation of the plant. The oil obtained from the various parts of asafoetida is also traded at premium prices (Moghaddam and Farhadi 2015; Hassanabadi et al. 2019).

6.4.3 Extraction Techniques

For the extraction of gum from the oleoresin, the crude sap is stirred with 90% ethanol for about 2 hours. The mixture obtained is filtered via Whatman No. 1 filter paper. The residue obtained is again washed with 90% ethanol (v/v) two times and then dried in vacuum for 12 hours at 40°C. After drying, the obtained powder is dissolved in distilled water at a temperature of 50°C and remained undisturbed for about 2 hours. Then, the solution is filtered using Whatman No. 1 filter paper. The filtrate obtained is concentrated in a vacuum at 40°C and further purified by dialysis at cut off 3500 Da. After filtration, the mixture is concentrated and purified by dialysis in the same way. Finally, the isolated gum is lyophilized at −40°C for 5 hours. Then, the vacuum of 10−6 Torr is employed and when it is ready, the temperature is maintained at 15°C. After 48 hours, the sample is ready (Figure 6.3) (Mohammadzadeh et al. 2007). The extraction of gum can also be done according to another method explained in Figure 6.4 (NIFTEM 2021a).

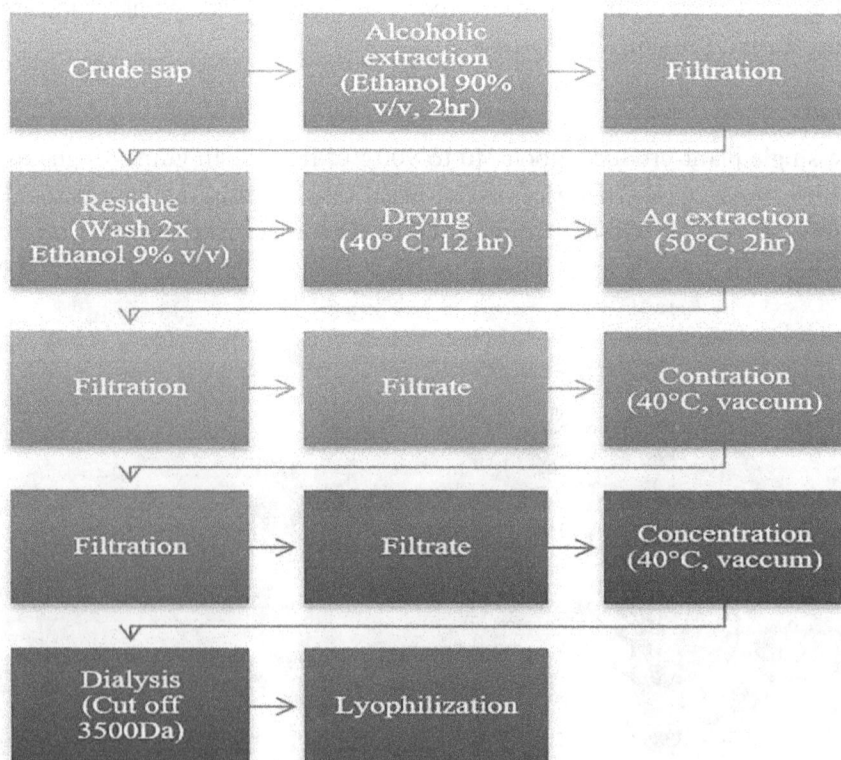

FIGURE 6.3 Schematic diagram for extraction and purification gum from oleoresin.

```
┌─────────────────────────────────────────────┐
│ Grind the yellowish-brown crude asafoetida   │
│           gum to obtain powder                │
└─────────────────────────────────────────────┘
                      ⬇
┌─────────────────────────────────────────────────────┐
│ Extraction of resins and volatile oil with ethanol (ethanol to crude gum ratio at │
│   35:1 w/w) at 75°C for 5 hrs under continuous stirring (200 rpm)                  │
└─────────────────────────────────────────────────────┘
                      ⬇
┌─────────────────────────────────────────────────────┐
│ Collect the ethanol insoluble gum after precipitation using a glass filter (100-160 │
│ μm). Then dissolve precipitate at x g/L in ultra-pure water for 30 min at 45 °C and  │
│              stir the content for 2 h at room temperature                            │
└─────────────────────────────────────────────────────┘
                      ⬇
┌─────────────────────────────────────────────────────┐
│ Then filter gum solution using cloth filter, centrifuge (at 1500 rpm for 15 min at 20 │
│   °C) and precipitate with 3 volumes of ethanol at 4 °C, overnight. Then collect      │
│ precipitate, dehydrate it in dry air, dissolve in 10-fold of water and precipitated again │
│           with 3 volumes of ethanol to increase the degree of purity                   │
└─────────────────────────────────────────────────────┘
                      ⬇
┌─────────────────────────────────────────────────────┐
│ Finally, collect the precipitate as described above, again │
│ resolved it in 5-fold of ultra-pure water and then freeze dried │
└─────────────────────────────────────────────────────┘
```

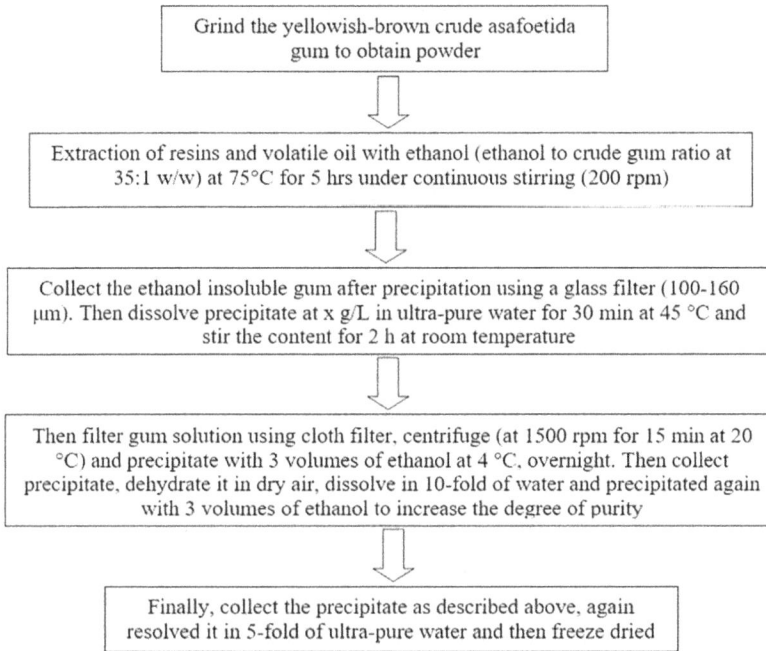

FIGURE 6.4   Extraction and purification gum from *Ferula* oleoresin.

6.4.4 Processing

The dried sap of asafoetida plant was tough to grate. Conventionally, it was crushed with stones or hammer (Ali 2019). Compounded asafoetida is the commonest form available. A fine powder of it contains about 30% asafoetida gum resin, along with Arabic gum rice or white wheat flour. It is mostly sold in compressed brick form. It is also available in powder and tablet forms (Giri et al. 2008) The processing of asafoetida to compounded asafoetida occurs in five steps viz. soaking, mixing, milling, tablet formation and packaging (Figure 6.5) (NIFTEM, 2021).

Usually, asafoetida is marketed in three forms viz. paste, tears and mass. Out of these three, mass is the commonest form in the bazaar, while lumps or tears are the purest forms of asafoetida (Table 6.4). Lumps or tears are flat or round, around 15–30 mm in diameter and have dull yellow or greyish colour, whereas the mass is agglutinated tears that are mixed with inessential matters. In contrast, the paste is semisolid and contains superfluous matter (Javaid et al. 2020).

6.5 CHARACTERIZATION

Usually, asafoetida occurs in nature as a soft rigid mass or uneven protuberances known as tears. It also occurs occasionally in semiliquid form. Tears are basically flattened or curved, 5–30 mm in diameter and have reddish-brown, dull yellow or greyish-white colour. Asafoetida mass always occurs with other impurities like fragments of root and fruits, sand and others. It is bitter and pungent in taste and has a strong garlic (alliaceous) like door. It gives a milky emulsion upon mixing and triturating with water. Pure asafoetida

Soak in Water
Soak the pasty mass of asafoetida oleoresin gum is in water

⬇

Mixing
Mixes the ingredients in the mandatory proportion using mixer grinder. Then add the slurry of soaked asafoetida and mix well to get compounded asafoetida

⬇

Milling
Covert the compounded asafoetida to the powder form using a milling machine

⬇

Tablet Form
Usually, asafoetida is in powder form but in addition, you can produce the compounded asafoetida tablet using tablet making machine

⬇

Packaging
After passing the compounded asafoetida or Hing powder is packed with the help of packaging machine. In order to maintain its moisture content and quality, polythene bags are mainly used for packaging purpose.

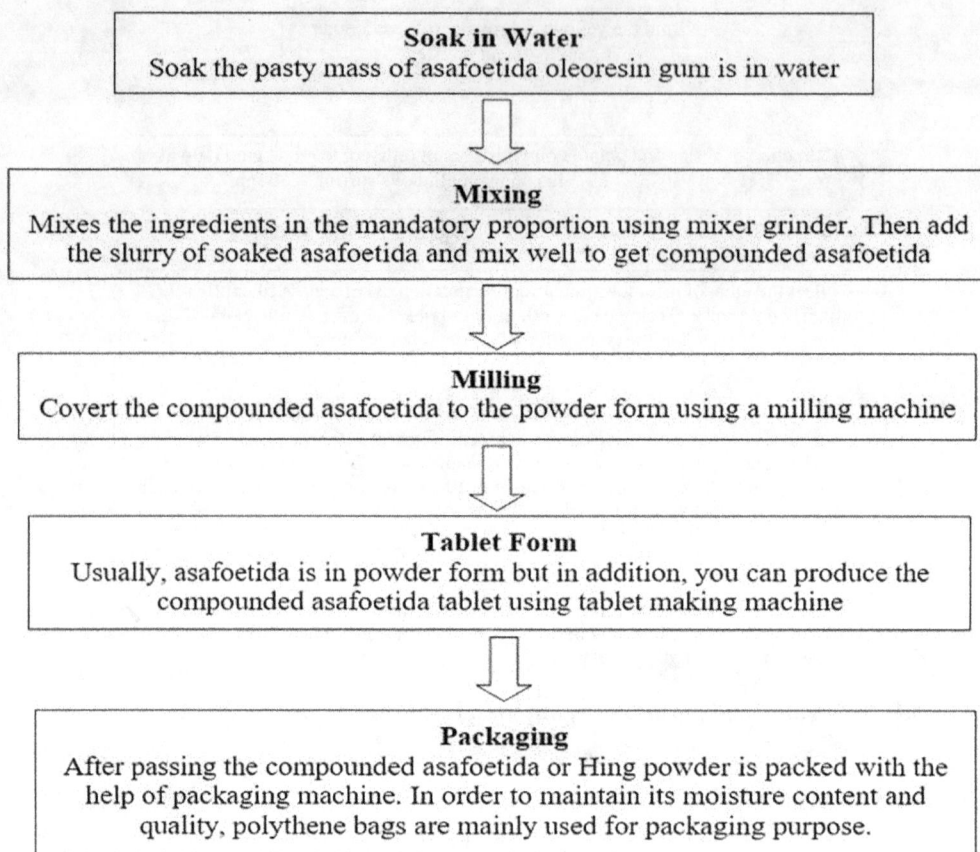

FIGURE 6.5 Compounded asafoetida manufacturing process from oleoresin gum (NIFTEM, 2021).

TABLE 6.4 Different Types of Asafoetida (NIFTEM 2021a)

Types	Characteristics
Tear asafoetida (bitter and sweet)	Secreted naturally from the plant. It is the best, rarest and the purest form of asafoetida. It is greyish or dull yellow in colour, flattened or rounded and 5–30 mm in diameter. It contained up to 15% of essential oil content.
Dried asafoetida (kokh)	Exudate is excreted after the first cut (incision) on the top of the root and is completely clean and dried.
Mass asafoetida (bitter and sweet)	It is a common and commercial form. Mainly available in two types of Paste and Shir. These are available in clean refined and unrefined forms. The percentage of sulphur-containing compounds is higher in bitter asafoetida as compared to sweet ones.
Keshteh asafoetida (bitter and sweet)	It is mainly composed of a thin layer of the upper part of the root and its secretions. It is the cheapest among all the types of asafoetida.

should have less than 15% of ash and 50% of insoluble matter in 90%. Fresh asafoetida has greyish-white colour; with age, it darkens to yellow, red and ultimately brown (Sood 2020; NIFTEM, 2021). Farhadi et al. (2019) characterized the oleoresin gum asafoetida obtained from different species of the *Ferula* genus growing in diverse parts of Iran using NMR-based metabolomic analysis. The results revealed that umbelliprenin, samarcandin, galbanic acid, farnesiferol B and farnesiferol C (Figure 6.6) were the significant metabolite that acts as markers to identify the purity of asafoetida samples and to differentiate the samples obtained from different species. Some physicochemical characteristics of asafoetida are given in Table 6.5.

Characteristics of pure asafoetida are as follows: Pure asafoetida progressively dissolves in water by forming a milky white solution without any deposit at the bottom. It burns without any scum. Further, pure asafoetida has a bitter taste, strong alliaceous and acrid odour (Gogate 2000).

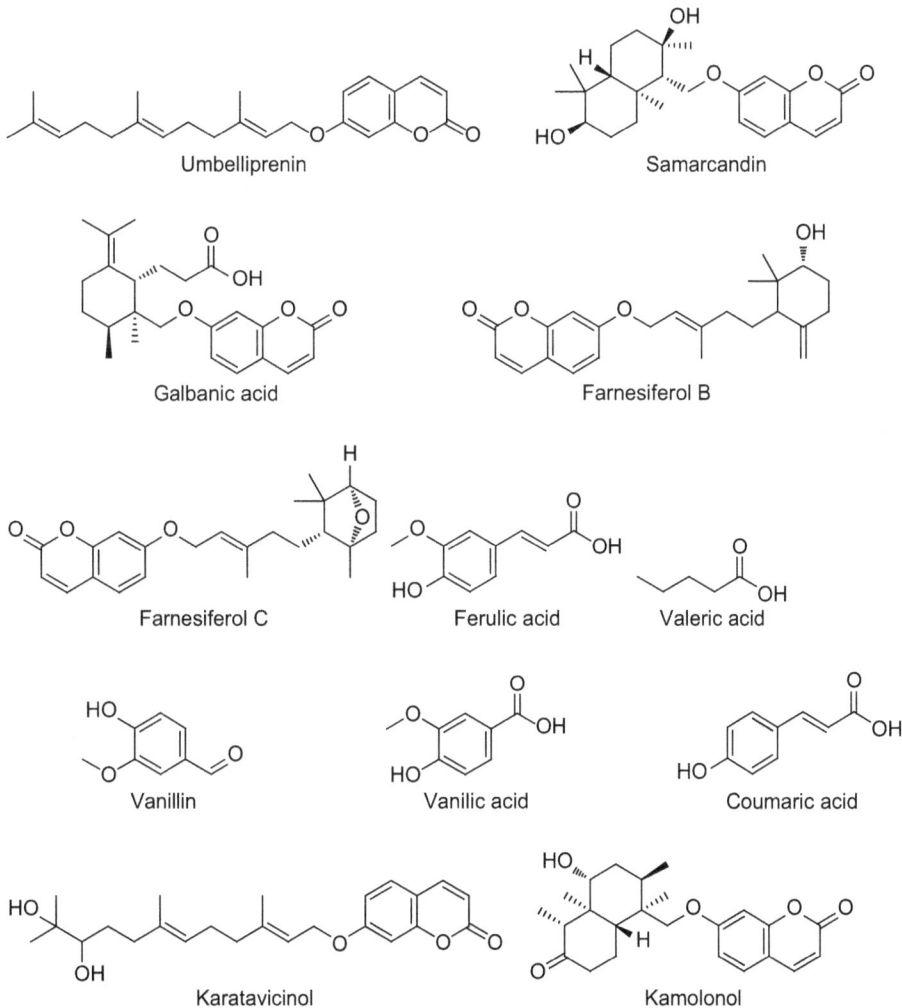

FIGURE 6.6 Structure of major non-volatile constituent of asafoetida.

TABLE 6.5   Physicochemical Characteristics of Asafoetida (NIFTEM, 2021)

Parameter	Remarks
Odour	Strong representative garlic like
Solubility	Insoluble in water, but soluble in oils and alcohol
Refractive index	1.493–1.518 @ 20°C
Optical rotation	−9°0′ to +9°18′ @ 20°C
Reactivity	Stable
Fire/explosion hazard	Flammable liquid
Flash point	65.5°C
Specific gravity	0.906–0.973 @ 20°C
Decomposition	Upon decomposition produces carbon monoxide smoke and acidic fumes
Toxicity	The liquid may irritate skin and eyes. Handling during pregnancy is not recommended

Characteristics of the impure asafoetida are as follows: Impure asafoetida easily dissolves in water or settles at the bottom. It never burns entirely on fire and completely differs in taste and smell as compared to the pure one (NIFTEM, 2021).

Adulteration and substitution: The usual adulterants used in asafoetida are sand, stones, acacia gum, gum Arabica, powdered gypsum, potato and barley or wheat flour. These adulterants are mixed in different proportions, with respect to the steadiness of the asafoetida (Ali 2019; Javaid et al. 2020).

Common chemical tests for the identification of asafoetida: Various chemical qualitative tests are conducted with the pure asafoetida or its aqueous extracts to recognize it (Nataraj and Gundakalle 2010).

1. When small amount of asafoetida is treated with sulphuric acid, it produces red colour, which on washing with water changes to violet.

2. On treatment with 50% of nitric acid, it produces the green colour.

3. On mixing with water, it forms an emulsion which is milky to yellowish-orange in colour.

4. 0.5 gm of sample is boiled with 5 mL of hydrochloric acid, then a small quantity of water is added to the mixture. Finally, the mixture is filtered and the filtrate is treated with an equivalent amount of ammonia, which resulted in a blue fluorescence owing to the presence of umbelliferone.

6.6 CHEMISTRY AND PROPERTIES OF OLEORESIN

Extravagant analysis of asafoetida revealed that per 100 gm, it mainly contains carbohydrates 67.8%, water 16.0%, minerals 7.0%, fibre 4.1%, proteins 4.0% and fat 1.1%. It has significant mineral and vitamin content that includes iron, calcium, phosphorus, as major mineral constituents, while carotene, riboflavin and niacin as vitamins. It has a substantially high calorific value of about 297, also contains ferulic acid resinous material of about 40–46%, and some highly valuable constituents *like* umbelliferone, asaresinotannols,

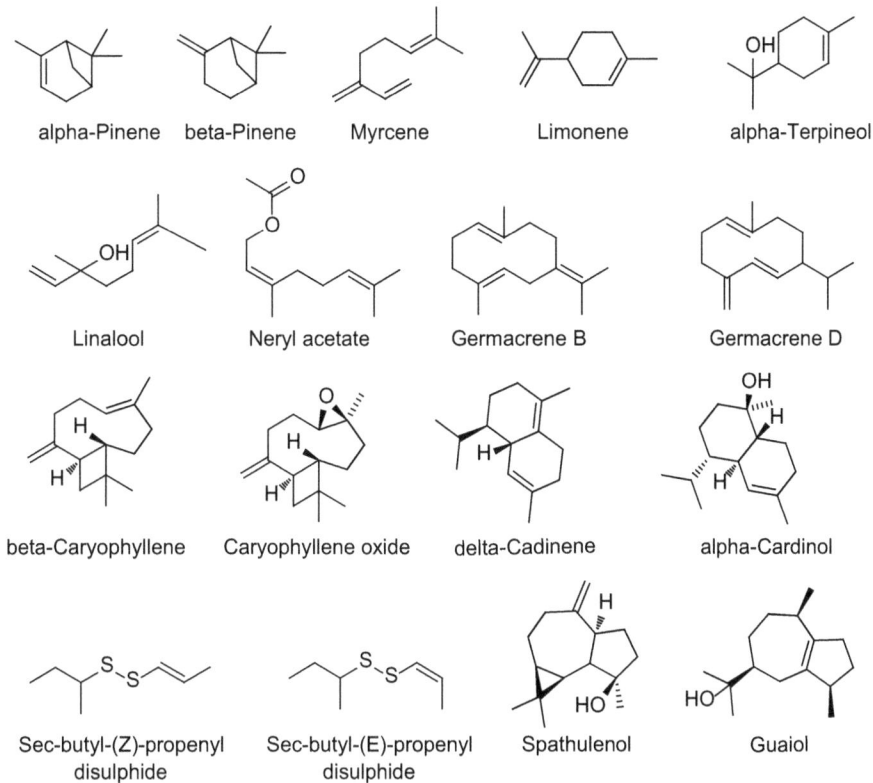

FIGURE 6.7   Chemical structure of main constituents present in the essential oil of *Ferula* species.

farnesiferols, etc. The second highest component after resin is gum (25%) that comprises rhamnose, glucose, l-arabinose, galactose and glucuronic acid. The third component is volatile oil (3–17%) that mainly containing disulphides (responsible for disagreeable odour) as its major components, notably α-pinene (2.04%–17.61%), 2-butyl propenyl disulphide (E-isomer 13.66–49.35% & Z-isomer 2.02–15.29%), β-pinene (1.06–21.18%), caryophyllene oxide, free ferulic acid, valeric acid, myrcene, α-terpineol, neryl acetate, β-caryophyllene, limonene, δ-cadinene, germacrene B, guaiol, α-cadinol, germacrene D, linalool and spathulenol and traces of vanillin (Figure 6.7) (Karimian et al. 2019; Sahebkar and Iranshahi 2010; Sood 2020).

One another study revealed that the fresh gum of *F. asafoetida* Linn. contained 10.54±0.75% moisture, 3.85±0.11% ash, 1.76±0.16% fat, 1.95±0.23% protein and 0.42±0.09% crude fibre. The total phenolic compounds and total flavonoids compounds composition of the hydroalcoholic extracts of gum is 9.67±0.45 mg GAE/g dried extract and 0.11±0.02B mg QE/g dried extract, respectively. Further, the mineral analysis (mg/ kg dried extract) of hydroalcoholic extracts of gum revealed the presence of barium (0.65±0.00), calcium (860.57±5.47), copper (3.55±0.05), iron (13.81±0.06), lithium (1.57±0.01), manganese (1.60±0.11), phosphorus (41.41±0.63), selenium (0.23±0.02), zinc (7.19±0.10) and sulphur (90.66±1.62) (Niazmand and Razavizadeh, 2020). The GC-MS analysis of hydroalcoholic extracts of gum revealed the presence of α-pinene (6.68±1.54%),

TABLE 6.6 Main Constituents of Asafoetida Responsible for Its Various Biological Properties

Name of the Pharmacological Activity	Phytochemicals
Anticancer	Luteolin, vanillin, umbelliferone, diallyl-disulphide, isopimpinellin, ferulic acid, α-pinene and α-terpineol
Antiseptic	Azulene, α-terpineol, β-pinene, diallyl-sulphide and umbelliferone
Antileukemic	Luteolin
Antioxidant	Luteolin and ferulic acid;
Antispasmodic	Luteolin, azulene, ferulic acid and umbelliferone
Antiinitrosaminic	Ferulic acid
Anti-inflammatory	α-pinene, azulene, β-pinene, isopimpinellin, ferulic acid, luteolin and umbelliferone
Antiviral	α-pinene, diallyl-disulphide, luteolin and ferulic acid
Anti-HIV	Luteolin and diallyl-disulphide
Antibacterial	Azulene, α-terpineol, α-pinene, diallyl-sulphide, diallyl-disulphide, luteolin, ferulic acid and umbelliferone
Antimutagenic	Diallyl-sulphide, umbelliferone, luteolin and ferulic acid
Hepatoprotective	Ferulic acid and luteolin
Antitumor	Diallyl-sulphide, diallyl-disulphide, luteolin and ferulic acid
Antitaggregant	Ferulic acid
Antineoplastic	Ferulic acid
Antiulcer	Azulene
Anticarcinogenic	Luteolin and ferulic acid
Sedative	α-Terpineol and α-pinene;

β-pinene (9.77±2.11%), α-phellandrene (7.23±0.97%), β-phellandrene (6.63±1.40%), (Z)-β-ocimene (20.91±3.33%), (E)-β-ocimene (17.27±2.89%), (Z)-1-propenyl sec-butyl disulphide (5.80±1.23%) and (E)-1-propenyl sec-butyl disulphide (17.62±3.21%) as key constituents (Figure 6.7), while the HPLC analysis revealed the presence of ferulic acid (3.72±1.09lµg/mg), vanilic acid (0.49±0.13 µg/mg), coumaric acid (0.29±0.07 µg/mg), umbelliprenin (1.02±0.10 µg/mg), galbanic acid (0.40±0.06 µg/mg), karatavicinol (0.37±0.08 µg/mg) and kamolonol (0.48±0.11 µg/mg) as major phenolic constituents in hydroalcoholic extracts of gum (Figure 6.6) (Niazmand and Razavizadeh, 2020). Saeidy et al. (2018) analysed the composition of metal cation (g/100 g ash) in asafoetida gum and found that calcium (66.76), magnesium (9.48), potassium (8.69), sodium (4.24), iron (1.44), aluminium (1.02), zinc (0.15) and manganese (0.12) were the main metal cations present in gum. Structures of some of the essential constituents are given in Figure 6.6. Further, Table 6.6 represents the main constituents of asafoetida responsible for its various biological properties.

6.7 APPLICATIONS (HEALTH AND MEDICINAL PROPERTIES)

6.7.1 Antidiabetic Activity

Diabetes is a growing global epidemic that is described as a recurrent, incurable disease caused by insulin deficiency that affects 10% of the population (Rabi et al. 2006). It appears to be shown that asafoetida affects the secretion of the pancreas directly through their association with the cell wall. Glut-2 transports glucose to the beta cell of the pancreatic islet Langerhans, where it is converted into adenosine triphosphate (ATP) during metabolism. The output of ATP then induces insulin secretion by changing the membrane potential, ensuring Ca++ ion flow into the cytoplasm. Calmodulin, which transports calcium in beta cells, is abundant in asafoetida (Illis 1998). Another secondary messenger for Ca++ also enhances the response of the beta cell. As this increases the tyrosine level, the enzyme activity of the tyrosine kinase is triggered, contributing to insulin secretion from the cell. This action was noted by oleo-gum resin boiling water extract at a dosage of 0.2 g/kg for 14 days in the case of Alloxan-induced diabetic rats (Abu-Zaiton 2010).

6.7.2 Antioxidant Activity

The reactive species and free radicals play a substantial part in different disease conditions. The various biochemical reactions going on in the body produce a variety of reactive species and free radicals, which are proficient in damaging various essential bio-molecules in the body. If these reactive species and free radicals are not effectually scavenged by cellular compounds, this leads to disease conditions (Halliwell et al. 1992; Bhardwaj et al. 2019; Sharma et al. 2020). Antioxidant chemicals can scavenge free radicals and cleanse the body, preventing them from doing any harm. The presence of essential oil in the plant was previously reported (Khajeh et al. 2005). The antioxidant potential of *F. asafoetida* essential oil components was investigated using *in vitro* nitric oxide (NO) and 1,1-diphenyl-2-picryl-hydrazyl (DPPH) radical scavenging test, reducing power test and iron ion chelation power assay. In all of the models investigated, the extract from the aerial portions of *F. asafoetida* had high antioxidant activity, though at varying degrees. These extracts demonstrated strong Fe++ chelation properties, as well as DPPH and nitric oxide radical scavenging abilities (Dehpour et al. 2009).

6.7.3 Anticancer Activity

In vitro growth, inhibitory assays on HEP-G2 cancer cell lines and breast cancer cell line (MCF-7) revealed that the asafoetida, ginger, cinnamon, and cardamom alcoholic and aqueous extracts, exhibited anticarcinogenic effects. Asafoetida, ginger, cinnamon and cardamom extracts were found to be effective against all these cancerous cells in both aqueous and alcoholic forms. Such aqueous extract and ethanolic extract reduced the number of HEP-G2 and MCF-7 cells in the body. Numerous researches have shown that asafoetida extracts administered orally reduce tumour growth in mice having Ehrlich ascites tumours after intraperitoneal transplantation (Upadhyay 2017). The cancer cell cytotoxicity might be owing to the massive proportion of poisonous essential oils in *F. asafoetida*, along with essential oils from diverse *Ferula* varieties (Kuete et al. 2012; Sahranavard et al. 2009). The bioactive constituents isolated from *F. asafoetida* include sesquiterpenes, coumarins, phenylpropanoids and disulphide compounds. All these were well known for their anticancer potential. Mogoltacin (a sesquiterpene coumarin isolated from *Ferula badrakema*) and stylosin (a monoterpene isolated from *Festuca ovina*) have been demonstrated to have cytotoxic activities against tumour cell lines by causing DNA damages and enhancing cell death (Mazzio and Soliman 2010). The prenylated coumarin derivative of sesquiterpene obtained from asafoetida showed antibacterial and cytotoxic activities against human cancer cells. The majority of sesquiterpene coumarins were found in the root, suggesting that they could be considered possible biological agents for the therapy of cancer (Kavoosi and Purfard 2013). Ferulic acid and farnesiferols present in *F. asafoetida* have been reported to retard the development of lung cancer in mice and angiogenesis (a vascular endothelial growth factor-accelerated process) (Kuete et al. 2012). The methanol extract was shown to be more cytotoxic than the ethanol extract in this investigation (Nazari and Iranshahi 2011). Aqueous and alcoholic extracts were also evaluated in vitro cytotoxicity assessments in several studies (Sultana et al. 2009). The findings revealed that the aqueous extracts were less cytotoxic as compared to the alcoholic extracts against cancer cells. Furthermore, because of the varied quantity of flavonoid and polyphenolic contents in aqueous extract as compared to alcoholic extract, the aqueous extract has a lower inhibitory effect against cancer cells than alcoholic extracts (Mohd et al. 2015; Vunjak and Freshney 2006).

6.7.4 Memory-Enhancing Activity

The key symptom of Alzheimer's disease in the majority of individuals worldwide is memory loss. The effect of extracts obtained from *F. asafoetida* on memory and learning in rats was tested by the researcher (Bagheri and Dashti-R 2015). After, the administration of two oral dosages (400 and 200 mg/kg) of aqueous extract isolated from *F. asafoetida* with rivastigmine as a supportive control, the researcher tested learning and memorization using the elevated plus-maze and passive avoidance paradigms. The extract significantly improved memory scores and transmission latency in an elevated plus-maze model. Additionally, they found a major increase in antioxidant potential and dose-based retardation of brain cholinesterase. *F. asafoetida's* memory-enhancing ability can be attributed to its acetylcholinesterase inhibitory and antioxidant potential. Bagheri et al. (2015) studied the impact of asafoetida on the prevention of dementia in mice, that might be triggered by $NaNO_2$ and D-galactose. The animals were grouped into four groups: dementia control (DC), normal control (NC), dementia treatment (DT) and dementia prophylactic (DP). The memory retention capabilities of the subgroups DP, NC and DT were better than those of the DC category. The occurrence of SMs comprising sulphur and sesquiterpene coumarins in asafoetida may account for its capacity to inhibit and cure amnesia (Platel and Srinivasan 1996; Upadhyay, P.K. 2017). Using the pentylenetetrazole (PTZ) kindling approach, the antioxidant and antiepileptic potential oleoresin gum extract of *F. asafoetida* was also assessed. The administration of plant extracts in treated groups resulted in a marked decrease in MDA and NO levels as well as an increase in SOD levels in comparison to the PTZ group. Because of its antioxidant characteristics, *F. asafoetida* gum extract is likely to reduce oxidative stress and lipid peroxidation. The advantages of hydroalcoholic oleoresin gum extracts of *F. asafoetida* on PTZ-induced seizures are most likely due to their antioxidant potential and lowering of oxidative stress (Platel and Srinivasan 1996; Upadhyay, 2017).

6.7.5 Antifertility Activity

Various extracts of *F. asafoetida* have been proven to have post-coital antifertility characteristics. Keshri et al. (1999) demonstrated that *F. asafoetida* resin gum methanolic extract at a concentration of 400 mg/kg daily prohibited post-coitus conception up to 80% in mature Sprague–Dawley rats from days 1 to 10. It has also been reported that when supplemented with polyvinylpyrrolidone, the above-mentioned dosage completely prevents conception across all rats (Keshri et al. 1999).

6.7.6 Hepatoprotective Effect

Dandagi et al. (2008) revealed that extracts of *Momordica charantia* Linn, *F. asafoetida* and *Nardostachys jatamansi* had hepatoprotective activity against induced model hepatotoxicity. The hepatoprotective activities of *M. charantia* Linn., *F. asafoetida* and *N. jatamansi* ethanol, benzene, petroleum ether, chloroform and aqueous extracts were tested in Wistar rats after carbon tetrachloride–induced liver toxicity. The above-mentioned extracts were made into polyhedral suspensions, and their hepatoprotective properties were assessed by measuring serum enzyme levels such as glutamate oxaloacetate transaminase, alkaline phosphatase and glutamate pyruvate transaminase. It was also reported that administering polyhedral suspension lowered the serum enzyme levels. Histopathological investigations of liver slices supplemented the biochemical findings. The experimental results demonstrate that polyhedral extract suspensions had potential action toward carbon tetrachloride–induced hepatotoxicity (Dandagi et al. 2008).

6.7.7 Anxiolytic Effect and Anthelmintic Activity

Alqasoumi (2012) investigated the anxiolytic, sedative and analgesic properties of asafoetida in rats by utilizing a hot plate, a motor activity meter and an elevated plus-maze. The typical anxiolytic agent, diazepam, was utilized. The findings indicate that asafoetida has a dose-based analgesic and anxiolytic potential along with a sedative effect at higher dosages. Asafoetida, on the other hand, appears to be a more promising treatment choice for anxiety disorders. Asafoetida at low dosages may be a viable therapeutic alternative to currently prescribed anxiolytic medications (Azizian et al. 2012; Alqasoumi 2012). Gundamaraju (2013) examined the anthelmintic activity of *F. asafoetida* aqueous extract (three different concentrations) against *Pheretima posthuma* by determining the period of worm paralysis and death. At a dosage of 100 mg/mL, the extract exhibited considerable anthelmintic effectiveness. Additionally, it demonstrated superior expressive activity than the conventional medication piperazine citrate (Gundamaraju 2013). Kumar and Singh (2014) evaluated the effect of *F. asafoetida* dried latex powder, dried powder of *Syzygium aromaticum* and *A. sativum* in the management of *Fasciola gigantica* (liver fluke). All three plants were also examined for their anthelmintic potential and the results were time- and concentration-dependent. The toxicity of ethanol extracts of these plants was higher than that of other organic extracts. *F. asafoetida* ethanol extract was highly toxic against liver fluke. These results revealed that the *F. asafoetida* dried root latex powder could be used as an efficient helminthicide agent.

6.8 SAFETY AND TOXICITY

The oleoresin of asafoetida is largely non-toxic as a dose of 15 g had no adverse effects on the human body. A case of methaemoglobinemia has been linked to the use of asafoetida (in milk) to cure colic in a 5-week-old baby. On foetal haemoglobin, but not on adult haemoglobin, asafoetida was discovered to have an oxidizing impact (Kelly et al. 1984). Toxic coumarin compounds from a closely similar plant, *F. communis*, have been shown to lower prothrombin levels and induce haemorrhaging in sheep. *F. galbaniflua* and *F. rubicaulis* are two more species that are said to have a rubefacient and irritant gum that can cause contact dermatitis in sensitive people. Asafoetida has been shown to have a modest sister chromatid exchange-inducing impact in clastogenicity and spermatogonia in mice spermatocytes. Coumarin components have been linked to chromosomal destruction caused by asafoetida (Walia 1973; Abraham and Kesavan 1984; Upadhyay et al. 2017).

Because of the oxidizing effects on foetal haemoglobin, asafoetida should not be administered to newborns, resulting in methaemoglobinaemia. So asafoetida should be avoided during breastfeeding due to its harmful effects on newborns (e.g., methaemoglobinaemia) (Al-Qahtani et al. 2020). Lactation and pregnancy are two of the most important aspects of a woman's life. Asafoetida has a legendary reputation as an emmenagogue and an abortifacient. However, usage of asafoetida during pregnancy is probably safe, as long as levels aren't higher than those found in food (Upadhyay et al. 2017).

6.9 CONCLUSION AND FUTURE PROSPECTIVE

Asafoetida is an oleoresin gum mainly isolated from the rhizome and roots exudates of *F. asafoetida*. It is widely used in traditional and modern systems of medicine owing to its variety of medicinal properties. Owing to its valuable aroma and biological properties, it is also extensively used all around the world as a flavouring and medicinal spice in various foodstuffs. The key bioactive constituents of the oleoresin gum are phenolic acids and their esters, flavonoids, coumarin, glycosides, terpenoids and sesquiterpene coumarins and their derivatives. While the volatile essential oils mainly contained sulphur compounds, monoterpenes and sesquiterpene. Owing to the presence of various bioactive phytoconstituents and essential oil, asafoetida is broadly used in traditional and modern herbalism for the cure of a variety of ailments such as hysteria, whooping cough, bronchitis, asthma, flatulent colic, infantile pneumonia, gastric eructation and some nervous conditions. Further, asafoetida oleoresin gum is also used as sedative, stimulant, carminative, expectorant, emmenagogue, laxative, vermifuge and antispasmodic. The scientific studies revealed that the asafoetida is also known to have a variety of pharmacological properties such as antioxidant, neuroprotective, antispasmodic, hepatoprotective, anticytotoxicity, anticancer, memory enhancing, anthelmintic, hypotensive, antibacterial, anti-obesity and antimicrobial. The functional and nutraceutical characteristics of asafoetida oleoresin gum and its volatile essential oil on gut health have been recognized recently. Although the asafoetida has very good nutraceutical and medicinal importance, comprehensive scientific studies are required to establish its pharmacology, safety and toxicology. Traditionally, *F. asafoetida* is cultivated on large scale in Iran and Afghanistan. In India, it is not cultivated traditionally. India largely depends upon other countries for their required need of asafoetida. But lately, it has been observed by the scientists of CSIR-IHBT (Council of Scientific and Industrial Research – Institute of

Himalayan Bioresource Technology), Himachal Pradesh, India that the cold desert areas of Leh-Ladakh, Lahaul and Spiti valley have great potential for the large-scale cultivation of *F. asafoetida*.

REFERENCES

Abraham, S.K. and Kesavan, P.C. 1984 Genotoxicity of garlic, turmeric and asafoetida in mice, *Mutation Research/Genetic Toxicology*, 136(1): 85–88.

Abu-Zaiton, A.S. 2010 Anti-diabetic activity of *Ferula assafoetida* extract in normal and alloxan-induced diabetic rats, *Pakistan Journal of Biological Sciences*, 13(2): 97–100.

Ali, A. 2019 On farm cultivation of economically important medicinal and aromatic plants for rural livelihood improvement in Chitral, Northern Pakistan, *Oceanography and Marine Biology*.

Al-Qahtani, S., Abusham, S. and Alhelali, I. 2020 Severe methemoglobinemia secondary to Ferula asafoetida ingestion in an infant: A case report, *Saudi Journal of Medicine & Medical Cciences*, 8(1): 56.

Alqasoumi, S. 2012 Anxiolytic effect of *Ferulaassafoetida L.* in rodents, *Journal of Pharmacognosy and Phytotherapy*, 4(6): 86–90.

Amalraj, A. and Sreeraj, G. 2017 Biological activities and medicinal properties of asafoetida: A Review, *Journal of Traditional and Complementary Medicine*, National Taiwan University. doi: 10.1016/j.jtcme.2016.11.004.

Amirhossein, S., Mehrdad, I. 2010b Biological activities of essential oils from the genus ferula (Apiaceae), *Asian Biomedicine*, 4: 835–847.

Amirhossein, S., Mehrdad, I. 2011a Volatile constituents of the genus ferula (Apiaceae): A review, *Journal of Essential Oil-Bearing Plants*, 14: 504–31.

Asili, J., Amirhossein, S., Bibi, S. F. B., Sirus, S., and Mehrdad, I. 2009 Identification of essential oil components of Ferula Badrakema Fruits by Gc-Ms and 13c-Nmr methods and evaluation of its antimicrobial activity, *Journal of Essential Oil-Bearing Plants*, 12: 7–15.

Asma, K., Arshiya, S., and Khaleequr, R. 2017 A single-blind randomized comparative study of Asafoetida vs Mefenamic acid in dysmenorrhea, associated symptoms and health-related quality of life, *Journal of Herbal Medicine*, 9: 21–31.

Azizian, H., Mohammad, E. R., Mansour E., and Seyyed M. B. 2012 Anti-obesity, fat lowering and liver steatosis protective effects of ferula Asafoetida Gum in Type 2 diabetic rats: Possible involvement of leptin, *Iranian Journal of Diabetes and Obesity*, 4: 120–6

Bagheri, S. M., and Mohammad, H. D. R. 2015 Influence of asafoetida on prevention and treatment of memory impairment induced by d -Galactose and NaNO2 in Mice, *American Journal of Alzheimer's Disease and Other Dementias*, 30: 607–12.

Barat, A.G. and Faravani, M. 2014 Effects of different cutting methods and times of cutting on growth performance and gum resin production of *Ferulaassafoetida*, *Journal of Agricultural Sciences(Belgrade)*, 59: 35–44.

Bayrami, G., Mohammad, H. B., Mehrdad, I. and Zahra, G. 2013 Relaxant effects of asafoetida extract and its constituent Umbelliprenin on guinea-pig tracheal smooth muscle, *Chinese Journal of Integrative Medicine*, 1–6.

Bellakhdar, J., Claisse, R., Fleurentin, J. and Younos, C. 1991 Repertory of standard herbal drugs in the Moroccan pharmacopoea, *Journal of Ethnopharmacology*, 35: 123–143.

Bhardwaj, P., Thakur, M.S., Kapoor, S., et al. 2019 Phytochemical screening and antioxidant activity study of methanol extract of stems and roots of Codonopsisclematidea from trans-Himalayan region, *Pharmacognosy Journal*, 11(3).

Bhatnager, R., Reena, R. and AmitaSuneja, D. 2021 Antibacterial activity of ferula asafoetida: A comparison of red and white type, *Journal of Applied Biology & Biotechnology*, 3: 18–021.

Bhattarai, N. K. 1992 Folk anthelmintic drugs of central Nepal, *Pharmaceutical Biology*, 30: 145–50.

Bonhage, F. and Mary, T. 2006 Handbook of medicinal plants, *Economic Botany*, 60(2): 196–196.

Buddrus, J. H. B., Abu, M. E., Khattab, A., Mishaal, S. et al. 1985 Foetidin, a Sesquiterpenoid Coumarin from FerulaAssa-Foetida, *Phytochemistry*, 24: 869–70.

Christensen, L. P., and Kirsten B. 2006 Bioactive polyacetylenes in food plants of the apiaceae family: Occurrence, bioactivity and analysis, *Journal of Pharmaceutical and Biomedical Analysis*. doi: 10.1016/j.jpba.2006.01.057.

Cragg, G.M., and Newman, D.J., 2013 Natural products: A continuing source of novel drug leads, *Biochimica et Biophysica Acta (BBA)*, 1830(6): 3670–3695.

Damanch, N.E. and Sharafatmandrad, M. 2017 Assessing the effects of different incision techniques on *Ferula asafoetida* properties, *Journal of Rangeland Science*, 7(1): 45–53.

Dandagi, P., Patil, M., Mastiholimath, V., Gadad, A. and Dhumansure, R. 2008 Development and evaluation of hepatoprotective polyherbal formulation containing some indigenous medicinal plants, *Indian Journal of Pharmaceutical Sciences*, 70: 265–68.

Dastan, D., Peyman, S., Atousa, A., Ahmad, R. G., Hossein, M. and Afshan, A. 2016 New coumarin derivatives from ferulapseudalliacea with antibacterial activity, *Natural Product Research*, 30: 2747–53.

Dehghan, G., Abbas, S., Mohammad, H. G., Susan, K. A., and Mohammad, A. 2007 Antioxidant potential of various extracts from *FerulaSzovitsiana* in relation to their phenolic content, *Pharmaceutical Biology*, 45: 691–99.

Dehpour, A. A., Mohammad, A. E., Nabavi, S. F. and Nabavi, S. M. 2009 Antioxidant activity of the methanol extract of *FerulaAssafoetida* and its essential oil composition, *Grasas y Aceites*, 60: 405–12.

Devanesan, S., Karuppiah, P., Mohamad, S. A. and Naif, A. A. 2020 Cytotoxic and antimicrobial efficacy of silver nanoparticles synthesized using a traditional phytoproduct, asafoetida gum, *International Journal of Nanomedicine*, 15: 4351–62.

Eftekhar, F., Morteza, Y. and Borhani, K. 2004 Antibacterial activity of the essential oil from *FerulaGummosa* seed, *Fitoterapia*, 75: 758–59.

Eigner, D. and Scholz, D. 1999 *Ferula Asafoetida* and *Curcuma Longa* in traditional medical treatment and diet in Nepal, *Journal of Ethnopharmacology*, 67: 1–6.

Elisabetsky, E., Wilsea, F., and Gregória, O. 1992 Traditional amazonian nerve tonics as antidepressant agent: ChaunochitonKappleri: A case study, *Journal of Herbs, Spices and Medicinal Plants*, 1: 125–162

El-Thaher, T. S., Matalka, K. Z., Taha, H. A. and Badwan, A. A. 2001 *FerulaHarmonis* 'zallouh' and enhancing erectile function in rats: Efficacy and toxicity study, *International Journal of Impotence Research*, 13: 247–51.

Farhadi, F., Asili, J., Iranshahy, M. and Iranshahi, M. 2019 NMR-based metabolomic study of asafoetida, *Fitoterapia*, 139: 104361.

Fatehi, M., Freshteh, F. and Zahra, F. H. 2004 Antispasmodic and hypotensive effects of *Ferula Asafoetida* gum extract, *Journal of Ethnopharmacology*, 91: 321–24.

Ford, P. W. 2003 Handbook of medicinal spices, *Journal of Natural Products*, 66: 732–33.

Fulder, S., Said, K. K., Fulder, S. and Azaizeh, H. 2003 Ethnopharmacological survey of medicinal herbs in Israel, the Golan Heights and the West Bank Region, *Journal of Ethnopharmacology*, 83: 251–65.

Gamal, E., Amira, M., and Hegazy, M. E.F. 2010 A crystal lapiferin derived from *FerulaVesceritensis* induces apoptosis pathway in MCF-7 breast cancer cells, *Natural Product Research*, 24: 246–57.

Ghasemi, Y., Faridi, P., Mehregan, I. and Mohagheghzadeh, A. 2005, *FerulaGummosa* fruits: An aromatic antimicrobial agent, *Chemistry of Natural Compounds*, 41: 311–14.

Gimlette, J. D. 1939 *A Dictionary of Malayan Medicine*. Humphrey Milford, Oxford University Press.

Giri, S.K., Prasad, N., Pandey, S.K., Prasad, M. and Babloo, B. 2008 Natural resins and gums of commercial importance- At a glance. Technical Bulletin, *Indian Institute of Natural Resins and Gums*, 35–36.

Gogate, V. M. 2000 Ayurvedic pharmacology and therapeutic uses of medicinal plants (Dravyagunavignyan), *Bharatiya Vidya Bhavan*, 1: 520.

Golmohammadi, F. 2016 *Ferulaassafoetida* as a main medicinal plant in East of Iran (Harvesting, main characteristics and economical importance), *Journal of Progressive Agriculture*, 7: 1–15.

Greater Kashmir 2021 Heeng cultivation: untapped agri-preneurship opportunity in J&K | https://www.greaterkashmir.com/news/opinion/heeng-cultivation-untapped-agri-preneurship-opportunity-in-jk/. (Accessed May 16, 2021).

Gundamaraju, R. 2013 Evaluation of anti-helmintic activity of FerulaFoetida 'Hing- a natural indian spice' Aqueous extract, *Asian Pacific Journal of Tropical Disease*, 3: 189–91.

Gurav, S. and Gurav, N. 2014 A comprehensive review: Bergenia ligulata Wall-A controversial clinical candidate, *International Journal of Pharmaceutical Sciences and Research*, 5: 1630–1642.

Hajimehdipoor, H., Somayeh, E., Azadeh, R., Morteza, J. A., and Mahmood, M. 2012 The cytotoxic effects of ferula Persica Var. Persica and FerulaHezarlalehzarica against HepG2, A549, HT29, MCF7 and MDBK Cell Lines, *Iranian Journal of Pharmaceutical Sciences Spring*, 8: 115–119. http://www.ijps.ir/article_1837.html.

Halliwell, B., John M.C., Gutteridge, and Carroll, E.C. 1992 Free radicals, antioxidants, and human disease: Where are we now?, *The Journal of Laboratory and Clinical Medicine*, 344: 721–724.

Hassanabadi, M., Mohsen Ebrahimi, Mostafa, F. and Ata, D. 2019 Variation in essential oil components among Iranian *Ferulaassafoetida L.* accessions, *Industrial Crops and Products*, 140: 111598.

Hassanabadi, M., Mohsen, E., Mostafa, F. and Ata, D. 2019 Variation in essential oil components among Iranian *Ferulaassafoetida L.* accessions, *Industrial Crops and Products*, 140.

Illis, L. S. 1998 Harrison's principles of internal medicine 14th Edition, *Spinal Cord*, 36: 665–665.

Iranshahi, M. 2013 Volatile constituents of the genus ferula (Apiaceae): A review biological activity of natural products and medicinal plants view project lime juice adulteration view project, *Article in Journal of Essential Oil-Bearing Plants*, 14: 504–31.

Iranshahi, M., Peyman, A., Mohammad, R., et al. 2007 Sesquiterpene coumarins from *FerulaSzowitsiana* and in vitro antileishmanial activity of 7-prenyloxycoumarins against promastigotes, *Phytochemistry*, 68: 554–61.

Iranshahy, M, and Mehrdad, I. 2011 Traditional uses, phytochemistry and pharmacology of asafoetida (FerulaAssa-Foetida Oleo-Gum-Resin) - A review, *Journal of Ethnopharmacology*, 8: 1–10.

James A. D., Edward S. A. 2021 Medicinal Plants of China. https://books.google.co.in/books/about/Medicinal_plants_of_China.html?id=hMNqAAAAMAAJ&redir_esc=y. (Accessed May 28, 2021).

Javaid, R., Javed, G., Anju, A. F. and Khan, A. A. (2020) Hing (Ferulafoetida Regel.): A potent Unani herb with its descriptive parameters of pharmacog-nosy and pharmacology: A review. *Journal of Drug Delivery and Therapeutics*, 10: 362–367.

John, D. 1984 One hundred useful raw drugs of the kani tribes of trivandrum forest division, Kerala, India, *Pharmaceutical Biology*, 22: 17–39.

Joshi, P. 1991 Herbal drugs used in guinea worm disease by the tribals of Southern Rajasthan (India), *Pharmaceutical Biology*, 29: 33–38.

Joshi, R., Prabodh, S., and Wiliam, S. 2016 Himalayan aromatic medicinal plants: A review of their ethnopharmacology, volatile phytochemistry, and biological activities, *Medicines*, 3: 6.

Kamboj, V. P. 2021 A review of Indian medicinal plants, (Accessed May 28, 2021).

Karimian, V., Parvin, R. and Jahanbakhsh, T. M. 2019 Chemical composition and biological effects of three different types (Tear, Paste, and Mass) of Bitter FerulaAssa-Foetida Linn, Gum, *Natural Product Research*.

Kartal, N, Munevver, S., Bektas, T., Dimitra, D., Moschos, P., and Atalay, S. 2007 Investigation of the Antioxidant Properties of ferulaorientalis L. Using a Suitable Extraction Procedure, *Food Chemistry*, 100: 584–89.

Kasaian, J., Milad, I., Milena, M., Sonia, P., Fatemeh, E., and Mehrdad, I. 2014 Sesquiterpene lactones from FerulaOopoda and their cytotoxic properties, *Journal of Asian Natural Products Research*, 16: 248–53.

Kavoosi, G. and Amin, M. P. 2013 Scolicidal effectiveness of essential oil from zataria multiflora and ferulaassafoetida: Disparity between phenolic monoterpenes and disulphide compounds, *Comparative Clinical Pathology*, 22: 999–1005.

Kazemi, F., Reza, M., Saeed, N., and Mohammad, N. S. 2020 Antihypertensive effects of standardized Asafoetida: Effect on hypertension induced by Angiotensin II, *Advanced Biomedical Research*, 9: 77.

Kelly, K.J., Neu, J., Camitta, B.M. and Honig, G.R. 1984 Methemoglobinemia in an infant treated with the folk remedy glycerited asafoetida, *Pediatrics (Evanston)*, 73(5): 717–719.

Keshri, G., Lakshmi, V., Singh, M.M. and Kamboj, V.P. 1999 Post-coital antifertility activity of Ferulaassafoetida extract in female rats, *Pharmaceutical biology*, 37(4): 273–276.

Keshri, G., Sudhir, K., Dinesh, K. K., Siron, M. R., and Man, M. S. 2008 Postcoital interceptive activity of wrightia tinctoria in sprague-dawley rats: A preliminary study, *Contraception*, 78: 266–70.

Khajeh, M., Yadollah, Y., Naader, B., Fatemeh, S., and Mohammad, R. P. 2005 Comparison of essential oils compositions of ferulaassa-foetida obtained by supercritical carbon dioxide extraction and hydrodistillation methods, *Food Chemistry*, 91: 639–44.

Kojima, K., Kimio, I., Purev, O., et al. 2000 Sesquiterpenoid derivatives from FerulaFerulioides IV, *Chemical and Pharmaceutical Bulletin*, 48: 353–56.

Kuete, V., Benjamin, W., Mohamed, E. F. H., et al. 2012 Antibacterial activity and cytotoxicity of selected egyptian medicinal plants, *Planta Medica*, 78: 193–99.

Kumar, A. 2017 From Afghanistan with Love. https://www.thedollarbusiness.com/magazine/from-afghanistan-with-love/46065 (accessed on June 16, 2021)

Kumar, P., Singh, D.K. 2014 In vitro anthelmintic activity of Allium sativum, Ferula asafoetida, Sizygiumaromaticum and their active components against Fasciola gigantica, *Journal of Biology and Earth Sciences*, 4: 57–65.

Lev, E., and Zohar, A. 2002 Ethnopharmacological survey of traditional drugs sold in the Kingdom of Jordan, *Journal of Ethnopharmacology*, 82: 131–45.

Maggi, F., Cinzia, C., Alberto, C., et al. 2009 Chemical Composition and Antimicrobial Activity of the Essential Oil from Ferula Glauca L. (F. Communis L. Subsp. Glauca) Growing in Marche (Central Italy), *Fitoterapia*, 80: 68–72.

Mahendra, P., and Shradha, B. 2012 FerulaAsafoetida : Traditional uses and pharmacological activity, *Pharmacognosy Reviews*. doi: 10.4103/0973–7847.99948.

Mandegary, A., Mandegary, A., Mohammad, S., et al. 2004 Antinociceptive and anti-inflammatory activity of the seed and root extracts of ferulaGummosaBoiss in mice and rats. *Journal of Pharmaceutical Sciences*. http://daru.tums.ac.ir/index.php/daru/article/view/201.

Marar, A. 2020 Explained: Why scientists are trying to cultivate asafoetida or heeng in the Indian Himalayas. https://indianexpress.com/article/explained/why-scientists-are-trying-to-cultivate-heeng-in-the-indian-himalayas-6792923/, (accessed on 16th June, 2021).

Mazzio, E. A., and Karam, F. A. S. 2010 *In Vitro* Screening of Tumoricidal Properties of International Medicinal Herbs: Part II, *Phytotherapy Research*, 24: 1813–24.

Moghaddam, M. and Farhadi, N. 2015 Influence of environmental and genetic factors on resin yield, essential oil content and chemical composition of Ferulaassafoetida L. populations, *Journal of Applied Research on Medicinal and Aromatic Plants*, 2: 69–76.

Mohammadzadeh, M.J., Emam, J.Z., Safari, et al. 2007 Physicochemical and emulsifying properties of Barijeh (Ferulagumosa) gum, *Iranian Journal of Chemistry and Chemical Engineering*, 26: 81–88.

Mohd, S., Mohd, A., Fathin, A. Y., et al. 2015 In Vitro cytotoxic activity of FerulaAssafoetida on Osteosarcoma Cell Line (Hos Crl), *JurnalTeknologi*, 77: 7–11.

Nataraj, H. R., and Gundakalle, M. B. 2010 Comparative pharmacognostic and phytochemical study of different market samples of Asafoetida (*Ferula narthex Bioss*), *International Journal of Research in Ayurveda and Pharmacy*, 1: 258–263.

Nazari, Z. E., and Mehrdad, I. 2011 Biologically active sesquiterpene coumarins from *Ferula* Species, *Phytotherapy Research*, 25: 315–23.

Newman, D.J. and Cragg, G.M. 2016 Natural products as sources of new drugs from 1981 to 2014, *Journal of natural products*, 79(3), 629–661.

Niazmand, R., and Razavizadeh, B. M. 2020 Ferula asafoetida: chemical composition, thermal behavior, antioxidant and antimicrobial activities of leaf and gum hydroalcoholic extracts. *Journal of Food Science and Technology*, 1–12.

NIFTEM. 2021 Handbook of asafetida processing. http://niftem.ac.in/newsite/wp-content/uploads/2021/01/Hing-Processing-Autosaved-converted.pdf (accessed on June 16, 2021)

NIFTEM. 2021a. Processing of asafoetida. http://niftem.ac.in/site/pmfme/processingnew/asafoetidaprocessing.pdf (accessed on June 16, 2021)

Omid, B., and Pirmoradei, M.R. 2006 A study of the effect of root diameter and incision time on gum yield in medicinal rangeland asafoetida (Ferula asafoetida L.) plant, *Iranian Journal of Natural Resources*, 59: 261–269.

Pimenov, M.G., and Leonov, M.V. 1993 *The Genera of the Umbelliferae: A Nomenclator.* https://www.cabdirect.org/cabdirect/abstract/19951608740.

Platel, K., and Srinivasan, K. 1996 Influence of dietary spices or their active principles on digestive enzymes of small intestinal mucosa in rats, *International Journal of Food Sciences and Nutrition*, 47: 55–59.

Rabi, D. M., Alun. L. E., Danielle, A. S., et al. 2006 Association of socio-economic status with diabetes prevalence and utilization of diabetes care services, *BMC Health Services Research*, 6: 1–7. doi: 10.1186/1472-6963-6-124.

Rashidi, F., Mahmood, K. M., Reza, R., and Hossein, N. V. 2013 The effects of essential oil of galbanum on caffeine induced-cleft palate in rat embryos, *Zahedan Journal of Research in Medical Sciences Journal*.

Saeidy, S., Nasirpour, A., Keramat, et al., 2018 Structural characterization and thermal behavior of a gum extracted from *Ferulaassafoetida L.*, *Carbohydrate Polymers*, 181: 426–432.

Sahebkar, A., and Iranshahi, M. 2010 Biological activities of essential oils from the genus ferula (Apiaceae). *Asian Biomedicine*. http://citeseerx.ist.psu.edu/viewdoc/download?doi=10.1.1.906.3560&rep=rep1&type=pdf

Sahranavard, S., Naghibi, M., Esmaeili, S., et al., 2009 Cytotoxic activities of selected medicinal plants from iran and phytochemical evaluation of the most potent extract. *Research in Pharmaceutical Sciences*, 4: 133–37.

Saleem, M., Aftab, A., and Sarwat, S. 2001 Asafoetida inhibits early events of carcinogenesis: A chemopreventive study, *Life Sciences*, 68: 1913–21.

Sayyah, M., Mandgary, A., and Kamalinejad, M. 2002 Evaluation of the anticonvulsant activity of the seed acetone extract of FerulaGummosaBoiss. Against seizures induced by pentylenetetrazole and electroconvulsive shock in mice, *Journal of Ethnopharmacology*, 82: 105–9.

Seetharam, K.A., Pasricha, J.S. 2021 Condiments and contact dermatitis of the finger-tips, *Europepmc. Org*. https://europepmc.org/article/med/28145344. (Accessed May 28, 2021)

Shah, N.C. and Zare, A. 2014 Asafoetida (Heeng): The well-known medicinal-condiment of India and Iran, *The Scitech Journal*, 1: 30–36.

Sharma, A., Bhardwaj, G., Gaba, J. and Cannoo, D.S. 2020 Natural Antioxidants: Assays and Extraction Methods/Solvents Used for Their Isolation. In Antioxidants in Fruits: Properties and Health Benefits. Springer.

Shweta, G., Ribadiya, C., Soni, J., Shah, N. and Jain, H. 2021 Herbal plants used as contraceptives, *International Journal of Current Pharmaceutical Review and Research*, 2: 47–53.

Singh, R. 2015 Medicinal plants: A review. *Journal of Plant Sciences*, 3: 50.

Singh, Y. N. 1986 Traditional medicine in Fiji: Some herbal folk cures used by Fiji Indians, *Journal of Ethnopharmacology*, 15: 57–88.

Sood, R. 2020 Asafoetida (Ferula asafoetida): A high-value crop suitable for the cold desert of Himachal Pradesh, India, *Journal of Applied and Natural Science*, 12(4): 607–617.

Srivastava, J., John, L., and Noel, V. 1996 Medicinal plants: an expanding role in development, *World Bank Technical Paper*.

Sultana, B., Farooq, A., and Muhammad, A. 2009 Effect of extraction solvent/technique on the antioxidant activity of selected medicinal plant extracts, *Molecules*, 14: 2167–80.

Tamemoto, K., Yoshihisa, T., Bei, C., Kazuyoshi, K., Hirofumi, S., Tomihiko, H., Gisho, H., et al. 2001 Sesquiterpenoids from the Fruits of FerulaKuhistanica and Antibacterial Activity of the Constituents of F. Kuhistanica, *Phytochemistry*, 58: 763–67.

Tiwari, K. C., Majumder, R., and Bhattacharjee, S. 1979 Folklore medicines from Assam and Arunachal Pradesh (District Tirap), *Pharmaceutical Biology*, 17: 61–67.

Upadhyay, P.K. 2017 Pharmacological activities and therapeutic uses of resins obtained from ferula asafoetida linn: A review, *International Journal of Green Pharmacy*, 11: 240.

Venkataraghavan, S., and Sundareesan, T.P. 1981 A short note on contraceptive in Ayurveda. https://www.sid.ir/en/journal/ViewPaper.aspx?ID=318700.

Vijayasteltar, L., Jismy, I. J., Ashil, J., Balu, M., Ramadasan, K., and Krishnakumar, I. M. 2017 Beyond the flavor: A green formulation of *Ferula Asafoetida* oleo-gum-resin with fenugreek dietary fibre and its gut health potential, *Toxicology Reports*, 4: 382–90.

Vunjak-Novakovic, G. and Freshney, R.I. 2006 Culture of cells for tissue engineering (Vol. 7). New York: Wiley-Liss.

Walia, K. 1973 Effect of asafoetida (7-hydroxycoumarin) on mouse spermatocytes, *Cytologia*, 38: 719–24.

Yaqoob, U., Irshad, A. N., and Mudasar, A. 2016 Phytochemical screening of the root tuber extracts of FerulaJaeschkeanaVatke, *Journal of Essential Oil-Bearing Plants*, 19: 208–11.

Yaqoob, U. 2016 Distribution and taxonomy of ferula L.: A review reproductivity biology, chemical profiling and biodiversity of MAP of Kashmir himalaya view project phytochemistry view project. *Researchgate.Net*. https://www.researchgate.net/publication/312590226.

Zimmerman, C. and Eric, Y. 2018 Herbal medicines for seizures, *Alternative and Complementary Therapies*, 24: 281–90.

Znati, M., Hichem, B. J., Sylvie, C., Jean, P. S., Féthia, et al. 2014 Antioxidant, 5-Lipoxygenase inhibitory and cytotoxic activities of compounds isolated from the ferula lutea flowers, *Molecules*, 19: 16959–75.

CHAPTER 7

Black Cumin Oleoresin

Characterization, Properties and Economic Importance

Sumera Mehfooz

National Institute of Unani Medicine Bangaluru

Imtiyaz Ahmad Mir

AYUSH, Government of Jammu & Kashmir

Ghulamudin Sofi and Najeeb Jahan

National Institute of Unani Medicine Bangaluru

CONTENTS

DOI: 10.1201/9781003186205-7

7.1 INTRODUCTION

Black cumin (*Nigella sativa*) is also known as "the herb from heaven" and has been described as a magical plant (Ahmad, et al. 2013). Black cumin, according to prophetic medicine, is a cure for all illnesses except death. *N. sativa* is an annual plant with blooms that are white, pale blue, or purple in colour. It belongs to the Ranunculaceae family. Natural habitats for *N. sativa* include Europe, North Africa, and Asia. Many countries cultivate it, including the Middle East Mediterranean region, South Europe, India, Pakistan, Syria, Turkey, and Saudi Arabia (Khare, 2004). Researchers at the Department of Pharmacology at King Faisal University, Saudi Arabia investigated black cumin seed extract for analgesic and anti-inflammatory properties in animal models in 2021. Black cumin seed extract was administered to animals; paw oedema (swelling) was reduced to a great extent in all inflammation-induced animals.

Black cumin oleoresin is made by extracting the seeds of black cumin using the supercritical fluid extraction technique. The oleoresin of black cumin is commonly used for culinary purposes as a spice and flavouring agent in a variety of foods, including bread, pickles, salads, yoghurt, and sauces. The oleoresin of black cumin seed has a protective effect on liver and renal disorders, as well as it induces apoptosis (programmed cell death) and possibly reduces tumour mass. Black seed oleoresin has also been reported to boost sperm motility, sperm count, and semen volume. More than 100 chemicals have been identified in *N. sativa*, some of which are yet to be properly characterized. Thymoquinone (TQ), dithymoquinone (DQ), thymohydroquinone (THQ), longifoline, α-thujene, β-pinine, carvone, carvacrol, limonene, p-cymene, and trans-anethole are some of the components found in black cumin oleoresin (*CO_2 Black Cumin Oleoresins Manufacturer, SCFE Oils Supplier from India*, n.d.). Because of the different therapeutic effects of the herbs and their ability to help maintain a healthy life, herbal medicine is gaining widespread favour among consumers in developing countries. Although traditional synthetic pharmaceuticals are commonly used to treat ailments, these treatments have substantial side effects. Natural products, such as *N. sativa*, are the best alternative for treating certain ailments or diseases without causing adverse effects in our bodies if ingested in accordance with scientific discoveries and studies (Abd Aziz, 2006).

7.2 BLACK CUMIN OLEORESIN'S CHEMICAL MAKEUP

Various scientific research and instrumental analysis have revealed that black cumin oleoresin contains a variety of chemicals. Major components of black cumin oleoresin were discovered using Gas Chromatography-Mass Spectrometry (GC-MS) analysis. The chemicals identified were cymene, thymoquinone, carvacrol, α-longipinene, longifolene, thymohydroquinone, palmitic acid, ethyl ester, linoleic acid, methyl ester, oleic acid, butyl ester, glyceryl palmitate, glyceryl linoleate, and sitosterol.

The effect of microencapsulation by spray drying on the chemical makeup of black cumin oleoresin was shown by GC-MS analysis of the volatile oil fraction which contains thymoquinone; thujene sp-cymene; trans-4-methoxythujane; Carvacrol; Longifolene; pinene. Microencapsulation reduced the amount of ingredient in the study, with the exception of thymoquinone.

Fixed oil (linoleic acid (omega-6), oleic acid, and palmitoleic acid are three types of fatty acids found in the oleoresin of the seeds of *Nigella*. Linolenic acid (omega-3), myristoleic acid, stearic acid, eicosadienoic acid, myristic acid, arachidic acid, behanic acid, linole, sterols (-sitosterol, avenasterol, stigmasterol, campesterol, and lanosterol), tocopherols and thymoquinone, retinol (vitamin A), and carotenoids (-carotene) account for 22%–38% of the total fixed oils present in it (Al-Jassir, 1992; Al-Saleh et al., 2006; A. A. Ansari et al., 1988; Atta-ur-Rahman et al., 1995; Gad et al., 1963; Hussein El-Tahir and Bakeet, 2006; Kamal et al., 2010; Muhammad, 2009; M. Sultan et al., 2009).

Glutamic acid, arginine, aspartic acid, leucine, glycine, valine, lysine, threonine, phenylalanine, isoleucine, histidine, and methionine estimates to 20.8%–31.2% as proteins. Glucose, rhamnose, xylose, and arabinose account for 24.9%–40% of total carbohydrates. Calcium, phosphorus, iron, potassium, sodium, zinc, magnesium, manganese, copper, and selenium are minerals found up to 3.7%–7%. Saponins like Hederin (melanthin), hederagenin constitutes 0.013%. Nigelicine, nigellimine, and nigellidine are alkaloids that constitutes 0.01% Vitamins not listed above include vitamin A, thiamin, riboflavin, pyridoxine, niacin, folacin, and vitamin C which account for 1%–4% of the total.

7.3 BLACK CUMIN'S ECONOMIC IMPORTANCE

As far as economic importance is concerned, it has been discovered that black cumin oleoresin is being sold for about $2500 per kg (OZONE Natural).

Black cumin is sold at a cost of 275–300 per kg in Pakistan (Mingora, Din, Peshawar, Pindi, Lahore, Gilgit and Astore) and 850–1000 per kg in the international market (Datta et al., 2012). Black cumin oil (1000 mL) is available in Germany for 23.90 EUR without delivery expenses (Datta et al., 2012). In the worldwide market, 100 capsules of black cumin seeds cost $9 and 20 bags of black cumin tea cost $6 (Datta et al., 2012). In the United States, Black Cumin cost varies as per product brand and product number as exemplified by the following market survey (Datta et al., 2012):

7.4 SCIENTIFIC CLASSIFICATION OF *NIGELLA SATIVA* (BLACK CUMIN)

Kingdom: Plantae

Clade: Tracheophyte

Division: Magnoliophyta

Order: Ranunculales

Family: Ranunculaceae

Genus: *Nigella*

Species: *sativa*

7.5 BLACK CUMIN BIOSAFETY AND POTENTIAL TOXICITY

According to several researches, *N. sativa* and thymoquinone have been found with a wide range of safety. The following are some of the most important studies on the biosafety and toxicity of black cumin and its constituents:

The enzymes and metabolites levels noticed in the liver and kidney of rats were unchanged after 5 days of 50 mg/kg intraperitoneal treatment of *N. sativa* (Junemann and Luetjohann, 1998). It was found that when seed powder of black cumin was fed orally to rabbits at a dose of 28 gm/kg, it had no harmful impact (Tissera, et al. 1997). The seed oil was found to be safe in rats when administered orally at a dose of 28.8 mL/kg (LD50 of 28.8 mL/kg) (Zaoui, et al. 2002). Oral thymoquinone (LD50 of around 1000 mg/kg) and intra-peritoneal thymoquinone (LD50 of around 100 mg/kg) caused no harm in mice and rats, respectively (Al-Ali, et al. 2008). Healthy individuals administered with *N. sativa* oil (5 mL/day) for 8 weeks reported no negative effects on the gastrointestinal tract, liver, or kidneys (Amini, et al. 2011; Fallah Huseini, et al. 2013). *N. sativa* seeds (3 g/day for 3 months) administered to 39 centrally obese individuals showed no discernible negative effects (HF Huseini, et al. 2010).

In ALL (Acute Lymphocytic Leukaemia), the most common childhood cancer, Hagag and colleagues found that giving *N. sativa* oil (80 mg/kg/day) to children receiving methotrexate treatment for 1 week reduced hepatotoxicity and enhanced survival rates in ALL kids (Adel, et al. 2015). Kolahdooz et al. found that giving infertile Iranian men 2.5 mL twice a day for 2 months raised semen parameters significantly in comparison to placebo-treated men, improved sperm morphology, semen volume, and kept pH of the seminal fluid to normal levels (Kolahdooz et al., 2014). Infertile men benefitted from the effects of Nigella sativa on Leydig cells, reproductive organs, and sexual hormones in another study (Mahdavi, et al. 2015).

7.6 IMPORTANT SCIENTIFIC STUDIES ON *NIGELLA SATIVA* AND ITS CONSTITUENTS

7.6.1 Anti-Tumour Action

The seed and oleo-gum-resin extracted from it are reported for various pharmacological actions. It has got potential to cure polycystic ovary as thymoquinone with olive oil showed a positive effect on NF-κB signalling pathway in the rats, where polycysts were induced in their ovary (Arif, et al. 2016). In human colon cancer cells, it induced apoptosis and arrested S phase of cell cycle (Khalife, et al. 2016). Essential oil nano-emulsion (20–50 nm diameter) at 20–80 μL/mL showed pronounced changes in the cell structure like blebbing in cell membrane, vacuolation, chromatin marginalization, and nuclear fragmentation in MCF-7 cells (Periasamy et al. 2016). Nano-particles (15.6–28.4 nm) inhibited A549 lung cancer cells lines (Manju, et al. 2016). Ethanol fractions and n-hexane showed cytotoxic activity in acute human renal adenocarcinoma and GP-293 (normal renal epithelial) cell lines (Shahraki, et al. 2016).

7.6.2 Nephroprotection

Thymoquinone developed nephroprotection in rats when administered at 50 mg/kg for 30 days, and it also showed protection in cadmium-induced toxicity (Erboga, et al. 2016).

7.6.3 Antimicrobial Action

Thymoquinone showed anti-methicillin resistant effect in *Staphylococcus aureus* (Hariharan, et al. 2016) and exhibited antimicrobial activity (Ramadan, 2016), and topical application was effective in the treatment of mastalgia in woman (Huseini, et al. 2016). Essential oil showed antifungal effect against various fungi at 10–200 μg/mL (Nadaf, et al. 2015) and antimicrobial effect after inducing infection by *Vibrio parahaemolyticus* (Manju, et al. 2016). 0.1 mg/disc extract showed antifungal activity against *Trichophyton mentagrophytes*, *Microsporum canis*, and *Microsporum gypseum* (Mahmoudvand, et al. 2014). There was normalization of immune reactions implicated in various conditions of hyperimmune response due to varied antigens by the essential oil of *Nigella* (Majdalawieh and Fayyad, 2015).

7.6.4 Antioxidant Action

Thymoquinone exhibited anti-inflammatory and antioxidant activities as it decreased inflammatory marker levels and increased activities of oxidant scavengers along with reduction in motor neuron apoptosis in rats (Gökce, et al. 2016). It strongly inhibited superoxide production and exocytosis in neutrophils (Boudiaf, et al. 2016). Seed oil showed significant antioxidant activity at 400 mg/kg intragastric in Wistar rats (Orhon, et al. 2016) and antioxidant effect in mice at 25–100 μg/mL (Adam, et al. 2016; Ramadan 2016). Seed oil ameliorated oxidative stress in the cortex and hippocampus, moreover enhancing remyelination in the hippocampus in autoimmune encephalomyelitis rats (Fahmy, et al. 2014). Essential oil exhibited antioxidant activity as it showed free radical scavenging action (Nadaf, et al. 2015). Aqueous extract of the resin oil showed strong reducing capacity in APAP-induced hepatotoxicity and it exhibited antioxidant activity in mice (Hamza and Al-Harbi, 2015). *Nigella* methanol extract administered orally in hyperlipidaemia rats showed antioxidant and hypolipidemic effects (Ahmad and Beg, 2016).

7.6.5 Anti-Diabetic Action

Thymoquinone showed protective action associated with the sensitivity of β-cell metabolic pathways under both normal and hyperglycaemia conditions in clonal β-cells and rodent islets (Gray, et al. 2016). Seed oil normalized glycaemic status and lipid profile when 3 g/day (three times a day) was given in type-2 diabetes mellitus patients (Heshmati et al., 2015). It was found effective in hypercholesterolemia (Sahebkar, et al. 2016). Lipid (4%) and volatile (3%) fractions of essential oil in streptozotocin-induced diabetes mellitus in Sprague Dawley rats reduced toxicological and adverse consequences of diabetes mellitus (Sultan, et al. 2014).

7.6.6 Effect on Thyroid Dysfunction

Seed oil when administered orally altered blood markers for Hashimoto's thyroiditis in humans favourably (Tajmiri, et al. 2016).

7.6.7 Hepatoprotection

Seed oil 2 mg/kg showed hepatoprotection by improving energy metabolism and strengthening antioxidant mechanism (Farooqui, et al. 2016). Hepato- and nephroprotective effects was noticed at 1 mg/kg administration in tramadol-induced male albino rats when administered for 30 days (Elkhateeb, et al. 2015), also increasing plasma transaminase activity, hepatic triglyceride, malondialdehyde (MDA) levels and decreased hepatic glutathione (GSH) levels in rats in a dose-dependent manner when oil was administered for 3 weeks (Develi, et al. 2014). Seed oil showed protection of liver against acetaminophen-induced hepatotoxicity (Adam, et al. 2016; Ramadan, 2016). Essential oil improved plasma lipid profile and antibody-mediated immunity when fed orally to chicken for 6 weeks (Ghasemi, et al. 2014).

7.6.8 Protection against Tissue Damage

Seed oil was shown to have protection against damage due to gamma radiation to jejunal mucosa in rats (Orhon, et al. 2016) and ameliorated the toxic changes caused in cornea in male albino rats (Salem, et al. 2016). It protected cortical neurons and myelinated axons against the damage caused by tramadol treatment in rats (Omar, 2016), prevented damage of hippocampal neurones accompanied with memory improvement in rats (Seghatoleslam et al., 2016).

7.6.9 Anti-Inflammatory Action

Seed oil modulated systemic inflammatory biomarkers when given 3 g/day in obese women for 8 weeks (Mahdavi, et al. 2015), lowered dyspepsia with 5 mL orally in patients with functional dyspepsia when given for 8 weeks (Mohtashami, et al. 2015). Anti-inflammatory, antioxidant, and immunomodulatory activities were reported for seed oil (Gholamnezhad, et al. 2015). Ethanol extract of seed oil in male Wistar rats stabilized cytokines (Gholamnezhad, et al. 2015). Methanolic extract 200 mg/kg (p.o.) administered to male albino Wistar rats for 2 months showed anti-inflammatory activity by down-regulation of the expression of ASC protein in pancreas to minimize the activation of caspase enzyme (Suguna, et al. 2014).

7.6.10 Action on Male Reproductive System

Seed oil altered abnormal semen quality without producing any adverse effect to normal when administered to infertile men for 2 months (Kolahdooz, et al. 2014). Oil was found as a good lead for male infertility treatment (Mahdavi, et al. 2015).

7.6.11 Psychopharmacological Action

Essential oil stabilize mood, relieves anxiety and improves cognition at a dosage of 500 mg in adolescent human males when given for 4 weeks (Bin Sayeed, et al. 2014). It produced anti-nitrosamine effects at 1 g/kg /day given intragastric in Wistar rats for 10 days (Ahlatci, et al. 2014). Hydro-alcoholic extract 100–400 mg/kg (p.o.) showed nootropic effect and decreased MDA concentration through anti-oxidation in rats when administered for 8 weeks (Beheshti, et al. 2016). Seed oil prevented hippocampal neural damage and it resulted in improvement in memory in experimental rats (Seghatoleslam, et al. 2016).

7.6.12 Anthelmintic Effect

Seed oil 0.5%–8% showed anthelminthic effect in *Ascaris suum* (Simalango and Utami, 2014).

7.6.13 Other Effects

N. sativa seeds at 250 mg/day are effective in seasonal allergic rhinitis with no side effects in 2 weeks (Ansari et al., 2010). Seed oil can be used as another option to the isotonic sodium chloride Seed oil can be used as another option to the isotonic sodium chloride in geriatric patients (Oysu et al., 2014), anti-diabetes mellitus potential (Heshmati and Namazi, 2015), oral health and hygiene (AlAttas et al., 2016).

7.7 BLACK CUMIN (*NIGELLA SATIVA*) AND ITS COMPONENTS HAVE DRUG INTERACTIONS

Drug interactions with other dietary supplements might be advantageous or dangerous. Black cumin, or *N. sativa*, has a number of favourable pharmacological, chemical, and biological interactions (Islam, et al. 2017).

Thymoquinone has got antagonistic interaction with doxycycline, omeprazole, cisplatin, collagen, co-trimoxazole, 5-flouorouracil, formaldehyde, OVA-antigen, garlic extract, oxytocin, oxytetracycline, antagonistic, paracetamol, streptozotocin, and tobramycin. Seed oil also acts as an antagonist to ethanol/NaOH/NaCl/indomethacin, erythromycin, Fe-NTA (ferric nitrilotriacetate), methicillin, methotrexate, methylene blue/diazepam, mupirocin, $NaNO_3$, nalidixic acid, nicotinamide, NO precursor/L-arginine, and seed extract for typhoid vaccine. However, thymoquinone acts as an agonist for curcumin/valproate ameliorate, cyclosporine A, 1, 2-dimethylhydrazine, and diesel exhaust particle.

An additive effect in patients when thymoquinone along with streptomycin, spectinomycin, and/or topotecan was reported. There is synergistic effect when given with doxorubicin, gentamycin, L-carnitine/α-lipoic acid, lincomycin, L-N (G)-nitroarginine methyl ester/N-acetylcysteine, parathormone, pilocarpine, and praziquantel. *Nigella* given with antibiotics decreases the bacterial resistance and increases the availability of amoxicillin.

7.8 CONCLUSION

Many beneficial effects have been found in oleoresin produced from black cumin seeds in various diseases. For millennia it has been demonstrated that black cumin seeds and their phytochemicals have been utilized to treat a variety of diseases. Black cumin oleoresin is a wonder medication as well as an essential flavouring agent when considering its economic value and therapeutic properties. In addition, the existence of several elements in black cumin oleoresin, which act primarily at distinct places, makes the black cumin oleoresin varied in its therapeutic efficacy. Medicinal plants are a gift from nature, and black cumin is one of the plants with amazing capabilities that need investigation for safer and more effective human medication. *N. sativa* seeds and oleoresin seem quite safe for human intake as shown by various studies. Black cumin oleoresin may be a cost-effective treatment for a variety of life-threatening illnesses, such as cancer and diabetes. However, more clinical and animal investigations are needed to rule out alternative effects and applications of black cumin oleoresin. COVID-19 is a persistent pandemic caused by SARS-CoV-2, a corona virus. Phytochemicals in home-grown remedies may be able to assist alleviate disease symptoms. *N. sativa* and its constituents have antiviral, antioxidant, immunomodulator, anti-inflammatory, antihistaminic, bronchodilator, and antitussive activities related to the causative organism and COVID-19 signs and symptoms, according to a number of randomized controlled trials, case reports, pilot studies, and in pre-clinical studies. Furthermore, active components of *N. sativa*, including nigellidine and α-hederin, have been discovered to be potential SARS-CoV-2 inhibitors. To treat COVID-19 patients, *N. sativa* can be utilized as an adjuvant therapy in addition to standard medications. However, randomized controlled trials are needed to confirm the potential effects of *N. sativa* as an alternative herbal treatment for COVID-19 patients.

REFERENCES

Abd Aziz, M. A. B. 2006 Extraction of nigella sativa using modern hydro distillation technique. Thesis: Faculty of Chemical and Natural Resources Engineering Technology University College of Engineering and Technology, Malaysia.

Adam, G. O., Rahman, Md. M., Lee, S.-J., Kim, G.-B., Kang, H.-S., Kim, J.-S., and Kim, S.-J. 2016 Hepatoprotective effects of Nigella sativa seed extract against acetaminophen-induced oxidative stress, *Asian Pacific Journal of Tropical Medicine*, 9(3): 221–227. https://doi.org/10.1016/j.apjtm.2016.01.039.

Adel A. H., Ahmed, M. A., Mohamed, S. E., Samir, M. H., and Enas, A. E. 2015 Therapeutic value of black seed oil in methotrexate hepatotoxicity in egyptian children with acute lymphoblastic Leukemia, *Infectious Disorders - Drug Targets*, 15(1): 64–71.

Ahlatci, A., Kuzhan, A., Taysi, S., Demirtas, O. C., Alkis, H. E., Tarakcioglu, M., Demirci, A., Caglayan, D., Saricicek, E., and Cinar, K. 2014 Radiation-modifying abilities of Nigella sativa and Thymoquinone on radiation-induced nitrosative stress in the brain tissue, *Phytomedicine*, 21(5): 740–744. https://doi.org/10.1016/j.phymed.2013.10.023.

Ahmad, A., Husain, A., Mujeeb, M., Khan, S. A., Najmi, A. K., Siddique, N. A., Damanhouri, Z. A., and Anwar, F. 2013 A review on therapeutic potential of Nigella sativa: A miracle herb, *Asian Pacific Journal of Tropical Biomedicine*, 3(5): 337–352. https://doi.org/10.1016/S2221-1691(13)60075-1.

Ahmad, S., and Beg, Z. H. 2016 Evaluation of therapeutic effect of omega-6 linoleic acid and thymoquinone enriched extracts from Nigella sativa oil in the mitigation of lipidemic oxidative stress in rats, *Nutrition*, 32(6): 649–655. https://doi.org/10.1016/j.nut.2015.12.003.

Al-Ali, A., Alkhawajah, A., Randhawa, M., and Shaikh, N. 2008 Oral and intraperitoneal LD50 of thymoquinone, an active principle of Nigella sativa, in mice and rats, *Journal of Ayub Medical College, Abbottabad: JAMC*, 20: 25–27.

AlAttas, S. A., Zahran, F. M., and Turkistany, S. A. 2016 Nigella sativa and its active constituent thymoquinone in oral health, *Saudi Medical Journal*, 37(3): 235–244. https://doi.org/10.15537/smj.2016.3.13006.

Al-Jassir, M. S. 1992 Chemical composition and microflora of black cumin (Nigella sativa L.) seeds growing in Saudi Arabia, *Food Chemistry*, 45(4): 239–242. https://doi.org/10.1016/0308-8146(92)90153-S.

Al-Saleh, I. A., Billedo, G., and El-Doush, I. I. 2006 Levels of selenium, dl-α-tocopherol, dl-γ-tocopherol, all-trans-retinol, thymoquinone and thymol in different brands of Nigella sativa seeds, *Journal of Food Composition and Analysis*, 19(2): 167–175. https://doi.org/10.1016/j.jfca.2005.04.011

Amini, M., Fallah Huseini, H., Mohtashami, R., Sadeqhi, Z., and Ghamarchehre, M. A. 2011 Hypolipidemic effects of Nigella sativa L. Seeds oil in healthy volunteers: A randomized, double-blind, placebo-controlled clinical trial, *Journal of Medicinal Plants*, 10(40): 133–138.

Ansari, A. A., Hassan, S., Kenne, L., Atta-Ur-Rahman, and Wehler, T. 1988 Structural studies on a saponin isolated from Nigella sativa, *Phytochemistry*, 27(12): 3977–3979. https://doi.org/10.1016/0031-9422(88)83062-0.

Ansari, M. A., Ansari, N. A., and Junejo, S. A. 2010 Montelukast versus nigella sativa for management of seasonal allergic rhinitis: A single blind comparative clinical trial, *Pakistan Journal of Medical Sciences*, 26(2): 249–254.

Arif, M., Thakur, S. C., and Datta, K. 2016 Implication of thymoquinone as a remedy for polycystic ovary in rat, *Pharmaceutical Biology*, 54(4): 674–685. https://doi.org/10.3109/13880209.2015.1072565.

Atta-ur-Rahman, Malik, S., Hasan, S. S., Choudhary, M. I., Ni, C.-Z., and Clardy, J. 1995 Nigellidine—A new indazole alkaloid from the seeds of Nigella sativa, *Tetrahedron Letters*, 36(12): 1993–1996. https://doi.org/10.1016/0040-4039(95)00210-4.

Beheshti, F., Hosseini, M., Vafaee, F., Shafei, M. N., and Soukhtanloo, M. 2016 Feeding of Nigella sativa during neonatal and juvenile growth improves learning and memory of rats, *Journal of Traditional and Complementary Medicine*, 6(2): 146–152. https://doi.org/10.1016/j.jtcme.2014.11.039.

Bin Sayeed, M. S., Shams, T., Fahim Hossain, S., Rahman, Md. R., Mostofa, A., Fahim Kadir, M., Mahmood, S., and Asaduzzaman, Md. 2014 Nigella sativa L. seeds modulate mood, anxiety and cognition in healthy adolescent males, *Journal of Ethnopharmacology*, 152(1): 156–162. https://doi.org/10.1016/j.jep.2013.12.050.

Boudiaf, K., Hurtado-Nedelec, M., Belambri, S. A., Marie, J.-C., Derradji, Y., Benboubetra, M., El-Benna, J., and Dang, P. M.-C. 2016 Thymoquinone strongly inhibits fMLF-induced neutrophil functions and exhibits anti-inflammatory properties in vivo, *Biochemical Pharmacology*, 104: 62–73. https://doi.org/10.1016/j.bcp.2016.01.006.

Co2 Black Cumin Oleoresins Manufacturer, SCFE Oils Supplier from India. (n.d.). Ozone Naturals. Retrieved October 16, 2021, from https://www.ozonenaturals.com/black-cumin-oleoresin.html

Datta, A., Saha, A., Bhattacharya, A., Mandal, A., Paul, R., and Sengupta, S. 2012 Black cumin (Nigella sativa L.) – A review, *Journal of Plant Development Sciences*, 4(1): 1–43.

Develi, S., Evran, B., Betül Kalaz, E., Koçak-Toker, N., and Erata, G Ö. 2014 Protective effect of Nigella sativa oil against binge ethanol-induced oxidative stress and liver injury in rats, *Chinese Journal of Natural Medicines*, 12(7): 495–499. https://doi.org/10.1016/S1875-5364(14)60077-7

Elkhateeb, A., El Khishin, I., Megahed, O., and Mazen, F. 2015 Effect of Nigella sativa Linn oil on tramadol-induced hepato- and nephrotoxicity in adult male albino rats, *Toxicology Reports*, 2: 512–519. https://doi.org/10.1016/j.toxrep.2015.03.002.

Erboga, M., Kanter, M., Aktas, C., Sener, U., Fidanol Erboga, Z., Bozdemir Donmez, Y., and Gurel, A. 2016 Thymoquinone ameliorates cadmium-induced nephrotoxicity, apoptosis, and oxidative stress in rats is based on its anti-apoptotic and anti-oxidant properties, *Biological Trace Element Research*, 170(1): 165–172. https://doi.org/10.1007/s12011-015-0453-x.

Fahmy, H. M., Noor, N. A., Mohammed, F. F., Elsayed, A. A., and Radwan, N. M. 2014 Nigella sativa as an anti-inflammatory and promising remyelinating agent in the cortex and hippocampus of experimental autoimmune encephalomyelitis-induced rats, *The Journal of Basic and Applied Zoology*, 67(5): 182–195. https://doi.org/10.1016/j.jobaz.2014.08.005.

Fallah Huseini, H., Amini, M., Mohtashami, R., Ghamarchehre, M. E., Sadeqhi, Z., Kianbakht, S., and Fallah Huseini, A. 2013 Blood pressure lowering effect of nigella sativa L. Seed oil in healthy volunteers: A randomized, double-blind, Placebo-controlled Clinical Trial. *Phytotherapy Research*, 27(12): 1849–1853. https://doi.org/10.1002/ptr.4944.

Gad, A. M., El–Dakhakhny, M., and Hassan, M. M. 1963 Studies on the chemical constitution of egyptian nigella sativa L. oil, *Planta Medica*, 11(2): 134–138. https://doi.org/10.1055/s-0028-1100226.

Ghasemi, H. A., Kasani, N., and Taherpour, K. 2014 Effects of black cumin seed (Nigella sativa L.), a probiotic, a prebiotic and a synbiotic on growth performance, immune response and blood characteristics of male broilers, *Livestock Science*, 164: 128–134. https://doi.org/10.1016/j.livsci.2014.03.014.

Gholamnezhad, Z., Rafatpanah, H., Sadeghnia, H. R., and Boskabady, M. H. 2015 Immunomodulatory and cytotoxic effects of Nigella sativa and thymoquinone on rat splenocytes, *Food and Chemical Toxicology*, 86: 72–80. https://doi.org/10.1016/j.fct.2015.08.028.

Gökce, E. C., Kahveci, R., Gökce, A., Cemil, B., Aksoy, N., Sargon, M. F., Kısa, Ü., Erdoğan, B., Güvenç, Y., Alagöz, F., and Kahveci, O. 2016 Neuroprotective effects of thymoquinone against spinal cord ischemia-reperfusion injury by attenuation of inflammation, oxidative stress, and apoptosis, *Journal of Neurosurgery: Spine*, 24(6): 949–959. https://doi.org/10.3171/2015.10.SPINE15612.

Gray, J. P., Zayasbazan Burgos, D., Yuan, T., Seeram, N., Rebar, R., Follmer, R. and Heart, E. A. 2016 Thymoquinone, a bioactive component of Nigella sativa, normalizes insulin secretion from pancreatic β-cells under glucose overload via regulation of malonyl-CoA, *American Journal of Physiology-Endocrinology and Metabolism*, 310(6): E394–E404. https://doi.org/10.1152/ajpendo.00250.2015.

Hamza, R. Z., and Al-Harbi, M. S. 2015 Amelioration of paracetamol hepatotoxicity and oxidative stress on mice liver with silymarin and Nigella sativa extract supplements, *Asian Pacific Journal of Tropical Biomedicine*, 5(7): 521–531. https://doi.org/10.1016/j.apjtb.2015.03.011.

Hariharan, P., Paul-Satyaseela, M., and Gnanamani, A. 2016 In vitro profiling of antimethicillin-resistant Staphylococcus aureus activity of thymoquinone against selected type and clinical strains, *Letters in Applied Microbiology*, 62(3): 283–289. https://doi.org/10.1111/lam.12544.

Heshmati, J., and Namazi, N. 2015 Effects of black seed (Nigella sativa) on metabolic parameters in diabetes mellitus: A systematic review, *Complementary Therapies in Medicine*, 23(2): 275–282. https://doi.org/10.1016/j.ctim.2015.01.013.

Heshmati, J., Namazi, N., Memarzadeh, M.-R., Taghizadeh, M., and Kolahdooz, F. 2015 Nigella sativa oil affects glucose metabolism and lipid concentrations in patients with type 2 diabetes: A randomized, double-blind, placebo-controlled trial, *Food Research International*, 70: 87–93. https://doi.org/10.1016/j.foodres.2015.01.030.

Huseini, H. F., Kianbakht, S., Mirshamsi, M. H., and Zarch, A. B. 2016 Effectiveness of topical nigella sativa seed oil in the treatment of cyclic Mastalgia: A randomized, triple-blind, active, and placebo-controlled clinical trial, *Planta Medica*, 82(04): 285–288. https://doi.org/10.1055/s-0035-1558208.

Hussein El-Tahir, K. E.-D., and Bakeet, D. M. 2006 The black seed nigella sativa linnaeus - a mine for multi cures: a plea for urgent clinical evaluation of its volatile oil, *Journal of Taibah University Medical Sciences*, 1(1, Supplement C): 1–19. https://doi.org/10.1016/S1658-3612(06)70003-8.

Islam, M., Guha, B., Hosen, S., Riaz, T., Shahadat, S., Sousa, L., Santos, J., Junior, J., Lima, R., Braga, A., Reis, A., Alencar, M., and Amélia, A. 2017 Nigellalogy: A review on nigella sativa, *MOJ Bioequivalence and Bioavailability* 3: 1–15. https://doi.org/10.15406/mojbb.2017.03.00056

Junemann, M., Luetjohann, S. 1998 Three great healing herbs: Tea tree, *St. Johns Wort, and Black Cumin*, Twin Lakes, WI: Lotus Light Publications.

Kamal, A., Ahmad, I., and Arif, J. 2010 Potential of Nigella sativa L. seed during different phases of germination on inhibition of bacterial growth, *E3 Journal of Biotechnology and Pharmaceutical Research*, 1(1): 9–13.

Khalife, R., Hodroj, M. H., Fakhoury, R., and Rizk, S. 2016 Thymoquinone from Nigella sativa seeds promotes the antitumor activity of noncytotoxic doses of topotecan in human colorectal cancer cells in vitro, *Planta Medica*, 82(04): 312–321. https://doi.org/10.1055/s-0035-1558289.

Khare C. P. 2004 Encyclopedia of Indian medicinal plants, *New York Springes-Verlag Berlin Heidelberg.*

Kolahdooz, M., Nasri, S., Modarres, S. Z., Kianbakht, S., and Huseini, H. F. 2014 Effects of Nigella sativa L. seed oil on abnormal semen quality in infertile men: A randomized, double-blind, placebo-controlled clinical trial, *Phytomedicine*, 21(6): 901–905. https://doi.org/10.1016/j.phymed.2014.02.006.

Mahdavi, R., Heshmati, J., and Namazi, N. 2015 Effects of black seeds (Nigella sativa) on male infertility: A systematic review, *Journal of Herbal Medicine*, 5(3): 133–139. https://doi.org/10.1016/j.hermed.2015.03.002.

Mahmoudvand, H., Sepahvand, A., Jahanbakhsh, S., Ezatpour, B., and Ayatollahi Mousavi, S. A. 2014 Evaluation of antifungal activities of the essential oil and various extracts of Nigella sativa and its main component, thymoquinone against pathogenic dermatophyte strains, *Journal de Mycologie Médicale*, 24(4): e155–e161. https://doi.org/10.1016/j.mycmed.2014.06.048.

Majdalawieh, A. F., and Fayyad, M. W. 2015 Immunomodulatory and anti-inflammatory action of Nigella sativa and thymoquinone: A comprehensive review, *International Immunopharmacology*, 28(1): 295–304. https://doi.org/10.1016/j.intimp.2015.06.023.

Manju, S., Malaikozhundan, B., Withyachumnarnkul, B., and Vaseeharan, B. 2016 Essential oils of Nigella sativa protects Artemia from the pathogenic effect of Vibrio parahaemolyticus Dahv2, *Journal of Invertebrate Pathology*, 136: 43–49. https://doi.org/10.1016/j.jip.2016.03.004.

Mohtashami, R., Fallah Huseini, H., Heydari, M., Amini, M., Sadeqhi, Z., Ghaznavi, H., and Mehrzadi, S. 2015 Efficacy and safety of honey based formulation of Nigella sativa seed oil in functional dyspepsia: A double blind randomized controlled clinical trial, *Journal of Ethnopharmacology*, 175: 147–152. https://doi.org/10.1016/j.jep.2015.09.022.

Muhammad T. S. 2009 Characterization of black cumin seed oil and exploring its role as a functional food. Faisalabad: University of Agriculture.

Nadaf, N. H., Gawade, S. S., Muniv, A. S., Waghmare, S. R., Jadhav, D. B., and Sonawane, K. D. 2015 Exploring anti-yeast activity of Nigella sativa seed extracts, *Industrial Crops and Products*, 77: 624–630. https://doi.org/10.1016/j.indcrop.2015.09.038

Omar, N. M. 2016 Nigella sativa oil alleviates ultrastructural alterations induced by tramadol in rat motor cerebral cortex, *Journal of Microscopy and Ultrastructure*, 4(2): 76–84. https://doi.org/10.1016/j.jmau.2015.12.001

Orhon, Z. N., Uzal, C., Kanter, M., Erboga, M., and Demiroglu, M. 2016 Protective effects of Nigella sativa on gamma radiation-induced jejunal mucosal damage in rats, *Pathology - Research and Practice*, 212(5): 437–443. https://doi.org/10.1016/j.prp.2016.02.017

Oysu, C., Tosun, A., Yilmaz, H. B., Sahin-Yilmaz, A., Korkmaz, D., and Karaaslan, A. 2014 Topical Nigella sativa for nasal symptoms in elderly, *Auris Nasus Larynx*, 41(3): 269–272. https://doi.org/10.1016/j.anl.2013.12.002

Periasamy, V. S., Athinarayanan, J., and Alshatwi, A. A. 2016 Anticancer activity of an ultrasonic nanoemulsion formulation of Nigella sativa L. essential oil on human breast cancer cells, *Ultrasonics Sonochemistry*, 31: 449–455. https://doi.org/10.1016/j.ultsonch.2016.01.035

Ramadan, M. F. 2016 Chapter 30—Black Cumin (Nigella sativa) Oils. In V. R. Preedy (ed.), *Essential Oils in Food Preservation, Flavor and Safety*, pp. 269–275. Academic Press. https://doi.org/10.1016/B978-0-12-416641-7.00030-4.

Sahebkar, A., Beccuti, G., Simental-Mendía, L. E., Nobili, V., and Bo, S. 2016 Nigella sativa (black seed) effects on plasma lipid concentrations in humans: A systematic review and meta-analysis of randomized placebo-controlled trials, *Pharmacological Research*, 106: 37–50. https://doi.org/10.1016/j.phrs.2016.02.008.

Salem, N. A., Mahmoud, O. M., Badawi, M. H. A., and Gab-Alla, A. A. 2016 Role of Nigella sativa seed oil on corneal injury induced by formaldehyde in adult male albino rats, *Folia Morphologica*, 75(4): 518–526. https://doi.org/10.5603/FM.a2016.0010

Seghatoleslam, M., Alipour, F., Shafieian, R., Hassanzadeh, Z., Edalatmanesh, M. A., Sadeghnia, H. R., and Hosseini, M. 2016 The effects of Nigella sativa on neural damage after pentylenetetrazole induced seizures in rats, *Journal of Traditional and Complementary Medicine*, 6(3): 262–268. https://doi.org/10.1016/j.jtcme.2015.06.003.

Shahraki, S., Khajavirad, A., Shafei, M. N., Mahmoudi, M., and Tabasi, N. S. 2016 Effect of total hydroalcholic extract of Nigella sativa and its n-hexane and ethyl acetate fractions on ACHN and GP-293 cell lines, *Journal of Traditional and Complementary Medicine*, 6(1): 89–96. https://doi.org/10.1016/j.jtcme.2014.11.018.

Simalango, D. M., and Utami, N. V. 2014 In-Vitro Antihelminthic effect of ethanol extract of black seeds (Nigella sativa) against ascaris suum, *Procedia Chemistry*, 13: 181–185. https://doi.org/10.1016/j.proche.2014.12.024.

Suguna, P., Geetha, A., Aruna, R., and Vijaiyan Siva, G. 2014. Nigella sativa Linn. Seed extract modulates the activity of ASC complex of NLRP3 inflammasome in rats subjected to experimental pancreatitis, *Biomedicine and Preventive Nutrition*, 4(2):113–120. https://doi.org/10.1016/j.bionut.2013.12.008.

Sultan, M., Butt, M., Anjum, F., Jamil, A., Akhtar, S., and Nasir, M. 2009. Nutritional profile of indigenous cultivar of Black cumin seeds and antioxidant potential of its fixed and essential oil, *Pakistan Journal of Botany*, 41: 1321–1330.

Sultan, M. T., Butt, M. S., Karim, R., Ahmad, A. N., Suleria, H. A. R., and Saddique, M. S. 2014. Toxicological and safety evaluation of Nigella sativa lipid and volatile fractions in streptozotocin induced diabetes mellitus, *Asian Pacific Journal of Tropical Disease*, 4: S693–S697. https://doi.org/10.1016/S2222-1808(14)60709-X.

Tajmiri, S., Farhangi, M. A., and Dehghan, P. 2016 Nigella sativa treatment and serum concentrations of thyroid hormones, transforming growth factor β (TGF-β) and interleukin 23 (IL-23) in patients with Hashimoto's Thyroiditis, *European Journal of Integrative Medicine*, 8(4): 576–580. https://doi.org/10.1016/j.eujim.2016.03.003.

Tissera, M., Chandrika, M., Serasinghe, P. and Tangavelu, R. 1997 Toxicity study of Kaluduru (oil of Nigella sativa), *Ayurveda Sameeksha*.

Zaoui, A., Cherrah, Y., Mahassini, N., Alaoui, K., Amarouch, H. and Hassar, M. 2002 Acute and chronic toxicity of Nigella sativa fixed oil, *Phytomedicine*, 9(1): 69–74. https://doi.org/10.1078/0944-7113-00084.

CHAPTER 8

Safety, Toxicity and Properties of Fennel Oleoresin

Vishakha Singh

Maharana Pratap University of Agriculture & Technology

Shweta Joshi

G.B. Pant University of Agriculture & Technology

CONTENTS

DOI: 10.1201/9781003186205-8

8.1 INTRODUCTION

India is among one of the recognized countries all over the world as "Home of Spices" for its exquisite quality of spices and medicinal plants (herbs). Both spices and herbs carry a wide range of pharmaceutical and physiological properties. Recently, medicinal herbs have gained popularity as compared to chemical drugs due to their fewer side effects and cost. These properties are well explored by biomedical research fields for development of nutraceutical and functional foods. The real amalgamation of both spices and herbs was started in India by Mughals in the 14th century. From then till now, Indian spices are known as the world's best spices. The by-products of spices and herbs have also been recognized worldwide for their wide application areas including meat processing, bakery, cosmetics and pharmaceuticals. Essential oil and oleoresins are some of the finest by-products explored worldwide for their therapeutic, culinary and pharmaceutical uses. Oleoresins are the resinous and concentrated product and show the complete profile of spices and herbs as compared to essential oil. Thus, they are designated as the true essence of spices. Oleoresins contain volatile and nonvolatile compounds. They are considered authentic extracts of spices, carrying their wholesome aroma and flavour. They are characterized by active compounds with high potency, thus are used in small doses. They are 8–20 times stronger in flavour than their respective spices. Therefore, oleoresins are the closest liquid extract of any spice. They are used at 0.1%–0.6% in the finished product.

Oleoresins obtained from the fennel plant are known as *Foeniculum vulgare* Mill. In the Middle Ages, fennel oleoresin was known as Fenkle, a name taken from Latin "foenum" which means "hay". In ancient times, it was believed that it gave longevity and strength and kept off the evil spirits. Fennel is one of the oldest and is one of the world's most dimensional condiments grown in arid and semiarid areas. Although it is considered indigenous to the Mediterranean Sea, it is of high economic importance due to its wide fields of application, especially its flavour. Fennel, as it is known globally, is an aromatic plant and belongs to the Apiaceae family. It is known as "Shmr" in Arabic, "Fenouil" in French, and "Razianeh" in French (Wesam, et al. 2015). In India, it has many local names. Some of them are mentioned here – Hindi: Motisaunf, Manipuri: Hop, Tamil: Sompu, Malayalam: Perumjeerakam, Telugu: Peddajilakarra, Kannada: Doddasompu, Bengali: Mauri and Sanskrit: Misreya, Madhurika. It is cultivated worldwide for its edible fruits and seeds. The dried fruit or the seeds of fennel are an important item of business. Various research studies have shown the efficacy of major phytochemical constituents present in fennel such as phenols and flavonoids to exhibit in vitro and in vivo medicinal properties such as anti-inflammatory, anti-pyretic, antithrombotic, anti-tumour, anti-mutagenic, anti-viral, hypoglycaemic and hypolipidemic properties (Barros, et al. 2010).

8.1.1 Uses of Fennel in Cookery

Fennel is a tremendously aromatic and flavourful condiment in cookery and medicative applications. The aroma of fennel seeds is similar to anise, and it's primarily used as flavouring agents in food, meat and fish dishes, alcoholic beverages, ice cream and herb/spice mixtures (Diaaz-Maroto, et al. 2005). The foliage, bulb and seeds of the fennel plant are extensively employed in numerous culinary cuisines across the globe. It is a major part of the Mediterranean cuisine, where its bulbs and leaves are used in raw and cooked forms in accompaniments, salads, pastas and vegetable dishes. Several cultures of the Indian sub-continent and the Middle East use fennel seeds in their cooking. Fennel is one of the major and widely used spices in Kashmiri Pandit and Gujarati cookery (Grieve, 1931).

8.1.2 Medicinal and Therapeutic Uses

Fennel has been reported to be antioxidant, antitumorous, chemopreventive, cytoprotective, hepatoprotective, hypoglycaemic and oestrogenic (Singh, 2008). It is mainly used as a purgative along with liquorice powder and also has carminative properties. To cure flatulence in infants, the custom of giving fennel water mixed with sodium bicarbonate and sweeteners as domestic "gripe water" exists in many cultures. Fennel tea, widely consumed as an antispasmodic, is prepared by pouring boiling water on a teaspoonful of bruised fennel seeds. The practice of eating raw fennel seeds, sometimes with a sweetener like table sugar, to improve digestion exists in the Indian subcontinent. Studies showed that the phytoestrogens present in fennel helps to promote the growth of breast tissue, thereby helping in milk secretion; traditionally this is considered one of the best galactagogues for lactating mothers (Agarwal, et al. 2008).

The main components of *F. vulgare* Mill. responsible for the medicinal and therapeutic properties are transanethole, fenchone, limonene, estragol and α-phellandrene (Figure 8.1). According to Bilia (2002), the relative concentration of these active components varies considerably due to the origin of the fennel and its phenological state. Agricultural practices, environment, ecological condition and genetics are major influencing factors affecting the yield and quality of the fennel oleoresins and their essential oils (Mona, et al. 2008).

The nutritional composition of fennel shows it to consist of moisture 6.3%, protein 9.5%, fat 10%, minerals 13.4%, fibre 18.5% and carbohydrates 42.3%. Major minerals and vitamins found in it are sodium, calcium, phosphorous, iron, potassium, thiamine, riboflavin, niacin and vitamin C. Its energy value is 370 (Bakhru, 1992). Volatile oil of fennel is a mixture of about a dozen of diverse chemicals and its main components are 40%–70% anethole (Bernath et.al. 1996), 1%–20% fenchone (Cosge, et al. 2008) and 2%–9% estragole (Raghavan, 2006).

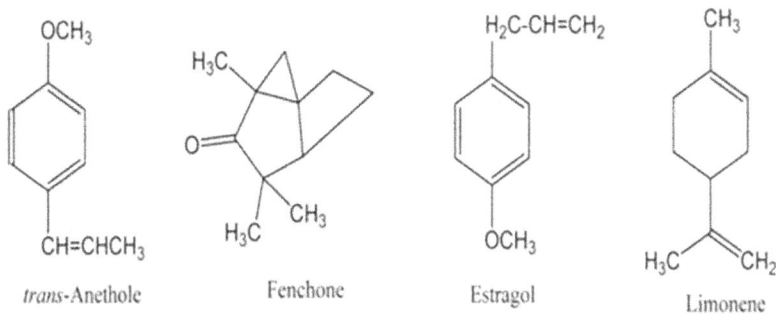

FIGURE 8.1   Major phytochemicals of fennel. (Miraldi, E. 1999. Comparison of the essential oils from ten Foeniculum vulgare Miller samples of fruits of different origin, *Flavour Fragrance Journal*, 14(6): 379–382.)

8.2 DISTRIBUTION, PRODUCTION AND ECONOMIC IMPORTANCE

The most common Indian name of Fennel is *Saunf.* Fennel is called "Marathon" by ancient Greeks as it is seen as a symbol of success in the battle which was fought and won by them in fennel field against Persians in 490 BC. In Rome, tender fennel shoots were used as food. In England, fennel was regarded as a royal spice during 13th century and was served alongside fruits to the kings.

It is widely cultivated throughout the world and the major growing countries are India, Germany, Russia, Romania, France, Italy and the United States. In India, the key fennel-producing states are Gujarat, Rajasthan, Karnataka, Maharashtra, Punjab, Uttar Pradesh and Bihar. Out of these Indian states, Rajasthan and Gujarat are major fennel producers. Both transplanting and direct sowing methods are used for the cultivation of fennel. It is a Rabi season (winter season) crop in India and is grown even at altitudes up to 6000 ft. Cold and dry weather is favourable for higher seed production with an optimum temperature of 15–20°C. But at the time of maturity, it needs a warm climate. In India, fennel is cultivated in about 1,00,000 ha area with the production to the tune of 1,43,000 MT and productivity of 1,430 kg/ha (Sharma, et al 2017).

The major importing countries of fennel are the United States, Vietnam, Middle East and East Asia. The area, production and export for fennel are given in Tables 8.1 and 8.2. It is native to Mediterranean region and south Europe which later spread to the east and north of Europe (Malhotra and Vashishtha, 2008). Fennel can be successfully cultivated on all types of soil except sandy soil. It grows well in loamy soil rich in lime and nutrients. The pH range of 6.5–8.0 is suitable for growth.

8.3 FENNEL OLEORESIN EXTRACTION METHOD

Extraction is the first step known for separation of the natural product that is desired from the raw materials. There are various extraction methods including steam distillation method, pressing, solvent extraction method and sublimation. Out of these, solvent extraction method is most commonly used.

TABLE 8.1　State-Wise Area and Production of Fennel in India

Major State	2016–17		2017–18		2018–19	
	Area (ha)	Production (Tons)	Area (ha)	Production (Tons)	Area (ha)	Production (Tons)
Gujarat	40910	87820	38130	79240	56416	117340
Rajasthan	45200	56240	24370	19950	30678	35290
Madhya Pradesh	1430	2520	1480	2720	1488	2760
West Bengal	1020	1020	1030	1050	1025	1050
Uttar Pradesh	690	760	730	800	708	790
Total (incl. others)	89540	148560	65810	103830	90392	157347

Source: Dheebisha, C. and Vishwanath, Y. C. 2020. Advances in cultivation of fennel. Journal of Pharmacognosy and Phytochemistry 2020; 9(2): 1295–1300.

TABLE 8.2   Major Importers of Fennel from India (2017–18)

Country	Quantity (MT)	Value (Rs. Lakhs)
Vietnam	18975.62	12245.42
USA	2314.59	2556.10
Malaysia	2298.54	1679.94
Saudi Arabia	1570.04	1193.80
UK	766.91	996.33
UAE	1183.52	967.62
Total (incl. others)	34550.00	25906.35

Source: Dheebisha, C. and Vishwanath, Y. C. 2020. Advances in the cultivation of fennel. Journal of Pharmacognosy and Phytochemistry 2020; 9(2): 1295–1300.

8.3.1 Solvent Extraction Method

Solvent extraction is the process based on relative solubilities of two different immiscible liquids. In this method, the difference in distribution coefficient and solubilities of two liquids that are immiscible when one compound transfers from one solvent to another are used as a method of extracting oleoresin. Solvent extraction method gives better separation results as compared to other methods of extraction used (Chen and Wang, 2017). If compared with the distillation method of separation, solvent extraction method is an easy and continuous process, uses less energy, has fast action, large capacity of production and has eased in automation. In simple words, solvent extraction is the act of removing or separating something which occurs over the course of two different immiscible phases. Through this method, a high amount of oleoresins can be obtained at a lower cost.

8.3.2 Major Steps in Solvent Extraction Method

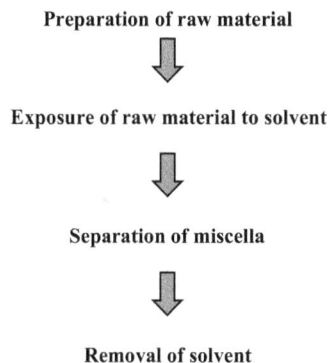

Preparation of raw material

⇩

Exposure of raw material to solvent

⇩

Separation of miscella

⇩

Removal of solvent

8.3.2.1 Preparation of Raw Material

It involves mainly two processes – cleaning and grinding of raw material. Cleaning is important for the quality of the product desired and to remove the hindrances affecting the separation process. Grinding ensures good solvent penetration. Smaller particle size results in high recovery of the desired material, but too fine particle size leads to slow percolation of solvent in the raw material and its difficult recovery.

8.3.2.2 Exposure of Material to the Solvent

There are three phases in this step, which are discussed in the following sections.

Addition of solvent to ensure even wetting of dry mass ⟹ **Allow absorption of solvent**

⟱

Continuous replacement of miscella with fresh solvent

8.3.2.3 Separation of a Miscella and Removal of Solvent

Fennel is a highly volatile compound, so low-temperature separation technique is used which help avoid loss and damage. High vacuum is used to reduce the side effect of high-temperature processing.

Vacuum evaporation is used for separating the solvent from micella. Vaporization from the surface of a liquid is called evaporation or vaporization of any liquid below its boiling point is called evaporation. This principle is used in vacuum evaporation method. In vacuum evaporation, pressure of the mixture is reduced below the vapour pressure of the solvent, causing it to evaporate at a lower temperature than normal, resulting in maximum up to 98% recovery of the desired compound.

8.4 ENCAPSULATION OF FENNEL OLEORESIN PRODUCTS

As oleoresins are liable to be damaged by light, heat, and oxygen (Shaikh, et al., 2006), they are encapsulated to be used in foods. Encapsulation is a common technique used to extend the shelf life of oleoresins obtained from herbs. For encapsulation, the first step involves preparing an oil-in-water emulsion that contains the encapsulating agent in the aqueous phase, which is then either spray dried or freeze-dried (Lim, et al. 2011). Encapsulation is of great significance and applicability in the food and flavouring industries due to its ability to protect sensitive food constituents against deteriorative reactions and loss of volatile compounds (Bringas-Lantigua, et al. 2011; Kadam, et al. 2011). Encapsulation is of utmost importance for fennel oil which is a well-known medical and spice herb. This kind of protective process is essential for its shelf stability and extended storage. In the processes of encapsulation, the appropriate encapsulating agent should be selected based on the physicochemical and drying properties of the agent. Along with the encapsulating agent (Gharsallaoui, et al. 2007), the process economics, the flavour release mechanisms, the expected product requirements for a specific application are considered very critical (Madene, et al. 2006).

Several encapsulating agents that belong to the categories of carbohydrate polymers, proteins, or lipids are available for applications in the food industry. Many encapsulating agents such as modified starch (MS), maltodextrin (MD), chitosan (CH) (Chranioti and Tzia 2012) and gum Arabic (Chranioti and Tzia 2014) have been tested in encapsulation of fennel oleoresin. Among all these, gum Arabic has been the most widely used agent as it is nontoxic, odourless, and tasteless, has tremendous emulsification capacity, low viscosity in aqueous solution, and very good volatile retention properties (Gabas et al., 2007). Many approaches have been focused on mixtures of different materials (Kaushik and Roos 2007).

8.5 CHEMISTRY AND PROPERTIES

Regarding its physico-chemical properties, it is pale yellow or light green in colour, soluble in water, and insoluble in oil, and its specific gravity is 0.953–0.975, optical rotation is 11.0–24.0, refractive index is 1.52800–1.54300 and flash point is 168.00 F. The oleoresin of fennel is obtained by the solvent extraction of its seeds. Fennel contains polyphenols, flavonoids, phytosterols, alkaloids, coumarins, tannins, as nonvolatile substances. The methanol extract is rich in flavonoids whereas its acetone extract has high amounts of polyphenol (Goswami and Chatterjee 2014). The nutritional composition of fennel includes carbohydrate (43%) protein (9.6%), fat (10%), fibre (18.4%) and minerals (13.8%) (Rather, et al. 2012). According to studies, among plant sources fennel contains high amounts of sodium, potassium, calcium and phosphorus. Fennel contains high level of nitrates which is considered a natural source of oestrogenic.

Fennel seeds contain 10%–12% of oil which is stored in its cotyledons. Oil obtained from fennel contain different fatty acids viz. linoleic acid (14%), palmitic acid (4%), petrocyclic acid (6%) and oleic acid (22%). According to Mimica (2003), the yield and qualitative composition of fennel essential oil and oleoresins depends upon the maturation stage of the plant and is significantly affected by the distillation method used. The essential oil of fennel contains 30 types of terpene compounds, the major one is anethole (80%) and other terpene compounds are limonene (5%) and fenshon (8%). These terpene compounds are responsible for various pharmacological and therapeutic effects (Salehi, 2006). Fennel is also rich in various flavonoids and phenolic compounds such as coumarin, tannin, hydroxycinnamic acids, rosmarinic acid, etc. Fennel essential oil and oleoresin are few of the major flavouring agents used in liquor, baking, cheese and cosmetic industry.

8.6 HEALTH AND MEDICINAL PROPERTIES OF FENNEL OLEORESINS

8.6.1 Antibacterial, Antimicrobial and Antifungal Properties

The fennel essential oil has been found effective against food-borne pathogens such as *Streptococcus aureus*, *Escherichia coli* and *Bacillus megaterium* (Mohsenzadeh, 2007). According to Mahady, et al. (2005), the oleoresins are also found effective against human pathogens like *Campylobacter jejuni* and *Helicopyroli*, whereas the antifungal property of *F. vulgare* essential oil is found against *Candida albicans*. The studies also suggest the synergistic activity of fennel oil and oleoresins with tetracycline and amoxicillin against strains of *B. subtilis* and *E. coli* (Akbar, 2018).

8.6.2 Anti-Inflammatory Activity

The anti-inflammatory activity of *F. vulgare* Mill. has been demonstrated by several studies. According to Wesam, et al. (2015), the inhibitory influence of fennel extract is due to lipoxygenase and cyclooxygenase pathways. The inhibitory effect also showed beneficial results in allergic reactions and various acute and subacute inflammatory conditions. Studies also suggest the decreased activity of superoxide dismutase and catalase enzymes responsible for causing oxidative damage in the body. It also helped in decreasing lipid peroxidation and was found to increase the plasma levels of HDL cholesterol in the body (Manzoor, et al. 2016).

8.6.3 Gastro and Hepatoprotective Activity

F. vulgare Mill. has significant gastroprotective effects. According to Alexandrovich, et al. (2003), the emulsion of fennel oil eliminated colic in 65% of infants. The fennel oil helps to reduce the mucosal lining of the stomach and showed a protective effect against gastric ulcer. These effects are attributed due to its antioxidant capacity. It has also been reported to possess a hepatoprotective effect. According to Ozbek et al. (2003), the hepatotoxicity created by carbon tetrachloride has been reduced by oleoresins of fennel by decreasing serum alkaline phosphatase (ALP) and bilirubin.

8.6.4 Heart Protective and Antidiabetic Effect

The hypolipidemic and anti-atherogenic effect of fennel l is well proved by various studies. It works by reducing the triglyceride level in fatty liver. It prevents the building up of fat deposits in arteries by facilitating the blood flow in coronary arteries (Wesam et al., 2015). The essential oil of fennel has anethole as a major component which works as an excellent antithrombotic effect by destabilizing clots and vasorelaxant and antiplatelet activity.

Various researches have also reported the hypoglycaemic effect of *F. vulgare*. Its continuous intake is also found in reducing the complications related to diabetes. El-Soud et al. (2011) in their study induced fennel essential oil in diabetic rats and the results showed hypoglycaemic effect by reducing the baseline value from 162.5 to 81.97 mg/dl.

8.6.5 Oestrogenic Activity

The oestrous inducing effect of various plant products came into light in 1926 owing to which medicinal properties of phytochemicals like saponins, isoflavonoids, flavonoids, essential oils, etc. have been isolated and extracted for the phytoestrogenic effect. According to Ostad, et al. (2001), fennel essential oil has been used for centuries as oestrous agent which is responsible for increasing milk secretion, facilitating birth, decreasing menstrual cramps and increasing sexual desire. Researchers have reported anethole (major component of fennel oil) polymers like dianthole and polyanthole as a causal agent for producing the desired effect (Lorand, et al. 2010).

8.6.6 Antioxidant Activity

Naturally occurring antioxidants have a major role to play in preventing oxidative stress damage in the human body, which, in turn, helps in preventing various degenerative diseases like cancer, diabetes, cardiovascular diseases, etc. Fennel contains a high amount of flavonoids and polyphenols owing to its high free radical scavenging activity thus known as an excellent source of antioxidant. Due to its high phenolic compounds, it has received the high attention of food scientists owing to its role in human health. Fennel by-products including its volatile oil also has strong antioxidant activity. According to Singh 2006, fennel oil showed high antioxidant activity in comparison to butylated hydroxytoluene and butylated hydroxyanisole (BHA). Diaz-Maroto, et al. 2005 also reported low antioxidant activity of ethanol extract of fennel as compared to its essential oil. This inhibitory mechanism of oil and ethanol extract was studied by monitoring peroxide accumulation in the emulsion during incubation using the ferric thiocyanate method (Manzoor, et al. 2016).

8.7 CLINICAL STUDIES ON TOXICITY AND SAFETY OF FENNEL OLEORESIN

Although herbal preparations show slight toxicity and side effects commonly, herbal preparations have been acknowledged as safe. Individual hypertoxicity of herbal preparations has been recognized as safe. Individual hypersensitivity is a common problem related to herbal preparations but it is controllable. The quantity of fennel that is consumed in food preparations is not noxious.

Various clinical studies suggest a certain level of toxicity of *F. vulgare*. According to Naga, et al. (2012), an oral dose of 3 g/kg of fennel extract was found nontoxic in mice but significant weight gain was observed in male mice after 90 days of administration, whereas Ostad, et al. (2001) in their study reported 1.32 g/kg as oral LD50 dose of essential oil in rats. Cuzzolin, et al. (2007) also stated potential drug–drug interaction in heart patients. Fennel intake increased the effect of Warfarin which increases the chances of bleeding.

Other preparations of fennel like its herbal tea have negligible antagonistic effects in therapeutic doses. But excess amount of fennel oil if consumed may cause nausea, vomiting and seizures.

Rather, et al. (2016) reported the growth of malignant tumours in mice. The compound responsible for this effect is estragole present in fennel. It is the major component of fennel oleoresin and oil. It becomes the basis to limit the use of this substance on recommendations given by the committee on the food of the European Union (Opinion of Scientific Committee 2001). To prove the genotoxicity and carcinogenicity of estragole in animals, a recent study was conducted by Paini, et al. (2010), whereas it was first proved by Drink water et al in 1976. The factor responsible for its carcinogenic effect is its metabolic activation leading to the formation of active free radicals and unstable molecules and damaging DNA, but its carcinogenicity is not proved in human samples. Side effects of anethole are also reported by Taylor (1964) causing mild lesions in rat liver if the dose administered is above 695 mg/kg. It has also shown teratogenicity above the concentration of 9.3 mg/mL.

Another compound, Bergapten (furanocoumarin), present in fennel essential oil also shows carcinogenic effect if exposed to the sun. Allergic reactions related to the skin and respiratory tract have been also reported but in rare cases. Fennel oil and oleoresins are not found safe for consumption by pregnant women due to their oestrogenic effects. Although a small amount if used as a spice is considered safe, its large doses cause uterine contraction. According to Shahmokhtar and Armand (2017), fennel is harmful in doses as small as 5 mL. Its seed oil can cause contact dermatitis in sensitive persons.

8.8 CONCLUSION

Fennel oleoresins have been found to have multidimensional uses in various sectors including pharmaceuticals, cosmetics, culinary, bakery, etc., which has increased its economic importance. Various studies have proved the health-promoting effects of fennel oleoresins due to the presence of various bioactive components. These bioactive components present in fennel oleoresins have been researched for treating various lifestyle diseases like diabetes, cardiovascular diseases and cancer. Due to its health-promoting effect, it is considerably attracting various nutraceutical industries for its potential use. The least side effects caused by using herbal ingredients or plant bioactive components has become the major reason for increasing their demand in various sector. Thus, there is a need to focus on the processing methods and preserving methods of fennel oleoresins so that its bioactive compounds remain intact and potent till its end use, and more studies and clinical trials should be done in this respect.

REFERENCES

Agarwal, R., Gupta, S.K., Agarwal, S.S., Srivastava, S. and Saxena, R. 2008 Oculohypotensive effects of *Foeniculum vulgare* in experimental models of Glaucoma, *Indian Journal of Physiology and Pharmacology*, 52: 77–83.

Akbar, S. 2018 "Fennel (Foeniculum vulgare Mill.): A common spice with unique medicinal properties, *Annals of Complementary and Alternative Medicine*, 1(1): 1–9.

Alexandrovich, I., Rakovitskaya, O., Kolmo, E., Sidorova, T. and Shushunov, S. 2003 The effect of fennel (*Foeniculum vulgare*) seed oil emulsion in infantile colic: a randomized, placebo-controlled study, *Alternative Therapies in Health and Medicine*, 9(4): 58–61.

Bakhru, H.K. 1992 *Herbs That Heal- Natural Remedies for Good Health*, Oriental Paperback: Vision Books Pvt. Ltd., New Delhi.

Barros, L., Carvalho, A.M., and Ferreira, C.F.R.I. 2010 The nutritional composition of fennel (*Foeniculum vulgare*): Shoots, leaves, stems and inflorescences, *LWT Food Science and Technology*, 43(5): 814–818.

Bernath, J., Nemeth, E., Kattaa, A., and Hethelyi, E. 1996 Morphological and chemical evaluation of Fennel (*Foeniculum vulgare* Mill.) population of different origin, *Journal of Essential Oil Research*, 8: 247–253.

Bilia, A.R., Flamini, G., Taglioli, V., Morelli, I. and Vincieri, F.F. 2002 GC–MS analysis of essential oil of some commercial Fennel teas, *Food Chemistry*, 76: 307–310.

Bringas-Lantigua, M., Exposito-Molina, I., Reineccius, G. A., Lopez-Hernandez, O., and Pino, J. A. 2011 Influence of spray-dryer air temperatures on encapsulated Mandarin oil, *Drying Technology*, 29: 520–526.

Chen, H., and Wang, L. 2017 *Post treatment Strategies for Biomass Conversion. In: Technologies for Biochemical Conversion of Biomass.* Elsevier Inc. pp. 197–217.

Chranioti, C., and Tzia, C. 2012 Binary mixtures of modified starch, maltodextrin and chitosan as efficient encapsulating agents of fennel oleoresin, *Food and Bioprocess Technology*, 6: 3238–3246. doi: 10.1007/s11947-012-0966-7.

Chranioti, C., and Tzia, C. 2014 Arabic gum mixtures as encapsulating agents of freeze-dried fennel oleoresin products, *Food and Bioprocess Technology*, 7: 1057–1065. doi: 10.1007/s11947-013-1074-z.

Cosge, B., Kiralan, M., and Gurbuz, B. 2008 Characteristics of fatty acids and essential oil from sweet fennel (*Foeniculum vulgare* Mill. var. dulce) and bitter fennel fruits (*F. vulgare* Mill. var. vulgare) growing in Turkey, *Natural Product Research*, 22: 1011–1016.

Cuzzolin, L., Francini-Pesenti, F., Zaffani, S., Brocadello, F., and Pengo, V. , Bassi, A., et al. 2007 Knowledge's about herbal products among subjects on warfarin therapy and patient-physician relationship: A pilot study, *Pharmacoepidemiology and Drug Safety*, 16(9): 1014–7.

Dheebisha, C. and Vishwanath, Y. C. 2020 Advances in cultivation of fennel, *Journal of Pharmacognosy and Phytochemistry*, 9(2): 1295–1300.

Diaaz-Maroto, M.C., Hidalgo, I.J.D., Saanchez-Palomo, E., and Pea rezCoello, M.S. 2005 Volatile components and key odorants of fennel (*Foeniculum vulgare* Mill.) and thyme (*Thymus vulgaris L.*) Oil extracts obtained by simultaneous distillation–extraction and supercritical fluid extraction, *Journal of Agriculture and Food Chemistry*, 53: 5385–5389.

Drinkwater, N.R., Miller, E.C., Miller, J.A., and Pitot, H.C. 1976 Hepatocarcinogenicity of estragole (1-allyl-4-methoxybenzene) and 1-hydroxyestragole in the mouse and mutagenicity of 1- acetoxyestragole in bacteria, *Journal of National Cancer Institute*, 57: 1323–1331.

El-Soud, N., El-Laithy, N., El-Saeed, G., Wahby, M., Khalil, M., and Morsy, F., et al. 2011 Antidiabetic activities of *Foeniculum vulgare* Mill. essential oil in streptozotocin-induced diabetic rats, *Macedonian Journal of Medical Science*, 4(2): 139–146.

Goswami, N. and Chatterjee, S. 2014 Assessment of free radical scavenging potential and oxidative DNA damage preventive activity of *Trachyspermumammil* (Carom) and *Foeniculum vulgare* Mill(fennel) seed extracts. *BioMed Research International*, 1–8.

Gabas, A. L., Telis, V. R. N., Sobral, P. J. A., and Telis-Romero, J. 2007 Effect of maltodextrin and arabic gum in water vapour sorption thermodynamic properties of vacuum dried pineapple pulp powder, *Journal of Food Engineering*, 82(2): 246–252.

Gharsallaoui, A., Saurel, R., Chambin, O., and Voilley, A. 2011 Pea (*Pisum sativum, L.*) protein isolate stabilized emulsions: a novel system for microencapsulation of lipophilic ingredients by spray drying, *Food and Bioprocess Technology*. doi: 10.1007/s11947-010-0497-z.

Grieve M. A. 1931 *Modern Herbal: the Medicinal, Culinary, Cosmetic and Economic Properties, Cultivation and Folk-lore of Herbs, Grasses, Fungi, Shrubs & Trees with their Modern Scientific Uses*. Brace & Company, Harcourt.

Kadam, M. L., Hashmi, S. I., and Kale, R. V. 2011 Studies on extraction of ginger oil and its microencapsulation, *Electronic Journal of Environmental, Agricultural and Food Chemistry*, 10: 2382–2390.

Kaushik, V., and Roos, Y. H. 2007 Limonene encapsulation in freeze drying of gum Arabic–sucrose–gelatin systems, *LWT- Food Science and Technology*, 40: 1381–1391.

Lim, H. K., Tan, C. P., Bakar, J., and Ng, S. P. 2011 Effects of different wall materials on the physicochemical properties and oxidative stability of spray-dried microencapsulated red-fleshed pitaya (*Hylocereus polyrhizus*) seed oil, *Food and Bioprocess Technology*, doi: 10.1007/s11947-011-0555-1.

Lóránd, T., Vigh, E. and Garai, J. 2010 Hormonal action of plant derived and anthropogenic nonsteroidal estrogenic compounds: Phytoestrogens and xenoestrogens, *Current Medicinal Chemistry*, 17(30): 3542–3574.

Mahady, G.B., Pendland, S.L., Stoia, A., Hamill, F.A., Fabricant, D., Dietz, B.M., Chadwick, L.R. (2005) In-vitro susceptibility of Helicobacter pylori to botanical extracts used traditionally for the treatment of gastro-intestinal disorders, *Phytotherapy Research*, 19: 988–999.

Malhotra, S.K. and Vashishtha, B.B. 2008 Package and Practices for production of seed spices, NRC on Seed Spices, Tabiji, Ajmer, p. 98.

Manzoor, A. R., Bilal, A. D., Shahnawaz, N. S., Bilal, A. B. and Mushtaq, A. Q. 2016 *Foeniculum vulgare*: A comprehensive review of its traditional use, phytochemistry, pharmacology, and safety, *Arabian Journal of Chemistry*, 9(2): 1574–1583.

Mimica-Dukic, N., Kujundzic, S., Sokovic, M. and Couladis, M. 2003 Essential oil composition and antifungal activity of *Foeniculum vulgare* Mill. obtained by different distillation conditions, *Phytotherapy Research*, 17(4): 368–71.

Miraldi, E. 1999 Comparison of the essential oils from ten *Foeniculum vulgare* Miller samples of fruits of different origin, *Flavour and Fragrance Journal*, 14(6): 379–382.

Mohsenzadeh, M. 2007 Evaluation of antibacterial activity of selected Iranian essential oils against Staphylococcus aureus and Escherichia coli in nutrient broth medium, *Pakistan Journal of Biological Sciences*, 10: 3693–3697.

Mona, Y., Kandil, M.A.M., Hend, M.F. and Swaefy, M.F. 2008 Effect of three different compost level on fennel and Salvia growth character and their essential oil, *Research Journal Agriculture and Biological Sciences*, 4: 34–39.

Naga, K. R., Anjaneyulu, N., Naga, G. M., and Sravya, N. 2012 Evaluation of anxiolytic activity of Ethanolic extract of *Foeniculum vulgare* in mice model, *International Journal of Pharmacy and Pharmaceutical Sciences*, 4: 584–586.

Ostad, S.N., Soodi, M., Shariffzadeh, M., Khorshidi, N., and Marzban, H. 2001 The effect of fennel essential oil on uterine contraction as a model for dysmenorrhea, pharmacology and toxicology study, *Journal of Ethnopharmacology*, 76(3): 299–304.

Ozbek, H., Ugras, S., Dulger, H., Bayram, I., Tuncer, I., Ozturk, G. and Ozturk, A. 2003 Hepatoprotective effect of *Foeniculum vulgare* essential oil *Fitoterapia*, 74: 317–319.

Paini, A., Punt, A., Viton, F., Scholz, G., Delatour, T., Marin- Kuan, M., Schilter, B., Van Bladeren, P.J., and Rietjens, I.M. 2010 A physiologically based biodynamic (PBBD) model for estragole DNA binding in rat liver based on in vitro kinetic data and estragole DNA adduct formation in primary hepatocytes, *Toxicology and Applied Pharmacology*, 245: 57–66.

Raghavan, S. 2006 *Handbook of Spices, Seasoning and Flavorings*. CRC Press Taylor and Francis Group, Boca Raton: New York

Rather, M.A., Dar, B.A., Sofi, S.N., Bhat, B.A., and Qurishi, M.A. 2016 *Foeniculum vulgare*: A comprehensive review of its traditional use, phytochemistry, pharmacology, and safety, *Arabian Journal of Chemistry*, 9: 1574–1583.

SalehiSurmaghi, H. 2006 Medicinal Plants and Phytotherapy. Donyaee Taghazie, Tehran, Iran, 59–63.

Shahmokhtar, M.K., and Armand, S. 2017 Phytochemical and biological studies of fennel (*Foeniculum vulgare* Mill.) from the south west region of Iran (Yasouj), *Natural Products Chemistry and Research*, 5: 4.

Sharma, S.K., Sharma, N.K. and Jakhar, R.R. 2017 Knowledge of recommended production technology of fennel cultivation by the farmers in Nagaur District of Rajasthan, India, *International Journal of Current Microbiology and Applied Sciences*, 6(3): 644–651.

Singh, G., Maurya, S., de Lampasona, M.P., and Catalan, C. 2006 Chemical constituents, antifungal and antioxidative potential of *Foeniculum vulgare* volatile oil and its acetone extract, *Food Control*, 17: 745–752.

Singh J. 2008 Spice and plantation crops, *Aavishkar Publishers and Distributors, Jaipur*, 58–60.

Taylor, J.M., Jenner, P.M., and Jones, W.I. 1964 A comparison of the toxicity of some allyl, propenyl, and propyl compounds in the rat, *Toxicology and Applied Pharmacology*, 6(4): 378–87.

Weiping, He and Baokang, H. 2011 A review of chemistry and bioactivities of a medicinal spice: *Foeniculum vulgare*, *Journal of Medicinal Plants and Research*, 5(16): 3595–3600

Wesam, K., Maryam, M., Sara, A.A., Naim, A.S., Majid, A.S., Damoon, A.L. 2015 Therapeutic and pharmacological potential of *Foeniculum vulgare* Mill: A review, *Journal of HerbMed Pharmacolgy*, 4(1): 1–9.

CHAPTER 9

Distribution, Production and Health Benefits of Ginger Oleoresin

Lisa F. M. Lee Nen That
RMIT University

Jessica Pandohee
Curtin University

CONTENTS

DOI: 10.1201/9781003186205-9

9.1 INTRODUCTION

Ginger, scientifically known as *Zingiber officinale* Roscoe, is a member of the Zingiberaceae family. As a perennial flowering plant, its distribution ranges mostly in tropical and subtropical countries (Shahidi and Hossain 2018). The underground stem, also known as the rhizome, has been used fresh, ground as a spice, or dried for the manufacture of oils and oleoresins (UNIDO and FAO 2005; Rasheed 2020). Its extensive application is mostly found in culinary and medicinal purposes, which makes it an important horticultural crop (Wannaprasert and Choenkwan 2021). Indeed, cultivation of ginger occurs in more than 35 countries. In 2019, production of ginger amounted to 4,081,374 tons globally and the top 10 producers were India, Nigeria, China, Nepal, Indonesia, Thailand, Cameroon, Bangladesh, Japan, and the Philippines (FAO 2021). Moreover, China was the top exporter with 537,826 tonnes followed by Thailand and the Netherlands.

The dried ginger rhizome is composed of fatty oils, proteins, carbohydrates, raw fibre, ash water and volatile oil. Ginger owes its pungent taste and aromatic flavour to the phenolic components found mostly in the essential oil and oleoresins (Wohlmuth et al., 2006; Panpatil et al., 2013; Mahboubi 2019). Maturity, location, processing methods and cultivar affect oleoresin and essential oil content (Bailey-Shaw et al., 2008; Kiran et al., 2013; EFSA Panel on Additives and Products or Substances used in Animal Feed (FEEDAP) et al., 2020). Ginger oleoresin is a viscous liquid obtained by solvent extraction and consists of essential oil and phenolic compounds, namely gingerols, shogaols and volatile compounds (Wohlmuth et al., 2006; EFSA Panel on Additives and Products or Substances used in Animal Feed (FEEDAP) et al., 2020). The most abundant component in oleoresin is gingerol (12.8% in the extract), and the total phenolic content of oleoresin was 52.4 ± 0.6 mg gallic acid equivalent (GAE) (Murthy, Gautam, and Naik 2015). However, gingerols content including 6-, 8- and 10-gingerol diminishes and converts to corresponding shogaols upon dehydration of ginger rhizome (Haniadka et al., 2012). This chapter provides an overview of the most recent findings regarding the extraction methods, characterisation and the applications of ginger oleoresin and its bioactive compounds.

9.2 EXTRACTION TECHNIQUES

Dry ginger is a primary product of ginger that is obtained by drying and grinding fresh ginger rhizomes. Ginger oleoresin is then produced from the extraction of powdered dry ginger together with a range of polar solvents such as alcohol and acetone or ethylene dichloride (Alfaro et al., 2003). The yield, flavour and pungency of the oleoresin depend on several factors, and these include the ginger cultivar used, ripeness of the rhizome, type of solvent used and the extraction techniques. Due to its economic importance in Asian countries and more recently in the health sector, several bodies of research have focused on the optimisation of oleoresin production in order to extract a wide range of bioactive compounds and flavour from ginger (Zancan et al., 2002; Elvianto Dwi 2011). In general, a yield of about 6.5% from the dry weight of ginger is considered within normal standards and can commercially contain up to 30% of volatile organic compounds.

Conventional purification methods in ginger manufacturing include active carbon stratum separation, macro-pore resin adsorption and solvent extraction (Cheng-Lun, Derong, and Le 2008). The latter has been the most common approach to extract the oleoresin from ginger as it is cheap and safe, but it is difficult and not efficient in producing refined oleoresin (Cheng-Lun, Derong, and Le 2008). Roy, Goto, and Hirose (1996) used supercritical carbon dioxide extraction and it has proven to be very efficient. However, specialised and costly technology is required, and therefore it is used in industrialised processes only. Moreover, the use of enzyme-assisted three-phase partitioning methods coupled with enzymes has been shown to result in increased efficiency in extraction of oleoresin and its phytochemical components (Varakumar, Umesh, and Singhal 2017). The bio-separation extraction takes advantage of partitioning of polar compounds, large molecules, such as proteins, and hydrophobic compounds followed by enzyme treatment. Other green technologies that have been developed are supercritical carbon dioxide (Said et al., 2015), ultrasound (Supardan et al., 2011), and enzymatic extractions (Nagendra chari et al., 2013).

9.3 CHARACTERISATION

To date, over 400 compounds, belonging to a wide range of chemical classes, such as phytochemicals, phenolic acid, organic acids and oil resins, have been detected at different concentrations in ginger (Feng et al., 2011). Of these, compounds unique to ginger showing bioactivity are gingerols, shogaols and zingerones. Ginger oleoresin consists mainly of gingerol (Murthy et al., 2015), however, the key pharmacologically active compound in ginger essential oil is 6-gingerol (Mahboubi 2019). One of the most comprehensive characterisations of ginger was carried out by Jiang et al. (2005), who identified 31 compounds with a gingerol moiety in methanol extracts of fresh ginger roots using liquid chromatography-electrospray ionisation tandem mass spectrometry in both positive and negative polarity modes. Some of the chemical classes they identified include gingerols, methyl-gingerols, gingerol acetates, shogaols, paradols, gingerdiols, mono- and diacetyl gingerols and dehydro-gingerdiones. Each class of ginger compounds exists as unbranched alkyl chain of increasing length. For instance, gingerol homologues exist as 4-, 6-, 8-, 10- and 12-gingerols, and shogaol homologues include 4-, 6-, 8-, 10- and 12-shogaols (Tao et al., 2009).

The flavour, aroma and taste of the ginger rhizome are highly attributed to the content of volatile organic compounds. The volatile compound classes include mono- and sesquiterpenes, camphene, beta-phellandrene, curcumin, cineole, geranyl acetate, terpineol, terpenes, borneol, geraniol, limonene, linalool, α-zingiberene, β-sesquiphellandrene, β-bisabolene and α-farnesene (Sivasothy, et al. 2011; Pang, et al. 2017). Yeh, et al. (2014) showed that there were more than 60 volatile organic compounds that contributed to the aroma and smell of ginger using gas chromatography mass spectrometry. The authors also reported the following as main volatile compounds present: camphene, sabinene, α-curcumene, zingiberene, α-farnesene, β-sesquiphellandrene, neral and geranial. Interestingly, while ginger essential oil consists of many volatile organic compounds, 30% has been characterised as zingiberene and other metabolites such as β-sesquiphellandrene and ar-curcumene are primary contributors to the gingery aroma. Although the volatile organic compounds make up less than 3% of the total content of ginger, they are highly potent, bioactive and contribute significantly to ginger's physical and chemical characteristics (Ekundayo, Laakso, and Hiltunen 1988).

9.4 CHEMISTRY AND PROPERTIES

Ginger is a spice known to be full of flavour and a source of "hotness" to food. The chemistry of ginger changes with its processing (whether it is a fresh rhizome, dried, powdered, extract or oleoresin). Therefore, ginger is a source of aroma and flavour due to the compounds present or that are being altered during cooking. The pungency of ginger is associated with gingerols, in particular 6-gingerol, which are volatile and highly labile, while zingiberene is responsible for its flavour. 6-Gingerol has a similar backbone to capsaicin and thus contributes to the spiciness and warmth of ginger. The use of heat, for instance during cooking, converts gingerols to zingerones and shogaols through a dehydration reaction. Zingerones and shogaols are less pungent than gingerols and therefore add a pleasant flavour to dishes (Table 9.1).

9.5 SAFETY AND TOXICITY

According to the US Food and Drug Administration (FDA), ginger, ginger essential oil and ginger oleoresin have been classified as "Generally Recognised as Safe" (GRAS) (Murthy, Gautam, and Naik 2015; U.S. Food and Drug Administration 2021). Ginger oleoresin is also non-toxic and was also considered to be safe as a remedy against nausea and vomiting during pregnancy as no adverse effects were incurred during pregnancy (Vilijoen, et al. 2014; Bodagh, Maleki, and Hekmatdoost 2018). Nevertheless, earlier studies have shown that ginger contained both mutagens and antimutagens, and among the bioactive compounds tested, 6-gingerol was a very strong mutagen (Nakamura and Yamamoto 1982, 1983; Soudamini, et al. 1995). However, the mutagenicity of 6-shogaol was 10^4 times lower, which implied that the hydroxylated aliphatic moiety was responsible for the mutagenicity of 6-gingerol. Further studies revealed that the mutagenicity is reduced in the presence of an antimutagen such as zingerone (Nagabhushan, Amonkar, and Bhide 1987).

Plants have numerous health benefits, and toxicity assays are important before examining the effectiveness of ginger and its compounds (Rahmani, Al shabrmi, and Aly 2014). The cytotoxicity of bioactive compounds has been examined in several studies. The 20% cytotoxic concentration (CC_{20}) for ginger essential oil was at 75.28 µg/mL in Madin-Darby bovine kidney (MDBK) cell line (Camero, et al. 2019). Chiaramonte et al. (2021) suggested that 6-gingerol could be toxic at high doses (50 & 100 µM) in sea urchins. At increasing doses, there is a rise in abnormal morphologies in embryos, and size of embryos was completely reduced at 100 µM of 6-gingerol. A maximum concentration of 300 µg/mL was not toxic to murine cells and instead exhibited anti-inflammatory effect (Liang, et al. 2018). The CC_{50} for 6-gingerol in human hepatocyte and lung adenocarcinoma was 0.2 mM (Halim, et al. 2021; Hayati et al., 2021). However, cytotoxicity of 6-gingerol could also differ across cell lines (Kumara et al., 2017; Mahomoodally et al., 2021). In a clinical study, administration of 5 mg of 6-gingerol (1.4% w/w of ginger extract) was considered to be safe for patients (Konmun, et al. 2017).

TABLE 9.1 List of Common Compounds That Have Been Characterised in Ginger

Compounds	Molecular Formula	Molecular Weight	Chemical Class	State at Room Temperature	Flavour Characteristics	Reference
4-Gingerol	$C_{15}H_{22}O_4$	266.3	Gingerol/Phenol	Solid		Jiang et al. (2005)
6-Gingerol	$C_{17}H_{26}O_4$	294.4	Gingerol/Phenol	Solid	Pungent	Yeh et al. (2014)
8-Gingerol	$C_{19}H_{30}O_4$	322.4	Gingerol/Phenol	Solid		Yeh et al. (2014)
10-Gingerol	$C_{21}H_{34}O_4$	350.5	Gingerol/Phenol	Solid		Yeh et al. (2014)
12-Gingerol	$C_{23}H_{38}O_4$	378.5	Gingerol/Phenol	Solid		Jiang et al. (2005)
Methyl-6-gingerol	$C_{18}H_{28}O_4$	308.4	Dimethoxybenzene	Solid		Jiang et al. (2005)
Methyl-8-Gingerol	$C_{20}H_{32}O_4$	336.4	Dimethoxybenzene	Solid		Jiang et al., 2005
Methyl-10-Gingerol	$C_{22}H_{36}O_4$	364.4	Dimethoxybenzene	Solid		Jiang et al. 2005
6-Shogaol	$C_{17}H_{24}O_3$	276.4	Shogaol/Phenol		Pungent, spicy-sweet	Yeh et al., 2014
8-Shogaol	$C_{19}H_{28}O_3$	304.4	Shogaol/Phenol			Yeh et al., 2014
10-Shogaol	$C_{21}H_{32}O_3$	332.5	Shogaol/Phenol			Yeh et al., 2014
12-Shogaol	$C_{23}H_{36}O_3$	360.5	Shogaol/Phenol			Yeh et al., 2014
6-Paradol	$C_{17}H_{26}O_3$	278.4		White powder	Spicy herbal aroma	Jiang et al. (2005)
1-Dehydro-6-Gingerdione	$C_{17}H_{22}O_4$	290.4				Jiang et al. (2005)
1-Dehydro-8-Gingerdione	$C_{19}H_{26}O_4$	318.4				Jiang et al. (2005)
1-Dehydro-10-Gingerdione	$C_{21}H_{30}O_4$	346.5				Jiang et al. (2005)
1-Dehydro-12-Gingerdione	$C_{23}H_{34}O_4$	374.5				Jiang et al. (2005)
Zingiberene	$C_{15}H_{24}$	204.35	Sesquiterpene			Jiang et al. (2005)
Camphene	$C_{10}H_{16}$	136.24	Terpene	Colourless crystalline solid	Mild, oil-camphoraceous aroma	JECFA (2006)
Sabinene	$C_{10}H_{18}O$	154.25			Terpineol odour	JECFA (2006)
α-Curcumene						
Zingiberene	$C_{15}H_{24}$	204.35	Sesquiterpene			JECFA (2006)
α-Farnesene	$C_{15}H_{24}$	204.35	Sesquiterpene	Colourless to pale-green liquid	Fruity aroma	JECFA (2006)
β-Sesquiphelladrene	$C_{15}H_{24}$	204.35	Sesquiterpene			JECFA (2006)
Geranial	$C_{10}H_{16}O$	152.23	Monoterpenoid	Yellow coloured liquid	Strong lemon smell	JECFA (2006)
α-Phellandrene	$C_{10}H_{16}$	136.23		Colourless to slightly yellow, mobile liquid	Peppery, woody, herbaceous aroma	JECFA (2006)
β-Phellandrene	$C_{10}H_{16}$	136.23				JECFA (2006)
Bisabolene	$C_{15}H_{24}$	204.35		Colourless slightly viscous oil	Pleasant, warm sweet-spicy-balsamic aroma	JECFA (2006)

9.6 APPLICATIONS

Ginger has been extensively studied for its nutraceutical value due to the high phenolic compound content in oleoresin (Semwal, et al. 2015; Kukula-Koch and Czernicka 2020). Biochemical and pharmacological properties of these phenolic compounds include anti-carcinogenic, antimutagenic, anti-apoptotic, antioxidant, anti-inflammatory, antipyretic, analgesic, cardio and hepatoprotective activities, which have had a positive effect on the different body systems (El Halawany, et al. 2017; Kim, et al. 2018). The antioxidant and anti-inflammatory activities have mostly contributed to the health applications of ginger oleoresin (Menon, et al. 2021). The antioxidant contents in ginger peel, unpeeled and peeled ginger extracts were $75.5\% \pm 0.7\%$, $73.01\% \pm 0.0\%$ and $51.01\% \pm 0.41\%$, respectively (Mbaeyi-Nwaoha, et al. 2013).

9.6.1 Effect on Cancer

Ginger is well known for its role in anticancer activity and both ginger extracts and their bioactive compounds have been extensively discussed (Mahomoodally, et al. 2021). In numerous studies examining different types of cancer *in vivo* and *in vitro*, the bioactive compounds have mostly reduced the growth of cancer cells in a dose-dependent manner and did not affect normal cells. This inhibition activity was possible due to their ability to modulate expression levels of compounds involved in apoptotic pathways.

6-Gingerol was reported to induce apoptosis and suppress tumours in several cancers (Rastogi et al. 2015). The metabolite inhibited growth and proliferation of three cervical cancer cell lines, namely HeLa (25.22%), CaSki (29.19%) and SiHa (35.48%) in both early and late apoptotic phases (Rastogi, et al. 2015). Treatment of 6-gingerol inhibited the proteasome involved in p53 degradation leading to reactivation of p53 apoptotic pathway. Furthermore, protein levels of p53 target genes including Bax, GADD45, Noxa, Puma and p21 were considerably diminished in 6-gingerol treated cells. 6-gingerol also bound to the β-5 subunit, which is specific for chymotrypsin activity and generated reactive oxygen species (ROS) in cancer cells. The DNA damage generated led to cell cycle arrest at G2/M cell cycle phases. The combined effect of 6-gingerol (50 μM) and cisplatin, a chemotherapeutic drug (2.5 μM), significantly enhanced the levels of ROS in cancer cells leading to increased oxidative stress. *In vivo* studies of 6-gingerol in HeLa xenografts in mice confirmed the above results tested *in vitro*.

The anticancer activity of 6-shogaol was also examined in HeLa cells as its inhibition on cell growth was dependent on increasing dosage (Liu, et al. 2012). Activation of caspase-3 and cleavage of downstream DNA repair enzyme PARP in 6-shogaols-treated cells led to a higher apoptosis rate (53%) than in control cells (8.8%). Cell cycle arrest occurred in G2 phase, and increasing levels of Annexin A1 promoted apoptosis and inhibition of the NF-κB. The anticancer role of 6-shogaol was further confirmed by Tan et al. (2013) as it inhibited proliferation in breast and colon cancer cells but not in normal cells. 6-Shogaol also showed more potency and was more selective at targeting cancer cells solely than 6-gingerol. This study established the role of 6-shogaol and provided further information on the mechanism of action. Cell cycle arrest was induced at the G2/M phase through the phosphorylation of Cdc2 and Cdc25C in both colon and breast cancer cells. Moreover, activation of caspase-3 and caspase-9 in a time-dependent manner (24, 48, 72 hours) led to apoptosis of the cancer cells. 6-Shogaol also suppressed the growth of all cell lines tested (leukaemia, colon cancer, melanoma, renal cancer, ovarian cancer, etc.) in the NCI-60 cell line panel. The 50% growth inhibition (GI_{50}) was between 100 nM and 10 μM. 6-Shogaol inhibited the NF-κB signalling pathway through the regulation of PPARγ signalling.

The anticancer activity of 6-, 8- and 10-gingerols was compared in mammary carcinoma cells (Bernard, McConnery, and Hoskin 2017), and they all inhibited the growth of both human and mouse mammary carcinoma cells. However, 8- and 10-gingerols showed higher potency than 6-gingerol. 8-Gingerol was more effective on human cell lines, namely MDA-MB-231 and MDA-MB-468 TNBC, while 10-gingerol showed more promising results on murine cell lines, namely 4T1 and E0771. The presence of longer unbranched alkyl side chains in 8-gingerol and 10-gingerol could allow better permeation in the tumour cell membrane. It was also reported that a different signalling pathway could be involved as 10-gingerol had no effect on p53 protein and inhibition of caspase 3. Ryu and Chung (2015) reported that proliferation of HCT116 human colon cancer cells was inhibited by 10-gingerol in a dose-dependent manner. The 50% inhibition concentration (IC_{50}) was 30 μM. It was suggested that 10-gingerol activated MAPK pathways, namely JNK, ERK and p38 leading to apoptosis. In a study looking at the effect of 10-gingerol in murine and human cell lines (4T1Br4, its isogenic line 4T1BM2, MDA-MB-231 and its brain-metastatic variant, MDA-MB-231BrM), the metabolite also inhibited metastasis to organs such as lung, bone and brain (Martin et al. 2017). However, the inhibition was mediated through a caspase-dependent apoptosis. The contradicting findings with Bernard, McConnery, and Hoskin (2017) could be due to differences in sensitivity of 10-gingerol among the cell lines used or the methodology employed. The two studies also differed in concentration of 10-gingerol required for MDA-MB-231 cells to accumulate in S-phase. Bernard, McConnery, and Hoskin (2017) suggested that treatment of 72 hour with a concentration of 200 μM would be effective, while Martin et al. (2017) found that the concentration rapidly led to apoptotic death in 4T1Br4 and MDA-MB-231BrM brain-metastatic variants. A recent study by Rasmussen, Murphy, and Hoskin (2019) suggested that 10-gingerol could have different effects in ovarian and breast cancer cells as there was no loss in cell viability when 10-gingerol (200 μM) was added to ovarian HEY cells for 24 hours.

Metabolites in ginger have also acted as adjuvant alongside chemotherapeutic drugs (Martin, et al. 2020). A recent study in breast cancer cells looked at the combined effect of 10-gingerol and doxorubicin, a chemotherapeutic drug (Martin et al., 2020). *In vitro* studies showed that their combined regimen had higher cytotoxic and synergistic effects on the cancer cells than doxorubicin alone. Both cell cycle arrest and cell death were induced by reducing the level of cyclin-dependent kinase. Inhibition of primary tumour growth and suppression of circulating tumour cells were observed in an orthotopic xenograft triple-negative breast cancer mouse model. The adjuvant activity of 10-gingerol was further confirmed as the combined regimen significantly reduced the tumour burden in all organs. Moreover, the metabolite suppressed some side effects caused by doxorubicin such as weight loss. The higher cholesterol levels and lipid rafts in cell membranes of cancer cells could promote the anticancer function of 10-gingerol (Mollinedo and Gajate 2020). These rafts are involved in regulating signalling pathways between the membrane and intracellular sites. Ediriweera, et al. (2020) reported that 10-gingerol suppressed the growth of MDA-MB-231/IR cells in dose- and time-dependent manner by targeting these lipid rafts. Moreover, the bioactive compound exhibited lesser toxicity to normal mammalian cells than docetaxel, a chemotherapeutic drug and also induced apoptosis through the PI3K/Akt signalling pathway.

9.6.2 Effect on Central Nervous System

Another health benefit of ginger that has been well-studied is the protective effect of its metabolites against Alzheimer's disease (AD), Parkinson's disease, epilepsy, and cerebral ischaemia (El Halawany, et al. 2017; Kim, et al. 2018; Han, Li, et al. 2019; Sapkota, Park, and Choi 2019; Ahmad et al. 2021; Rashid, et al. 2021). Moreover, it has been newly demonstrated that this protective effect was possible as 6-gingerol, 8-gingerol and 6-shogaol could penetrate the blood–brain barrier by passive diffusion (Simon, et al. 2020). In a study conducted by Kim, et al. (2018), scopolamine-induced mice treated with 6-gingerol improved memory impairment and cognitive dysfunction. Addition of 6-gingerol led to an increase in expression levels of BDNF which is involved in neurone survival. This was mediated by Akt/CREB pathway and CREB is a transcription factor which plays a role in neural functions. Han, Li, et al. (2019); Sapkota, Park, and Choi (2019) have demonstrated that bioactive compounds, namely 6-gingerol, 6-shogaol and 6-paradol exhibited anti-neuroinflammatory effect in mice induced with experimental autoimmune encephalomyelitis (EAE). A reduction in demyelination in the spinal cord, astrogliosis, microglial activation and lower levels of proinflammatory cells including IL-17 and TNF-α were observed. It was reported that 6-gingerol alleviated the severity of EAE by modulating the NF-κB and MAPK signalling. A study by El Halawany, et al. (2017) showed that gingerol had neuroprotective and anti-inflammatory effect in streptozotocin-induced mice exhibiting symptoms of AD. Gingerol improved cognitive, behavioural impairment and pathology in streptozotocin-induced mice. Moreover, the injection of gingerol suppressed the activity of Aβ-42, β-secretase, APH1a which are involved in amyloidogenic pathway and COX-2 and contribute to neuropathology of AD. Zingerone was reported to improve histological symptoms such as reduction in seizure activity, hippocampal damage in mice suffering from epilepsy (Rashid, et al. 2021). The metabolite demonstrated antioxidant and anti-inflammatory properties as it reduced neural cell death and suppressed proinflammatory cytokines such as TNF-α, IL-6, IL-1β by down-regulation of NF-κB. An increase in expression of Bcl-2 which generated an increase in neuron survival and a decrease in caspase-3-activated cells suggested that it regulated the mitochondrial intrinsic apoptotic pathway. The neuroprotective effect of 6-gingerol was observed in hypoxia-treated cells as it regulated the levels of miR-103/BNIP3 (Kang, et al. 2019). Cerebral ischaemia is a disorder in the CNS caused by ischaemia and hypoxia. 6-Gingerol reduced apoptosis and autophagy in these cells by up-regulating levels of miR-103 and down-regulation of BNIP3 by inhibition of p38 MAPK and JNK pathways. miR-103 is involved in ischaemic stroke angiogenesis, while Bcl2/adenovirus EIB 19kD-interacting protein 3 (BNIP3), which regulates autophagy and induces apoptosis, is associated with cerebral ischaemia.

9.6.3 Effect on Lipid Metabolism

The bioactive compounds have played a role in inhibition of adipogenesis. Addition of 6-gingerol (15 µg/mL) in 3T3-L1 cells reduced the intracellular lipid accumulation and inhibited differentiation of preadipocytes (Tzeng and Liu 2013). The reduction of protein levels of PPARγ, C/EBPα, FAS and aP2 was also observed as 6-gingerol was added in a concentration-dependent manner. Tzeng and Liu (2013) suggested that adipogenesis occurred through Akt signalling as phosphorylation of Akt in 3T3-L1 cells was observed upon treatment with 6-gingerol. Indeed, studies by H.H. Zhang, et al. (2009) have demonstrated that substrate GSK3β, a component in the Akt signalling pathway, could regulate PPARγ and C/EBPα, which, in turn, affects the regulation of FAS and aP2. These proteins are involved in adipogenesis and fatty acid synthesis. However, Suk et al. (2016) demonstrated that instead of 6-gingerol, 40 µM of 6-shogaol suppressed adipogenesis of 3T3-L1 preadipocytes by down-regulating the protein expression of PPARγ, C/EBPα and FAS. Moreover, 6-shogaol stimulates lipid breakdown. In other studies by Suk, et al. (2017), gingerenone A (40 µM) had the most potent inhibitory effect among a group of compounds including 6-gingerol, 8-gingerol and 10-gingerol and did not affect cell viability in MDI-induced adipogenesis. Moreover, gingerenone A inhibited lipid accumulation in preadipocyte cells in a dose-dependent manner by suppressing the protein expression levels of transcription factors involved in adipogenesis and lipogenesis. Adipocyte lipid accumulation is suppressed by regulation of fatty acid metabolism through AMPK activation. Activation of AMPK can be used to treat obesity as it inhibits anabolic pathways as well as promotes catabolic pathways. The oral administration of gingerenone A in high-fat diet mice attenuated their weight gain and led to a reduction of adipocyte size by AMPK activation in epididymal white adipose tissue. Gingerenone A suppressed adipocyte hypertrophy suggesting a possible role of gingerenone A in reducing inflammation in adipose tissue and macrophages. Moreover, the bioactive compound could protect against adipose tissue inflammation by inhibiting the recruitment of macrophage to adipocytes and reducing the expression levels of proinflammatory cytokine *TNF*.

9.6.4 Hepatoprotective Effect

Bioactive compounds in ginger oleoresin have demonstrated hepatoprotective activity on carbon tetrachloride and dimethyl nitrosamine-induced liver injuries in rats. Cheong et al. (2015) showed that administration of zingerone orally (10 mg/kg) suppressed abnormalities in liver histology such as necrotic areas and inflammatory cell infiltration. Moreover, the zingerone metabolite suppressed proinflammatory cytokines, such as TNF-α, IL-1β, which activate the NF-κB signalling pathway. This, is turn, regulated expression of inflammatory proteins including COX-2 and iNOS. Zingerone also protected against cell damage caused by *t*-BHP, a cytotoxic agent and reduced lipid peroxidation. There was a decrease in the phosphorylation of JNK, ERK and p38, which are usually activated by many cellular stressors such as oxidative stress. In a study by Khatri, et al. (2018), treatment with ginger oleoresin (300, 600mg/kg) in carbon tetrachloride–induced rats improved conditions including loss of body weight and liver swelling. Ginger oleoresin also reduced lipid peroxidation and oxidative stress by increasing the levels of antioxidant enzymes and markers such as superoxide dismutase, catalase and glutathione. Moreover, disruption of calcium homeostasis was restored, and ginger oleoresin protected the liver against pathological changes.

9.6.5 Gastroprotective Effect

Metabolites of ginger have exerted a positive effect on the digestive system as the accumulation of ginger usually occurs in the digestive tract (Bode and Dong 2011). Indeed, in a study by Wang, et al. (2011), the effect of ginger was tested on aspirin-induced gastric ulcers in rats. Ginger inhibited ulcer formation and protected against histopathological features such as distorted gastric glands and damaged mucosal epithelium in the rats. Ginger also restored nitric oxide level by reducing the iNOS activity to its normal level. Both 6-gingerol and 6-shogaol suppressed the activity of proinflammatory cytokines TNF-α and IL-1β. F. Zhang, et al. (2017) also demonstrated the therapeutic effects of 6-, 8-, 10- gingerols in rats suffering from colitis. The three metabolites (30 mg/kg/day) exhibited anti-inflammatory activity by reducing the levels of TNF-α and IL-1β. They also alleviated colitis symptoms and mucosal injuries and reduced oxidative stress. Zingerone was also reported to have a gastroprotective effect on ethanol-induced gastric ulcers in rats (Karampour, et al. 2019). The effect of zingerone was compared to ranitidine, a drug used for the treatment of peptic ulcers. Zingerone decreased the number of ulcers greatly as the dosage was increased (50, 100, 200 mg/kg). It also reduced lipid peroxidation and had free radical scavenging activity leading to a protective effect on gastrointestinal tract. Moreover, zingerone could play a role in the nitric oxide pathway as it restored the level of nitric oxide to its normal level.

9.6.6 Antibacterial, Antifungal, Antiviral and Anthelmintic Effects

Several studies have examined the antimicrobial effect of ginger oleoresin and have had inconsistent results. Mbaeyi-Nwaoha, et al. (2013) evaluated the antibacterial properties of ginger oleoresin obtained from ginger peels, peeled ginger and unpeeled extracts. The bacteria tested were *Escherichia coli*, *Staphylococcus aureus*, *Salmonella typhimurium*, *Aspergillus niger* and *Bacillus subtilis*. Although the inhibition zone for *B. subtilis* and *A. niger* and zone of inhibition increased in a dose-dependent manner (0.5–1.5 mL of oleoresin), the addition of ginger oleoresin was ineffective for *S. aureus*, *S. typhimurium* and *E. coli*. The authors suggested that the dose of oleoresin could be too low or the uneven diffusion of extracts through agar medium could lead to unequal contact with microorganisms. Other studies by Bellik (2014) reported that both ginger oleoresin and essential oil inhibited the growth of *E. coli*, *B. subtilis*, *S. aureus* and *Penicillium* spp. The minimum inhibitory concentration (MIC) for oleoresin and essential oil was 2 mg/mL and 869.2 mg/mL, respectively. Ginger oleoresin and essential oil were less effective against *Bacillus cereus* and *A. niger*. Murthy, Gautam, and Naik (2015) reported that oleoresin exhibited antimicrobial activity against foodborne bacteria, namely *E. coli*, *S. aureus*, *Pseudomonas aeruginosa*, *Listeria monocytogenes*, *B. cereus*, *Yersinia enterocolitica* and *B. subtilis*, and fungi, including *A. niger*, *Aspergillus flavus*, *Aspergillus oryzae*, *Aspergillus ochraceus*, *Fusarium oxysporum*, *Rhizopus oryzae* and *Penicillium chrysogenum*. The highest zone of inhibition for bacteria and fungi were *E. coli* (20 mm) and *F. oxysporum* (23 mm). The range of inhibition zone was 16–20 mm for bacteria and 13–23 mm for fungi.

Studies have also evaluated the antimicrobial activity of bioactive compounds. Park, Bae, and Lee (2008) demonstrated that out of the five bioactive compounds, namely 10-gingerol; 12-gingerol; 5-acetoxy-6-gingerol; 3,5-diacetoxy-6-gingerdiol; and galanolactone, only 10- and 12-gingerol were effective in inhibiting growth of periodontal bacteria such *Porphyromonas gingivalis*, *Porphyromonas endodontalis* and *Prevotella intermedia*. The MIC range was 6–14 µg/mL, and the minimum bactericidal concentration (MBC) was 4–14 µg/mL. The antibacterial activity of 10-gingerol was higher than 12-gingerol which could be due to the length and modification of alkyl side chains in gingerols. A study by Chiaramonte, et al. (2021) showed that 6-gingerol did not have any antimicrobial effect on *E. coli*, *B. subtilis* and *Micrococcus roseus*. Other studies suggested that zingerone could affect the virulence of *P. aeruginosa* (Kumar, et al. 2015). Indeed, zingerone suppressed the biofilm-forming capacity, the motility phenotypes and the production of virulence factors.

The inconsistent findings in the antibacterial effect of ginger oleoresin and its bioactive compounds could be due to many factors. Bellik (2014) argued that the botanical origin of plant material could affect the biological properties of the phytochemicals. Indeed, essential oil, oleoresin and 6-gingerol contents vary depending on maturity, location and cultivar (Bailey-Shaw, et al. 2008; Kiran, et al. 2013). Moreover, ginger oleoresin consists of different phenolic compounds, which adds to its complexity and renders it difficult to determine which compound may be conferring antibacterial activity.

Ginger has also demonstrated antifungal activities. A study by Hussein and Joo (2018) tested ginger essential oil for its antifungal effect and analysed six pathogenic fungi causing ginseng root rot disease, namely *Alternaria panax*, *Botrytis cinerea*, *Cylindrocarpon destructans*, *F. oxysporum*, *Sclerotinia sclerotiorum* and *Sclerotinia nivalis*. The MIC of ginger essential oil to suppress the growth of all fungi was 0.3% (v/v). The antifungal activity of ginger oleoresin also was investigated against *Pestalotiopsis microspora* in harvested Chinese olive (Chen, et al. 2018). Ginger oleoresin inhibited growth in a concentration-dependent manner ($EC_{50} = 2.04$ µL of ginger oleoresin per mL of propylene glycol, $EC_{90} = 8.87$ µL/mL). Inhibition of spore germination was also in a dose-dependent manner, and the 100% inhibition rate was achieved at a concentration of 8 µL of ginger oleoresin/mL propylene glycol. The addition of ginger oleoresin led to increase in cell membrane permeability and imbalance in intracellular and extracellular electrolytes. There was also a change in fatty acid composition as ginger oleoresin enhanced the degradation or peroxidation of unsaturated fatty acids which led to increased membrane fluidity.

The antiviral activity of ginger essential oil was also evaluated in MDBK cells against caprine alphaherpesvirus-1 (Camero, et al. 2019). Ginger essential oil inhibited viral activation at a concentration of 1396 and 139.6 µg/mL after 8 hours. It was suggested that time of contact was important for the inactivation of virus. Bioactive compounds such as 6-gingerol have also been evaluated for their antiviral activities. Halim, et al. (2021) reported that 6-gingerol exhibited antiviral activity in 4 dengue virus serotypes. The IC_{50} for DENV-1, DENV-2, DENV-3 and DENV-4 was 14.7, 14.17, 78.76 and 112.84 µM, respectively. The effect of 6-gingerol was also investigated on Chikungunya virus (Hayati et al., 2021). The findings suggested that 6-gingerol had limited virucidal activity but inhibited viral activity in a dose-dependent manner at 0.1 and 0.15 mM. The IC_{50} for post-treatment and full treatment of 6-gingerol was 0.038 and 0.031 mM, respectively, which suggested that 6-gingerol inhibited the virus by suppression of viral replication.

Ginger compounds are also effective in exhibiting anthelmintic activities. A study by Lin et al. (2010) investigated the effects of 6-gingerol, 10-gingerol, 6-shogaol, 10-shogaol and hexahydrocurcumin against *Angiostrongylus cantonensis*, a nematode parasite. They all exhibited 95–100% larvicidal activity in a dose-dependent fashion. 10-gingerol and hexahydrocurcumin suppressed mobility in the worm to a greater extent compared to the other ginger compounds or antiparasitic drugs such as mebendazole and albendazole. Lin et al. (2014) demonstrated that the bioactive compounds namely gingerenone A, 6-dehydrogingerdione, 6-gingerol, 10-gingerol, 5-hydroxy-6-gingerol, 4-shogaol, 6-shogaol, 10-shogaol, hexahydrocurcumin, 3R, 5S-6-gingerdiol and 3S, 5S-6-gingerdiol reduced mobility of oscillation (10%–100%) and peristalsis (35%–40%) against cestode *Hymenolepis nana*. 10-Shogaol and 10-gingerol exhibited the maximum lethal efficacy and the cestode experienced the greater loss of oscillation and peristalsis activity.

9.6.7 Effects on Cardiovascular System

Ginger and its metabolites have demonstrated their protective effect in several studies looking at cardiovascular diseases. Indeed, Ma, et al. (2021) showed that 6-gingerol alleviated the pressure and suppressed myofibroblast differentiation caused by cardiac remodelling in mice after they were subjected to transverse aortic constriction (TAC). Moreover, the metabolite exhibited anti-inflammatory properties by suppressing the production of pro-inflammatory cytokines, namely IL-6, TNF-α, and MCP-1. 6-Gingerol has a cardioprotective effect by modulating the MAPK p38 pathway. The metabolite also prevented cardiac complications in streptozotocin-induced diabetic rats (El-Bassossy, et al. 2016). It alleviated blood glucose levels and improved the cardiac dysfunction caused by diabetes. Research by Han, Zhang et al. (2019) demonstrated that 6-gingerol had a cardioprotective effect against ischaemia–reperfusion injury in rats which could be caused by excess Ca^{2+}. The administration of the metabolite caused a decrease in the L-type Ca^{2+} contractility in both normal and ischaemic ventricular myocytes by 58.17%±1.05% and 55.22%±1.34%, respectively. A decrease in the cell shortening (48.87%±5.44%) and the transients (42.5%±9.79%) were also observed.

Wang, et al. (2018) reported the potential of 6-gingerol as a therapeutic agent in the treatment of atherosclerosis. Apolipoprotein E-deficient mice suffering from atherosclerosis were subjected to chronic mild stress and 6-gingerol improved behavioural changes such as increased plaque formation, elevation of plasma total cholesterol and atherosclerotic lesions, reduced inflammation and regulated lipid metabolism through AMPK pathway.

9.6.8 Effect on Nausea and Vomiting

Ginger has a key role in alleviating nausea and vomiting and several clinical studies have examined the anti-emetic effect of ginger and its compounds. In a clinical trial conducted by Adib-Hajbaghery and Hosseini (2015), ginger essence had a positive effect on post-operative nausea and vomiting. The mean nausea intensity decreased after 1 hour post-surgery at every 30 min interval. Moreover, an increasing amount of ondansetron, a medication to alleviate vomiting and nausea was given to the control group. Lee and Shin (2017) examined the effectiveness of aromatherapy using ginger essential oil to alleviate nausea and vomiting in abdominal surgery patients. The level of nausea and vomiting was measured at 6, 12 and 24 hours post aromatherapy using Korean version of index of nausea, vomiting and retching. The scores for the test group were significantly lower and nausea and vomiting decreased remarkably in the first 6 hour. Another study by Sritoomma et al. (2014) compared the effect of Swedish massage with aromatic ginger oil and traditional Thai massage in older patients suffering from chronic low back pain. Previously, the two massages did not have any significant differences in a clinical trial and reduced the pain intensity considerably (Chatchawan, et al. 2005). However, addition of ginger essential oil to Swedish massage had a more noticeable effect than Thai massage in both the short-term and long-term period. The anti-emetic activity of 6-gingerol was demonstrated in a randomised, double-blind, placebo-controlled phase II study (Konmun, et al. 2017). Administration of 5 mg of 6-gingerol orally to patients who had highly emetogenic chemotherapy improved their appetite and quality of life. The metabolite also enhanced the overall complete response rate in patients receiving anti-emetic drug.

The mechanism by which ginger compounds alleviated nausea and vomiting has been investigated. Studies have suggested that ginger compounds may be targeting 5-HT3 receptors which are involved in nausea and vomiting caused by chemotherapy and post-operative surgery (Abdel-Aziz, et al. 2005; Abdel-Aziz, et al. 2006). Gingerol had a protective effect on rats and minks from chemotherapy-induced nausea and vomiting (Tian, et al. 2020). Pre-treatment with gingerol was shown to reduce the number of retching and vomiting in rats and minks in a dose-dependent manner for 72 hours. There was a reduction in the number of abnormal neurons in the area postrema and an increase in the content of Nissl granules. Gingerol also suppressed loss of villi, epithelial cells and inflammatory cell infiltration. The bioactive compound modulated the central and peripheral 5-HT system, substance P system and dopamine system by regulating the expression levels of the proteins involved, namely neurokinin-1 receptor, preprotachykinin, dopamine, dopamine D2 receptor, tyrosine hydroxylase, 5-HT and substance P. Further studies demonstrated that 6-gingerol, 6-shogaol and zingerone inhibited 5-HT responses in a dose-dependent manner (Walstab, et al. 2013; Jin, et al. 2014). They all had the ability to antagonise the 5-HT3 receptors non-competitively. This highlighted the role of ginger as an adjunct in massage therapy.

9.7 FUTURE SCOPE AND CONCLUSION

In recent years, there have been advances in research looking at health applications in ginger oleoresin and its metabolites. Some studies have supplemented information on the well-known benefits of ginger. Current progress has also highlighted the beneficial role of ginger oleoresin due to its pharmacological properties. Indeed, these properties such as antioxidant and anti-inflammatory activities have been observed in the different body systems.

These recent studies have not only given more insight into the health benefits but also raised new questions into the mechanism of action of ginger compounds, and potential benefits not yet explored. Further research is still necessary and the focus of health benefits in the previous section has been mostly focused on only a handful of metabolites. The complexity of ginger oleoresin renders it difficult to determine the pharmacological properties and the mechanisms of action of ginger in different body systems. Therefore, on-going research should look at determining whether lesser-known bioactive compounds could have other beneficial effects. Moreover, factors including the composition of fresh and dry ginger, differences in bioactivities in ginger products, molecular target of gingerols and shogaols and metabolism of each bioactive compound have affected the efficacy of bioactivities of ginger (Sang et al. 2020). These factors contribute to the inconsistent findings in clinical trials and other studies in determining the efficacy of ginger. For example, in the previous section, the antibacterial activity of ginger was still unclear, and in clinical trials, ginger products and dosage were not consistent. This emphasised the importance of understanding and identifying all the bioactive compounds. Moreover, standardisation of several factors such as the type of ginger, metabolite, and dosage for each health application would optimise and maximise the efficacy of ginger and its metabolites (Sang, et al. 2020).

REFERENCES

Abdel-Aziz, H.A., Nahrstedt, F., Petereit, T., Windeck, M., Ploch and Verspohl, E. J. 2005 5-HT3 receptor blocking activity of arylalkalanes isolated from the rhizome of *Zingiber officinale*, *Planta Medica*, 71: 609–616.

Abdel-Aziz, H.A., Windeck, T., Ploch, M. and Verspohl, E. J. 2006 Mode of action of gingerols and shogaols on 5-HT3 receptors: Binding studies, cation uptake by the receptor channel and contraction of isolated guinea-pig ileum, *European Journal of Pharmacology*, 530: 136–143.

Adib-Hajbaghery, M. and Hosseini, F. S. 2015 Investigating the effects of inhaling ginger essence on post-nephrectomy nausea and vomiting, *Complementary Therapies in Medicine*, 23: 827–831.

Ahmad, N., Ahmad, R., Amir, M., Alam, M.A., Almakhamel, M.Z., Ali, A., Ahmad, A., and Ashraf, K. 2021 Ischemic brain treated with 6-gingerol loaded mucoadhesive nanoemulsion via intranasal delivery and their comparative pharmacokinetic effect in brain, *Journal of Drug Delivery Science and Technology*, 61: 102130.

Alfaro, M., Jacqueline, J., Bélanger, M.R., Padilla, F.C. and Jocelyn Paré, J.R. 2003 Influence of solvent, matrix dielectric properties, and applied power on the liquid-phase microwave-assisted processes (MAP™) extraction of ginger (*Zingiber officinale*), *Food Research International*, 36(-5): 499–504.

Bailey-Shaw, Y. A., Williams, L. A. D., Junior, G. O., Green, C. E., Hibbert, S. L., Salmon, C. N. A. and Smith, A. M. 2008 Changes in the contents of oleoresin and pungent bioactive principles of Jamaican ginger (*Zingiber officinale* Roscoe.) during maturation, *Journal of Agricultural and Food Chemistry*, 56: 5564–5571.

Bellik, Y. 2014 Total antioxidant activity and antimicrobial potency of the essential oil and oleoresin of *Zingiber officinale* Roscoe, *Asian Pacific Journal of Tropical Disease*, 4(1): 40–44.

Bernard, M. M., McConnery, J. R. and Hoskin, D. W. 2017 (10)-Gingerol, a major phenolic constituent of ginger root, induces cell cycle arrest and apoptosis in triple-negative breast cancer cells, *Experimental and Molecular Pathology*, 102: 370–376.

Bodagh, M. N., Maleki, I., and Hekmatdoost, A. 2018 Ginger in gastrointestinal disorders: A systematic review of clinical trials, *Food Science & Nutrition*, 7: 96–108.

Bode, A. M., and Dong, Z. 2011 The amazing and mighty ginger. In Herbal Medicine: Biomolecular and Clinical Aspects, edited by I. F. F., Benzie and S., Wachtel-Galor. Boca Raton (Florida): CRC Press/ Taylor & Francis.

Camero, M., Lanave, G., Catella, C., Capozza, P., Gentile, A., Fracchiolla, G., Britti, D., Martella, V., Buonavoglia, C. and Tempesta, M. 2019 Virucidal activity of ginger essential oil against caprine alphaherpesvirus-1, *Veterinary Microbiology*, 230: 150–155.

Chatchawan, U., Thinkhamrop, B., Kharmwan, S., Knowles, J. and Eungpinichpong, W. 2005 Effectiveness of traditional Thai massage versus Swedish massage among patients with back pain associated with myofascial trigger points, *Journal of Bodywork and Movement Therapies*, 9: 298–309.

Chen, T., J. Lu, B. Kang, M. Lin, L. Ding, L. Zhang, G. Chen, S. Chen, and H. Lin. 2018. Antifungal activity and action mechanism of ginger oleoresin against *Pestalotiopsis microspora* isolated from Chinese olive fruits, *Frontiers in Microbiology*, 9: 2583.

Cheng-Lun, L., Tang, D., and Li, L. 2008 Research on the extracting and anti-oxidation dynamic characteristics of ginger oleoresin, *International Journal of Food Science & Technology*, 43(3): 517–525.

Cheong, K. O., Shin, D., Bak, J., Lee, C., Kim, K.W., Je, N.K., Chung, H.Y., Yoon, S. and Moon, J. 2015 Hepatoprotective effects of zingerone on carbon tetrachloride- and dimethylnitrosamine-induced liver injuries in rats, *Archives of Pharmacy Research*, 39: 279–291.

Chiaramonte, M., Bonaventura, R., Costa, C., Zito, F. and Russo, R. 2021 [6]-Gingerol dose-dependent toxicity, its role against lipopolysaccharide insult in sea urchin (*Paracentrotus lividus Lamarck*), and antimicrobial activity, *Food Bioscience*, 39: 100833.

Ediriweera, M. K., Moon, J.Y., Nguyen, Y.T., and Cho, S.K. 2020 10-gingerol targets lipid rafts associated P13K/Akt signaling in radio-resistant triple negative breast cancer cells, *Molecules*, 25: 3164.

EFSA Panel on Additives and Products or Substances used in Animal Feed (FEEDAP), Bampidis, V., Azimonti, G., Bastos, M.L., Christensen, H., Kos Durjava, M., Kouba, M., López-Alonso, M., López Puente, S., Marcon, F., Mayo, B., Pechová, A., Petkova, M., Ramos, F., Sanz, Y., Villa, R.E., Woutersen, R., Brantom, P., Chesson, A., Westendorf, J., Gregoretti, L., Manini, P., and Dusemund, B. 2020 Safety and efficacy of essential oil, oleoresin and tincture from Zingiber officinale Roscoe when used as sensory additives in feed for all animal species, *EFSA Journal*, 18(6): e06147.

Ekundayo, O., Laakso, I., and Hiltunen, R. 1988 Composition of ginger (Zingiber officinale roscoe) volatile oils from Nigeria, *Flavour and Fragrance Journal*, 3(2): 85–90.

El-Bassossy, H. M., Elberry, A.A., Ghareib, S.A., Azhar, A., Banjar, Z.M., and Watson, M.L. 2016 Cardioprotection by 6-gingerol in diabetic rats, *Biochemical and Biophysical Research Communications*, 477(4): 908–914.

El Halawany, A. M., El Sayed, N.S., Abdallah, H.M. and El Dine, R.S. 2017 Protective effects of gingerol on streptozotocin-induced sporadic Alzheimer's disease: Emphasis on inhibition of β-amyloid, COX-2, alpha-, beta - secretases and APH1a, *Scientific Reports*, 7: 2902.

Elvianto Dwi, D. 2011 Oleoresin from ginger using extraction process with ethanol solvent. *Jurnal Teknik Kimia UPN Veteran Jatim* 6(1).

FAO 2021 Crops. Accessed 9 May 2021. http://www.fao.org/faostat/en/#data/QC/visualize.

Halim, J. A. N., Halim, S.N., Denis, D., Haryanto, S., Dharmana, E., Hapsari, R., Sasmono, R.T., and Yohan, B. 2021 Antiviral activities of curcumin and 6-gingerol against infection of four dengue virus serotypes in A549 human cell line *in vitro*, *Indonesian Journal of Biotechnology*, 26(1): 41–47.

Han, J., Li, X., Ye, Z., Lu, X., Yang, T., Tian, J., Wang, Y., Zhu, L., Wang, Z. and Zhang, Y. 2019 Treatment with 6-gingerol regulates dendritic cell activity and ameliorates the severity of experimental autoimmune encephalomyelitis, *Molecular Nutrition and Food Research*, 63: 1801356.

Han, X., Zhang, Y., Liang, Y., Zhang, J., Li, M., Zhao, Z., Zhang, X., Xue, Y., Zhang, Y., Xiao, J. and Chu, L. 2019 6-Gingerol, an active pungent component of ginger, inhibits L-type Ca^{2+} current, contractility, and Ca^{2+} transients in isolated rat ventricular myocytes, *Food Science & Nutrition*, 7: 1344–1352.

Haniadka, R., Rajeev, A.G., Palatty, P.L., Arora, R., and Baliga, M.S. 2012 *Zingiber officinale* (Ginger) as an anti-emetic in cancer chemotherapy: A review, *The Journal of Alternative and Complementary Medicine*, 18(5): 440–444.

Hayati, R. F., Better, C.D., Denis, D., Komarudin, A.G., Bowolaksono, A., Yohan, B., and Sasmono, R.T. 2021 [6]-gingerol inhibits Chikungunya virus infection by suppressing viral replication, *BioMed Research International*, 2021: 6623400.

Hussein, K. A. and Joo, J.H. 2018 Antifungal activity and chemical composition of ginger essential oil against ginseng pathogenic fungi, *Current Research in Environmental & Applied Mycology*, 8(2): 194–203.

Jin, Z., Lee, G., Kim, S., Park, C., Park, Y.S. and Jin, Y. 2014 Ginger and its pungent constituents non-competitively inhibit serotonin currents on visceral afferent neurons, *Korean Journal of Physiology and Pharmacology*, 18: 149–153.

Kang, C., Kang, M., Han, Y., Zhang, T., Quan, W., and Gao, J. 2019 6-Gingerols (6G) reduces hypoxia-induced PC-12 cells apoptosis and autophagy through regulation of miR-103/BNIP3, *Artificial Cells*, 47(1): 1653–1661.

Karampour, N. S., Arzi, A., Rezaie, A., Pashmforoosh, M. and Kordi, F. 2019 Gastroprotective effect of zingerone on ethanol-induced gastric ulcers in rats, *Medicina*, 55: 64.

Khatri, R., Bhardwaj, K., Sharma, A., Tamang, S., Chettri, K.U. and Sharma, A. 2018 Evaluation of ginger oleoresin in carbon tetrachloride induced hepatotoxicity in rats, *Journal of Pharmaceutical Technology, Research and Management*, 6(2): 93–113.

Kim, C., Seo, Y., Lee, C., Park, G.H. and Jang, J. 2018 Neuroprotective effect and molecular mechanism of [6]-gingerol against scopolamine-induced amnesia in C57BL/6 Mice, *Evidence-Based Complementary and Alternative Medicine*, 2018.

Kiran, C. R., Chakka, A.K., Amma, K.P.P., Menon, A.N., Kumar, M.M.S. and Venugopalan, V. V. 2013 Influence of cultivar and maturity at harvest on the essential oil composition, oleoresin and [6]-gingerol contents in fresh ginger from Northeast India, *Journal of Agricultural and Food Chemistry*, 61: 4145–4154.

Konmun, J., Danwilai, K. Ngamphaiboon, N., Sripanidkulchai, B., Sookprasert, A. and Subongkot, S. 2017 A phase II randomized double-blind placebo-controlled study of 6-gingerol as an anti-emetic in solid tumor patients receiving moderately to highly emetogenic chemotherapy, *Medical Oncology*, 34: 69.

Kukula-Koch, W., and Czernicka, L. 2020 Gingerols and shogaols from food. In Handbook of Dietary Phytochemicals, edited by J., Xiao, S. D., Sarker and Y., Asakawa, 1–31. Singapore: Springer

Kumar, L., Chhibber, S., Kumar, R., Kumar, M. and Harjai, K. 2015 Zingerone silences quorum sensing and attenuates virulence of *Pseudomonas aeruginosa*, *Fitoterapia*, 102: 84–95.

Kumara, M., Shylajab, M. R., Nazeemc, P. A. and Babu, T. 2017 6-gingerol is the most potent anti-cancerous compound in ginger (*Zingiber officinale Rosc.*), *Journal of Developing Drugs*, 6(1): 1000167.

Lee, Y. R., and Shin, H.S. 2017 Effectiveness of ginger essential oil on post-operative nausea and vomiting in abodominal surgery patients, *The Journal of Alternative and Complementary Medicine*, 23(3): 196–200.

Liang, N., Sang, Y., Liu, W., Yu, W. and Wang, X. 2018 Anti-inflammatory effects of gingerol on lipopolysaccharide-stimulated RAW 264.7 cells by inhibiting NF-κB signaling pathway, *Inflammation*, 41(3): 835–845.

Lin, R., Chen, C., Chung, L. and Yen, C. 2010 Larvicidal activities of ginger (*Zingiber officinale*) against *Angiostrongylus cantonensis*, *Acta Tropica* 115: 69–76.

Lin, R., Chen, C., Lu, C., Ma, Y., Chung, L., Wang, J., Lee, J. and Yen, C. 2014 Anthelmintic constituents from ginger (*Zingiber officinale*) against *Hymenolepis nana*, *Acta Tropica*, 140: 50–60.

Liu, Q., Y. Peng, L. Qi, X. Cheng, X. Xu, L. Liu, E. Liu, and P. Li. 2012 The cytotoxicity mechanism of 6-shogaol-treated HeLa human cervical cancer cells revealed by label-free shotgun proteomics and bioinformatics analysis, *Evidence-Based Complementary and Alternative Medicine*, 2012.

Ma, S., Z. Guo, F. Liu, S. Hasan, D. Yang, N. Tang, P. An, M. Wang, H. Wu, Z. Yang, D. Fan, and Q. Tang. 2021 6-gingerol protects against cardiac remodeling by inhibiting the p38 mitogen-activated protein kinase pathway, *Acta Pharmacologica Sinica*.

Mahboubi, M. 2019 *Zingiber officinale* Rosc. Essential oil, a review on its composition and bioactivity, *Clinical Phytoscience*, 5: 6.

Mahomoodally, M. F., Aumeeruddy, M.Z., Rengasamy, K.R.R., Roshan, S., Hammad, S., Pandohee, S., Hu, X., and Zengin, G. 2021 Ginger and its active compounds in cancer therapy: From folk uses to nano-therapeutic applications, *Seminars in Cancer Biology*, 69: 140–149.

Martin, A. C. B. M., Fuzer, A.M., Becceneri, A.B., da Silva, J.A., Tomasin, R., Denoyer, D., Kim, S., McIntyre, K.A., Pearson, H.B., Yeo, B., Nagpal, A., Ling, X., Selistre-de-Araújo, H.S., Vieira, P.C., Cominetti, M.R., and Pouliot, N. 2017 10-gingerol induces apoptosis and inhibits metastatic dissemination of triple negative breast cancer *in vivo*, *Oncotarget*, 8(42): 72260–72271.

Martin, A. C. B. M., R. Tomasin, L. Luna-Dulcey, A. E. Graminha, M. A. Naves, R. H. G. Teles, V. D. da Silva, J. A. da Silva, P. C. Vieira, B. Annabi, and M. R. Cominetti 2020 10-gingerol improves doxorubicin anticancer activity and decreases its side effects in triple negative breast cancer models, *Cellular Oncology*, 43: 915–929.

Mbaeyi-Nwaoha, I. E., Ifeanyi, O.G., and Apochi, O.V. 2013 Production of oleoresin from ginger (*Zingiber officinale*) peels and evaluation of its antimicrobial and antioxidative properties, *African Journal of Microbiology Research*, 7(42): 4981–4989.

Menon, V., Elgharib, M., El-awady, R., and Saleh, E. 2021 Ginger: From serving table to salient therapy, *Food Bioscience*, 41: 100934.

Mollinedo, F., and Gajate, C. 2020 Lipid rafts as signaling hubs in cancer cell survival/death and invasion: Implications in tumor progression and therapy, *Journal of Lipid Research*, 61: 611–635.

Murthy, P. S., Gautam, R., and Naik, J.P. 2015 Ginger oleoresin chemical composition, bioactivity and application as bio-preservatives, *Journal of Food Processing and Preservation*, 39: 1905–1912.

Nagabhushan, M., Amonkar, A.J., and Bhide, S.V. 1987 Mutagenicity of gingerol and shogaol and antimutagenicity of zingerone in *Salmonella* microsome assay, *Cancer Letters* 36: 221–233.

Nagendra chari, K. L., Manasa, D., Srinivas, P. and Sowbhagya, H.B. 2013 Enzyme-assisted extraction of bioactive compounds from ginger (*Zingiber officinale* Roscoe), *Food Chemistry*, 139(1): 509–514.

Nakamura, H., and Yamamoto, T. 1982 Mutagen and anti-mutagen in ginger, *Zingiber officinale*, *Mutation Research Letters*, 103(2): 119–126.

Nakamura, H., Yamamoto, T. 1983 The active part of the [6]-gingerol molecule in mutagenesis, *Mutation Research*, 122: 87–94.

Pang, X., Cao, J., Wang, D., Qiu, J., and Kong, F. 2017 Identification of ginger (*Zingiber officinale* Roscoe) volatiles and localization of aroma-active constituents by GC-olfactometry, *Journal of Agricultural and Food Chemistry*, 65(20): 4140–4145.

Panpatil, V. V., S. Tattari, N. Kota, C. Nimgulkar, and K. Polasa. 2013 *In vitro* evaluation on antioxidant and antimicrobial activity of spice extracts of ginger, turmeric and garlic. *Journal of Pharmacognosy and Phytochemistry* 2 (3): 143–148.

Park, M., J. Bae, and D. Lee. 2008 Antibacterial activity of [10]-gingerol and [12]-gingerol isolated from ginger rhizome against periodontal bacteria. *Phytotherapy Research* 22: 1446–1449.

Rahmani, A. H., F. M. Al shabrmi, and S. M. Aly. 2014 Active ingredients of ginger as potential candidates in the prevention and treatment of diseases via modulation of biological activities. *International Journal of Physiology, Pathophysiology and Pharmacology* 6(3): 125–136.

Rasheed, N. 2020 Ginger and its active constituents as therapeutic agents: Recent perspectives with molecular evidences. *International Journal of Health Sciences* 14(6): 1–3.

Rashid, S., A. F. Wali, S. M. Rashid, R. M. Alsaffar, A. Ahmad, B. L. Jan, B. A. Paray, S. M. A. Alqahtani, A. Arafah, and M. U. Rehman. 2021 Zingerone targets status epilepticus by blocking hippocampal neurodegeneration via regulation of redox imbalance, inflammation and apoptosis. *Pharmaceuticals* 14: 146.

Rasmussen, A., K. Murphy, and D. W. Hoskin. 2019 10-gingerol inhibits ovarian cancer cell growth by inducing G2 arrest *Advanced Pharmaceutical Bulletin* 9(4): 685–689.

Rastogi, N., S. Duggal, S. K. Singh, K. Porwal, V. K. Srivastava, R. Maurya, M. L. B. Bhatt, and D. P. Mishra. 2015. Proteasome inhibition mediates p53 reactivation and anticancer activity of 6-Gingerol in cervical cancer cells. *Oncotarget* 6 (41): 43310–43325.

Roy, Bhupesh C., Motonobu Goto, and Tsutomu Hirose. 1996 Extraction of Ginger Oil with Supercritical Carbon Dioxide: Experiments and Modeling. *Industrial and Engineering Chemistry Research* 35: 607–612.

Ryu, M. J., and H. S. Chung. 2015 (10)-Gingerol induces mitochondrial apoptosis through activation of MAPK pathway in HCT116 human colon cancer cells. *In Vitro Cellular & Developmental Biology* 51: 92–101.

Said, P.P., O.P. Arya, R.C. Pradhan, R.S. Singh, and B.N. Rai. 2015 Separation of Oleoresin from Ginger Rhizome Powder Using Green Processing Technologies. *Journal of Food Process Engineering* 38 (2): 107–114.

Sang, S., H. D. Snook, F. S. Tareq, and Y. Fasina. 2020 Precision research on ginger: The type of ginger matters. *Journal of Agricultural and Food Chemistry* 68: 8517–8523.

Sapkota, A., S. J. Park, and J. W. Choi. 2019 Neuroprotective effects of 6-shogaol and its metabolite, 6-paradol, in a mouse model of multiple sclerosis. *Biomolecules & Therapeutics* 27 (2): 152–159.

Semwal, R. B., D. K. Semwal, S. Combrinck, and A. M. Viljoen. 2015 Gingerols and shogaols: Important nutraceutical principles from ginger. *Phytochemistry* 117: 554–568.

Shahidi, F., and A. Hossain. 2018. Bioactives in spices, and spice oleoresins: Phytochemicals and their beneficial effects in food preservation and health promotion. *Journal of Food Bioactives* 3: 8–75.

Simon, A., A. Darcsi, Á. Kéry, and E. Riethmüller. 2020 Blood-brain barrier permeability study of ginger constituents. *Journal of Pharmaceutical and Biomedical Analysis* 177: 112820.

Sivasothy, Yasodha, Wong Keng Chong, Abdul Hamid, Ibrahim M. Eldeen, Shaida Fariza Sulaiman, and Khalijah Awang. 2011 Essential oils of *Zingiber officinale* var. *rubrum Theilade* and their antibacterial activities. *Food Chemistry* 124 (2): 514–517.

Soudamini, K. K., M. C. Unnikrishnan, K. Sukumaran, and R. Kuttan. 1995 Mutagenicity and anti-mutagenicity of selected spices. *Indian Journal of Physiology and Pharmacology* 39 (4): 347–353.

Sritoomma, N., W. Moyle, M. Cooke, and S. O'Dwyer. 2014 The effectiveness of Swedish massage with aromatic ginger oil in treating chronic low back pain in older adults: A randomized controlled trial. *Complementary Therapies in Medicine* 22: 26–33.

Suk, S., G. T. Kwon, E. Lee, W. J. Jang, H. Yang, J. H. Kim, N. R. Thimmegowda, M. Chung, J. Y. Kwon, S. Yang, J. K. Kim, J. H. Y. Park, and K. W. Lee. 2017 Gingerenone A, a polyphenol present in ginger, suppresses obesity and adipose tissue inflammation in high-fat diet-fed mice. *Molecular Nutrition and Food Research* 61 (10): 1700139.

Suk, S., S. G. Seo, J. G. Yu, H. Yang, E. Jeong, Y. J. Jang, S. S. Yaghmoor, Y. Ahmed, J. M. Yousef, K. O. Abualnaja, A. L. Al-Maliki, T. A. Kumosani, C. Y. Lee, H. J. Lee, and K. W. Lee. 2016 A bioactive constituent of ginger, 6-shogaol, prevents adipogenesis and stimulates lipolysis in 3T3-L1 adipocytes. *Journal of Food Biochemistry* 40: 84–90.

Supardan, Muhammad Dani, Anwar Fuadi, Pocut Nurul Alam, and Normalina Arpi. 2011 Solvent extraction of ginger oleoresin using ultrasound. *Makara Sains* 15 (2): 163–167.

Tan, B. S., O. Kang, C. W. Mai, K. H. Tiong, A. S. Khoo, M. R. Pichika, T. D. Bradshaw, and C. Leong. 2013 6-Shogaol inhibits breast and colon cancer cell proliferation through activation of peroxisomal proliferator activated receptor γ (PPARγ). *Cancer Letters* 336: 127–139.

Tao, Yi, Wenkui Li, Wenzhong Liang, and Richard B. Van Breemen. 2009 Identification and quantification of gingerols and related compounds in ginger dietary supplements using high-performance liquid chromatography-tandem mass spectrometry. *Journal of Agricultural and Food Chemistry* 57 (21): 10014–10021.

Tian, L., W. Qian, Q. Qian, W. Zhang, and X. Cai. 2020 Gingerol inhibits cisplatin-induced acute and delayed emesis in rats and minks by regulating the central and peripheral 5-HT, SP, and DA systems. *Journal of Natural Medicines* 74: 353–370.

Tzeng, T., and M. Liu. 2013 6-Gingerol prevents adipogenesis and the accumulation of cytoplasmic lipid droplets in 3T3-L1 cells. *Phytomedicine* 20: 481–487.

UNIDO, and FAO. 2005 *Herbs, spices and essential oils.* FAO.

U.S. Food and Drug Administration. 2021. Food and Drugs. Accessed 11 May 2021 https://www.ecfr.gov/cgi-bin/text-idx?SID=dfc2dae5c6f384d423719ba6d29c7c1b&mc=true&node=se21.3.182_120&rgn=div8.

Varakumar, S., K. V. Umesh, and R. S. Singhal. 2017 Enhanced extraction of oleoresin from ginger (*Zingiber officinale*) rhizome powder using enzyme-assisted three phase partitioning. *Food Chemistry* 216: 27–36.

Vilijoen, E., J. Visser, N. Koen, and A. Musekiwa. 2014 A systematic review and meta-analysis of the effect and safety of ginger in the treatment of pregnancy-associated nausea and vomiting. *Nutrition Journal* 13 (1): 20.

Walstab, J., Krüger, D., Stark, T., Hofmann, T., Demir, I.E., Ceyhan, G.O., Feistel, B., Schemann, M., and Niesler, B. 2013 Ginger and its pungent constituents non-competitively inhibit activation of human recombinant and native 5-HT3 receptors of enteric neurons, *Neurogastroenterology & Motility*, 25: 439–e302.

Wang, S., Tian, M., Yang, R., Jing, Y., Chen, W., Wang, J., Zheng, X., and Wang, F. 2018 6-Gingerol ameliorates behavioral changes and atherosclerotic lesions in ApoE−/− mice exposed to chronic mild stress, *Cardiovascular Toxicology*, 18: 420–430.

Wang, Z., Hasegawa, J., Wang, X., Matsuda, A., Tokuda, T., Miura, N., and Watanabe, T. 2011 Protective effects of ginger against aspirin-induced gastric ulcers in rats, *Yonago Acta Medica*, 54: 11–19.

Wannaprasert, P., and Choenkwan, S. 2021 Impacts of the COVID-19 pandemic on ginger production: Supply chains, labor, and food security in Northeast Thailand, *Forest and Society*, 5(1): 120–135.

Wohlmuth, H., Smith, M.K., Brooks, L.O., Myers, S.P. and Leach, D.N. 2006 Essential oil composition of diploid and tetraploid clones of ginger (*Zingiber officinale* Roscoe) grown in Australia, *Journal of Agricultural and Food Chemistry*, 54: 1414–1419.

Zancan, K.C., Marcia, O.M., Marques, A.J., Petenate, J. and Meireles, M.A.A. 2002 Extraction of ginger (*Zingiber officinale* Roscoe) oleoresin with CO_2 and co-solvents: a study of the antioxidant action of the extracts, *The Journal of Supercritical Fluids*, 24(1): 57–76.

Zhang, F., Ma, N., Gao, Y., Sun, L., and Zhang, J. 2017 Therapeutic effects of 6-gingerol, 8-gingerol, and 10-gingerol on dextran sulfate sodium-induced acute ulcerative colitis in rats, *Phytotherapy Research*, 31: 1427–1432.

Zhang, H. H., Huang, J., Düvel, K., Boback, B., Wu, S., Squillace, R.M., Wu, C. and Manning, B.D. 2009 Insulin stimulates adipogenesis through the Akt-TSC2-mTORC1 pathway, *PLoS One*, 4(7): e6189.

CHAPTER 10

Applications of Garlic Oleoresin

Gargee Dey and Tridip Boruah

Madhab Choudhury College, Barpeta

CONTENTS

DOI: 10.1201/9781003186205-10

10.1 INTRODUCTION

Garlic (*Allium sativum*) belongs to the family Liliaceae and is close to the genus of onion. It is a perennial flowering plant, which is native to Central Asia. It is a monocot with flat leaves, long-beaked spathes and heads (Shree and Kumari 2019). Almost every cultivated *Allium* species has a chromosome number of 8. With low GC content and a large amount of repetitive sequence, garlic has 32.7 pg of DNA per 2C nucleus. Garlic has a very partial genetic variability, which further restricts the breeding availability of newer cultivars. Nowadays it is cultivated all over the world for its rich flavoured and high phytopharmaceutical value (Singha, et al. 2019). It has been reported, that allicin thiosulfinates is one of the main components in garlic that attributes to the biological function (Leontiev et al., 2018); the allicin is a viable compound and decays spontaneously. Commonly the Garlic species can be further classified into four groups: *Allium longicuspis, Allium ophioscorodon, Allium sativum, Allium pekinense* sub-group, and *Allium subtropical.* The *ophioscorodon* group is distributed in Central Asia, the *sativum* group is spread over the Mediterranean zone and the *subtropical* is distributed in the south and southeast of Asia and the *Pekingese* group is spread all over the east of Asia. In the year 1800, Bentham and Hooker classified Allium under the family Liliaceae, and tribe Alliaceae due to its superior ovary. In the year 1987, Taktajan placed this under the family order Amaryllidales, family Alliaceae, subfamily Alloideae and tribe Allieae. After molecular analysis of the plastid DNA of garlic, Klass, et al. (1998) established the phylogenetic positioning for the large subunit of ribulose-1–5-bis-phosphate carboxylase.

Garlic oleoresin extracted from *A. sativum* mainly possesses antimicrobial (Kyung, et al. 2002), anticancer (Mousa 2001) and antioxidant (Wu, et al. 2001) biological activities. It can also increase immunity (Kang, et al. 2001). Garlic is one of the oldest spices that humans are consuming for several thousand years (Block 2010). Some of the earliest references of the use of garlic oleoresin are in Avesta during the sixth century BC. During the early Olympics in Greece, it has been recorded that garlic oleoresin was supplied to the athletics in order to increase their stamina (Lawson and Bauer 1998). Ancient India and China recommended the medicinal use of garlic in curing respiration-related diseases. Seventy-six percent of the total production and supply of garlic is done by China, so a major part of garlic oleoresin also comes from this place.

10.2 DISTRIBUTION, PRODUCTION AND ECONOMIC IMPORTANCE

It is very important to comprehend and report the origin of a species to maintain its geographical authenticity. The garlic develops through sterile propagation of the clove by the cultivars and hence is morphologically similar. Vvedensky (1964) reported that all the domestic type of garlic has progressed from the wild type *Allium longicuspis* which is mainly confined to the Central region of Asia. Various techniques and experiments have been carried out in order to identify the geographical origin of garlic. High-resolution magic angle spinning-nuclear magnetic resonance (HRMAS-NMR) spectroscopy is based on the principle of metabolomics which analyses the component of the species biochemically and classifies the information of the sample (Jo, et al. 2020). An electronic nose system is developed concerning the principal component analysis to identify the origin of the species. This system is established by using Amplified Fragment Length Polymorphisms (AFLP) and GC-MS. High-resolution mass spectrometry is another method that helps to determine the origin by comparing the trace metal profile of the sample (Hrbek, et al. 2018). Stable isotopic composition using isotope ratio mass spectrometer (IRMS) is a highly sensitive analytical technique that distinguishes the geographical origin and reflects the cultivation environment (Ariyama, et al. 2006). RAPD technique is also used to compare the genetic variability and further classification of the origin of the species. For this technique, various species of garlic have been collected and the relatable potential was high in *Allium longicuspis* and *Allium ophioscorodon* (Manzum, et al. 2014). Graphite furnace atomic absorption and quadrupole ICPMS and inductively coupled plasma (ICP) emission is also used to study the phytogeographical origin of the species (Smith 2005). It has been reported that two botanical varieties have evolved from the wild type *A. ophioscorodon* and *A. sativum.* Due to climatic and environmental variation, these two types show evidence of a difference in shape, size, colour and the number of cloves, they have different maturation periods too. Few morphological similar traits have been found between them, which will further help in classifying their groups (Ovesná, et al. 2011). The phylogenetic relation between *A. longicuspis* and *A. sativum* is very complex, based on the relative level of variation. The secondary diversity of the garlic species was distributed to the Caucasus and Mediterranean in ancient times.

China is the largest garlic oleoresin producer with more than 66% of the total production. Every year India produces over 1.1 million metric tons of seasoning herbs containing garlic oleoresin. In India, although garlic is mainly cultivated in the northern part, reports suggest that Rajasthan has the highest amount of garlic oleoresin production followed by Gujarat and Orissa as per the statistics of 2018. Although garlic is mainly used to enhance the flavour of the food, the extracts from garlic are used as medicine for the treatment of many diseases. Garlic oleoresin is used in pharmaceutical industries in order to produce supplements. The USA is referred to as the world's largest garlic oleoresin importing country followed by Germany, Indonesia, Australia, France, and Brazil. Garlic extract and oil of garlic are widely used in pharmaceutical industries and also a broad range of researches are going on to produce modified better versions of the essential oil (Khezri, et al. 2021). Again, from an economical point of view, it is very important to extract oleoresin essential oil from the surplus garlic in order to minimize the wastage along with maximizing the valuation of raw garlic utilizing it as a very reliable source for income generation.

10.3 EXTRACTION TECHNIQUE

Garlic has a high content of organic as well as inorganic components that plays a crucial role in its medicinal as well as has nutritional value. Garlic oleoresin extracted from garlic has a wide array of therapeutic values. In order to extract the components, numerous techniques are being used. It has been found that garlic oleoresin mainly consists of organosulfur compound as a major component, particularly thiosulfinate allicin. The major preparation of garlic for the scientific studies is done from the raw garlic homogenate. After crushing or cutting the garlic, the allinase enzyme gets activated and reacts with the alliin, which remains intact in the inner side of the garlic to produce allicin (Lanzotti, et al. 2014). The major compounds that are present in the garlic oleoresin are S-allylcysteine and S-allylmercaptocysteine (Rabinkov, et al. 2000). Garlic oleoresin contains chemicals like dimethyl mono to hexa sulfides, diallyl, and allyl methyl. The extraction of garlic oleoresin is preceded by hydrodistillation of the raw garlic homogenate. As oil is nonpolar in nature, it does not get attracted to the polarity of the water and hence gets separated easily (Melgar-Lalanne, et al. 2017). To extract the solvent of garlic, there are various types of extraction procedures, broadly classified into the classical distillation solvent extraction of garlic oleoresins and the ultrasound-assisted extraction of garlic oleoresins. Dimethyl trisulfide (DMTS), methyl allyl trisulfide (MATS), diallyl trisulfide (DATS), 2-vinyl-[4H]-1,3-dithiin (2-VDT), and 3-vinyl-[4H]-1,2-dithiin (3-VDT) are some of the common compounds that are widely present in the garlic oleoresins (Rohani, et al. 2011). Few of the widely used extraction techniques of garlic oleoresins are described briefly.

10.3.1 Simultaneous Distillation Solvent Extraction (SDE)

This type of extraction is carried out through Lickens–Nickerson apparatus (in low-density configuration). Diethyl ether is taken as the solvent and deionized water is used to treat with the sample flask for each batch of garlic cloves. The micro-SDE is carried out for around 2 hours. The steam is then condensed with the solution of glacial water-glycol. The solvent is evaporated with a gentle nitrogen blowdown stream in order to evaporate the solvent and further determination of garlic oleoresin is carried out (Kimbaris, et al. 2006). GC analysis is conducted to assure the absence of the solvent. The remaining volatile oil is then weighed on an analytical scale.

10.3.2 Microwave-Assisted Hydrodistillation Extraction (MWHD)

This type of extraction is initiated by preparing a setup for a power household microwave oven that mainly consists of a steam condenser, flask, and a pressure-equalizing dropping funnel. Diethyl ether is taken as a solvent. Along with diethyl ether, deionized water is used to treat with the sample flask for each batch of garlic cloves (Yalavarthi and Thiruvengadarajan, 2013). For the isolation of the garlic oleoresin, distillation is carried out for 30 minutes at maximum power. By blow downing nitrogen, the solvent is evaporated from the extraction. A syringe filter is used in order to determine the yield of garlic oleoresin.

10.3.3 Ultrasound-Assisted Extraction (USE)

This extraction method is performed in an ultrasound-cleaning bath at a fixed frequency of 35 kHz against indirect sonication, and the temperature is maintained at 25°C. Diethyl ether is used to treat with the sample flask for each batch of garlic cloves. The sonication is continued for 30 minutes. The organic layer that is formed after the sonication is then transferred to the flask containing NaCl, and this method is repeated three times for the proper separation of extracted oil. Gas chromatography, HPLC, and liquid chromatography have also been used to extract and distinguish various chemical components present in the garlic oleoresins (Sadeghi, et al. 2016).

10.3.4 Encapsulation

Thiosulfinate allicin is mainly responsible for a wide range of bioactivities in oleoresins. However, allicin is a temperature-sensitive compound, and it gets decayed spontaneously at high temperatures (Shen, et al. 2002). The chemical compounds are being coated or entrapment within another carrier material, that is, encapsulation of the garlic bioactive compounds like wall material, membrane, carrier or shell to protect them next to unfavourable environmental conditions, such as heat, pH, light, oxygen moisture content, etc. The encapsulation techniques can be conducted through mechanical processes, chemical processes, and physicochemical processes (Otunola, et al. 2017).

10.4 CHARACTERIZATION

The characterization of garlic oleoresin extracts can be conducted through several structural, physiochemical, microscopic, spectroscopic and thermogravimetric means using techniques such as scanning electron microscopy (SEM), atomic force microscopy (AFM), transmission electron microscopy (TEM), Fourier transform infrared spectroscopy (FTIR), and thermogravimetric analysis (TGA).

10.4.1 Scanning Electron Microscopy (SEM)

SEM is used to study the morphology of the surface of oil extracts of garlic oleoresins. The powder obtained by molecular inclusion of garlic oleoresin using β-cyclodextrin presented irregular surfaces with different forms (Tavares, et al. 2019). The samples after placing at aluminium stub are then incubated at 60°C. With the help of a vacuum sputter coater, the specimen is coated with gold. Morphological changes such as cell elongation can be observed under SEM micrographs. SEM also helped in the analysis of whether lignin, hemicelluloses and other waxy compounds were replaced by $NaClO_2$ and further treated with alkali.

10.4.2 Atomic Force Microscopy (AFM)

The modern-day scientists prefer characterization techniques based on nanoemulsions because it provides a fair idea of all the active ingredients responsible for protection against degradation and oxidation of essential oils such as garlic oleoresins. Getting a clear image of interface morphology along with proper measurement of interfacial interaction systems of the droplets of nanoemulsions are also considered a crucial task for designing systems that are fully based on nanoemulsions (Ho, et al. 2021). Due to the loopholes in the traditional characterization techniques, the young researchers prefer AFM for the characterization of the challenging interface of garlic oleoresins.

10.4.3 Transmission Electron Microscopy (TEM)

TEM is used to investigate the size and division of the elementary compounds present in the garlic oleoresin. The liposomes present in the garlic oleoresin can also be identified with the help of TEM (Pinilla, et al. 2019). Condensation of cytoplasmic materials, structural integrity, and disintegrated membranes can be observed under TEM. This method is initiated by preparing a diluted nanoemulsion of garlic oleoresin which is then subjected to a carbon coating followed by staining with phosphotungstic acid. The sample is now kept to dry at 27°C, and now it is subjected to accelerating voltage of 80k and visualized under a transmission electron microscope.

10.4.4 Fourier Transforms Infrared Spectroscopy (FTIR)

Garlic oleoresin obtained from steam distillation can be studied with FTIR spectroscopy. The sulphur-containing compounds present in the oil such as methyl ally trisulphide and diallyl trisulphide were identified using this spectroscopic method. According to Rajam, et al. (2013), through FTIR, the protective film of Fe^{2+} on allicin can also be detected. Some precautions are recommended before using the instrument; it is needed to clean properly with the help of sterilized cotton which is soaked in acetone and n-hexane before drying the instrument to a level where obtaining background air spectrum will not be an issue to measure. The FTIR spectrum must be obtained in the 4000–6000 cm^{-1} region to get a proper graph from the garlic oleoresin extracts.

10.4.5 Thermogravimetric Analysis (TGA)

TGA is used to analyse the thermal property of fibre and cellulose of garlic oleoresin. The TGA mainly exhibits the degradation of fibres that initiates around the temperature of 100°C mainly responsible due to the evaporation of moisture from the extract. The formation of cellulose microfibers leads to an increase in the thermal stability of the garlic oleoresin (Reddy and Rhim 2018). One of the major advantages of this method is that it requires a very small amount of sample for analysis. Approximately 5 mg sample is needed to be heated up to 600°C from the existing room temperature conditions under the flow of nitrogen (50 cm^3/min) with a heating rate of not less than 10°C/min to acquire the thermogravimetric data.

10.5 CHEMISTRY AND PROPERTIES

Maximum compounds present in the garlic oleoresin are polar compounds because of their steroidal and phenolic origin. Sulphur-containing compounds, saponins, flavonoids, enzymes, and Maillard reaction products are the major ones. The blue-green colour of garlic clove after chopping, cooking, or pickling is mainly due to the excessive dominance of sulphur content in the garlic as the alliin reacts with amino acids and products into a cluster of carbon-nitrogen ring namely, pyrroles, links together, and form polypyrrole that further absorbs some precise wavelength of the light. The total flavonoid, phenolic compound, and phenolic acid present in garlic oleoresin is about 3.4 mg garlic acid equivalents (GAE)/g of dry weight to 10.5 mg (GAE)/g of dry weight; the two major types of phenolic acid present in garlic oleoresin is caffeic acid and ferulic acid (Beato, et al. 2011). Garlic oleoresin contains 31% carbohydrate, 5%–6% protein, and 0.2% fat, potassium (1.0–1.2 mg/g) phosphorous (3.9–4.6 mg/g), and calcium (0.5–0.9 mg/g) precisely. The sharp flavour of garlic oleoresin is due to the phytochemicals present in the cell, the crushing of the cloves leads to the breakdown of the cell and enzymes present in the cell vacuoles degrades resulting in strong taste and smell of the garlic (Jones, et al. 2004). The allicin, a lipid-soluble sulphur compound is responsible for the burning sense of heat in unprocessed garlic extracts containing oleoresin as it opens the transient receptor potential channel but the compound undergoes reaction and gets reduced when the temperature is increased, and hence after flavouring the garlic the burning sensation also decreases (Amarakoon, et al. 2017). The degrading allicin results in diallyl disulphide (DADS) and DATS, and these two compounds are responsible for the characteristic strong odour in garlic oleoresin. Garlic oleoresin as a whole contains 82% of sulphur content; the sulphur-containing compounds include ajoenes (E-ajoene, Z-ajoene), sulfides DADS, DATS, thiosulfinates, vinyldithiins (2-vinyl-(4H)-1,3-dithiin, 3-vinyl-(4H)-1,2-dithiin), etc. (Al-Snafi 2013). The main odoriferous molecules of garlic oleoresins are allicin and S-methyl cysteine sulfoxide (MCSO).

10.6 APPLICATION (HEALTH AND MEDICINAL PROPERTIES)

Garlic oleoresin is utilized in many ways due to its active biological activities including antidiabetic, renoprotective, antiatherosclerotic, antifungal, antibacterial, anticarcinogenic, antioxidant, and antihypertensive activities (Rahman and Lowe 2006; Davis 2005). Garlic oleoresin is also used in the cure of urinary and respiratory tract, indigestion, and cardiac disorders as it shows diuretic, aphrodisiac, antipyretic, and sedative effects (Gupta, 2010).

10.6.1 Antifungal Application

Garlic oleoresin exhibits a broad spectrum of fungal resistivity against *Aspergillus*, *Rhodotorula*, *Trichosporon*, *Cryptococcus*, etc. Pârvu, et al. (2019) stated that the garlic extract also provides resistivity against *Meyerozyma guilliermondii* and *Rhodotorula mucilaginosa* by inhibiting their growth and germination process. Petroleum ether, and methanolic and ethanolic compounds present in the garlic oleoresin provide resistivity against the human fungal pathogen, for example *Rhizopus stolonifer*, *Trichophyton mentagrophytes*, *Trichophyton verrucosum*, *Penicillium expansum*, *Candida* species, *Botrytis cinerea*, *Aspergillus niger*, and *T. rubrum* (Fufa 2019). The chemical compounds present in the garlic oleoresin attack the fungal cell wall, which results in irreversible ultrastructural changes in the cell of the pathogen and the germination ability gets affected. The cytoplasmic content is also affected leading to cell death.

10.6.2 Antibacterial Application

Allicin is one of the major components present in the garlic oleoresin that provides resistivity against a wide variety of microbial activity that includes both Gram-positive and Gram-negative bacteria, for example *Staphylococcus aureus*, *Streptococcus faecalis*, *Streptococcu mutans*, *Pseudomonas aeruginosa*, *Klebsiella aerogenes*, *Vibrio mycobacteria*, *Enterococcus faecalis* (Wallock-Richards, et al. 2014). The garlic oleoresin crude extract due to the presence of methanolic, ethanolic, and aqueous extract inhibits the growth of various degrees of susceptibility. According to Meriga, et al. (2012), the aqueous extract of garlic shows antibacterial activities toward the Gram-negative and Gram-positive strains. The garlic oleoresin also provides resistivity against intestinal bacteria, the main causative agent of diarrhoea in animals and humans. It also provides resistivity against the toxins produced by a bacterial infection (El-Saber Batiha, et al. 2020). The allicin interacts with the enzyme that contains thiol and by oxidizing protein cysteine or glutathione residues, it undergoes conformational changes and can inhibit the pathogenic activity in the host body.

10.6.3 Antiviral Application

The garlic oleoresin provides resistivity against vesicular stomatitis virus, human rhinovirus type 2, influenza B, human cytomegalovirus, Herpes simplex types 1 and 2, Parainfluenza virus type 3, and vesicular virus; garlic extraction contains many phytochemicals like ajoene, allyl methyl thiosulfinate, allicin, and methyl allyl thiosulfinate (Sawai, et al. 2008). The phytochemical allicin prevents adhesion interaction and fusion of leukocytes. DATS, present in garlic oleoresin, inhibits the viral replication and also inhibits the immediate early gene expression and further increases the activity of natural killer cell that will kill the virus cell.

10.6.4 Antioxidant and Anti-Inflammatory Applications

Repetitive ingestion of garlic oleoresin increases the inner antioxidant activities and reduces oxidative unfavourable effects (Asdaq, et al. 2011). It also provides resistivity against gentamycin, an antibiotic that endorses hepatic damage through increasing the aspirate transaminase and lowering the plasma albumin level (Wallock-Richard, et al. 2014).

The phytochemicals present in garlic oleoresin are also effective in possessing anti-inflammatory activities. Khodakaram-Tafti, et al. (2013) have stated that this phytochemical compound of garlic extract weakens the liver inflammation and damage caused by the pathogen *Eimeria papillata* infection. The emigration of neutrophilic granulocytes into epithelia can be inhibited by the anti-inflammatory application of garlic oleoresin (Hobauer, et al. 2000).

10.6.5 Anticancer Application

The garlic oleoresin inhibits cell growth, regulates carcinogenic metabolites, and reduces the anticancer agent by declining the invasion, angiogenesis, and migration. Gruhlke, et al. (2017) stated in their reports that in the year 1960, allicin solution, a derivative of oleoresin, has the ability to kill the tumour cells if dipped into it. Allicin also has the ability to restrain colorectal cancer metastasis by increasing immunity by resisting the formation of tumour cells. It can also suppress cancer cell proliferation by inverting gene silencing (Chhabria and Desai, 2018). Garlic oleoresin has the ability to decrease the propagation of colon, breast, stomach, lung and prostate types of cancer.

10.6.6 Effect on Diabetes Mellitus and Obesity

Medicinal derivatives of garlic oleoresin are effective against hyperlipidaemia and type II diabetes; they also have the ability to decrease cholesterol and blood sugar level. Cysteine sulfoxide, allyl propyl disulphide, and allicin suppress the glucose level in blood as these compounds enhance the secretion of insulin from the pancreas (Faroughi, et al. 2018).

Obesity nowadays is one of the major health problems that can result in cardiovascular disorder, hypertension, and metabolic syndrome. Garlic extracts including garlic oleoresin have the ability to reduce body weight by down-regulating the gene expressions and up-regulating the protein expression of the mitochondrial inner membrane. Anti-obesity is mainly achieved by stimulating the AMP-activated protein kinase and increasing of thermogenesis with the help of garlic extract (Lee, et al. 2011). Ajoene has the ability to achieve apoptosis, by decreasing the fat accumulation in adipocytes, due to which drastic declination in body weight is also observed.

10.7 SAFETY, TOXICITY, AND FUTURE SCOPE

Garlic extracts are being used safely in cooking as an accepted condiment and for flavouring reasons. Even though the US Food and Drug Administration (FDA) has reported that the presence of too many volatile compounds in the garlic extracts is harmless for human health, few experiments have shown positive results when looking for some side effects like vomiting, dizziness, tachycardia, insomnia, diarrhoea, sweating, etc. (Rana, et al. 2011). Due to its antithrombotic properties, raw garlic extracts containing oleoresin have negative effects on the pharmacokinetics of protease inhibitors. Garlic also has the ability to prolong the bleeding time so many doctors suggest stopping the intake of garlic-containing products 78–10 days prior to operation. Garlic oleoresin also has some cardiovascular effects such as irreversible antiplatelet activity, anticoagulant, fibrinolytic activity, and excessive decrement in the count of platelet (Borrelli, et al. 2007). Intake of allicin, a derivative of garlic oleoresin, at a concentration of more than 200 gm/mL causes cell damage in rat liver.

Due to the large genomic size of garlic, there is a major hindrance in the development of biological tools, tagging and mapping of genes for molecular studies. But since the last few years, new genetic tools have developed such as SSRs, RAPDs, AFLPs, and isozymes are some of the few markers that are being used in the mapping. In India, new researches are going on the extraction of garlic oleoresin from long day garlic, and it has been estimated that in the upcoming years, India will produce on an average 30 lakh tonnes of long day garlic (Gupta 2015). The research on essential oil is still in the infant stage in the Indian subcontinent, but looking at the high and ever-increasing demand for garlic oleoresin on the world stage, it is inevitable for the young researchers of this region to take this field of research seriously in the near future.

10.8 CONCLUSION

Garlic is one of the oldest authenticated herbaceous, aromatic spices which is broadly spread all over the world. It is mainly grown in mild climates and needs to be drained of loamy soil to grow. It is estimated that the origin of the species is from the Central part of Asia. China produces more than 50% of the world's total production of garlic. Garlic oleoresins contain a high amount of organosulfur, saponins, flavonoids, enzymes, etc., which plays an essential role in nutritional as well as medicinal value. The main sulphur-containing compounds present in garlic oleoresins are allicin, ajoenes, DADS, DATS, etc. The chemicals are characterized by using SEM, AFM, TEM, FTIR, and TGA. The chemicals can be extracted by various technologies like SDE, MWHD, USE, chromatography, etc. Garlic oleoresin has s high therapeutic index. It has the ability to provide resistance against bacteria, fungus, viruses, diabetes, obesity, cancer, cardiovascular disease, and so on. A high intake of garlic-derived products including garlic oleoresin can lead to several diseases and has many side effects too. Nowadays, many researches are going on in order to improve the quality of garlic and also to introduce new breeding variants for the production of high-quality garlic oleoresin.

REFERENCES

Al-Snafi, A.E. 2013 Pharmacological effects of Allium species grown in Iraq-An overview, *International Journal of Pharmaceutical and Health Care Research*, 1(4): 132–147.

Amarakoon, S., and Jayasekara, D. 2017 A review on garlic (*Allium sativum* L.) as a functional food, *Journal of Pharmacognosy and Phytochemistry*, 6(6): 1777–1180.

Ariyama, K., Nishida, T., Noda, T., Kadokura, M., and Yasui, A. 2006 Effects of fertilization, crop year, variety, and provenance factors on mineral concentrations in onions, *Journal of Agricultural and Food Chemistry*, 54(9): 3341–3350.

Asdaq, S.M.B., and Inamdar, M.N. 2011 Pharmacodynamic and pharmacokinetic interactions of propranolol with garlic (*Allium sativum*) in rats, *Evidence-Based Complementary and Alternative Medicine*, 1: 1–11.

Beato, V.M., Orgaz, F., Mansilla, F., and Montaño, A. 2011 Changes in phenolic compounds in garlic (*Allium sativum* L.) owing to the cultivar and location of growth, *Plant Foods For Human Nutrition*, 66(3): 218–223.

Block, E. 2010 Allium botany and cultivation, ancient and modern. In *Garlic and Other Alliums: The Lore and The Science*, ed. E. Block. Cambridge: The Royal Society of Chemistry, 1–32.

Borrelli, F., Capasso, R., and Izzo, A.A. 2007 Garlic (*Allium sativum* L.): Adverse effects and drug interactions in humans, *Molecular Nutrition & Food Research*, 51(11): 1386–1397.

Chhabria, S., and Desai, K. 2018 Purification and characterisation of alliinase produced by Cupriavidus necator and its application for generation of cytotoxic agent: Allicin, *Saudi Journal of Biological Sciences*, 25(7): 1429–1438.

Davis, S.R. 2005 An overview of the antifungal properties of allicin and its breakdown products–the possibility of a safe and effective antifungal prophylactic, *Mycoses*, 48(2): 95–100.

El-Saber Batiha, G., Magdy Beshbishy, A.G., Wasef, L., Elewa, Y.H., Al-Sagan, A., El-Hack, A., Mohamed, E., Taha, A.E., M Abd-Elhakim, Y., and Prasad Devkota, H. 2020 Chemical constituents and pharmacological activities of garlic (*Allium sativum* L.): A review, *Nutrients*, 12(3): 872.

Faroughi, F., Charandabi, S.M.A., Javadzadeh, Y., and Mirghafourvand, M. 2018 Effects of garlic pill on blood glucose level in borderline gestational diabetes mellitus: a randomized controlled trial, *Iranian Red Crescent Medical Journal*, 20(5): e60675.

Fufa, B.K. 2019 Anti-bacterial and anti-fungal properties of garlic extract (*Allium sativum*): A review, *Microbiology Research Journal International*, 28(3): 1–5.

Gruhlke, M.C., Nicco, C., Batteux, F., and Slusarenko, A.J. 2017 The effects of allicin, a reactive sulfur species from garlic, on a selection of mammalian cell lines, *Antioxidants*, 6(1): 1.

Gupta, M. 2010 Pharmacological properties and traditional therapeutic uses of important Indian spices: A review, *International Journal of Food Properties*, 13(5): 1092–1116.

Gupta, R.P. 2015 A step towards increasing garlic productivity, *Current Science*, 108(8): 1414–1415.

Ho, T.M., Abik, F., and Mikkonen, K.S. 2021 An overview of nanoemulsion characterization via atomic force microscopy, *Critical Reviews in Food Science and Nutrition*, 2021(1): 1–21.

Hobauer, R., Frass, M., Gmeiner, B., Kaye, A.D., and Frost, E.A. 2000 Garlic extract (*Allium sativum*) reduces migration of neutrophils through endothelial cell monolayers, *Middle East Journal of Anaesthesiology*, 15(6): 649–658.

Hrbek, V., Rektorisova, M., Chmelarova, H., Ovesna, J., and Hajslova, J. 2018 Authenticity assessment of garlic using a metabolomic approach based on high resolution mass spectrometry, *Journal of Food Composition and Analysis*, 67(3): 19–28.

Jo, S., Song, Y., Jeong, J.H., Hwang, J., and Kim, Y. 2020 Geographical discrimination of Allium species (garlic and onion) using 1H NMR spectroscopy with multivariate analysis, *International Journal of Food Properties*, 23(1): 241–254.

Jones, M.G., Hughes, J., Tregova, A., Milne, J., Tomsett, A.B., and Collin, H.A. 2004 Biosynthesis of the flavour precursors of onion and garlic, *Journal of Experimental Botany*, 55(404): 1903–1918.

Kang, N.S., Moon, E.Y., Cho, C.G., and Pyo, S. 2001 Immunomodulating effect of garlic component, allicin, on murine peritoneal macrophages, *Nutrition Research*, 21(4): 617–626.

Khezri, Z., Shekarchizadeh, H., and Fathi, M. 2021 Stability enhancement of garlic essential oil using new opopanax gum/gelatin nanofibres, *International Journal of Food Science & Technology*, 56(5): 2255–2263.

Khodakaram-Tafti, A., Hashemnia, M., Razavi, S.M., Sharifiyazdi, H., and Nazifi, S. 2013 Genetic characterization and phylogenetic analysis of Eimeria arloingi in Iranian native kids, *Parasitology Research*, 112(9): 3187–3192.

Kimbaris, A.C., Siatis, N.G., Daferera, D.J., Tarantilis, P.A., Pappas, C.S., and Polissiou, M.G. 2006 Comparison of distillation and ultrasound-assisted extraction methods for the isolation of sensitive aroma compounds from garlic (*Allium sativum*), *Ultrasonics Sonochemistry*, 13(1): 54–60.

Klaas, M. 1998 Applications and impact of molecular markers on evolutionary and diversity studies in the genus Allium, *Plant Breeding*, 117(4): 297–308.

Kyung, K.H., Kim, M., Park, M., and Kim, Y.S. 2002 Alliinase-independent inhibition of Staphylococcus aureus B33 by heated garlic, *Journal of Food Science*, 67(2): 780–785.

Lanzotti, V., Scala, F., and Bonanomi, G. 2014 Compounds from Allium species with cytotoxic and antimicrobial activity, *Phytochemistry Reviews*, 13(4): 769–791.

Lawson L.D., and Bauer R. 1998 Garlic: A review of its medicinal effects and indicated active compounds. In *Phytomedicines of Europe-Chemistry and Biological Activity*, Washington DC: American Chemical Society, 176–209.

Lee, M.S., Kim, I.H., Kim, C.T., and Kim, Y. 2011 Reduction of body weight by dietary garlic is associated with an increase in uncoupling protein mRNA expression and activation of AMP-activated protein kinase in diet-induced obese mice, *The Journal of Nutrition*, 141(11): 1947–1953.

Leontiev, R., Hohaus, N., Jacob, C., Gruhlke, M.C., and Slusarenko, A.J. 2018 A comparison of the antibacterial and antifungal activities of thiosulfinate analogues of allicin, *Scientific Reports*, 8(1): 1–19.

Manzum, A.A., Sultana, S.S., Warasy, A.A., Begum, R., and Alam, S.S. 2014 Characterization of four specimens of *Allium sativum* L. by differential karyotype and RAPD analysis, *Cytologia*, 79(3): 419–426.

Melgar-Lalanne, G., Hernández-Álvarez, A.J., Jiménez-Fernández, M., and Azuara, E. 2017 Oleoresins from *Capsicum spp.*: Extraction methods and bioactivity, *Food and Bioprocess Technology*, 10(1):51–76.

Meriga, B., Mopuri, R., and MuraliKrishna, T. 2012 Insecticidal, antimicrobial and antioxidant activities of bulb extracts of *Allium sativum*, *Asian Pacific Journal of Tropical Medicine*, 5(5): 391–395.

Mousa, A.S. 2001 Discovery of angiogenesis inhibition by garlic ingredients: Potential anti-cancer benefits, *Faseb Journal*, 15(4): A117.

Otunola, G.A., Afolayan, A.J., Ajayi, E.O., and Odeyemi, S.W. 2017 Characterization, antibacterial and antioxidant properties of silver nanoparticles synthesized from aqueous extracts of *Allium sativum*, Zingiber officinale, and Capsicum frutescens, *Pharmacognosy Magazine*, 13(Suppl 2): 201.

Ovesná, J., Kučera, L., Horníčková, J., Svobodová, L., Stavělíková, H., Velíšek, J., and Milella, L. 2011 Diversity of S-alk (en) yl cysteine sulphoxide content within a collection of garlic (*Allium sativum* L.) and its association with the morphological and genetic background assessed by AFLP, *Scientia Horticulturae*, 129(4): 541–547.

Pârvu, M., Moţ, C.A., Pârvu, A.E., Mircea, C., Stoeber, L., Roşca-Casian, O., and Ţigu, A.B. 2019 *Allium sativum* extract chemical composition, antioxidant activity and antifungal effect against Meyerozyma guilliermondii and Rhodotorula mucilaginosa causing onychomycosis. *Molecules*, 24(21): p3958.

Pinilla, C.M.B., Thys, R.C.S., and Brandelli, A. 2019 Antifungal properties of phosphatidylcholine-oleic acid liposomes encapsulating garlic against environmental fungal in wheat bread, *International Journal of Food Microbiology*, 293(6): 72–78.

Rabinkov, A., Miron, T., Mirelman, D., Wilchek, M., Glozman, S., Yavin, E., and Weiner, L. 2000 S-Allylmercaptoglutathione: The reaction product of allicin with glutathione possesses SH-modifying and antioxidant properties, *Biochimica et Biophysica Acta (BBA)-Molecular Cell Research*, 1499(1–2): 144–153.

Rahman, K., and Lowe, G.M. 2006 Significance of garlic and its constituents in cancer and cardiovascular disease, *The Journal of Nutrition*, 136(3 suppl): 736S–40S.

Rajam, K., Rajendran, S., and Saranya, R. 2013 *Allium sativum* (Garlic) extract as nontoxic corrosion inhibitor, *Journal of Chemistry*, 2013(1): 1–4.

Rana, S.V., Pal, R., Vaiphei, K., Sharma, S.K., and Ola, R.P. 2011 Garlic in health and disease, *Nutrition Research Reviews*, 24(1): 60–71.

Reddy, J.P., and Rhim, J.W. 2018 Extraction and characterization of cellulose microfibers from agricultural wastes of onion and garlic, *Journal of Natural Fibers*, 15(4): 465–473.

Rohani, S.M.R., Moradi, M., Mehdizadeh, T., Saei-Dehkordi, S.S., and Griffiths, M.W. 2011 The effect of nisin and garlic (*Allium sativum* L.) essential oil separately and in combination on the growth of Listeria monocytogenes, *LWT-Food Science and Technology*, 44(10): 2260–2265.

Sadeghi, M., Nematifar, Z., Fattahi, N., Pirsaheb, M., and Shamsipur, M. 2016 Determination of bisphenol A in food and environmental samples using combined solid-phase extraction–dispersive liquid–liquid microextraction with solidification of floating organic drop followed by HPLC, *Food Analytical Methods*, 9(6): 1814–1824.

Sawai, T., Itoh, Y., Ozaki, H., Isoda, N., Okamoto, K., Kashima, Y., Kawaoka, Y., Takeuchi, Y., Kida, H., and Ogasawara, K. 2008 Induction of cytotoxic T-lymphocyte and antibody responses against highly pathogenic avian influenza virus infection in mice by inoculation of apathogenic H5N1 influenza virus particles inactivated with formalin, *Immunology*, 124(2): 155–165.

Shen, C., Xiao, H., and Parkin, K.L. 2002 In vitro stability and chemical reactivity of thiosulfinates, *Journal of Agricultural and Food Chemistry*, 50(9): 2644–2651.

Shree, S., and Kumari, A. 2019 Postharvest Handling, Diseases and Disorders in Bulb Vegetables. In *The Vegetable Pathosystem*, ed. M. Ansar, and A. Ghatak. Boca Raton: Apple Academic Press.

Singha, R.N., Kumara, N., and Kumarb, P. 2019 Garlic (*Allium sativum*): Mankind's Health Superstar, *Interdisciplinary Journal of Contemporary Research*, 6(6): 93–98.

Smith, R.G. 2005 Determination of the country of origin of garlic (*Allium sativum*) using trace metal profiling, *Journal of Agricultural and Food Chemistry*, 53(10): 4041–4045.

Tavares, L., Barros, H.L.B., Vaghetti, J.C.P., and Noreña, C.P.Z. 2019 Microencapsulation of garlic extract by complex coacervation using whey protein Isolate/Chitosan and gum Arabic/Chitosan as wall materials: Influence of anionic biopolymers on the physicochemical and structural properties of microparticles, *Food and Bioprocess Technology*, 12(12): 2093–2106.

Vvedensky, A.I. 1964 The genus Allium in the USSR, *Herbertia*, 11(1964): 65–218.

Wallock-Richards, D., Doherty, C.J., Doherty, L., Clarke, D.J., Place, M., Govan, J.R., and Campopiano, D.J. 2014 Garlic revisited: Antimicrobial activity of allicin-containing garlic extracts against Burkholderia cepacia complex, *PLoS One*, 9(12): p.e112726.

Wu, C.C., Sheen, L.Y., Chen, H.W., Tsai, S.J., and Lii, C.K. 2001 Effects of organosulfur compounds from garlic oil on the antioxidation system in rat liver and red blood cells, *Food and Chemical Toxicology*, 39(6): 563–569.

Yalavarthi, C., and Thiruvengadarajan, V.S. 2013 A review on identification strategy of phyto constituents present in herbal plants, *International Journal of Research in Pharmaceutical Sciences*, 4(2): 123–140.

CHAPTER 11

Characterization and Extraction Techniques of Nutmeg Oleoresin

Tahira Mohsin Ali, Natasha Abbas Butt and Marium Shaikh

University of Karachi

CONTENTS

DOI: 10.1201/9781003186205-11

11.1 INTRODUCTION

The evergreen nutmeg tree (*Myristica fragrans*) is the most famous member of the plant family Myristicaceae and is characterized by moderate height (10–20) m, dark green leaves, and grayish brown bark. Its ripe fruit is a source of two commercially important spices, nutmeg and mace. The nutmeg is derived from the pit of a drupe-like fruit, while mace belongs to the reddish dried web of threads or aril surrounding the seed. The Myristicaceae family is also called "nutmeg family" reflecting the popularity of nutmeg. The term nutmeg originated from the Latin word "*Nux muscatus*," which means "musky nut." The hard nutmeg seed inside the fruit is somewhat ovular in shape with (20–30) mm length and (15–18) mm width. The average dried weight of a single seed is about 12.5 g. Whole nutmeg is usually crushed or ground prior to its use in any food as it quickly loses its aroma when stored in powdered form. Its value-added products are essential oil, oleoresin, and nutmeg butter (Duke 2002).

Apart from nutmeg's use as spice, it has extraordinary medicinal properties because of which it is used in therapeutic drugs since ancient times. The oleoresin from nutmeg in contrast to essential oil contains both the volatile and non-volatile components of the seed. The characteristic aroma of nutmeg oleoresin is sweet, spicy clove like. Preference of nutmeg oleoresin over whole seed has various advantages such as ease of use, more uniform and standardized flavor profile, more hygienic, longer shelf life and cuts down freight charges being less in bulk volume/weight. Being liquid, it can be easily homogenized into any product giving real flavor and aroma of original nutmeg spice. The usage level of oleoresins is between 0.1% and 0.5% (Suderman 2011). Nutmeg oleoresin consists of various phytoconstituents that imparts a wide scope application with respect to biological, medicinal, pharmaceutical, and nutritional effects (Bamidele et al. 2011). The oleoresin is extracted in organic solvents that must be removed prior to its packaging. The three main active components of nutmeg oleoresin are myristicin, elemicin, and safrole. But overall nutmeg oleoresin is a mixture of monoterpene hydrocarbons, sesquiterpene alcohols, esters, ketones, oxides, aromatics, and acids. The oleoresin has strong antimicrobial, antioxidant, analgesic, antidiarrheal, aphrodisiac, antidepressant, and hepatoprotective activities.

11.2 PRODUCTION, DISTRIBUTION AND ECONOMIC IMPORTANCE OF NUTMEG

Nutmeg is native to Spice Islands of Indonesia. In the early 16th century, these Islands gained popularity because of the growth of important spice crops such as nutmeg, mace, and cloves. Today, Indonesia is the largest producer of nutmeg spice and contributes more than 75% of the world's total production (Sharangi, Bhutia, Raj, and Sreenivas 2018). The second largest producer of nutmeg was once Grenada (West Indies) with a total global market share of 20%. In 2002 and 2004, the disastrous hurricanes, Ivan and Emily, destroyed more than 90% nutmeg trees of the country. However, till 2011, Grenada started producing nutmeg spice again with almost double rate but the recovery from preharvest volumes is still less than 15%. Other major nutmeg cultivating countries of the world are Sri Lanka, India, Guatemala, Malaysia, and Nepal. Based on the country of cultivation, nutmeg is also classified as East Indian nutmeg (produced in Indonesia) and West Indian nutmeg (produced in Grenada). Both varieties differ in their color and flavor profile. The East Indian type is darker and more aromatic while the West Indian variety is characterized by a mild flavor and lighter appearance (Peter 2012). The FAOSTAT data available for global nutmeg production are compiled with mace and cardamom, which shows Indonesia on top of the list with annual production of 43,970 tons in 2019 (FAOSTAT 2019).

The distribution of whole nutmeg around the globe could be assessed in terms of major nutmeg exporting countries. The percent export share in terms of value in the world market contributed by different countries is listed in Table 11.1. Indonesia has always been the prime exporter of nutmeg and stands topmost in the international trade. In 2019, Indonesia exported 13,312 tons of nutmeg contributing to the global market share of 57.7% followed by Sri Lanka and India. Even though Grenada is among the major nutmeg producers, its annual export value in 2019 was only 572 tons (ITC 2019a), which could be related to the aftermath of 2002 and 2004 hurricanes.

The Netherlands is said to be a re-exporter as it first imports nutmeg from Indonesia and then sells it to other countries with the United States and European Union being the major buyers. Some of the important importers of nutmeg are China, India, Vietnam, United Arab Emirates, and Germany. In 2019, the top three importers, China, India, and Vietnam, imported 2373, 1636, and 1339 tons of nutmeg, respectively (ITC 2019a). Nutmeg is considered an economically important crop with widespread spice, condiment, perfumery, and pharmaceutical uses. The total world export market of nutmeg was worth 111,132 thousand USD in 2019 with an average growth in value of 7% between 2018 and 2019 (ITC 2019a). Nutmeg butter, ground nutmeg, essential oil, and oleoresins are some of the important value-added products derived from nutmeg. In 2019, the world's total exports

TABLE 11.1   Percent Share in Value in 2019 by Different Countries in World's Nutmeg Exports

Exporters	Percent Share
Indonesia	57.7
Sri Lanka	10.7
India	8.8
United Arab Emirates	5.9
Netherlands	5.2
Grenada	4.3

Source: ITC (2019a)

of oleoresin/essential oils and other allied products was worth 962,770 thousand USD with 5% (p.a.) growth of world imports between 2015 and 2019 (ITC 2019b).

11.3 NUTMEG OLEORESIN

Nutmeg oleoresins are defined as semisolid extracts composed of gummy, resinous, waxy, and oily/fatty material that are extracted from nutmeg using organic solvents that may be polar or non-polar but should be non-aqueous. However, it should not be mingled with essential oils that involves steam distillation or supercritical extraction. Some components might be the same, but essential oils are mainly composed of aromatic compounds. Therefore, as opposed to essential oils, oleoresins are more dense/heavier and are less volatile and contains both volatile and non-volatile flavor notes. Table 11.2 elaborates the physical characteristics of nutmeg oleoresin.

11.4 EXTRACTION OF OLEORESIN FROM NUTMEG

Solvent-based extraction methods are used for extracting oleoresin from nutmeg, which include organic solvents such as ethanol, hexane, petroleum ether, isopropanol, and ethyl acetate. Later, these solvents must be removed through evaporation. The different techniques that have been used so far for nutmeg oleoresin extraction are as follows:

Soxhlet method
Maceration method
Steam distillation combined with maceration method
Ultrasound-assisted extraction method

11.4.1 Soxhlet Method

The simplest and oldest method has been reported by Borges and Pino (1993) for the extraction of nutmeg oleoresin using Soxhlet apparatus whereby 95% (v/v) ethanol at a temperature of 75°C–85°C for 3–5 hours was used. The extract was then filtered, and solvent was removed using rotary evaporator. Depending upon particle size, the 18.0–25.4% oleoresin yield was obtained using this method with a volatile content ranging from 10.5 to 16.5%. The extraction time of 5 hours with finely ground particle size (0.21–0.42 mm) resulted in significantly higher yields. Gas liquid chromatography has shown the presence of around 15 different compounds using Soxhlet method. The higher concentration was observed for sabinene (40%) followed by terpinen-4-ol (22%) and (E)-sabinene hydrate (7.3%) in volatile oil portion of the oleoresin. However, steam-distilled essential oil portion of nutmeg showed higher concentration of sabinene (56.5%) followed by α-pinene (10.4%) and

TABLE 11.2   Physical Characteristics of Nutmeg Oleoresin

Physical Characteristics of Nutmeg Oleoresin		References
Specific gravity at 25°C	0.885	Rodianawati et al. (2015)
Refractive index at 25°C	1.489	Rodianawati et al. (2015)
Aroma	Sweet, spicy clove-like aroma	Morsy (2016)
Color	Light brown	Rodianawati et al. (2015)

β-pinene (8.0%). The recovery of volatiles using this method was only (67%) of the amount present in raw nutmegs, which indicates that volatile compounds were reduced during solvent evaporation stage, which can make oleoresin deficient in aromatic compounds. Kapoor et al. (2013) also used Soxhlet method for oleoresin extraction using ethyl acetate, ethanol, and isopropyl alcohol as solvent regimes and obtained 2.5–3.8% yield while 16% yield was reported by Pashapoor, Mashhadyrafie, and Mortazavi (2020) using petroleum ether.

11.4.2 Maceration Method

In maceration method, described by Assagaf et al. (2011), nutmeg powder (20 mesh) was combined with 96% (v/v) ethanol in the ratio of 1:5. The flask containing solvent and nutmeg flour were macerated in a water bath set at a temperature of 54°C with continuous shaking. After 4 hours of extraction, the mixture was filtered, and the filtrate was cooled to separate fat from nutmeg. The solvent was then evaporated at 40°C at a pressure of 172 mbar to obtain oleoresin. The remaining nutmeg powder was once again extracted with ethanol using the same procedure and the extracts were then combined. This method resulted in 15.17% oleoresin yield. Oleoresin profile conducted through Gas Chromatography-Mass Spectroscopy (GC-MS) showed the presence of 39 components. The highest percent relative area was observed for methyl eugenol followed by myristicine, cis-methyl isoeugenol, elemicin, and isocoumarin.

11.4.3 Steam Distillation Combined with Maceration Method

The maceration and Soxhlet methods essentially require the removal of solvent after extraction, which may result in a loss of volatiles. The loss of volatiles can be reduced if steam distillation is performed prior to solvent extraction. Rodianawati et al. (2015) described a combination of distillation and maceration methods, where, first, the essential oil-containing volatiles were recovered from the nutmeg flour after 5 hours of steam distillation in a Clevenger apparatus. Water was removed from the distillate (essential oil) by the addition of anhydrous sodium sulfate. The residual flour of steam distillation after drying to 10–15% moisture was then subjected to maceration using ethanol (96%, v/v) at 40°C for 2.5 hours on a hot plate. After which it was filtered and cooled to 4°C to easily separate the nutmeg butter. The ethanol filtrate was then concentrated by removal of the solvent using a rotary evaporator at 40°C and 175 mbar pressure. The maceration step was repeated once again, and the ethanol filtrates were combined. This filtrate (resin) was then mixed with essential oils to obtain oleoresin. The yield obtained through this method was found to be 13.61%. The components analyzed through GC-MS for this oleoresin showed the highest percentage peak area for sabinene followed by α-pinene and β-pinene. Myristicin, the most active component of nutmeg oleoresin, was found to have a 5.46% peak area (Rodianawati et al. 2015). A total of 27 different components were detected using this method. The specific gravity of this oleoresin was found to be 0.885 with a refractive index of 1.489 at 25°C. Almost similar procedure has also been reported by Assagaf et al. (2011), where steam distillation was performed before solvent maceration and resulted in 58 different components. The higher number of components in the method reported by Assagaf et al. (2011) could be because of higher temperature of (54°C) and longer extraction time of 4 hours during maceration period.

11.4.4 Ultrasound-Assisted Extraction Method

The ultrasonic waves utilized in this method allows higher mass transfer efficacy. Ultrasound waves are known for their cavity formation capability. These cavities on interaction with solid particles collapse/burst leading to high-speed jet entry of solvent into the particles. These cavities may also expand the pores present in the cell wall, which subsequently allow higher infusion of solvent into the solute particles (Ji et al. 2006; Vardanega, Santos, and Meireles 2014). The process begins with a crushing/size reduction of nutmeg. The flour and solvent are then placed in an Erlenmeyer tube (Ananingsih, Soedarini, and Karina 2020). The tube is tightly sealed with aluminum foil to prevent the escape of solvent followed by its placement into an ultrasonic bath where it is exposed to waves at a preset frequency of 45 kHz. This method can be used with different solid to solvent ratio, temperature, and time of exposure to ultrasonic waves. Response surface methodology showed that optimum yield can be obtained after 60 minutes of extraction at a temperature of 52°C using 1:20 ratio of solids to solvent. After extraction with solvent in an ultrasonic bath, the conventional steps of filtration and concentration through a rotary evaporator are employed to obtain oleoresin. Hexane was used by Ananingsih et al. (2020); however, it is not allowed in food and ethanol is therefore a better choice. Morsy (2016) used absolute ethanol and an ultrasound technique to obtain nutmeg oleoresin. Oleoresin yield (8.26%) obtained by UAE (120 W energy) using absolute ethanol as solvent for 10 minutes was close to the yield (9.63%) obtained by maceration under similar conditions. However, exposure to 120 W for longer extraction times reduced the yield, which could be attributed to degradation of compounds. Thus, longer times at lower intensity are preferred for higher extraction yields using ultrasonic waves (Morsy 2016). Thus, this method allows higher extraction yields in shorter times and seems to be commercially more feasible as conventional methods such as Soxhlet or Clevenger apparatus can pose higher fabrication costs and longer extraction times.

11.5 FACTORS AFFECTING NUTMEG OLEORESIN EXTRACTION

11.5.1 Quality of Nutmeg Fruit

The seeds of sound nutmeg fruit aged 5–9 months have been reported for oleoresin extraction (Assagaf et al. 2011; Rodianawati, Hastuti, and Cahyanto 2015). The substandard quality of nutmeg kernels will have lower volatile content, which will subsequently result in an inferior flavor profile of oleoresin extracted therefrom. According to FAO (1994), nutmeg is characterized into three quality standards: (a) sound nutmegs, (b) substandard nutmeg, and (c) low-quality nutmegs. Sound nutmegs are defined as wholesome and unbroken seeds without any stalk contamination and must be rich in oil content. The presence of woody, brittle nutmegs and adulteration with sand reduces the oleoresin yield and overall flavor profile of oleoresin. Also, substandard ground nutmeg may be adulterated with other genus members of *M. fragrans*, spices, dried fruit pulp of nutmeg, coffee husks, etc. (Van Ruth et al. 2019). Flow Infusion Electrospray Ionization Mass Spectroscopy analysis of nutmeg compounds showed a significantly higher amount of flavor-contributing compounds, i.e., myristicin, eugenol, elemicin, and isoeugenol, in higher quality nutmeg grades as opposed to substandard grades for which cumulated intensity was only 40% to that of premium nutmegs. Similarly, Proton Transfer Reaction Mass Spectroscopy analysis of volatile compounds suggested that though the profile of volatile compounds is same in high- and low-quality nutmeg grades, but the intensity of the latter is only 10% to that of higher grade nutmegs. Thus, a higher concentration of volatile compounds will subsequently result in a richer aroma and flavor quality of nutmeg oleoresin.

11.5.2 Grinding Temperature Used for Nutmeg Powder

Grinding, being an energy/shear intensive procedure, produces heat, which may result in the release of oil from nutmeg. The oil expulsion from seeds causes caking and agglomeration phenomena, which subsequently affects the efficacy of grinding by reducing the functional surface area. The nutmeg is known to have (7–16%)oil content. McKee, Thompson, and Harden (1993) compared ambient grinding (25°C) with chilled grinding (4°C) and liquid nitrogen grinding and found insignificant difference in moisture content (6.8–6.9%). In terms of yield, more consistent percent oleoresin content (34.2–34.7%)was obtained when liquid nitrogen grinding was used for three different batches of nutmeg followed by chilled/refrigerated grinding (22.3–33.3%) and ambient grinding (20.1–46.3%). The most inconsistent yield in latter could be attributed to more pronounced clumping/agglomeration of oils and resin in nutmeg powder under ambient conditions. Also, the liquid nitrogen-based grinding method resulted in higher intensity oleoresin color equivalents (0.969 g/100 mL) compared to powders ground under chilled or ambient conditions. Thus, if initially nutmegs are ground under liquid nitrogen, the oleoresin extracted therefrom will have higher yield, higher antioxidant capacity, and more intense color, which may reduce its percent dosage in food and non-food products and can, therefore, offset the higher input cost because of the use of liquid nitrogen (McKee et al. 1993).

11.5.3 Particle Size of Nutmeg Powder

Because of high oil content, nutmeg cannot be ground into fine particle size. Usually, the medium size particles varying in mesh (14–28) mm are used for oleoresin extraction (McKee et al. 1993; Rodianawati et al. 2015). Like any other extraction procedure, fine particle size is preferred for oleoresin extraction (Nagy and Simándi 2008). Borges and Pino (1993) found that fine size of nutmeg powder ranging from 0.21 to 0.42 mm resulted in higher oleoresin yield compared to coarsely ground (0.59–1.00 mm) nutmeg powder. Fine particle size ruptures flavor cells and exposes larger surface area to solvent, which subsequently increases the extraction yield. The volatile content (%) was also found to be higher for finely ground nutmeg.

11.5.4 Choice of Solvents for Extraction

Solvents vary in their polarity, which can also have a significant impact on the yield and composition of oleoresin (Said et al. 2015). The most commonly used solvents for nutmeg oleoresin are ethanol, hexane, ethyl acetate, petroleum ether, and isopropyl alcohol. The

TABLE 11.3 Effect of Different Solvents on Nutmeg Oleoresin Extraction Yield, Total Number of Components Detected in GC-MS along with Extraction Yields of Myristicin, Elemicin, and Myristic Acid

Extraction Solvent	Oleoresin Yield (%)	Total Number of Components	Myristicin (%)	Elemicin (%)	Myristic Acid (%)
Ethanol	3.8	40	4.2	9.3	7.3
Ethyl acetate	3.2	51	5.0	11.5	5.0
Isopropyl alcohol	2.5	37	8.1	17.8	5.3

Source: Kapoor et al. (2013).

solvent to solid ratio used for oleoresin extraction ranges from 1:4 to 1:20. Because of the use of different conditions of temperature, time and nutmeg/solvent ratio, inter-comparison of yields is difficult. Under similar conditions of extraction, using Soxhlet apparatus, Kapoor et al. (2013) conducted a study that extracted nutmeg oleoresin separately from ethyl acetate, ethanol, and isopropanol. The order of polarity of these solvents is ethanol > isopropanol > ethyl acetate. Table 11.3 shows that ethanol is a more effective solvent choice because of the presence of relatively more polar compounds in nutmeg. Being more polar, ethanol may also prevent too much extraction of nutmeg butter in oleoresin. The number of compounds and their yields also change depending upon the polarity of the solvent, which can subsequently affect antioxidant and iron-chelating properties. The ethanol extracted oleoresin showed the highest activity in mustard oil compared to EA (ethyl acetate)- and IPA (isopropanol)-based oleoresin. The ethanol-based oleoresin significantly delayed and reduced the formation of primary and secondary oxidation products assessed through peroxide value, TBA and anisidine values. The study by Kapoor et al. (2013) deduced higher antioxidant capacity of ethanol-derived oleoresin, which could be because of synergistic action of two or more compounds present in oleoresin, which amplified the antioxidant capacity manifold. Ethanol is also considered a green solvent as it is recyclable, does not leave any residue in food and has no adverse impact on environment (Chemat et al. 2015; Morsy 2016). The extraction temperatures used for nutmeg oleoresin range from ambient to 85°C.

11.6 CHARACTERIZATION OF NUTMEG OLEORESIN

Major and minor chemical components of nutmeg oleoresin are determined mainly by GC-MS.

Gas Chromatography Quadrupole-Time-of-Flight Mass Spectrometry

Near Infrared Spectroscopy

Nuclear Magnetic Resonance Spectroscopy

Ultraviolet Spectroscopy

Though major nutmeg compounds identified using different extraction regimes are same, however, some differences in terms of minor compounds can be seen depending upon the polarity and percent purity of solvents used. Asika et al. (2016) characterized dichloromethane and water extracts of nutmeg seed using GC-MS, which revealed presence of 18 compounds of biological interest in dichloromethane extracts as compared to 6 in aqueous one with antimicrobial, fumigant, antitoxic, and anesthetic properties (Berdyshev et al.

2011; Jadhav, Kalase, and Patil 2014; Liu, Chu, and Liu 2010; Purwantiningsih and Chan 2011; Sermakkani and Thangapandian 2012). In another study, Arshad, Ali, and Hasnain (2020) identified 23 different compounds with highest percentage of α-terpinolene (44.51%) in its oleoresin. However, percentage and chemical constituents may differ based on agro-climatic conditions of different regions across the globe. Variation in chemical components in nutmeg oleoresin is found, as liberation of chemical constituents from secretory cells of nutmeg, which is temperature, pressure, and solvent dependent. Extraction treatment and temperature also affects the compositional profile, and properties of nutmeg oleoresin. As soon as the heating temperature during extraction is increased, percentage of bioactive compounds is also increased as analyzed through GC-MS (Rodianawati, Hastuti, and Cahyanto 2015).

Phenylpropenes, including eugenol, allylphenols, chavicol, and isoeugenol, are produced by plants as a defense against microbes and herbivores. Because of their strong aroma, these are also considered floral attractants for pollination. However, humans have been using phenylpropenes for food preservation and flavoring (Koeduka et al. 2006). Various biochemical pathways have also been studied for the synthesis of phenylpropenes, including eugenol and isoeugenol present in nutmeg (Koeduka et al. 2006).

11.6.1 Compounds Identified in Nutmeg Oleoresin

Several compounds have been identified in nutmeg oleoresin, which range from 18 to 53 using different techniques (Arshad et al. 2020; Asika et al. 2016; Morsy 2016; Rodianawati et al. 2015). Variation in the number of components might be due to differences in extraction treatment, solvent ratio, variety of species, and techniques used for identification. However, some of the major and minor components along with their chemical structures that are so far identified in nutmeg oleoresin are presented in Tables 11.4 and 11.5, respectively.

The constituents of nutmeg oleoresin can be majorly characterized into ***monoterpene hydrocarbons*** (α-thujene, α-pinene, camphene, sabinene, β-pinene, β-myrcene, ʟ-phellandrene, Δ³-carene, α-terpinene, ρ-cymene, limonene, γ-terpinene, (E)-sabinene hydrate, α-terpinolene, and (Z)-trans-sabinene hydrate), ***oxides*** (1,8-cineole), ***sesquiterpene hydrocarbons*** (α-copaene, trans- β-caryophyllene, trans-α-bergamotene, β-sesquiphellandrine, germacrene-D, bicyclogermacrene, β-bisabolene), ***aromatics*** (safrole, eugenol, methyl eugenol, chavibetol, methyl isoeugenol, myristicin, elemicin, methoxyeugenol, trans-isoelemicin), ***monoterpene alcohols*** (linalool, p-menth-2-en-1-ol, cis ρ-2-menthen-1-ol, terpinen-4-ol, α-terpineol, piperitol isomer and geranyl linalool isomer), ***sesquiterpene alcohols*** (guaiol), ***esters*** (trans-sabinene hydrate acetate, Cis-sabinene hydrate acetate, endobornyl acetate, α-terpinyl acetate, citronellyl acetate, neryl acetate, tetradecanoic acid, ethyl ester, 9-octadecanoic acid, ethyl ester), ***ketones*** (α-ionone), and ***acids*** (dodecanoic acid, myristic acid, pentadecanoic acid, oleic acid). The monoterpene hydrocarbons and oxygenated compounds comprise the major portion of nutmeg oleoresin (Morsy 2016). The molecular formulas and physical characteristics of some major compounds present in nutmeg oleoresin are presented in Table 11.6.

TABLE 11.4　Major Compounds and Their Structures Identified in Nutmeg Oleoresin

Compound Name	Percentage	Structures	References
Cadinene	0.09–1.1		(Arshad, Ali, and Hasnain 2020; Asika et al. 2016; Rodianawati, Hastuti, and Cahyanto 2015)
Cymene	0.54–15.2		(Asika et al. 2016; Morsy 2016)
Carvacrol	4.89		(Arshad, Ali, and Hasnain 2020)

(Continued)

TABLE 11.4 (*Continued*) Major Compounds and Their Structures Identified in Nutmeg Oleoresin

Compound Name	Percentage	Structures	References
Elemicin	0.35–17.8		(Arshad, Ali, and Hasnain 2020; Assagaf et al. 2011; Fernando and Senevirathne 2019)
Myrcene	0.10–2.93		(Fernando and Senevirathne 2019; Morsy 2016, Rodianawati, Hastuti, and Cahyanto 2015; Wahyuni and Bermawie 2020)
Myristic acid	0.80–19.38		(Assagaf et al. 2011; Morsy 2016; Wahyuni and Bermawie 2020)
Myristicin	0.74–14.84		(Arshad, Ali, and Hasnain 2020; Asika et al. 2016; Fernando and Senevirathne 2019)

(*Continued*)

TABLE 11.4 *(Continued)* Major Compounds and Their Structures Identified in Nutmeg Oleoresin

Compound Name	Percentage	Structures	References
Sabinene	7.91–41.92		(Asika et al. 2016; Fernando and Senevirathne 2019; Hasmita, Redha, and Junaidy 2019; Wahyuni and Bermawie 2020)
Safrole	0.83–43.37		(Arshad, Ali, and Hasnain 2020; Asika, Fernando, and Senevirathne 2019; Hasmita, Redha, and Junaidy 2019; Wahyuni, and Bermawie 2020)
α-Pinene	0.58–15.8		(Arshad, Ali, and Hasnain 2020, Asika et al. 2016; Morsy 2016; Wahyuni and Bermawie 2020)
Limonene	2.09–12.28		(Arshad, Ali, and Hasnain 2020; Hasmita, Redha, and Junaidy 2019; Wahyuni and Bermawie 2020)

TABLE 11.5 Minor Compounds and Their Structures Identified in Nutmeg Oleoresin

Compound Names	Percentage	Structures	References
Austrobailignan-7	0.4		(Kapoor et al. 2013)
Camphene	0.12–0.25		(Morsy 2016; Rodianawati, Hastuti, and Cahyanto 2015)
Carene	0.14–1.7		(Arshad, Ali, and Hasnain 2020; Fernando and Senevirathne 2019; Morsy 2016, Rodianawati, Hastuti, and Cahyanto 2015)
Caryophyllene	0.23–4.17		(Arshad, Ali, and Hasnain 2020; Asika et al. 2016)

(Continued)

TABLE 11.5 (*Continued*) Minor Compounds and Their Structures Identified in Nutmeg Oleoresin

Compound Names	Percentage	Structures	References
Cineole	2.3		(Morsy 2016)
Citronellyl acetate	0.08–0.5		(Kapoor et al. 2013, Morsy 2016)
Copaene	0.45–1.04		(Arshad, Ali, and Hasnain 2020; Fernando and Senevirathne 2019; Rodianawati, Hastuti, and Cahyanto 2015)
Cubenene	0.06–0.62		(Arshad, Ali, and Hasnain 2020; Fernando and Senevirathne 2019)
Dodecanoic acid	0.39–0.69		(Asika et al. 2016; Morsy 2016)

(*Continued*)

TABLE 11.5 (*Continued*) Minor Compounds and Their Structures Identified in Nutmeg Oleoresin

Compound Names	Percentage	Structures	References
Farnesene	0.44		(Hasmita, Redha, and Junaidy 2019)
Fragransin D3	0.5–1.2		(Kapoor et al. 2013)
Germacrene	0.11–0.96		(Fernando and Senevirathne 2019; Morsy 2016; Rodianawati, Hastuti, and Cahyanto 2015)
Geranyl acetate	1.5		(Asika et al. 2016; Kapoor et al. 2013)

(Continued)

TABLE 11.5 (*Continued*) Minor Compounds and Their Structures Identified in Nutmeg Oleoresin

Compound Names	Percentage	Structures	References
Glycerine-1,3-dimyristate	1.2–29.6		(Kapoor et al. 2013)
Guaiacin	0.3–2.6		(Ha et al. 2020; Kapoor et al. 2013)
Guaiol	0.12–0.24		(Asika et al. 2016; Morsy 2016)

(*Continued*)

TABLE 11.5 (*Continued*) Minor Compounds and Their Structures Identified in Nutmeg Oleoresin

Compound Names	Percentage	Structures	References
Humulene	0.45		(Rodianawati, Hastuti, and Cahyanto 2015)
Isoeugenol	0.90–0.55		(Asika et al. 2016; Fernando and Senevirathne 2019)
Licarin C	0.3–0.8		(Kapoor et al. 2013)
Linalool	0.15–1.46		(Hasmita, Redha, and Junaidy 2019, Kapoor et al. 2013; Morsy 2016)

(*Continued*)

TABLE 11.5 (*Continued*) Minor Compounds and Their Structures Identified in Nutmeg Oleoresin

Compound Names	Percentage	Structures	References
Methoxyeugenol	0.36–1.4		(Kapoor et al. 2013)
Neryl acetate	0.15–0.69		(Morsy 2016)
Oleic acid	0.19–3.33		(Asika et al. 2016; Fernando and Senevirathne 2019; Morsy 2016)
Palmitic acid	5.02–0.6		(Asika et al. 2016; Fernando and Senevirathne 2019)

(*Continued*)

TABLE 11.5 (*Continued*) Minor Compounds and Their Structures Identified in Nutmeg Oleoresin

Compound Names	Percentage	Structures	References
α-Phellandrene	0.01–2.7		(Arshad, Ali, and Hasnain 2020; Fernando and Senevirathne 2019; Morsy 2016; Rodianawati, Hastuti, and Cahyanto 2015)
Vaccenic acid	7.46		(Asika et al. 2016)
Virolongin B	0.7–1.2		(Kapoor et al. 2013)

(*Continued*)

TABLE 11.5 (*Continued*) Minor Compounds and Their Structures Identified in Nutmeg Oleoresin

Compound Names	Percentage	Structures	References
α-Ionone	0.16–0.8		(Morsy 2016)
α-Thujene	0.99–7.63		(Morsy 2016; Rodianawati, Hastuti, and Cahyanto 2015)
α-Terpinyl acetate	0.10–0.74		(Arshad, Ali, and Hasnain 2020; Kumar et al. 2005, Shahidi and Hossain 2018)

(*Continued*)

TABLE 11.5 (*Continued*) Minor Compounds and Their Structures Identified in Nutmeg Oleoresin

Compound Names	Percentage	Structures	References
α-Terpinene	0.83–10.65		(Hasmita, Redha, and Junaidy 2019; Morsy 2016; Rodianawati, Hastuti, and Cahyanto 2015; Wahyuni and Bermawie 2020)
α-Terpineol	0.26–4.27		(Arshad, Ali, and Hasnain 2020; Hasmita, Redha, and Junaidy 2019; Morsy 2016; Wahyuni and Bermawie 2020)
Tridecanoic acid	7.20		(McKee 1990)
β-Pinene	2.98–11.29		(Arshad et al. 2020; Fernando and Senevirathne 2019; Hasmita et al. 2019; Morsy 2016)

TABLE 11.6 Physical Characteristics of Major Compounds Identified in Nutmeg Oleoresin

Compound Name	Molecular Formula	Odor	State and Color	Density (g/cm³) (20°C)	Refractive Index (20°C)	Boiling Point (°C)	Melting Point (°C)	References
Carvacrol	$C_{10}H_{14}O$	Thymol, spicy odor	Colorless to pale yellow liquid	0.974–0.979	1.521–1.528	237.7	1.0	(Andersen 2006; De Vincenzi et al. 2004; Mazza et al. 1993; Pirbalouti et al. 2011; Ultee et al. 2000, Weast 1972)
ρ-Cymene	$C_{10}H_{14}$	Mild pleasant	Colorless liquid	0.857	1.484–1.491	177.3	−67.7	(Bennett et al. 1982; Eggersdorfer 2000; Favre and Powell 2013; Kirk et al. 1983)
Elemicin	$C_{12}H_{16}O_3$	Spicy, floral	Colorless to pale liquid	1.0	1.497	279.8	–	(Parthasarathy et al. 2008; Solheim and Scheline 1980)
Eugenol	$C_{10}H_{12}O_2$	Medium spicy	Liquid	1.089–1.095	1.548–1.552	254	−12	(Brown 1994; O'Neil et al. 2006)
Isoeugenol	$C_{10}H_{12}O_2$	Spicy clove like	Pale yellow liquid	1.143–1.145	–	276.5	–	(Hammoud et al. 2019; Lewis 2016; National Toxicology Program 2010)
Limonene	$C_{10}H_{16}$	Citrusy like odor	Colorless liquid	0.842	1.4744	176.0	−86.43	(Gobato et al. 2015; Hammerschmidt et al. 2003; Mann et al. 1994; Pakdel et al. 2001; Wang et al. 2009)
Myrcene	$C_{10}H_{16}$	Pleasant terpene like	Yellow oily liquid	0.789–0.793	1.466–1.471	167	≤10	(Behr and Johnen 2009; Booth et al. 2017; Eggersdorfer 2000; Marongiu et al. 2004)
Myristic acid	$C_{14}H_{28}O_2$	Faint	Oily white crystalline solid	0.844	–	163.6	–	(Acid 1987; Cox and Nelson 2008; Stephen 1964)
Myristicin	$C_{11}H_{12}O_3$	Woody aroma	Colorless clear liquid	0.862	1.472	326.2	53.9	(Beyer et al. 2006; Clark et al. 1996; Rahman et al. 2015; Shulgin 1966)
Sabinene	$C_{10}H_6$	Terpene, citrus	Colorless to pale yellow liquid	1.095–1.099	1.537–1.540	234.5	11.2	(Shulgin et al. 1967)
Safrole	$C_{10}H_{10}O_2$	Sassafras	Colorless slightly yellow oil	–	–	–	–	(Beyer, Ehlers, and Maurer 2006; Hickey 1948; Perkin and Poleck 1886)
α-Pinene	$C_{10}H_{16}$	Resinous Pine like	Colorless liquid	0.855–0.860	1.463–1.468	155	−64	(Gobato, Gobato, and Fedrigo 2015)
α-Terpene	$C_{10}H_{16}$	Citrus-woody	Colorless oily liquid	0.833–0.838	1.475–1.480	175	<25	(Eggersdorfer 2000)

11.7 CHEMISTRY AND PROPERTIES OF MAJOR COMPOUNDS IDENTIFIED IN NUTMEG OLEORESIN

11.7.1 Eugenol

It is the major phenolic compound of nutmeg oleoresin and belongs to aromatics because of its strong characteristic odor. It has a wide range of herbal and medicinal activities. It is considered non-mutagenic and carries GRAS status by the FDA (Upadhyay et al. 2017). The compound is light sensitive and that is why nutmeg oleoresins are recommended to be stored in the dark to prevent degradation of some important compounds. In aqueous formulations, eugenol exhibits poor solubility (Nuchuchua et al. 2009). Besides nutmeg, eugenol is also a key bioactive molecule present naturally in clove, basil, thyme, cinnamon, bay, and turmeric. Many derivatives of eugenol have been reported that have unlocked new paths in research fields (Khalil et al. 2017).

11.7.1.1 Characterization

The IR spectrum of eugenol showed characteristic peaks at 2870 and 2960 cm^{-1} (-CH$_3$ stretching), 1370 & 1450 cm^{-1} (-CH$_3$ bending), 1514 cm^{-1} (aromatic -C=C- stretching), 2860 and 2930 cm^{-1} (-CH$_2$- stretching), 1465 and 720 cm^{-1} (-CH$_2$- bending), 910 and 990 cm^{-1} (C=CH$_2$ bending), and 3300 and 3550 cm^{-1} (CO-H stretching). The ^{1}HNMR spectrum: H$_a$ (δ 3.258 ppm), H$_b$ (δ 3.733 ppm), H$_c$ (δ 5.02 ppm), H$_d$ (δ 5.4 ppm), H$_e$ (δ 5.91 ppm), H$_f$ (δ 6.572 ppm), H$_g$ (δ 6.721 ppm) (Yang 2005). The DSC thermograph of eugenol displayed an endothermic peak at 258.8°C, which corresponds to its volatilization (Pramod et al. 2015).

11.7.1.2 Properties

Eugenol is considered a strong antioxidant because of its radical-scavenging property (Gülçin 2011). It has been used as dental antiseptic and possess antigenotoxic, anticonvulsant, antifungal, bacteriostatic, and bactericidal properties (Tai et al. 2002; Walsh et al. 2003; Zheng, Kenney, and Lam 1992). However, a high concentration of eugenol acts as a pro-oxidant and may cause allergic and inflammatory reactions (Bertrand et al. 1997).

11.7.2 Methoxy Eugenol

Like eugenol, methoxy eugenol is also a phenolic component of aromatics. Methoxy eugenol is a commonly used food additive that attributes the scent of smoke and is used to preserve white and red meat. However, the maximum allowable limit in food is 5 ppm (Sudradjat et al. 2018).

11.7.2.1 Characterization

The ^{1}HNMR spectrum: δ 3.31 (2H, H-7), δ 3.87 (6H, s, -OCH$_3$,2), δ 5.08 (m, 2H, H-9), δ 5.39 (s, 1H, -OH), δ 5.9 (m, 1H, H-8), δ 6.4 (s, 2H, H-2,6) (Lee et al. 2006).

11.7.2.2 Properties

Methoxyeugenol is a potent compound found in nutmeg oleoresin and oil, which possesses anti-inflammatory, antifungal, and antimicrobial activities (Agnihotri, Wakode, and Ali

2012; López et al. 2015; Paul et al. 2013). The anticancer activity of this compound against endometrial cancer has also been identified by Paul et al. (2013).

11.7.3 Isoeugenol

Isoeugenol, an aromatic compound, is an isomer of eugenol. The olefinic double bond conjugates with the benzene ring. Therefore, isoeugenol is less flexible as compared to eugenol (Chen, Wang, Hu, and Wang, 2012). It is used in perfumery on a large scale and is made by isomerization with sodium or potassium salt by heating. Commercially isoeugenol is available in two forms: cis-isomers and trans isomers, with the latter being more thermodynamically stable. Isoeugenol has been used to produce vanillin from *B. fusiformis* CGMCC1347 cells (Zhao et al. 2005).

11.7.3.1 Characterization

FTIR spectra showed maximum absorption at: 3503, 3057, 3014, 2936, 2930, 2843, 1603, 1506, 1367, 1030, 963 cm^{-1}. The ^{1}HNMR (400.1 MHz, CDCl$_3$): δ 1.86 ppm (3H, dd, CH$_3$); δ 3.90 ppm (3H, s, OCH$_3$); δ 5.55 ppm (1H, s, OH); δ 6.08 ppm (1H, dq, H2'); δ 6.32 ppm (1H, dd, H1'); δ 6.85 ppm (3H, m, H3, H5, and H6) (Carrasco et al. 2008).

11.7.3.2 Properties

Isoeugenol and their isomers have shown antifungal activities against strains of *Cryptococcus neoformans* (Pinheiro et al. 2017). Isoeugenol, when incorporated in films, has proven to have antibacterial and antifungal activities as well. These edible films have been used for wrapping food items such as vegetables and meat products (Chen et al. 2012).

11.7.4 Myristicin

Myristicin, with the chemical name 1-allyl-5-methoxy-3,4 methylene-dioxybenzene, is the principal component of nutmeg oleoresin ranging from 0.74 to 14.84%. It also belongs to aromatic group of compounds characterized with high boiling point. It is a derivative of safrole with a methoxy group located on C4. This methoxy group imparts sedative effect to the whole compound (Subarnas, Apriyantono, and Mustarichie 2010). It is soluble in organic solvents but insoluble in water (Hasmita et al. 2019). Increase in temperature and pressure yields higher myristicin content in nutmeg oleoresin (Sudradjat et al. 2018).

11.7.4.1 Characterization

The UV spectroscopy of myristicin showed maximum absorptions at 210 nm, 232 nm, and 280 nm (Dighe and Charegaonkar 2009). The IR spectrum showed characteristic peaks at 1431 cm^{-1} (-CH$_2$), 1631 cm^{-1} (C=C), 1131 & 1090 cm^{-1} (C-O-C).The ^{1}HNMR spectrum δ 3.29 (d, -CH$_2$-, J=6.5Hz), δ 3.87 (s, -OCH$_3$-), δ 5.08 (d,=CH$_2$), δ 5.89 (m, -CH=J=6.5Hz), δ 5.91 (s, -OCH$_2$O-), δ 6.32 (s, -H$_1$-Ar-), δ 6.35 (s, -H$_6$-Ar-) (Sohilait and Kainama 2015).

11.7.4.2 Properties

Locomotor activity as examined on mice after inhalation of nutmeg oil revealed interesting outcomes. The blood plasma was run on GC-MS for identification of chemical components. The first component detected in blood plasma after half an hour of inhalation was found to be myristicin. Locomotor activity is dose dependent. Higher dose and longer times resulted in increased locomotor inhibition, which is attributed to increased myristicin levels in blood plasma after inhalation (Subarnas et al. 2010). Higher dose of myristicin may cause health problems mainly related to brain, as myristicin causes hallucinogenic effects. Symptoms might occur within 3–6 hours after ingesting it. Intoxication dose is 1–2 mg of myristicin/kg body weight. Therefore, its dose must be adjusted to minimize its euphoric effects. Several intoxications have been reported internationally after myristicin exposure (Rahman et al. 2015).

11.7.5 Sabinene

Sabinene is a bicyclic monoterpene hydrocarbon that acts as a plant metabolite and is identified in almost all nutmeg oleoresins. Its amount typically varies between 7.91% and 41.92%. It is used as biofuel, flavoring and perfume additive. The complicated ring structure of sabinene makes it chemical synthesis difficult. Therefore, microbial synthesis is gaining importance that serves as an alternative to conventional routes (Yamasaki et al. 2007; Zaidlewicz and Gimiñska 1997).

11.7.5.1 Characterization

^{1}HNMR (CDCl$_3$ at 400 MHz): H1 (4.662 ppm), H2 (4.573 ppm), H3 (0.866 ppm), H4 (0.322 ppm), H5 (−0.070 ppm), H6 (2.081 ppm), H7 (1.739 ppm), H8 (1.696 ppm), H9 (0.274 ppm), H10 (0.776 ppm), H11 (0.776 ppm), H12 (0.776 ppm), H13 (0.883 ppm), H14 (0.883 ppm), H15 (0.883 ppm), H16 (2.202 ppm) (Abraham and Mobli 2008).

11.7.5.2 Properties

Sabinene has shown antifungal, anti-inflammatory, and antioxidant effects (Cao et al. 2018; Yamasaki et al. 2007). Use of magnesium alumino metasilicate as excipient during extraction increased the amount of sabinene up to 9.41 times. Black pepper spicy terpenic odor is mainly due to sabinene (Chatterjee, Gupta, and Variyar 2015) and thus may also impart characteristic flavor to nutmeg oleoresin.

11.7.6 Safrole

Safrole belongs to benzodioxol class of compounds. Its structure possesses aromatic compounds, i.e., allylbenzene and propyl benzene (Yang et al. 2018). It is a plant metabolite found naturally in several plants like cinnamon, black pepper and nutmeg. Safrole can also be identified qualitatively as well as quantitatively by HPTLC. Various mobile phases for safrole identification used for TLC include ethyl acetate, toluene, and formic acid (Dighe and Charegaonkar 2009).

11.7.6.1 Characterization

The maximum UV absorption wavelength for safrole is found to be 200 nm and 290 nm (Dighe and Charegaonkar 2009). FTIR spectra of safrole gives characteristic peaks at (2977–2842) cm^{-1} (=Csp^2-H (aliphatic/aromatic)), 1639 cm^{-1} (C=C aliphatic absorption),

1608 cm^{-1} (C=C aromatic), 1432 cm^{-1} (–CH$_2$-), 1246 cm^{-1} and 1034 cm^{-1} (C-O-C). ^{1}HNMR spectra: (500 MHz, CDCl$_3$, ppm), δ 3.32 ppm (d –CH$_2$-), δ 5.06 ppm (d, =CH$_2$), δ 5.92 ppm (s, -OCH$_2$O-), δ 5.95 ppm (m, -CH=), δ 6.67 ppm (d, H-C5Ar), δ 6.74 ppm (s, C3-Ar), δ 6.84 ppm (d, H-C6-Ar) (Sohilait and Kainama 2016).

11.7.6.2 Properties
Safrole has been reported to inhibit bacterial and fungal growth in vivo mode. Catechols can also be synthesized from safrole that is responsible for antiproliferative activity in breast cancer cells (Madrid Villegas et al. 2011). In the past, it has also been used to cure urinary tract infections and skin issues. However, later, it was discontinued because of toxic and hepatocarcinogenic effects of safrole (Abel 1997; Buchanan 1978; Ioannides, Delaforge, and Parke 1981; Kemprai et al. 2020).

11.7.7 Elemicin
Elemicin is a herbicidal olefinic compound also identified as 5′-metoxy eugenol. It is a naturally occurring phenylpropene (belongs to a class of anisoles) containing a methoxybenzene, which is a constituent of oleoresin and essential oils of different plant species mainly elemi, mace, and nutmeg. Elemicin is a weak basic spice and flower tasting compound. The molecule of elemicin is composed of total 31 bonds out of which 15 are non-hydrogen bonds, 7 are multiple bonds, 6 are aromatic bonds, 5 rotatable bonds, 3 ether bonds, 1 six-membered ring, and 1 double bond. Generally, elemicin occurs in different foods such as carrots, wild carrots, banana, parsley, blackberries, tarragon, and sweet bay (Rossi et al. 2007). It could be used as food additive to decrease the microbial load in poultry (Rossi et al. 2007).

11.7.7.1 Characterization
The ^{1}HNMR spectrum (CDCl$_3$,400 MHz): δ 3.832 (H1,H2,H3), δ 7.388 (H4), δ 3.260 (H5,H6), δ 5.974 (H7), δ 5.460 (H8), δ 5.329 (H9), δ 7.388 (H10), δ 3.832 (H11,H12,H13), δ 3.854 (H14,H15,16) (Abraham and Mobli 2008).

11.7.7.2 Properties
Elemicin is a bioactive compound that acts as an antidepressant, antihistaminic, antibacterial, and fungicide, and possesses anti-HSV effects (Sajjadi et al. 2012; Duke and Bogenschutz 1994; Rossi et al. 2007). Essential oils/oleoresin contains considerable amount of elemicin compound. It has been studied that oils that contain high amount elemicin showed stronger antifungal activity and no cytotoxic effects at 0.16–0.64 μL/mL (max. 24 h) (Tavares et al. 2008).

11.7.8 Myrcene
Myrcene is an acyclic monoterpene that is abundantly used in industrial processes. Because of its reactive diene structure, it is stored in cool place. However, it can be stabilized by addition of 4-(tert-butyl) catechol (0.1%). Myrcene also serves as an intermediate in terpene alcohol production. It also finds applications in fragrances, cosmetics, pharmaceuticals, dyes, and varnishes, etc. (Eggersdorfer 2000).

This compound is classified as GRAS by Flavor Extract Manufacturers' Association (FEMA) (Behr and Johnen 2009). It has also been included in list of artificial flavoring substance. It is obtained by β-pinene pyrolysis.

11.7.8.1 Characterization
Myrcene shows maximum UV absorption at 225 nm (Weast 1979). The IR spectrum displayed maximum peaks at (1672, 1634, 1597, 997, 900, 893) cm^{-1}. The ^{1}HNMR spectrum (CDCl$_3$,400 MHz): δ 1.719 (H1,H2,H3), δ 5.147 (H4), δ 2.385 (H5,H6), δ 2.467 (H7,H8), δ 4.678 (H9), δ 4.871 (H10), δ 6.215 (H11), δ 5.037 (H12), δ 5.030 (H13), δ 1.709 (H14,H15,16) (Abraham and Mobli 2008).

11.7.8.2 Properties
Myrcene has shown low dermal and oral toxicity (Behr and Johnen 2009; Opdyke 1979; Paumgartten et al. 1998).

11.7.9 Pinene
Pinene, a bicyclic monoterpene, is the most widely occurring terpenoid in nature. As its name implies, it has the fragrance of pine tree. It contains a four-membered ring. Pinene has two active isomers, namely α- and β-pinene (Silva et al. 2012).

11.7.9.1 Characterization
^{1}HNMR shifts of β-pinene (400 MHz): H-1 (2.514 ppm), H-3s (2.213 ppm), H-3a (2.515 ppm), H-4s (1.857 ppm), H-4a (1.811 ppm), H-5 (1.914 ppm), H-7a (1.418 ppm), H-7s (2.281 ppm), H-10s (4.731 ppm), H-10a (4.767 ppm) (Kolehmainen et al. 1997).

11.7.9.2 Properties
α- and β-pinene enantiomers biological activities (antimicrobial and antifungal) have been widely studied. However, only positive enantiomers were active against agar diffusion test. Negative enantiomers do not give any activity (Silva et al. 2012; Tabanca et al. 2007; Yang et al. 2011).

11.8 HEALTH AND MEDICINAL PROPERTIES OF NUTMEG OLEORESIN

11.8.1 Antioxidant Property
Nutmeg is an antioxidant rich seed, which is frequently added to food as seasoning. The antioxidant property of nutmeg is exploited to increase the shelf life of meat and oils (Acosta et al. 2016; Tomaino et al. 2005) through prevention of oxidative rancidity and it also carries therapeutic significance. Consumption of antioxidants is known to reduce the risk of cancer, cardiovascular diseases, aging, and inflammation. All spices are rich source of antioxidants including nutmeg. The antioxidant activity of nutmeg is derived from phenolic and flavonoid compounds, which act as oxygen donors to free radicals (Acosta et al. 2016; Arshad, Ali, and Hasnain 2018). The oleoresin extracted using petroleum ether was found to have an IC$_{50}$ value of 123.36 µg/mL to scavenge DPPH free radicals in diabetic rats (Pashapoor et al. 2020). The common reductones present in nutmeg are trans-isoeugenol,

methyl eugenol, terpene-4-ol, elemicin, and transmethyl eugenol (Kapoor et al. 2013). These antioxidants donate oxygen to reactive oxygen species (ROS) and thereby reduces oxidative stress in human body (Zehiroglu and Sarikaya 2019). Also, compounds like beta-caryophyllene and eugenol are known to stimulate the activity of catalase, superoxide dismutase, and glutathione peroxidase (Gupta, Bansal, Babu, and Maithil 2013). The ROS produced in the body can injure cell membranes and may initiate or further proliferate many diseases, including atherosclerosis, diabetes, cancers, inflammation, and neuro-disorders (Dröge and Schipper 2007).

11.8.2 Antimicrobial Property

Antimicrobial activity of oleoresin may vary depending upon the choice of organic solvent used for extraction (Gupta et al. 2013). Nutmeg extracts/oleoresins are extensively reported for their antifungal and antibacterial properties (Acosta et al. 2016; Figueroa-Lopez, Andrade-Mahecha, and Torres-Vargas, 2018a, 2018b; Rodianawati et al. 2015; Shafiei et al. 2012). The antimicrobial activity against bacteria and fungi is mostly related to the presence of myristic acid, trimyristicin, β-pinene, ρ-cymene, β-caryophyllene, and carvacrol (Narasimhan and Dhake 2006). The nutmeg oleoresin have shown antibacterial property against *Bacillus subtilis*, *Staphylococcus aureus*, *Pseudomonas putida*, *Pseudomonas aeruginosa*, and *Escherichia coli O157*. β-Pinene is found to be very potent against *E. coli O157* (Takikawa et al. 2002). Figueroa-Lopez et al. (2018a) reported that minimum inhibitory concentration (MIC) of nutmeg oleoresin extract was lower for gram-positive bacteria. The mechanism of antibacterial activity is mostly related to disruption of cellular membranes by these lipophilic compounds, which in turn inactivate cellular enzymes and may also damage the cytoplasmic content. The functional groups responsible for antibacterial activity are carboxylic (COOH), -COOR (ester), amine ($-NH_2$), and (-SH) sulphydryl groups, which are known to penetrate the cell wall of microorganisms. Narasimhan et al. (2004) associated the unsaturated side chain on aromatic ring structure of myristicin to be responsible for the antibacterial activity. Many compounds present in oleoresin can work synergistically to inhibit microbial growth for, e.g., cymene works synergistically with carvacrol to expand/destabilize the cellular membrane. The concentration of 1% is found to inhibit sporulation/germination and mycelia growth. Interestingly, Rodianawati et al. (2015) found no difference in antifungal activity of nutmeg oleoresin against *Aspergillus niger*, *Fusarium oxysporum*, *Penicillium glabrum*, *Rhizopus oryzae*, and *Mucor racemosus* when it was heated from 100 to 180°C, which suggest that oleoresin can remain active against fungi during thermal processing of food. The nutmeg components responsible for antibacterial and antifungal activity are listed in Table 11.7.

Because of antibacterial property possessed by nutmeg, it has long been used for the treatment of various ailments such as diarrhea, oral infections, skin infections, indigestion, and gastric problems (Abourashed and El-Alfy 2016; Grover et al. 2002). Thus, nutmeg oleoresin in future may also find use in drugs/medicine as a natural cure for many ailments as consistent use of synthetically developed antibiotics is leading to drug-resistant bacterial strains worldwide, which then require development of stronger antibiotics with more harsh side effects. Besides its use in medicines, the antimicrobial property of nutmeg

TABLE 11.7   Compounds in Nutmeg Oleoresin Responsible for Antibacterial and Antifungal Activities

Active Constituents of Nutmeg Oleoresin	Antibacterial Activity	Antifungal Activity	References
Sabinene	√		(Ultee, Bennik, and Moezelaar 2002)
α-Pinene	√		(Dorman and Deans 2004)
β-Pinene	√		(Dorman and Deans 2004; Takikawa et al. 2002)
Trimyristin	√		(Narasimhan and Dhake 2006)
Myristic acid	√		(Narasimhan and Dhake 2006)
Myristicin	√		(Narasimhan and Dhake 2006)
ρ-Cymene	√		(Ultee et al. 2002)
Carvacrol	√		(Ultee et al. 2002)
Citronellol	√		(Dorman and Deans 2004)
Geraniol	√		(Dorman and Deans 2004)
Limonene	√		(Dorman and Deans 2004)
Menthone	√		(Dorman and Deans 2004)
Myrcene	√		(Dorman and Deans 2004)
α-Phellandrene	√		(Dorman and Deans 2004)
Terpinolene	√		(Dorman and Deans 2004)
δ-3-Carene	√		(Dorman and Deans 2004)
Linalool	√		(Dorman and Deans 2004)
α-Terpineol	√		(Dorman and Deans 2004)
Terpinen-4-ol	√		(Dorman and Deans 2004)
β-Caryophyllene		√	(Sabulal et al. 2006; Ultee et al. 2002)
Erythro-austrobailignan-6		√	(Cho et al. 2007)
Meso-dihydroguaiaretic acid		√	(Cho et al. 2007)
Nectandrin-B		√	(Cho et al. 2007)
Isoeugenol	√	√	(Pinheiro et al. 2017)
Elemicin		√	(Tavares et al. 2008)
Eugenol	√		(Walsh et al. 2003)
Methoxy eugenol	√	√	(Agnihotri, Wakode, and Ali 2012)

is also exploited to replace synthetic food preservatives and for the development of active packaging material.

11.8.3 Hypolipidemic Property

Nutmeg is known since ancient times to have fat-lowering properties. Pashapoor et al. (2020) found that 100–200 mg/kg of nutmeg oleoresin obtained using petroleum ether extraction significantly reduced total cholesterol, triglycerides, and LDL levels in diabetic rats but increased HDL-C levels suggesting improvement in HDL to LDL ratio on consumption of nutmeg. The hypolipidemic activity of nutmeg oleoresin is due its high phenolic and flavonoid content, which is assumed to (a) inhibit HMB CoA reductase activity, which reduces cholesterol levels, and (b) stimulate effects of glucose utilization in the peripheral tissues (Bhaskar and Kumar 2012). Antihyperlipidemic effects of nutmeg are also proven in the study of Arulmozhi et al. (2007).

11.8.4 Antidepressant Property

Depression and anxiety are common neuro-disorders these days and are considered chronic illnesses. The medicines related to depression have many side effects, because of which patients in general show reluctance in their consumption. The hexane extract of nutmeg (10 mg/kg) administered orally for 3 days has been reported to show antidepressant activity in rats and had higher efficacy compared to fluoxetine and imipramine, which are synthetic drugs used for the treatment of mental disorders. The efficacy of extract is assumed to be related to the serotonergic mechanism and through the ability of extract to interfere with 1-adrenoceptors or dopamine D_2 receptors (Dhingra and Sharma 2006).

11.8.5 Aphrodisiac Property

The 50% ethanolic extract up to 500 mg/kg was found to improve aphrodisiac activity in male rats, while no adverse effects were observed up to a dose of 4000 ppm. The aphrodisiac activity was improved in terms of mounting frequency, mating performance, libido, frequency of penile reflexes, intromission frequency, and ejaculatory latency, but decreased post-ejaculatory level, which indicates sustainable improvement in sexual activity (Ahmad, Latif, and Qasmi 2003; Ahmad, Latif, Qasmi, and Amin 2005). Since oleoresins are also prepared through ethanol extractions, therefore it could be used in therapeutic drugs to treat sexual disorders in male.

11.8.6 Hepatoprotective Property

Liver toxicity is very common worldwide because of sedentary lifestyle, exposure to various drugs, and immense consumption of fat-loaded fast foods (Bruha, Dvorak, and Petrtyl 2012; Simon et al. 2020). Myristicin is one of the major components of nutmeg oleoresin irrespective of the solvent used for extraction. Morita et al. (2003) in their detailed study on different spice powders found that nutmeg had the highest hepatoprotective efficacy and was mainly guided through myristicin present in the seed extract. This was further confirmed in mice model where oral administration of myristicin had a dose-dependent impact in controlling increase of serum ALT and AST activity on lipopolysaccharide/D-galactosamine induced liver toxicity. The intake of myristicin is also found to reduce DNA fragmentation by suppressing the elevation of tumor necrosis factor alpha (TNF α). Autoimmune diseases, chemicals, drugs, viruses, and alcohol consumption are the major reasons of liver damage among many (Ansari 2010; Ganesan et al. 2019; Huang et al. 2019; Jaeschke and Ramachandran, 2020; Parvez and Rishi 2019). Thus, therapeutic drugs containing active ingredients of nutmeg may assist in the treatment/prevention of hepatotoxicity.

11.8.7 Anticancer Property

As yet, no research has been conducted on the anticancer activity of nutmeg oleoresin. However, active components in nutmeg seed/essential oils /aqueous extracts associated with anticancer activity like methyl eugenol and myrislignan are also found in nutmeg oleoresin (Kapoor et al. 2013; Lu et al. 2017; Yi et al. 2015). The anticancer activity was due to the ability of these compounds to induce apoptosis and cell cycle arrest (Lu et al. 2017). Thus, it may be used in treatment of different types of cancers. The National Cancer Institute has reported that almost 19% of Myrsinaceae extracts exhibited anti-leukemic activity when compared to almost 90 other plant species (Beckerman and Persaud 2019; Cragg, Newman, and Yang 2006).

11.8.8 Antidiarrheal Property

The petroleum ether extracts of nutmeg are known to reduce the frequency of loose stools and increases the latency period, and therefore, it has long been used by herbalists to treat the condition of diarrhea (Grover et al. 2002). Besides extract, nutmeg powder is also used for household treatment for diarrhea.

11.8.9 Analgesic Property

Zhang et al. (2016) have reported analgesic effects for nutmeg oil, which contains many monoterpenes. These compounds are also present in varying amounts in nutmeg oleoresin. Therefore, it could be speculated that oleoresin from nutmeg can also have analgesic effects as reported for its oil. The analgesic activity is attributed to the ability of monoterpenes to inhibit expression of COX-2 and blood substance P-level. Similarly, the 95% alkaloid extracts of nutmeg also reduced acetic acid induced writhing in rat models with an LD_{50} value of 5.1 g/kg (Hayfaa, Sahar, and Awatif 2013), and thus it may find uses in pain-relieving drugs.

11.9 APPLICATIONS/USES OF NUTMEG OLEORESIN

11.9.1 Use of Nutmeg Oleoresin in Probiotic Yogurt

Yogurt is an important probiotic, which has many health benefits because of the presence of microorganisms beneficial for gut health. Nutmeg oleoresins being a rich source of antioxidants is also explored for utilization in probiotic yogurt in encapsulated form at 0.5%w/v in two yogurt mixes prepared with *Lactobacillus acidophilus* strain 5(LA5) and *Bifidobacterium animalis* ssp. Lactis (Bb12), respectively. The encapsulated form of nutmeg prevents the loss of flavor and aroma on exposure to different environmental and processing conditions. Yogurt enriched with nutmeg oleoresins were found to be insignificantly different from the control yogurt in terms of overall consumer acceptability while probiotic count also remained at acceptable levels even after 4 weeks of cold storage (Illupapalayam, Smith, and Gamlath 2014).

11.9.2 Use of Nutmeg Oleoresin in Biocomposite Films

Nutmeg oleoresins, known for its antimicrobial property, are also explored for the development of biodegradable gelatin/microcrystalline cellulose films. The inclusion of oleoresin in polymeric matrix not only confers surface barrier properties to films but also extends the shelf life of food products (Acosta et al. 2016). Nutmeg oleoresin incorporated films are though found to be active against both gram-positive and gram-negative bacteria, but MIC is found to be lower for gram-positive ones. Moreover, the incorporation of oleoresin also significantly reduced the solubility and water-vapor permeability of biocomposites placed under different relative humidity conditions (2–90%), making it more suitable for film fabrication (Figueroa-Lopez et al. 2018b). Nutmeg oleoresins being hydrophobic interacts with hydrophobic molecules of the film and subsequently reduces the hydrophilic region available for absorption and desorption of water. The light barrier properties were enhanced, and oil permeability also reduced on addition of oleoresin in gelatin/microcrystalline cellulose matrix, which are considered desirable traits for the food wrapping films. Figueroa-Lopez et al. (2018a) also reported an increase in the seal strength by 8% on incorporation of nutmeg oleoresin as oils are considered a better medium for heat transfer and allow better fusion of biocomposites.

11.9.3 Use of Nutmeg Oleoresins for Bread Preservation

Nutmeg oleoresin as previously discussed can be used as a component of active packaging material to extend the shelf life of food products. Nutmeg oleoresin is explored as an additive in biocomposites prepared from gelatin/microcrystalline cellulose and has been found to improve the barrier, seal, and solubility properties of films. The same biocomposite film, when used as a sealed packaging material for breads, has been found to reduce the moisture loss from the bread. Loss of moisture is known to reduce the shelf life of bread as it makes bread harder. Also, after 9 days' storage, the bread packed in oleoresin-containing film showed a lower CFU count per gram for *S. aureus*, molds, and yeasts compared to control bread packed in reference film without any nutmeg oleoresin (Figueroa-Lopez et al. 2018a). The microbial growth in breads packed in reference film also showed reduced pH because of microbiological reactions. Sensory results have shown that the breads packed in nutmeg oleoresin-based gelatin films were less hard as compared to control bread. Thus, it seems that nutmeg oleoresin-containing biocomposites can be used to extend the shelf life without physically adding any preservative into the bread.

11.9.4 Use of Nutmeg Oleoresin Encapsulates in Donuts

Donut is a deep-fried food product very popular in the western world as a breakfast meal. Arshad, Ali, and Hasnain (2019) studied the effect of nutmeg oleoresin on the physical and functional properties of deep-fried donuts. The microcapsules of oleoresin were prepared in native/modified sorghum starches along with gum arabic. The nutmeg enriched donuts had higher flavonoid and phenolic content and correspondingly higher antioxidant capacity in finished product with more intense crust color, as evident by increase in a* and decrease in L* values. Sensory attributes of nutmeg oleoresin were also in the acceptable range and were not disliked by panelists. Interestingly, the presence of microcapsules of oleoresin did not significantly affect the specific volume of donuts.

11.9.5 Use of Nutmeg Oleoresin for the Synthesis of Silver Nanoparticles

Pranati et al. (2019) reported the synthesis of nanoparticles using 10% of commercially available oleoresin in 1 mM solution of silver nitrate. The nanoparticles were prepared at room temperature and were recovered from the salt solution through centrifugation. The synthesized silver nanoparticles were found to have concentration dependent antibacterial activity against oral pathogens like *S. aureus*, *Streptococcus mutans*, *Enterococcus faecalis*, and *Pseudomonas*. However, the most pronounced activity was observed against *Pseudomonas*. Silver nanoparticles are frequently used in biomedical applications and in packaging materials.

11.9.6 Use of Nutmeg Oleoresin as Natural Antioxidant in Oil

Synthetic antioxidants are expensive and toxic, and may have lower efficacy compared to natural antioxidants. Because of some reports (Carocho and Ferreira 2013; Mut-Salud et al. 2016) related to toxicity of synthetic antioxidants, their cut-off limit by Food and Drug Administration, USA, and European Food Safety Authority has been set, which is limiting their frequent use in food products. Kapoor et al. (2013) used nutmeg oleoresin at a 200 ppm level in mustard oil and compared it to synthetic antioxidants BHA, BHT, and propyl gallate at the same level. The oleoresin from nutmeg exhibited higher efficacy compared to BHA and BHT and thus can play a promising role in future by replacing synthetic antioxidants in food chain. The oleoresin has been found to delay the formation of both primary and secondary oxidation products and thus can extend the shelf life of oil and oil-based products.

11.9.7 Use of Nutmeg Oleoresin as Food Seasoning

Nutmeg oleoresin being liquid has more widespread applications compared to ground/ whole nutmeg. It can be used to impart nutmeg flavor to breads, pie fillings, meat products, snacks, sauces, and beverages. Oleoresins are concentrated forms of spices that give a more standardized and consistent product in terms of both color and flavor.

11.10 TOXICITY

Nutmeg oleoresin-directed safety and toxicity assessment has not been conducted hitherto. However, studies regarding toxicity of nutmeg seed and essential oils have been reported in literature to some extent (Beckerman and Persaud 2019; Manier et al. 2021). Nutmeg is commonly eaten in the form of all spice powder in food products and beverages with apparently no signs of toxicity. The common routes of toxicity in humans are oral and respiratory, while parenteral are reported only in animal models during experiments. Conflicting research have been reported on mutagenic activity of nutmeg oleoresin. Damhoeri et al. (1985) reported a low level of dose-dependent mutagenic activity in the order of (103–104) RPG (revertant per plate per gram sample) against two streptomycin dependent strains using salmonella/mammalian microsome. Myristicin present in nutmeg is known to be responsible for mutagenicity as it has a structure similar to a known mutagen called safrole. However, an earlier study conducted by Buchanan, Goldstein, and Budroe (1982) neither reported mutagenic activity for nutmeg oleoresin nor for myristicin.

A 10-year retrospective study conducted by Ehrenpreis et al. (2014) also reported ocular exposure in children less than 13 years of age. Common symptoms that may appear because of nutmeg intoxication are listed in Table 11.8. However, none of the nutmeg intoxications, whether intentional or unintentional, resulted in death during a study conducted between

TABLE 11.8   Clinical Effects and Their Symptoms because of Nutmeg Intoxication

Clinical Effects	Symptoms	References
Cardiovascular	Tachycardia, hypertension, hypotension	(Demetriades et al. 2005; Ehrenpreis et al. 2014; Gupta and Rajpurohit 2011; Van Lennep et al. 2015)
Gastrointestinal	Diarrhea, vomiting, nausea, pain in abdomen, disturbed electrolyte, and fluid balance because of excessive vomiting and diarrhea	(Shaund 2011; Van Lennep et al. 2015)
Psychiatric and neurological	Sweating for several hours, unconsciousness, hallucinations, color distortion, convulsions, headaches, drowsiness, euphoria, sedation, numbness, muscular excitation, psychosis, seizures, tingling in toes and fingers, hysteria, belligerence, dry mouth	(Brenner, Frank, and Knight 1993; Demetriades et al. 2005; Ehrenpreis et al. 2014; Gupta and Rajpurohit 2011; Van Lennep et al. 2015)
Hepatic	Hepatic necrosis and fatty degradation of liver	(IPCS 1997; Xia 2021)
Dermatological	Flushing of skin	(Shaund 2011)
Urinary	Temporary increase of albumin in urine and urine retention	(Ghosh and Ghosh 2010)
Allergenic reactions	Temporary fever, edema of eyelids and face itching, facial flushing	(Gupta and Rajpurohit 2011)
Ocular	Blurred vision, mydriasis, and ocular dysfunction	(Ehrenpreis et al. 2014)
Respiratory	Depression	(Ehrenpreis et al. 2014)
Gynecological effects	Abortion	(Gupta and Rajpurohit 2011)

1998 and 2004 in Texas (Forrester 2005), where around 64.7% cases were reported because of intentional exposure that involved male gender. Other studies have also reported moderate to minor clinical effects that are treatable after nutmeg intoxication (Ehrenpreis et al. 2014; Shaund 2011). The literature to this date shows two deaths on nutmeg abuse (Demetriades et al. 2005; Stein, Greyer, and Hentschel 2001). The major causes of nutmeg intoxication are because of intentional or unintentional abuse, or polypharmaceutical/combined drug exposure. Most of the intentional exposures are found to be common in adolescents/adults (Ehrenpreis et al. 2014; Shaund 2011; Stein et al. 2001). Because of the ability of nutmeg to cause hallucinations, it is considered a cheap narcotic and recreational drug.

11.10.1 Major Components Responsible for Psychotropic Effects and Their Mode of Actions

The major components responsible for nutmeg intoxication are myristicin, elemicin, and safrole (IPCS, 1997), which are said to be responsible for different clinical effects on high dose exposure. The psychotropic effects of nutmeg can be associated with myristicin, which is metabolized to 3-methoxy-4,5 methylenedioxyamphetamine (MMDA), through the addition of amine group to the allyl side chain (Quin, Fanning, and Plunkett 1998). The MMDA is known to imitate the effects of endogenous agonists of central nervous system, which in turn induces hallucinations. Besides MMDA formation, myristicin is also an inhibitor of monoamine oxidase, which may also cause euphoric effects. Intoxications have been reported on intake of 5 g of nutmeg, which corresponds to intake of 1–2 mg/kg of myristicin based on body weight. An old study has also reported $LD_{50}>1$ mg/kg in rats (Truitt et al. 1961). The psychotropic effect of elemicin and safrole is attributed to its converted metabolite TMA (3,4,5-trimethoxy amphetamine) through oxidation of their oleficin side chain followed by transamination (IPCS 1997). However, TMA is three times less potent than MMDA as a psychotropic drug. Interestingly, neither nutmeg ingredients (elemicin, myristicin or safrole) nor their amphetamine metabolites are traced in the urine of (Manier et al. 2021) nutmeg abusers, which make diagnosis of nutmeg intoxication difficult. The further breakdown of metabolites of myristicin, elemicin, and safrole were identified by Beyer, Ehlers, and Maurer (2006) and Manier et al. (2021) in the urine through use of advanced techniques.

11.10.2 Diagnosis and Treatment

The diagnosis of nutmeg toxicity may pose a challenge to health care professionals as initially it may cause symptoms such as alcohol drinking or other narcotic drugs. Therefore, till now history of patient and urine analysis is necessary to confirm nutmeg intoxication. The treatment for nutmeg intoxication is supportive and may not necessarily require hospitalization depending upon the extent of toxicity. It is usually treated with medicines such as benzodiazepines, which counter the effects of amphetamine while antiemetics may be used to treat nausea and vomiting. Other drugs used for treatment may include cannabis, antihistamine, acetaminophen, duloxetine, clonazepam, diphenhydramine, K2, and lisdexamfetamine. Oral administration of activated charcoal may also be used to adsorb the excess drug. Treatments may also involve oxygen support/ventilator in case of higher dose toxicity. Polypharmacy overdose exposure of nutmeg is harsh and requires more careful treatment by health care professionals (Beckerman and Persaud 2019; Ehrenpreis et al. 2014).

11.11 SAFETY

There are conflicting reports on the safety dose of nutmeg. And currently, not a single research has been conducted on safety related to nutmeg oleoresin. Barceloux (2009) reported no side effects on consumption of less than 10 g nutmeg. Table 11.9, however, indicates that the consumption dose on safer side must be less than 3 g as unintentional polypharmaceutical exposure can lead to adverse effects. The recreational dose reported for nutmeg is between 5 and 30 g (Barceloux 2009).

11.12 FUTURE SCOPE

The research on safety, toxicity, and causes of intoxication because of nutmeg and derived products such as oleoresins, extracts, and essential oils is still scanty. Minimum safety dose of nutmeg oleoresin is yet to be established. It is still unknown whether the breakdown metabolites of myristicin, elemicin, and safrole detected in urine because of nutmeg intoxication/overdose are also present on low consumption doses of nutmeg or not. Safety alert levels for the guidance of laboratory personnel and health care professionals must be established in order to confirm the cases of nutmeg intoxication. Future research must

TABLE 11.9   Nutmeg Doses Reported for Different Clinical Effects in Humans[a]

Nutmeg Dose	Clinical Effects	References
3–5 g	Hallucination	(Beyer, Ehlers, and Maurer 2006; Brenner et al. 1993)
3 nutmeg whole seeds	Stupor	(Mazurak 2018)
28 g of nutmeg	Tachycardia, paranoia, miosis, hallucinations	(Abernethy and Becker 1992)
14 g grated nutmeg	Flushing, dry mouth, sense of impending doom	(Johnson-Arbor and Smolinske 2020; Payne 1963)
2 nutmeg seeds (14 g)	Death	(Cushny 1908)

[a] Typically, one nutmeg seed corresponds to 7 g (Abernethy and Becker 1992).

also focus on the LD_{50} value of nutmeg oleoresin's active components. From a commercial point of view, the research must also focus on the methods to optimize/improve the yield of oleoresin from nutmeg.

11.13 CONCLUSION

Nutmeg oleoresin is a mixture of volatile and non-volatile components of nutmeg seed and can thus be used in place of ground nutmeg powder as it can impart the same characteristic taste and aroma. The oleoresin being available in liquid form can have more versatile application in food, beverages, perfumes, toiletries, cosmetics, and in therapeutic drugs because of its ease of blending with other ingredients. Various studies on organic extracts of nutmeg have also confirmed its strong antibacterial, antifungal, antioxidant, anti-inflammatory, and aphrodisiac activities, and thus, it can be used to develop nutraceutical products and may also find application as a natural antioxidant and bio-preservative.

ACKNOWLEDGMENT

We would like to thank Dr. Nasima Khatoon of Industrial Analytical Centre, HEJ, University of Karachi, for her guideline in writing nutmeg oleoresin characterization.
    GC-MS, Gas Chromatography-Mass Spectroscopy.

REFERENCES

Abel, G. 1997 "Safrole–Sassafras albidum", *In Adverse Effects of Herbal Drugs*, 123–127. Springer-Verlag.

Abernethy, M. K., and Becker, L. B. 1992 Acute nutmeg intoxication, *The American Journal of Emergency Medicine*, 10: 429–430. doi: 10.1016/0735-6757(92)90069-A.

Abourashed, E. A., and El-Alfy, A.T. 2016 Chemical diversity and pharmacological significance of the secondary metabolites of nutmeg (Myristica fragrans Houtt), *Phytochemistry Reviews*, 15: 1035–1056. doi: 10.1007/s11101-016-9469–x.

Abraham, R. J., and Mobli, M. 2008 *Modelling¹H NMR Spectra of Organic Compounds: Theory, Applications and NMR Prediction Software*. UK: John Wiley & Sons.

Acid, L. 1987 Final report on the safety assessment of oleic acid, lauric acid, palmitic acid, myristic acid, and stearic acid, *Journal of the American College of Toxicology*, 6: 321–401. doi: 10.3109/10915818709098563.

Acosta, S., Chiralt, A., Santamarina, P., Rosello, J., González-Martínez, C., and Cháfer, M. 2016 Antifungal films based on starch-gelatin blend, containing essential oils, *Food Hydrocolloids*, 61: 233–240. doi: 10.1016/j.foodhyd.2016.05.008.

Agnihotri, S., Wakode, S., and Ali, M. 2012 Essential oil of Myrica esculenta Buch. Ham.: composition, antimicrobial and topical anti-inflammatory activities, *Natural Product Research*, 26: 2266–2269. doi: 10.1080/14786419.2011.652959.

Ahmad, S., Latif, A., Qasmi, I.A., and Amin, K.M.Y. 2005 An experimental study of sexual function improving effect of Myristica fragrans Houtt.(nutmeg), *BMC Complementary and Alternative Medicine*, 5: 1–7. doi: 10.1186/1472-6882-5-16.

Ahmad, S., Latif, A., and Qasmi, I.A. 2003 Aphrodisiac activity of 50% ethanolic extracts of Myristica fragrans Houtt.(nutmeg) and Syzygium aromaticum (L) Merr. & Perry.(clove) in male mice: a comparative study, *BMC Complementary and Alternative Medicine*, 3. doi: 10.1186/1472-6882-3-6.

Ananingsih, V. K., Soedarini, B., and Karina, E. 2020 Separation of oleoresin from nutmeg using ultrasound assisted extraction and hexane as solvent, *Proceedings of the IOP Conference Series: Materials Science and Engineering*, 012029. doi: 10.1088/1757-899X/854/1/012029.

Andersen, A. 2006 Final report on the safety assessment of sodium p-chloro-m-cresol, p-chloro-m-cresol, chlorothymol, mixed cresols, m-cresol, o-cresol, p-cresol, isopropyl cresols, thymol, o-cymen-5-ol, and carvacrol, *International Journal of Toxicology*, 25: 29–127. doi: 10.1080/10915810600716653.

Ansari, J. 2010 Therapeutic approaches in management of drug-induced hepatotoxicity, *Journal of Biological Sciences*, 10: 386–395. doi: 10.3923/ijp.2011.579.588.

Arshad, H., Ali, T.M., and Hasnain, A. 2018 Native and modified Sorghum starches as wall materials in microencapsulation of nutmeg oleoresin, *International Journal of Biological Macromolecules*, 114: 700–709. doi: 10.1016/j.ijbiomac.2018.03082.

Arshad, H., Ali, T.M., and Hasnain, A. 2019 Physical and functional properties of fried donuts incorporated with nutmeg microcapsules composed of gum-arabic and sorghum starch as wall materials, *Journal of Food Measurement and Characterization*, 13: 3060–3068. doi: 10.1007/s11694-019-00228-y.

Arshad, H., Ali, T.M., and Hasnain, A. 2020 Bioactive properties and oxidative stability of nutmeg oleoresin microencapsulated by freeze drying using native and OSA sorghum starches as wall materials, *Journal of Food Measurement and Characterization*, 14: 2559–2569. doi: 10.1007/s11694-020-00502-4.

Arulmozhi, D., Kurian, R., Veeranjaneyulu, A., and Bodhankar, S.. 2007 Antidiabetic and anti-hyperlipidemic effects of Myristica fragrans. In animal models, *Pharmaceutical Biology*, 45: 64–68. doi: 10.1080/13880200601028339.

Asika, A.O., Adeyemi, O.T., Anyasor, G.N., Gisarin, O., and Osilesi, O. 2016 GC-MS determination of bioactive compounds and nutrient composition of myristica fragrans seeds, *Journal of Herbs, Spices & Medicinal Plants*, 22: 337–347. doi: 10.1080/10496475.2016.1223248.

Assagaf, M., Hastuti, P., Hidayat, C., and Yuliani, S. 2011 Comparison of seed nutmeg oleoresin extraction (Myrictica Houtt fragrans) origin of north maluku and maceration method using combined distillation–Maceration, *Proceedings of the Proceeding ICBB (The International Conference on Bioscience and Biotechnology)*.

Bamidele, O., Akinnuga, A., Alagbonsi, I., Ojo, O., Olorunfemi, J. and Akuyoma, M. 2011. Effects of ethanolic extract of Myristica fragrans Houtt.(nutmeg) on some heamatological indices in albino rats, *International Journal of Medicine and Medical Sciences*, 3: 215–218.

Barceloux, D. G. 2009 Nutmeg (Myristica fragrans Houtt), *Disease-a-Month*, 55: 373–379. doi: 10.1016/j.disamonth.2009.03.007.

Beckerman B., and Persaud, H. 2019 Nutmeg overdose: spice not so nice, *Complementary Therapies in Medicine*, 46: 44–46. doi: 10.1016/j.ctim.2019.07.011.

Behr, A., and Johnen, L. 2009 Myrcene as a natural base chemical in sustainable chemistry: A critical review, *ChemSusChem: Chemistry & Sustainability Energy & Materials*, 2: 1072–1095. doi: 10.1002/cssc.200900186.

Bennett, M., Huang, T.N., Matheson, T., Smith, A., Ittel, S., and Nickerson, W. 1982 "(η6-Hexamethylbenzene) ruthenium complexes". In Inorganic Syntheses. USA: John Wiley & Sons.

Berdyshev, E. V., Goya, J., Gorshkova, I., Prestwich, G.D., Byun, H.S., Bittman, R., and Natarajan, V. 2011 Characterization of sphingosine-1-phosphate lyase activity by ESI-LC/MS/MS quantitation of (2E)-hexadecenal, *Analytical Biochemistry*, 408: 12–18. doi: 10.1016%2Fj.ab.2010.08.026.

Bertrand, F., Basketter, D.A., Roberts, D.W., and Lepoittevin, J.P. 1997 Skin sensitization to eugenol and isoeugenol in mice: possible metabolic pathways involving ortho-quinone and quinone methide intermediates, *Chemical Research in Toxicology*, 10: 335–343. doi: 10.1021/tx960087v.

Beyer, J., Ehlers, D., and Maurer, H.H. 2006 Abuse of nutmeg (Myristica fragrans Houtt.): Studies on the metabolism and the toxicologic detection of its ingredients elemicin, myristicin, and safrole in rat and human urine using gas chromatography/mass spectrometry. *Therapeutic Drug Monitoring*, 28: 568–575. doi: 10.1097/00007691-200608000-00013.

Bhaskar, A., and Kumar, A. 2012 Antihyperglycemic, antioxidant and hypolipidemic effect of Punica granatum L flower extract in streptozotocin induced diabetic rats, *Asian Pacific Journal of Tropical Biomedicine*, 2: 1764–1769. doi: 10.1016/S2221-1691(12)60491-2.

Booth, J. K., Page, J.E., and Bohlmann, J. 2017 Terpene synthases from Cannabis sativa, *Plos One*, 12: 0173911. doi: 10.1371/journal.pone.0173911.

Borges, P., and Pino, J. 1993 Preparation of nutmeg oleoresin by alcohol extraction, *Food/Nahrung*, 37: 280–282. doi: 10.1002/food.19930370315.

Brenner, N., Frank, O., and Knight, E. 1993 Chronic nutmeg psychosis, *Journal of the Royal Society of Medicine*, 86: 179–180. https://www.ncbi.nlm.nih.gov/pmc/articles/PMC1293919/pdf/-jrsocmed00100-0067.pdf.

Brown, K. N. 1994 *Synthesis and Properties of Expanded Cage Complexes of Pt (IV), Pt (II), Co (III) and Cr (III)*. Thesis, Australian National University.

Bruha, R., Dvorak, K., and Petrtyl, J. 2012 Alcoholic liver disease, *World Journal of Hepatology*, 4: 81. doi: 10.4254%2Fwjh.v4.i3.81.

Buchanan, R. L. 1978 Toxicity of spices containing methylenedioxybenzene derivatives, *Journal of Food Safety*, 1: 275–293. doi: 10.1111/j.1745-4565.1978.tb00281.x.

Cao, Y., Zhang, H., Liu, H., Liu, W., Zhang, R., Xian, M., and Liu, H. 2018 Biosynthesis and production of sabinene: Current state and perspectives, *Applied Microbiology and Biotechnology*, 102: 1535–1544. doi: 10.1007/s00253-017-8695-5.

Carocho, M., and Ferreira, I.C. 2013. A review on antioxidants, prooxidants and related controversy: natural and synthetic compounds, screening and analysis methodologies and future perspectives, *Food and Chemical Toxicology*, 51: 15–25. doi: 10.1016/j.fct.2012.09.021.

Carrasco, A. H., Espinoza, C.L., Cardile, V., Gallardo, C., Cardona, W., Lombardo, L., Catalán, M.K., Cuellar, F.M., and Russo, A. 2008. Eugenol and its synthetic analogues inhibit cell growth of human cancer cells (Part I), *Journal of the Brazilian Chemical Society*, 19: 543–548. doi: 10.1590/S0103-50532008000300024.

Chatterjee, S., Gupta, S., and Variyar, P.S. 2015. Comparison of essential oils obtained from different extraction techniques as an aid in identifying aroma significant compounds of nutmeg (Myristica fragrans), *Natural Product Communications*, 10: 1443–1446. doi: 10.1177%2F1934578X1501000833.

Chemat, F., Rombaut, N., Fabiano-Tixier, N.S., Pierson, J.T., and Bily, A. 2015 "Green extraction: from concepts to research, education, and economical opportunities". In *Green Extraction of Natural Products*. Wiley-VCH Verlag GmbH & Co. KGaA. doi: 10.1002/9783527676828.ch1.

Chen, M., Wang, Z.W., Hu, C.Y., and Wang, J.L. 2012 Effects of temperature on release of eugenol and isoeugenol from soy protein isolate films into simulated fatty food, *Packaging Technology and Science*, 25: 485–492. doi: 10.1002/pts.995.

Cho. J. Y., Choi, G.J., Son, S.W., Jang, K.S., Lim, H.K., Lee, S.O., Sung, N.D., Cho, K.Y., and Kim, J.C. 2007 Isolation and antifungal activity of lignans from Myristica fragrans against various plant pathogenic fungi, *Pest Management Science: Formerly Pesticide Science*, 63: 935–940. doi: 10.1002/ps.1420.

Clark, C. R., DeRuiter, J., and Noggle, F.T. 1996 Analysis of 1-(3-methoxy-4, 5-methylenedioxyphenyl)-2-propanamine (MMDA) derivatives synthesized from nutmeg oil and 3-methoxy-4, 5-methylenedioxybenzaldehyde, *Journal of Chromatographic Science*, 34: 34–42. doi: 10.1093/chromsci/34.1.34.

Cragg, G. M., Newman, D.J., and Yang, S.S. 2006 Natural product extracts of plant and marine origin having antileukemia potential. The NCI experience, *Journal of Natural Products*, 69: 488–498. doi: 10.1021/np0581216.

Cushny, A. R. 1908 Nutmeg poisoning, *Proceedings of the Royal Society of Medicine*, 1: 39–44. https://www.ncbi.nlm.nih.gov/pmc/articles/PMC2045778/pdf/procrsmed00847-0043.pdf.

De Vincenzi, M., Stammati, A., De Vincenzi, A.T., and Silano, M. 2004 Constituents of aromatic plants: carvacrol, *Fitoterapia*, 75: 801–804. doi: 10.1016/j.fitote.2004.05.002.

Demetriades, A. K., Wallman, P., McGuiness, A. and Gavalas, M. 2005 Low cost, high risk: Accidental nutmeg intoxication, *Emergency Medicine Journal*, 22: 223–225. 10.1136/emj.2002.004168.

Dhingra, D., and Sharma, A. 2006 Antidepressant-like activity of n-hexane extract of nutmeg (Myristica fragrans) seeds in mice, *Journal of Medicinal Food*, 9: 84–89. doi: /10.1089/jmf.2006.9.84.

Dighe, V. V., and Charegaonkar, G.A. 2009 HPTLC analysis of Myristicin and Safrole in seed powder of Myristica fragrans Houtt, *JPC–Journal of Planar Chromatography–Modern TLC* 22: 445–448. doi: 10.1556/JPC.22.2009.6.11.

Dorman, H. D., and Deans, S.G. 2004 Chemical composition, antimicrobial and in vitro antioxidant properties of Monarda citriodora var. citriodora, Myristica fragrans, Origanum vulgare ssp. hirtum, Pelargonium sp. and Thymus zygis oil, *Journal of Essential Oil Research*, 16: 145–150. doi: 10.1080/10412905.2004.9698679.

Dröge, W., Schipper, H.M. 2007 Oxidative stress and aberrant signaling in aging and cognitive decline, *Aging Cell*, 6: 361–370. doi: 10.1111/j.1474-9726.2007.00294.x.

Duke, J., and M. J. Bogenschutz. 1994 Dr. Duke's phytochemical and ethnobotanical databases: USDA, Agricultural Research Service. https://phytochem.nal.usda.gov/phytochem/ethnoPlants/show/207?qlookup=Nutmeg&offset=0&max=20&et=. (Accession date: 26th April 2021)

Duke, J. A., Bogenschutz-Godwin, M.J., Du-Cellier, J., and Duke, P.K. 2002 CRC *Handbook of Medicinal Spices*. Boca Raton: CRC press.

Eggersdorfer, M. 2000 "Terpenes". In *Ullmann's Encyclopedia of Industrial Chemistry*. Wiley-VCH Verlag GmbH & Co. KGaA. doi: 10.1002/14356007.a26_205.

Ehrenpreis, J. E., DesLauriers, C., Lank, P., Armstrong, P.K., and Leikin, J.B. 2014 Nutmeg poisonings: A retrospective review of 10 years experience from the Illinois Poison Center. 2001–2011, *Journal of Medical Toxicology*, 10: 148–151. doi: 10.1007/s13181-013-0379-7.

FAO. 1994 Nutmeg and Derivatives. Food and Agriculture Organization of United Nations. Italy, Rome. http://www.fao.org/3/v4084e/v4084e.pdf.

FAOSTAT. 2019. http://www.fao.org/faostat/en/#data/QC/visualize. (Accession Date: 26th April, 2021)

Favre, H. A., and Powell, W.H. 2013 *Nomenclature of Organic Chemistry: IUPAC Recommendations and Preferred Names 2013*. UK: The Royal Society of Chemistry.

Fernando, A., and Senevirathne, W. 2019 Raw Material from Nutmeg (Myristica fragrans) as Effective Fungicide against Fusarium oxysporum and the Oleoresin Profile of Nutmeg, *Journal of Applied Life Sciences International*, 22: 1–10. doi: 10.9734/jalsi/2019/v22i430133.

Figueroa-Lopez, K.J., Andrade-Mahecha, M.M., and Torres-Vargas, O.L. 2018a Development of antimicrobial biocomposite films to preserve the quality of bread, *Molecules*, 23: 212. doi: /10.3390/molecules23010212.

Figueroa-Lopez, K.J., Andrade-Mahecha, M.M., and Torres-Vargas, O.L. 2018b Spice oleoresins containing antimicrobial agents improve the potential use of bio-composite films based on gelatin, *Food Packaging and Shelf Life*, 17: 50–56. doi: 10.1016/j.fpsl.2018.05.005.

Forrester, M.B. 2005 Nutmeg intoxication in Texas, 1998–2004, *Human and Experimental Toxicology*, 24: 563–566. doi: 10.1191/0960327105ht567oa.

Ganesan, M., New-Aaron, M., Dagur, R.S., Makarov, E., Wang, W., Kharbanda, K.K., Kidambi, S., Poluektova, L.Y., and Osna, N.A. 2019 Alcohol metabolism potentiates HIV-induced hepatotoxicity: Contribution to end-stage liver disease, *Biomolecules*, 9: 851. doi: 10.3390/biom9120851.

Ghosh, A., and Ghosh, T. 2010 Herbal drugs of abuse, *Systematic Reviews in Pharmacy*, 1: 141–145.

Gobato. R., Gobato, A., and Fedrigo, D.F.G. 2015 Molecular electrostatic potential of the main monoterpenoids compounds found in oil Lemon Tahiti-(Citrus Latifolia Var Tahiti), *Parana Journal of Science and Education*, 1: 1–10.

Grover, J., Khandkar, S., Vats, V., Dhunnoo, Y., and Das, D. 2002 Pharmacological studies on Myristica fragrans--antidiarrheal, hypnotic, analgesic and hemodynamic (blood pressure) parameters, *Methods and Findings in Experimental and Clinical Pharmacology*, 24: 675–680. doi: 10.1358/mf.2002.24.10.802317.

Gülçin, İ. 2011 Antioxidant activity of eugenol: A structure-activity relationship study, *Journal of Medicinal Food*, 14: 975–985. doi: 10.1089/jmf.2010.0197.

Gupta, A. D., Bansal, V.K., Babu, V., and Maithil, N. 2013 Chemistry, antioxidant and antimicrobial potential of nutmeg (Myristica fragrans Houtt), *Journal of Genetic engineering and Biotechnology*, 11: 25–31. doi: 10.1016/j.jgeb.2012.12.001.

Gupta, A. D., and Rajpurohit, D. 2011 "Antioxidant and antimicrobial activity of nutmeg (Myristica fragrans)." In *Nuts and Seeds in Health And Disease Prevention*. UK: Academic Press (Elsevier). doi: 10.1016/B978-0-12-375688-6.10098-2.

Ha, M. T., Vu, N.K., Tran, T.H., Kim, J.A., Woo, M.H., and Min, B.S. 2020 Phytochemical and pharmacological properties of Myristica fragrans Houtt: An updated review, *Archives of Pharmacal Research*, 43: 1067–1092. doi: 10.1007/s12272-020-01285-4.

Hammerschmidt, F. J., Panten, J., Pickenhagen, W., Schatkowski, D., Bauer, K., Garbe, D., and Surburg, H. 2003 "Flavors and Fragrances". In *Ullmann's Encyclopedia of Industrial Chemistry*, Wiley-VCH Verlag GmbH & Co. KGaA.

Hammoud Z., Gharib, R., Fourmentin, S., Elaissari, A. and Greige-Gerges, H. 2019 New findings on the incorporation of essential oil components into liposomes composed of lipoid S100 and cholesterol, *International Journal of Pharmaceutics*, 561: 161–170. doi: 10.1016/j.ijpharm.2019.02.022.

Hasmita, I., Redha, F., and Junaidy, R. 2019 Enhancement of quality of nutmeg oil using rotary vaccumm evaporator, *Proceedings of the Journal of Physics: Conference Series*, 1232: IOP Publishing. doi: 10.1088/1742-6596/1232/1/012039.

Hayfaa, A. A. S., Sahar, A.M. A.S. and Awatif, M.A.S. 2013 Evaluation of analgesic activity and toxicity of alkaloids in Myristica fragrans seeds in mice, *Journal of Pain Research*, 6: 611. doi: 10.2147%2FJPR.S45591.

Hickey, M. J. 1948 Investigation of the chemical constituents of Brazilian sassafras oil, *The Journal of Organic Chemistry*, 13: 443–446.

Huang, Y., Wu, C., Ye, Y., Zeng, J., Zhu, J., Li, Y., Wang, W., Zhang, W., Chen, Y., and Xie, H. 2019 The increase of ROS caused by the interference of DEHP with JNK/p38/p53 pathway as the reason for hepatotoxicity, *International Journal of Environmental Research and Public Health*, 16: 356. doi: 10.3390/ijerph16030356.

Illupapalayam, V. V., Smith, S.C., and Gamlath, S. 2014 Consumer acceptability and antioxidant potential of probiotic-yogurt with spices, *LWT-Food Science and Technology*, 55: 255–262. doi: 10.1016/j.lwt.2013.09.025.

Ioannides, C., Delaforge, M., and Parke, D. 1981 Safrole: its metabolism, carcinogenicity and interactions with cytochrome P-450, *Food and Cosmetics Toxicology*, 19: 657–666. doi: 10.1016/0015-6264(81)90518-6.

IPCS. 1997 Myristica fragrans Houtt. (PIM 355). In International Programme on Chemical Safety. http://www.inchem.org/documents/pims/plant/pim355.htm (Accession date: 24th April 2021)

ITC. 2019a International Trade Centre. Product 090811, Nutmeg neither ground nor crushed. https://www.trademap.org/Country_SelProduct_TS.aspx?nvpm=1%7c%7c%7c%7c%7c090811%7c%7c%7c6%7c1%7c1%7c2%7c2%7c1%7c2%7c4%7c1%7c1 (Accession date: 26th April, 2021).

ITC. 2019b International Trade Centre. Product 330190, Extracted oleoresins; concentrates of essential oils in fats, fixed oils, waxes and the like, obtained by enfleurage or maceration; terpenic by-products of the deterpenation of essential oils; aromatic aqueous distillates and aqueous solutions of essential oils. https://www.trademap.org/Country_SelProduct.aspx?nvpm=1%7c%7c%7c%7c%7c330190%7c%7c%7c6%7c1%7c1%7c2%7c1%7c1%7c2%7c1%7c1%7c1B (Accession date: 26th April, 2021).

Jadhav, V., Kalase, V., and Patil, P. 2014 GC-MS analysis of bioactive compounds in methanolic extract of Holigarna grahamii (wight) Kurz, *International Journal of Herbal Medicine*, 2: 35–39. https://www.florajournal.com/archives/2014/vol2issue4/PartA/2-3-26.1.pdf

Jaeschke, H., and Ramachandran, A. 2020. Mechanisms and pathophysiological significance of sterile inflammation during acetaminophen hepatotoxicity, *Food and Chemical Toxicology*, 138: 111240. doi: 10.1016/j.fct.2020.111240.

Ji, J. B., Lu, X.H., Cai, M.Q., and Xu, Z.C. 2006 Improvement of leaching process of Geniposide with ultrasound, *Ultrasonics Sonochemistry*, 13: 455–462. doi: 10.1016/j.ultsonch.2005.08.003.

Johnson-Arbor, K., and Smolinske, S., 2020 Stoned on spices: a mini-review of three commonly abused household spice, *Clinical Toxicology*, 59: 101–105. doi: 10.1080/15563650.2020.1840579.

Kapoor, I., Singh, B., Singh, G., De Heluani, C.S., De Lampasona, M., and Catalan, C.A. 2013 Chemical composition and antioxidant activity of essential oil and oleoresins of nutmeg (Myristica fragrans Houtt.) fruits, *International Journal of Food Properties*, 16: 1059–1070. doi: 10.1080/10942912.2011.576357.

Kemprai, P., Protim Mahanta, B., Sut, D., Barman, R., Banik, D., Lal, M., Proteem Saikia, S., and Haldar, S. 2020 Review on safrole: identity shift of the 'candy shop'aroma to a carcinogen and deforester, *Flavour and Fragrance Journal*, 35: 5–23. doi: 10.1002/ffj.3521.

Khalil, A. A., Rahman, U., Khan, M.R., Sahar, A., Mehmood, T., and Khan, M. 2017 Essential oil eugenol: sources, extraction techniques and nutraceutical perspectives, *RSC Advances*, 7: 32669–32681. doi: 10.1039/C7RA04803C.

Kirk, R. E., Othmer, D.F., Grayson, M., and Eckroth, D. 1983 *Encyclopedia of Chemical Technology*. NJ: John Wiley and Sons.

Koeduka, T., Fridman, E., Gang, D.R., Vassão, D.G., Jackson, B.L., Kish, C.M., Orlova, I., Spassova, S.M., Lewis, N.G. and Noel, J.P. 2006 Eugenol and isoeugenol, characteristic aromatic constituents of spices, are biosynthesized via reduction of a coniferyl alcohol ester, *Proceedings of the National Academy of Sciences*, 103: 10128–10133. doi: 10.1073/pnas.0603732103.

Kolehmainen, E., Laihia, K., Laatikainen, R., Vepsäläinen, J., Niemitz, M., and Suontamo, R. 1997 Complete Spectral Analysis of the 1H NMR 16-Spin System of β-Pinene, *Magnetic Resonance in Chemistry*, 35: 463–467.

Kumar, A., Tandon, S., Ahmad, J., Yadav, A., and Kahol, A. 2005 Essential oil composition of seed and fruit coat of Elettaria cardamomum from South India, *Journal of Essential Oil Bearing Plants*, 8: 204–207. doi: 10.1080/0972060X.2005.10643446.

Lee, J. W., Choi, Y.H., Yoo, M.Y., Choi, S.U., Hong, K.S., Lee, B.H., Yon, G.H., Kim, Y.S., Kim, Y.K., and Ryu, S.Y. 2006 Inhibitory effects of the seed extract of Myristicae semen on the proliferation of human tumor cell lines (II), *Korean Journal of Pharmacognosy*, 37: 206–211. https://www.koreascience.or.kr/article/JAKO200603041324072.pdf

Lewis, R. A. 2016 *Hawley's Condensed Chemical Dictionary*. NJ: John Wiley & Sons.

Liu, Z. L., Chu, S.S., and Liu, Q.R. 2010. Chemical composition and insecticidal activity against Sitophilus zeamais of the essential oils of Artemisia capillaris and Artemisia mongolica, *Molecules*, 15: 2600–2608. doi: 10.3390/molecules15042600.

López, V., Gerique, J., Langa, E., Berzosa, C., Valero, M.S., and Gómez-Rincón, C. 2015 Antihelmintic effects of nutmeg (Myristica fragans) on Anisakis simplex L3 larvae obtained from Micromesistius potassou, *Research in Veterinary Science*, 100: 148–152. doi: 10.1016/j.rvsc.2015.03.033.

Lu, X., Yang, L., Chen, J., Zhou, J., Tang, X., Zhu, Y., Qiu, H., and Shen, J. 2017 The action and mechanism of myrislignan on A549 cells in vitro and in vivo, *Journal of Natural Medicines* 71: 76–85. doi: 10.1007/s11418-016-1029-6.

Madrid, V. A., Espinoza, C.L., Montenegro, V.I., Villena, G.J., and Carrasco, A.H. 2011 New catechol derivatives of safrole and their antiproliferative activity towards breast cancer cells, *Molecules*, 16: 4632–4641. doi: 10.3390/molecules16064632.

Manier, S. K., Wagmann, L., Weber, A.A., and Meyer, M.R. 2021 Abuse of nutmeg seeds: Detectable by means of liquid chromatography-mass spectrometry techniques?, *Drug Testing and Analysis*. In press. doi: 10.1002/dta.3027.

Mann, J., Davidson, R.S., Hobbs, J.B., Banthorpe, D., and Harborne, J.B. 1994 *Natural Products: Their Chemistry and Biological Significance*. UK: Longman Publishing Group

Marongiu, B., Piras, A., and Porcedda, S. 2004. Comparative analysis of the oil and supercritical CO_2 extract of Elettaria cardamomum (L.) Maton, *Journal of Agricultural and Food Chemistry*, 52: 6278–6282. doi: 10.1021/jf034819i.

Marzuki, I., Joefrie, B., Aziz, S.A., Agusta, H., and Surahman, M. 2014 Physico-chemical characterization of Maluku nutmeg oil, *International Journal of Science and Engineering*, 7: 61–64. doi: 10.12777/ijse.7.1.61-64.

Nelson, D. L. and Cox, M.M. 2008 *Lehninger Principles of Biochemistry*. NY: W.H Freeman.

Mazurak, M., and Kusa, J. 2018 Jan Evangelista Purkinje: A passion for discovery, *Texas Heart Institute Journal*, 45: 23–26. doi: 10.14503%2FTHIJ-17-6351.

Mazza, G., Kiehn, F., and Marshall, H. 1993 *Monarda: A Source of Geraniol, Linalool, Thymol and Carvacrol-Rich Essential Oils*. New crop Wiley, New York. 628–631.

McKee, L., Thompson, L., and Harden, M. 1993 Effect of three grinding methods on some properties of nutmeg, *LWT-Food Science and Technology*, 26: 121–125. doi: 10.1006/fstl.1993.1026.

McKee, L. H. 1990. *"Composition, Antioxidant Properties and Microbiology of Nutmeg Ground by Three Procedures"*. Ph.D diss., Texas Tech University.

Morita, T., Jinno, K., Kawagishi, H., Arimoto, Y., Suganuma, H., Inakuma, T., and Sugiyama, K. 2003 Hepatoprotective effect of myristicin from nutmeg (Myristica fragrans) on lipopolysaccharide/d-galactosamine-induced liver injury, *Journal of Agricultural and Food Chemistry*, 5: 1560–1565. doi: 10.1021/jf020946n.

Morsy, N. F. 2016 A comparative study of nutmeg (Myristica fragrans Houtt.) oleoresins obtained by conventional and green extraction techniques, *Journal of Food Science and Technology*, 53: 3770–3777. doi: 10.1007/s13197-016-2363-0.

Mut-Salud, N., Álvarez, P.J., Garrido, J.M., Carrasco, E., Aránega, A., and Rodríguez-Serrano, F. 2016 Antioxidant intake and antitumor therapy: toward nutritional recommendations for optimal results, *Oxidative medicine and Cellular Longevity* Article ID 6719534. doi: 10.1155/2016/6719534.

Nagy, B., and Simándi, B. 2008 Effects of particle size distribution, moisture content, and initial oil content on the supercritical fluid extraction of paprika, 46: 293–298. doi: 10.1016/j.supflu.2008.04.009.

Narasimhan, B., Belsare, D., Pharande, D., Mourya, V., and Dhake, A. 2004 Esters, amides and substituted derivatives of cinnamic acid: synthesis, antimicrobial activity and QSAR investigations, *European Journal of Medicinal Chemistry*, 39: 827–834. doi: 10.1016/j.ejmech.2004.06.013.

Narasimhan, B., and Dhake, A.S. 2006 Antibacterial principles from Myristica fragrans seeds, *Journal of Medicinal Food*, 9: 395–399. doi: 10.1089/jmf.2006.9.395.

Nuchuchua, O., Saesoo, S., Sramala, I., Puttipipatkhachorn, S., Soottitantawat, A., and Ruktanonchai, U. 2009 Physicochemical investigation and molecular modeling of cyclodextrin complexation mechanism with eugenol, *Food Research International*, 42: 1178–1185. doi: 10.1016/j.foodres.2009.06.006.

O'Neil, M. J., Heckelman, P., Koch, C., and Roman, K. 2006 *An Encyclopedia of Chemicals, Drugs and Biologicals*. Whitehouse Station. NJ: Merck & Co.

Opdyke, D. L. 1979. Monographs on fragrance raw materials, *Food and Cosmetics Toxicology*, 17: 509–533. doi: 10.1016/0015-6264(79)90012-9.

Pakdel, H., Pantea, D.M., and Roy, C. 2001 Production of dl-limonene by vacuum pyrolysis of used tires, *Journal of Analytical and Applied Pyrolysis*, 57: 91–107. doi: 10.1016/S0165-2370(00)00136-4.

Parthasarathy, V. A., Chempakam, B., and Zachariah, T.J. 2008 "Nutmeg and Mace". In *Chemistry of Spices*. Cabi. doi: 10.1079/9781845934057.0000.

Parvez, M. K., and Rishi, V. 2019 Herb-drug interactions and hepatotoxicity, *Current Drug Metabolism*, 20: 275–282. doi: 10.2174/1389200220666190325141422.

Pashapoor, A., Mashhadyrafie, S., and Mortazavi, P. 2020 The antioxidant potential and antihyperlipidemic activity of myristica fragrans seed (nutmeg) extract in diabetic rats. *Journal of Human, Environment, and Health Promotion*, 6: 91–96

Paul, S., Hwang, J.K., Kim, H.Y., Jeon, W.K., Chung, C., and Han, J.S. 2013 Multiple biological properties of macelignan and its pharmacological implications, *Archives of Pharmacal Research*, 36: 264–272. doi: 10.1007/s12272-013-0048-z.

Paumgartten, F. J. R., De-Carvalho, R., Souza, C., Madi, K., and Chahoud, I. 1998 Study of the effects of ß-myrcene on rat fertility and general reproductive performance, *Brazilian Journal of Medical and Biological Research*, 31: 955–965. doi: 10.1590/S0100-879X1998000700012.

Payne, R.B. 1963 Nutmeg intoxication, *New England Journal of Medicine*, 269: 36–38. doi: 10.1056/NEJM196307042690108.

Perkin, W. H., and Trikojus, V. M. 1927 CCXII.—A synthesis of safrole and o-safrole, *Journal of the Chemical Society (Resumed)*, 1663–1666. doi: 10.1039/JR9270001663.

Peter, K. V. 2012 *Handbook of Herbs and Spices*. Wood Head Publishing: Elsevier. doi: 10.1016/B978-0-85709-039-3.50031-1.

Pinheiro, L., Sousa, J., Barreto, N., Dantas, T., Menezes, C., Lima, A. and Silva, A. 2017 Eugenol and isoeugenol in association with antifungal against cryptococcus neoformans, *International Journal of Pharmacognosy and Phytochemical Research*, 9: 596–599. doi: 10.25258/phyto. v9i2.8133.

Pirbalouti, A., Rahimmalek, M., Malekpoor, F., and Karimi, A. 2011 Variation in antibacterial activity, thymol and carvacrol contents of wild populations of' Thymus daenensis subsp. Daenensis' Celak, *Plant Omics*, 4: 209–214.

Poleck, T. 1886 Ueber die chemische Structur des Safrols, *Berichte der deutschen chemischen Gesellschaft*, 19: 1094–1098. doi: 10.1002/cber.188601901243.

Pramod, K., Suneesh, C.V., Shanavas, S., Ansari, S.H. and Ali, H. 2015 Unveiling the compatibility of eugenol with formulation excipients by systematic drug-excipient compatibility studies, *Journal of Analytical Science and Technology*, 6: 1–14. doi: 10.1186/s40543-015-0073-2.

Pranati, T., Anitha, R., Rajeshkumar, S., Lakshmi, T. 2019 Preparation of silver nanoparticles using nutmeg oleoresin and its antimicrobial activity against oral pathogens. *Research Journal of Pharmacy and Technology*, 12: 2799–2803. doi: 10.5958/0974-360X.2019.00471.2.

Purwantiningsih, H. A., and Chan, K. 2011. Free radical scavenging activity of the standardized ethanolic extract of Eurycoma longifolia (TAF-273), *International Journal of Pharmacy and Pharmaceutical Sciences*, 3: 343–347.

Quin, G., Fanning, N., and Plunkett, P. 1998 Nutmeg intoxication, *Journal of Accident and Emergency Medicine*, 15: 287. doi: 10.1136%2Femj.15.4.287-d.

Rahman, N., Fazilah, A., and Effarizah, M. 2015 Toxicity of nutmeg (myristicin): A review, *International Journal of Advanced Science Engineering and Information Technology*, 5: 61–64. https://core.ac.uk/download/pdf/194425327.pdf

Rodianawati, I., Hastuti, P. and Cahyanto, M.N. 2015 Nutmeg's (Myristica fragrans Houtt) oleoresin: Effect of heating to chemical compositions and antifungal properties, *Procedia Food Science*, 3: 244–254. doi: 10.1016/j.profoo.2015.01.027.

Rossi, P. G., Bao, L., Luciani, A., Panighi, J., Desjobert, J.M., Costa, J. Casanova, J., Bolla, J.M. and Berti, L. 2007 (E)-Methylisoeugenol and elemicin: Antibacterial components of Daucus carota L. essential oil against Campylobacter jejuni, *Journal Of Agricultural and Food Chemistry*, 55: 7332–7336. doi: 10.1021/jf070674u.

Sabulal, B., Dan, M., Kurup, R., Pradeep, N.S., Valsamma, R.K., and George, V. 2006 Caryophyllene-rich rhizome oil of Zingiber nimmonii from South India: Chemical characterization and antimicrobial activity, *Phytochemistry*, 67: 2469–2473. doi: 10.1016/j.phytochem.2006.08.003.

Said, P., Arya, O., Pradhan, R., Singh, R., and Rai, B. 2015 Separation of oleoresin from ginger rhizome powder using green processing technologies, *Journal of Food Process Engineering* 38: 107–114. doi: 10.1111/jfpe.12127.

Sajjadi, S., Shokoohinia, Y., Hemmati, S., Gholamzadeh, S. and Behbahani, M. 2012 Antivirial activity of elemicin from Peucedanum pastinacifolium, *Research in Pharmaceutical Sciences*, 7: 784.

Sangalli, B. C., Sangalli, B., and Chiang, W. 2000 Toxicology of nutmeg abuse, *Journal of Toxicology: Clinical Toxicology*, 38: 671–678. doi: 10.1081/CLT-100102020.

Sermakkani, M., and Thangapandian, V. 2012 GC-MS analysis of Cassia italica leaf methanol extract, *Asian Journal of Pharmaceutical and Clinical Research*, 5: 90–94. https://asset-pdf. scinapse.io/prod/2186275073/2186275073.pdf

Shafiei, Z., Shuhairi, M.N., Md Fazly Shah Yap, N., Harry Sibungkil, C.A., and Latip, J. 2012 Antibacterial activity of Myristica fragrans against oral pathogens, *Evidence-Based Complementary and Alternative Medicine*, 12: 825362. doi: 10.1155/2012/825362.

Shahidi, F., and Hossain, A. 2018 Bioactives in spices, and spice oleoresins: Phytochemicals and their beneficial effects in food preservation and health promotion, *Journal of Food Bioactives*, 3: 8–75. doi: 10.31665/JFB.2018.3149.

Sharangi, A. B., Bhutia, P. H., Raj, A. C., and Sreenivas, M. 2018 *Underexploited Spice Crops: Present Status, Agrotechnology, and Future Research Directions*. Newyork: CRC Press.

Shaund, D. C. F., and Lee, C. 2011 The spice of life: An analysis of nutmeg exposures in California, *Clinical Toxicology*, 49: 177–180. doi: 10.1155/2012/825362.

Shulgin, A. T., Sargent, T., and Naranjo, C. 1967 The chemistry and psychopharmacology of nutmeg and of several related phenylisopropylamines, *Psychopharmacol Bulletin*, 4: 13.

Shulgin, A. T. 1966 Possible implication of myristicin as a psychotropic substance, *Nature*, 210: 380–384.

Silva, A. C. R., Lopes, P.M., De-Azevedo, M.M.B., Costa, D.C.M., Alviano, C.S., and Alviano, D.S. 2012 Biological activities of a-pinene and β-pinene enantiomers, *Molecules*, 17: 6305–6316. doi: 10.3390/molecules17066305.

Simón, J., Casado-Andrés, M., Goikoetxea-Usandizaga, N., Serrano-Maciá, M., and Martínez-Chantar, M.L. 2020 Nutraceutical properties of polyphenols against liver diseases, *Nutrients*, 12: 3517. doi: 10.3390/nu12113517.

Sohilait H. J., and Kainama, H. 2015 Synthesis of Myristicin Ketone (3, 4-Methylenedioxy-5-Methoxyphenyl)-2-Propanone from Myristicin, *Science*, 3: 62–66. doi: 10.11648/j. sjc.20150303.15.

Sohilait, H. J., and Kainama, H. 2016 Synthesis of 1-(3, 4-methylenedioxyphenyl)-1-butene-3-one from safrole, *European Journal of Pure and Applied Chemistry*, 3: 66–70

Solheim, E., and Scheline, R. 1980 Metabolism of alkenebenzene derivatives in the rat III. Elemicin and isoelemicin, *Xenobiotica*, 10: 371–380. doi: 10.3109/00498258009033770.

Stein, U., Greyer, H., and Hentschel, H. 2001 Nutmeg (myristicin) poisoning—report on a fatal case and a series of cases recorded by a poison information centre, *Forensic Science International*, 118: 87–90. doi: 10.1016/S0379-0738(00)00369-8.

Stephen, H. 1964 Solubilities of inorganic and organic compounds, *Ternary and Multicomponent Systems*, 2: 100–101.

Subarnas, A., Apriyantono, A., and Mustarichie, R. 2010 Identification of compounds in the essential oil of nutmeg seeds (Myristica fragrans Houtt.) that inhibit locomotor activity in mice, *International Journal of Molecular Sciences*, 11: 4771–4781. doi: 10.3390/ijms11114771.

Suderman, D. R. 2011 *Effective Use of Flavorings and Seasonings in Batter and Breading Systems*, Manhatttan USA: AACC International.

Sudradjat, S. E., Timotius, K.H., Mun'im, A., and Anwar, E. 2018 The isolation of myristicin from nutmeg oil by sequences distillation, *Journal of Young Pharmacists* 10: 20–23. doi: 10.5530/jyp.2018.10.6.

Tabanca, N., Demirci, B., Crockett, S., Başer, K.H.C. and Wedge, D.E. 2007 Chemical composition and antifungal activity of Arnica longifolia, Aster hesperius, and Chrysothamnus nauseosus essential oils, *Journal of Agricultural and Food Chemistry*, 55: 8430–8435. doi: 10.1021/jf071379c.

Tai, K. W., Huang, F.M., Huang, M.S., and Chang, Y.C. 2002 Assessment of the genotoxicity of resin and zinc-oxide eugenol-based root canal sealers using an in vitro mammalian test system, *Journal of Biomedical Materials Research: An Official Journal of The Society for Biomaterials and The Japanese Society for Biomaterials*, 59: 73–77. doi: 10.1002/jbm.1218.

Takikawa, A., Abe, K., Yamamoto, M., Ishimaru, S., Yasui, M., Okubo, Y., and Yokoigawa, K. 2002 Antimicrobial activity of nutmeg against Escherichia coli O157, *Journal Of Bioscience and Bioengineering*, 94: 315–320. doi: 10.1016/S1389-1723(02)80170-0.

Tavares, A. C., Gonçalves, M.J., Cavaleiro, C., Cruz, M.T., Lopes, M.C., Canhoto, J., and Salgueiro, L.R. 2008 Essential oil of Daucus carota subsp. halophilus: composition, antifungal activity and cytotoxicity, *Journal of Ethnopharmacology*, 119: 129–134. doi: 10.1016/j.jep.2008.06.012.

Tomaino, A., Cimino, F., Zimbalatti, V., Venuti, V., Sulfaro, V., De Pasquale, A., and Saija, A. 2005 Influence of heating on antioxidant activity and the chemical composition of some spice essential oils, *Food Chemistry*, 89: 549–554. doi: 10.1016/j.foodchem.2004.03.011.

National Toxicology Program 2010 *Toxicology and Carcinogenesis Studies of Isoeugenol (CAS No. 97-54-1) in F344/N rats and B6C3F1 mice (Gavage Studies)*. Technical Report Series: National Toxicology Program.

Truitt E. B., Callaway, M., Braude, M.C., and Krantz, J.C. 1961 The pharmacology of myristicin. A contribution to the psychopharmacology of nutmeg, *Journal of Neuropsychiatry*, 2: 205–210.

Ultee, A., Bennik, M., and Moezelaar, R. 2002 The phenolic hydroxyl group of carvacrol is essential for action against the food-borne pathogen Bacillus cereus, *Applied and Environmental Microbiology*, 68: 1561–1568. doi: 10.1128/AEM.68.4.1561-1568.2002.

Ultee, A., Slump, R., Steging, G., and Smid, E. 2000 Antimicrobial activity of carvacrol toward Bacillus cereus on rice, *Journal of Food Protection*, 63: 620–624. doi: 10.4315/0362-028X-63.5.620.

Upadhyay, A., Arsi, K., Wagle, B.R., Upadhyaya, I., Shrestha, S., Donoghue, A.M., and Donoghue, D.J. 2017 Trans-cinnamaldehyde, carvacrol, and eugenol reduce Campylobacter jejuni colonization factors and expression of virulence genes in vitro, *Frontiers in Microbiology*, 8: 713. doi: 10.3389/fmicb.2017.00713.

Van Lennep, J. R., Schuit, S., Van Bruchem-Visser, R., and Özcan, B. 2015 Unintentional nutmeg autointoxication. Letter to the Editor, *The Netherland Journal of Medicine*, 73. http://www.njmonline.nl/getpdf.php?id=1536

Van Ruth, S. M., Silvis, I.C., Alewijn, M., Liu, N., Jansen, M., and Luning, P.A. 2019 No more nutmegging with nutmeg: Analytical fingerprints for distinction of quality from low-grade nutmeg products, *Food Control*, 98: 439–448. doi: 10.1016/j.foodcont.2018.12.005.

Vardanega, R., Santos, D.T., and Meireles, M.A.A. 2014 Intensification of bioactive compounds extraction from medicinal plants using ultrasonic irradiation, *Pharmacognosy Reviews*, 8: 88–95. doi: 10.4103%2F0973-7847.134231.

Wahyuni, S., and Bermawie, N. 2020 Yield and fruit morphology of selected high productive Papua nutmeg trees (Myristica argentea Warb), *Proceedings of the IOP Conference Series: Earth and Environmental Science: IOP Publishing*. doi: 10.1088/1755-1315/418/1/012032.

Walsh, S. E., Maillard, J.Y., Russell, A., Catrenich, C., Charbonneau, D., and Bartolo, R. 2003 Activity and mechanisms of action of selected biocidal agents on Gram-positive and-negative bacteria, *Journal of Applied Microbiology*, 94: 240–247. doi: 10.1046/j.1365-2672.2003.01825.x.

Wang, Y., Xiao, J., Suzek, T.O., Zhang, J., Wang, J., and Bryant, S.H. 2009 PubChem: a public information system for analyzing bioactivities of small molecules, *Nucleic Acids Research*, 37: 623–633. doi: 10.1093/nar/gkp456.

Weast, R. C. 1972 *Hand book of Chemistry and Physics*. Boca Raton: CRC Press.

Xia, W., Cao, Z., Zhang, X., and Gao, L. 2021 A proteomics study on the mechanism of nutmeg-induced hepatotoxicity, *Molecules*, 26: 1748. doi: 10.3390/molecules26061748.

Yamasaki, Y., Kunoh, H., Yamamoto, Y.H., and Akimitsu, K. 2007 Biological roles of monoterpene volatiles derived from rough lemon (Citrus jambhiri Lush) in citrus defense, *Journal of General Plant Pathology*, 73: 168–179. doi: 10.1007/s10327-007-0013-0.

Yang, A. H., Zhang, L., Zhi, D.X., Liu, W.L., Gao, X., and He, X. 2018 Identification and analysis of the reactive metabolites related to the hepatotoxicity of safrole, *Xenobiotica*, 48: 1164–1172. doi: 10.1080/00498254.2017.1399227.

Yang, Y. 2005 Study on the inclusion compounds of eugenol with α-, β-, γ-and heptakis (2, 6-di-O-methyl)-β-cyclodextrins, *Journal of Inclusion Phenomena and Macrocyclic Chemistry*, 53: 27–33. doi: 10.1007/s10847-005-0247-4.

Yang, Z., Wu, N., Zu, Y., and Fu, Y. 2011 Comparative anti-infectious bronchitis virus (IBV) activity of (-)-pinene: Effect on nucleocapsid (N) protein, *Molecules*, 16: 1044–1054. doi: 10.3390/molecules16021044.

Yi, J. L., Shi, S., Shen, Y.L., Wang, L., Chen, H.Y., Zhu, J., and Ding, Y. 2015 Myricetin and methyl eugenol combination enhances the anticancer activity, cell cycle arrest and apoptosis induction of cis-platin against HeLa cervical cancer cell lines, *International Journal of Clinical and Experimental Pathology*, 8: 1116.

Zaidlewicz, M., and Gimiñska, M. 1997 Syntheses with organoboranes—VIII. Transformation of (1S, 6R)-(+)-2-carene into (1S, 6R)-(+)-3 (10)-carene and (1R, 5R)-(–)-α-thujene into (1R, 5R)-(+)-sabinene, *Tetrahedron: Asymmetry*, 8: 3847–3850. doi: 10.1016/S0957-4166(97)00589-2.

Zehiroglu, C., and Sarikaya, S.B.O. 2019 The importance of antioxidants and place in today's scientific and technological studies, *Journal of Food Science and Technology*, 56: 4757–4774. doi: 10.1007/s13197-019-03952-x.

Zhang, W. K., Tao, S.S., Li, T.T., Li, Y.S., Li, X.J., Tang, H.B., Cong, R.H., Ma, F.L., and Wan, C.J. 2016 Nutmeg oil alleviates chronic inflammatory pain through inhibition of COX-2 expression and substance P release in vivo, *Food and Nutrition Research*, 60: 30849. doi: 10.3402/fnr.v60.30849.

Zhao, L. Q., Sun, Z.H., Zheng, P., and Zhu, L.L. 2005 Biotransformation of isoeugenol to vanillin by a novel strain of Bacillus fusiformis, *Biotechnology Letters*, 27: 1505–1509. doi: 10.1007/s10529-005-1466-x.

Zheng, G. Q., Kenney, P.M., and Lam, L.K. 1992 Sesquiterpenes from clove (Eugenia caryophyllata) as potential anticarcinogenic agents, *Journal of Natural Products*, 55: 999–1003. doi: 10.1021/np50085a029.

CHAPTER 12

Health and Medicinal Properties of Rosemary Oleoresin

Laura Natali, Afanador-Barajas, and
Adriana Patricia Diaz-Morales
Universidad Central

Edgar Vázquez-Núñez
Universidad de Guanajuato

Sergio Rubén Peréz-Ríos, Marycarmen Cortés-Hernández,
and Gabriela Medina-Peréz
Universidad Autónoma del Estado de Hidalgo. Av. Universidad s/n Tulancingo

Cecilia Bañuelos
Centro de Investigación y de Estudios Avanzados del Instituto Politécnico Nacional

CONTENTS

DOI: 10.1201/9781003186205-12

12.1 INTRODUCTION

Rosemary is an evergreen perennial plant from the Mediterranean district. This plant is grown throughout the world. Currently, people consume it as a spice, a seasoning in cooking, and therapeutic purposes. Furthermore, because of its cell reinforcement properties, rosemary extract has generally been used in the food industry to improve the shelf life of different products (Senanayake 2018).

Rosemary is now classified as *Salvia rosmarinus* (L.) similar to *Rosmarinus officinalis* L. (Schleid, 1852) and belongs to the family Lamiaceae with a taxonomic classification (Drew et al., 2017):

Streptophyta (phylum)

Magnoliopsida (class)

Lamiales (order)

Lamiaceae (family)

Salvia (genus)

rosmarinus (species)

Rosemary plants are propagated by seeds, cuttings, layering, or root division. Depending on the geographical area and the use given to the plant material, rosemary leaves are harvested three to four times a year (Ribeiro-Santos et al., 2015). Since the dried product includes only leaves, the crop is cut regularly before flowering (Senanayake 2013). When destined for the spice market, the plant is cut as often as possible at a juvenile stage, as it is used in different culinary and meat applications. Only the leaves, or the concentrates obtained from the leaves, are typically used as culinary spices because of their antioxidant and food-enhancing properties (Senanayake 2018).

Rosemary oleoresins (ROs) are characterized by being a light green fluid; their aroma is characteristic of rosemary. This oleoresin is extracted conventionally by maceration with an organic diluent such as ethanol, hexane, or acetone. Another method used is pressurized liquid extraction (PLE), which is a traditional method to obtain oleoresins. Oleoresins can also be extracted using supercritical fluid extraction (SFE) (Lee et al., 2019; Carvalho et al., 2005). Sánchez-Camargo et al. (2016) studied two procedures in rosemary, super-critical antisolvent fractionation (SAF) and PLE, which were coordinated to isolate and enhance phenolic compounds for antioxidant bioactivity.

The main compounds involved in the antioxidant activity of rosemary extracts are phenolic diterpenes, such as rosmanol, carnasol, carnosic acid, isorosmanol, and epirosmanol (Loussouarn et al., 2017). Initial studies on the subject carried out by Okamura et al. (1994) reported that the highest concentration of phenolic compounds was extracted from rosemary leaves. Different phenolic compounds, such as rosmaric acid, carnosic acid, and carnosol, have been identified in oleoresins in rosemary (Lee et al., 2019). In addition, several RO components such as rosmanol, rosmariquinone, rosmariridiphenol, and carnasol are effective antioxidants (Nieto, Ros, and Castillo, 2018). Sánchez-Camargo et al. (2016) showed the correlation between the bioactivity of rosemary and the contents of phenolic diterpenes (carnosol and carnosic acid) and phenolic acids (rosmarinic acid). The therapeutic and cooking properties of *S. rosmarinus* oleoresin have been well identified. This chapter aims to present a detailed review of the literature on extraction methods and the chemical composition of oleoresin from *S. rosmarinus* to highlight potential applications. Figure 12.1 shows the main procedures and applications in ROs. Rosemary has been widely used in various sectors as a food ingredient for flavoring and traditional medicine because of its health benefits, such as antimicrobial, analgesic, and antirheumatic effects. Several groups have reported its anticancer (Moore, Yousef, and Tsiani 2016), anti-inflammatory (Hamidpour 2017), and antioxidant (Rašković et al., 2014) activities.

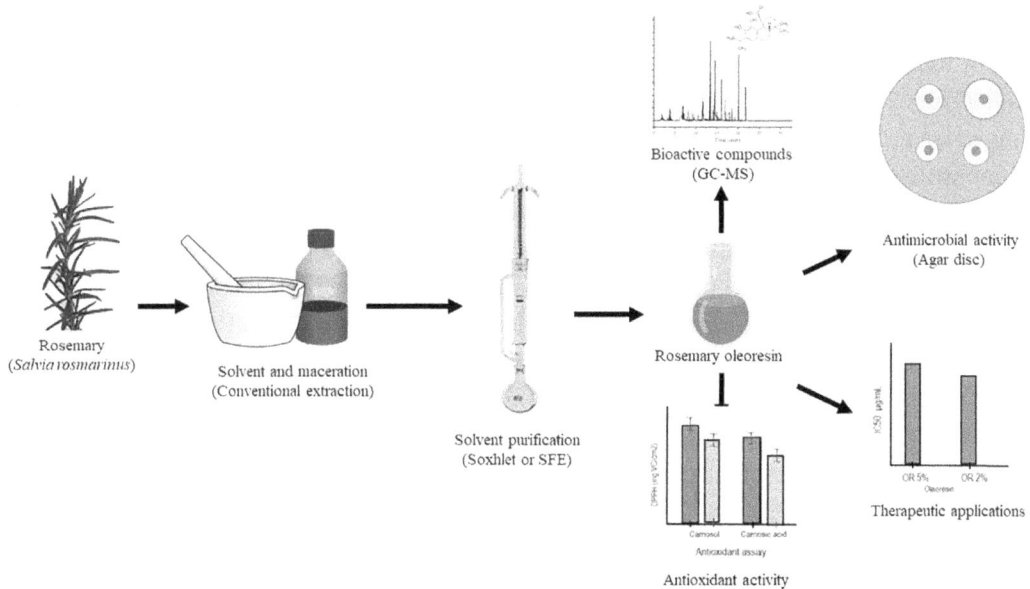

FIGURE 12.1 Representation of the *S. rosmarinus* oleoresin extraction, bioactive compounds, and therapeutic, antimicrobial, and antioxidant applications.

12.2 ROSEMARY EXTRACTION OLEORESIN

Regarding the extraction of rosemary's oleoresin, several researchers have evaluated different methods to prove the most effective in terms of yield, profitability, and reduction of the loss of some volatile compounds, among others. Several conventional methods exist to extract the essential oil, such as water distillation or steam distillation (Boutekedjiret et al., 2003). However, new methods have been tried, for example, microwave-assisted hydrodistillation (MAHD) (Moradi, Fazlali, and Hamedi 2018), organic solvent extraction (OSE) (Presti et al., 2005), microwave hydrodiffusion and gravity (MHDG) (Ferreira et al., 2020), high-pressure microwave extraction (solvent-free) (HPSFM) (Filly et al., 2014), supercritical CO_2 extraction (SCE) (Conde-Hernández et al., 2017), ultrasound extraction (EU) (Rodríguez-Rojo et al., 2012), and solvent-less microwave extraction (SFME) (Filly et al., 2014). The physicochemical characteristics of the extracted essential oils depend on the extraction method applied, and these extracts can vary significantly between them. Table 12.1 details the principles of the methods of extraction used to obtain essential oils.

12.2.1 Hydrodistillation and Steam Distillation

Hot water or steam is used to carry out this extraction process so that bioactive compounds can be released from the plant matrix, and this solvent is the medium that carries the compounds out. It is indirectly cooled to condense the mixture's steam, produce oil, and separate the biocompounds to facilitate separation from the water. Anhydrous sodium sulfate is widely used as a drying agent in the final step of the process (Aramrueang, Asavasanti, and Khanunthong 2019). The duration of the extraction with this method ranges from 1 to 10 hours; several factors condition the amount of oil extracted, such as distillation time, temperature, pressure, and plant material. Plant biomass is exposed to boiling water or steam during distillation to increase essential oil release through evaporation (Stratakos and Koidis 2016). Some drawbacks are found in this method. For instance, long-term boiling water might create artifacts due to the water's high temperatures or acidity, then the composition of the volatile oils can be found. When oils have a high concentration of esters, the hydrolysis of these compounds to acids and alcohols can be observed (Mejri et al., 2018).

The most common methods to extract essential oils are water and steam distillation; this method has been used to extract oils from diverse plant species, i.e., *Origanum onites* (Ozel and Kaymaz 2004), *Cannabis indica* and *Cannabis sativa* (Naz et al., 2017), *Ocimum basilicum* L. (Pagano et al., 2018), *Citrus auranticum* L. (Kusuma, Putra, and Mahfud 2016), and *S. rosmarinus* L. (Reverchon and Senatore 1992), among others. Several variables are essential to consider as crucial, such as contact time, which has been extensively studied as an essential factor in evaluating the quality of the process and oil extracted itself.

12.2.2 Microwave-Assisted Extraction

The microwave-assisted extraction (MAE) method involves three steps: (a) detachment of the solutes from the active sites of the solid matrix based on the higher pressure and temperature in the system; (b) diffusion of a solvent through the matrix of plant material; and (c) solutes released from the matrix to the solvent (Delazar et al., 2012).

TABLE 12.1   Methods to Extract Phytochemicals from Plant Extracts

Method	Principle	Reference
Hydrodistillation	It can be performed as (a) water distillation, (b) direct steam distillation, and (c) water and steam distillation. There are involved three physicochemical processes: hydrodiffusion, hydrolysis, and decomposition by heat. Uses water (liquid or steam) as an extraction solvent to recover volatile or polar plant material components.	Azmir et al. (2013)
Steam distillation	The process consists of separating substances taking advantage of their temperature sensitivity; the separation principle involves heating the mixture of undissolved liquids (two or more). Therefore, it is of paramount importance to ensure the contact of the surface of the liquids with the atmosphere.	Azmir et al. (2013)
Microwaved-assisted extraction	Nonionizing radiation waves with frequencies from 200 MHz to 300 GHz and wavelengths from 1 cm to 1 m heat facilitate the separate selectively the targeted material.	Ferreira et al. (2020)
Organic solvent extraction	This chemical extraction method is suitable for solvent extraction of oil from vegetables, oilseeds, and seeds. In addition, plant biomolecules as waxes and pigments can be extracted by applying other suitable processes.	Presti et al. (2005)
Microwave hydrodiffusion and gravity	Microwaves are applied for hydrodiffusion of essential oils from the inner to the outer sides of plant materials to extract and separate. This method is carried out at atmospheric pressure and without the use of any solvent.	Karakaya et al. (2014)
Pressure solvent extraction	This method promotes various phenomena (phase transition, change in reaction dynamics, or molecular structure, among others), inducing both directions reaction, decreasing the volume, and improving extraction efficiency.	Conde-Hernández et al. (2017)
Ultrasound extraction	The use of ultrasound produces a cavitation effect, increasing the frequency and speed of the molecules and thus improving the distribution and access of the solvent, resulting in a more remarkable recovery of target compounds.	Rodríguez-Rojo et al. (2012)
Solvent-free microwave extraction	Dry distillation using microwaves to facilitate extraction from a fresh plant matrix without adding water or organic solvent.	Chemat et al. (2015)
Supercritical fluid extraction	This technique is commonly applied for solid and liquid matrices. The most used supercritical fluid is CO_2. However, this process may be modified by the use of co-solvents such as ethanol or methanol.	Zermane et al. (2016)

Microwave radiation is used to increase the temperature of the solvent. Therefore, the solvent must have a high dielectric constant (Rodríguez-Rojo et al., 2012). In addition, the polarity of the compounds is also important; for example, for the rosemary oil extraction, it has been used with ethanol, methanol, or acetone separately or as a mixture, which could increase the dielectric constant (Liu et al., 2018).

In some experiments, they have evaluated the use of water only, and it was found that reduced or similar amounts of phenolic compounds are obtained using the hydrodistillation method because of localized overheating. On the other hand, acetone proved to be an excellent alternative in extracting phenolic compounds from diverse plant tissues when the extraction was assisted with microwaves; this result can be attributed to the better absorption of microwave energy. Thus, the inner cell temperature increases, causing the breakdown of cell walls and the release of compounds into the surrounding solvent (Liu et al., 2011).

12.2.3 Organic Solvent Extraction

Solvent extraction is a procedure to separate soluble and insoluble components from a solid matrix (plant) to a liquid solvent, preferably the organic ones (Lao and Giusti 2018).

There are four stages in the process, that is, (a) the solid components of the plant are expanded because of the solvent, (b) the dissolution of the solute in the solvent, (c) the solute diffusion in the solid phase; Fick's second law describes this step, and the last step, and (d) the diffusion through the outer layers of solid particles; phenolic compounds are distinguished as the color change of the solution is perceived (Cömert and Gökmen 2018).

It has been reported that the temperature, the composition of the solvent, the solid–liquid ratio, the pH, the particle size of the biomass, and/or the number of stages to complete the extraction are the factors that can affect the extraction efficiency (Liyana-Pathirana and Shahidi 2005).

12.2.4 Microwave Hydro-Diffusion and Gravity

This method of green extraction combines microwave-assisted heating and Earth's gravity to an atmosphere of pressure. This technique was developed to be applied on an industrial and laboratory scale to extract essential oils from various aromatic plants. First, the plant biomass is put in a microwave reactor without the addition of solvents. Next, the high temperature inside the biomass relaxes the plant cells, causing oil release from receptacles. The extract is later transferred from the interior to the exterior of the plant material (Vian et al., 2008).

The phenomenon mentioned above is known as hydro-diffusion and is reported to allow the extraction and separation of liquid phase components. The extract is passed through a perforated disk, then cooled, and finally separated in a container. An essential advantage of this method is that is not required a distillation or evaporation process, resulting in a reduction of energy and operation cost (Chemat et al., 2015).

12.2.5 Pressure Solvent Extraction

It is a solid–liquid technique alternative to other methods, such as percolation, extraction, maceration, or Soxhlet reflux, offering advantages, such as extraction time, solvent consumption, and reproducibility. In this method, the synergic effect of organic solvents under pressure and high temperature is exploited (Schügerl 1994). It has been reported that the increase in temperature accelerates the extraction of oils; at the same time, the elevated pressure keeps the solvent in a liquid state, resulting in fast and safe extractions. In addition, the high pressure forces the solvent to enter the pores of the matrix of the plant material and facilitates the extraction of analytes; the elevated temperature decreases the viscosity of the liquid solvent, allowing better penetration of the matrix and weakening the solute–matrix interactions (Sapkale et al., 2010).

A sample is placed in an extraction cell (stainless steel) and filled with solvent; the sample is heated (50°C –200°C) in an oven. The increase in temperature generates the expansion of the solvent and, therefore, the pressure in the extraction cell (500–3000 psi). The solvent that escapes during this ventilation is collected in a vial. A static extraction stage of approximately 5–10 minutes is followed by pumping fresh solvent through the system to rinse the sample and tube. All the solvent present in the system is then purged with compressed gas, and the total amount of solvent is collected in the vial (Mandal, Mandal, and Das 2015).

12.2.6 Ultrasonic Assisted Extraction

This method includes two types of physical phenomena: (a) diffusion through cell walls and (b) washing of cell contents once the walls are broken (Tiwari 2015). During the process, the sample is exposed to ultrasound waves with frequencies from 20 to 2000 kHz. The reduction in the size of plant material might increase the number of cells exposed to ultrasound-induced cavitation.

Ultrasound causes swelling of the cell wall pores, facilitating the diffusion, which influences the mass transfer. Cavitation also destroys plant material causing problems in solid–liquid separation (Oreopoulou, Tsimogiannis, and Oreopoulou 2019). This extraction process improves extraction performance and the use of safe solvents and improves the extraction of sensitive components exposed to these conditions, significantly improving the yield extraction (Dzah et al., 2020). This method has been applied to extract plant components, especially phenolic acids, such as carnosic and rosmarinic acids from *S. rosmarinus*. Rodríguez-Rojo et al. (2012) and Zu et al. (2012) reported a significant improvement in phenolic content when the plant samples were extracted using ethanol for 15–45 min. These methods showed a better performance than the traditional ones.

12.2.7 Solvent-Free Microwave Extraction

The application of this method considers the placement of plant material in a microwave reactor in the absence of solvents (Filly et al., 2014). The increase in temperature of the extraction setup leads to the extraction of oils from the ruptured glands. This process enhances the release of the oils (mediated by water evaporation) by azeotropic distillation. The steam passes through a condenser outside the microwave cavity, where it condenses. The excess water is refluxed into the extraction vessel. Finally, the essential oil is collected and dried (Ferreira et al., 2020; Filly et al., 2014; Li et al., 2013). As it can be observed, the solvent-free microwave extraction combines the dry distillation and microwave heating methods performed at atmospheric pressure (Lucchesi, Chemat, and Smadja 2004).

12.2.8 Supercritical Fluid Extraction

This method is rapid, automatable, selective, and avoids large amounts of toxic solvents. Because of its critical conditions, CO_2 has been widely used as a supercritical fluid, allowing easy separation from solutes; additionally, this fluid reduces the negative environmental impact, is non-flammable, and is not expensive. McHugh and Krukonis (1994) reported conditions for supercritical CO_2, such as critical temperature above 31°C and a critical pressure of 1000 psi; the authors also reported the need for high-pressure conditions, i.e., 6000—10000 psi.

SFE is recommended for treating thermolabile compounds because of its adequate operative circumstances, i.e., low temperature, which provide favorable conditions for thermosensitive compounds (Lesellier, Lefebvre, and Destandau 2021). Table 12.2 lists the experimental setups, where the methods mentioned above are described; as explained, some factors and conditions are crucial to succeed in the oil extraction, so these aspects are explained.

Finally, Conventional methods, such as steam and water distillation and solvent maceration, are exhaustive and time- and power-consuming, and may use some toxic substances as solvents. New emerging extraction methods can improve the performance of essential oil extraction in many ways; these new methods can also be optimized and adapted for specific biological compounds.

To sum up, modern methods are easily automatized, and several parameters can be controlled at a time. Therefore, it is highly recommended to select the extraction method properly to achieve the desirable physicochemical characteristics of the extracts, the higher yield, and the optimal quality. Furthermore, new trends are currently being developed to study the implementation of efficient green extraction processes and their full impact on the environment and the fulfillment of the customer's requirements to meet the challenges of this century.

12.3 BIOACTIVE COMPOUNDS IN OLEORESIN OF ROSEMARY

The main components of rosemary include polar or nonpolar chemicals: some are more soluble in water and some are related to oil. Many compounds have been separated from *S. rosmarinus*, counting diterpenes, flavones, triterpenes, and steroids. The antioxidant action of rosemary extracts has been related to two phenolic diterpenes: carnosic acid and carnosol (Genena et al., 2008; Frankel et al., 1996).

For example, carnosol, egrosmanol, rosmaridiphenol, and rosmariquinone have been detected in RO, also other phenolic acids, such as p-hydroxybenzoic acid, rosmarinic acid, and flavonoids, such as genkawanin, cirsimaritin, and tetrahydroxyflavone. In addition, phenolic diterpenes, carnosic acid, carnosol, and methyl carnosate were identified in significant quantities (Upadhyay and Mishra 2014; Babovic et al., 2010; Santoyo et al., 2005; Cuvelier, Richard, and Berset 1996; Richheimer et al., 1996; Genena et al., 2008). Figure 12.2 shows the main bioactive compounds of ROs.

Etter (2004) reviewed the rosemary components in the rosemary plant, RO, and rosemary extracts to use as antioxidant particles. The compounds were borneol, caffeic acid, carnosic acid, carnosol, epirosmaniol, isorosmanol, methiepyrosmanol, rosmanol, rosmanidiphenol, rosmarinic acid, rosmariquinone, and ursolic acid in the plant material. On the other hand, the essential oil extracted from rosemary comprises 1.8 cineole, camphor, α-pinene, β-pinene, and β-caryophyllene (Ait-Ouazzou et al., 2011). Similarly, Santoyo et al. (2005) found some compounds in rosemary essential oil, such as α-pinene, 1,8-cineole, camphor, verbenone, and borneol, that showed antimicrobial activity. They found that borneol was the most effective, followed by camphor and verbenone.

TABLE 12.2 Experimental Setups to Extract Phytochemical Compounds of Rosemary Plant Material

Method	Aim of the Study	Conditions of Extraction	Results	Reference
Superciritical extraction Hydrodistillation Steam distillation	To obtain the chemical composition and determine the antioxidant activity of the essential oil of rosemary cultivated in Mexico via supercritical fluid extraction (CO_2), hydrodistillation, and steam distillation methods.	SCE: The supercritical fluid-extraction equipment was integrated by feeding section, extraction section, and outlet section. Dried ground rosemary (25 g; particle size of $600 \pm 50\,\mu m$) were submitted to extraction at 40 and 50°C and pressures of 10.34 and 17.24 MPa, respectively. HD and SD: The extraction processes were performed by using conventional apparatus.	A higher yield and antioxidant activity were observed in the CO_2-SCE, SD, and HD, respectively. It was estimated that SCE was 14 times higher than obtained by SD and HD regarding the antioxidant activity. The predominant components in the extracted oils were camphor and eucalyptol.	Conde-Hernández et al. (2017)
Microwave-assisted hydrodistillation	To compare the rosemary oil obtained by microwave-assisted hydrodistillation with those by conventional hydrodistillation.	MAHD: The extraction was performed in and multimode oven at 2450 MHz and 900 W. A 100 g sample of rosemary was heated in 300 mL of water for 30 min. HD: 100 g of rosemary leaves were extracted in a conventional apparatus.	The MAHD resulted efficiently in the ratio energy/extraction time (30 min compared to 90 min in HD). In addition, it was observed an increase of 17% of oxygenated compounds in the MAHD method.	(Moradi, Fazlali, and Hamedi 2018)
Microwave-assisted hydrodistillation Hydrodistillation Steam distillation	To find an optimal extraction method (MAHD, HD, and SD) based on techno-economical aspects and quality-wise parameters of extracts.	MAHD: The extraction oil was performed at atmospheric pressure for 40 W for 30 min and 70 and 100 W for 20 min. HD: Dried leaves (100 g) of S. rosmarinus were extracted with 1 liter of water for 180 min. SD: Dried leaves (100 g) of rosemary were submitted to steam distillation with 2 L of water for 120 min.	MAHD offers significant advantages over traditional WD and SD, shorter extraction times for 440 W 30 min and for 770 and 1100 W 20 min against 3 h for HD and SD, better yields for MAHD with 440 W 0.45% and 770 W 0.50% and 1100 W 0.55% for WD 1.30% and SD 0.54%, respectively.	(Jaimand, Rezaee, and Homami 2018)
Organic solvent extraction	To establish optimal extraction conditions for rosemary oil and determine the antioxidant properties of the extracts.	Powder from dry leaves was submitted to an organic solvent extraction under the following conditions: 1:20 w/v (g dry leaves/mL solvent), ultrasonic bath (40 kHz), 50°C, vacuum filtration, and evaporation to remove the ethanol.	There were no found differences in yields, ranging from 16 to 19%; however, when the samples were treated at different proportions of ethanol, it was found to affect the concentration of total phenolic, flavonoid, and condensed tannin, respectively. In addition, a higher 2,2-diphenyl-1-picrylhydrazyl scavenging ability was found when used with 80% ethanol solution.	Wang et al. (2018)

(Continued)

TABLE 12.2 (*Continued*)   Experimental Setups to Extract Phytochemical Compounds of Rosemary Plant Material

Method	Aim of the Study	Conditions of Extraction	Results	Reference
Solvent-free microwave hydrodiffusion and gravity.	To propose a multiple-benefit process to extract essential oil and aqueous extract rich in phenolic compounds.	The extraction was carried out using MHDG in multimode microwave equipment (2450 MHz and 900 W). All experiments were performed at atmospheric. Plant samples were soaked in water for 1 h to allow the adsorption of the liquid. The HD was carried out by using a conventional apparatus. First, samples were extracted by using water for 3 h. Then, rosemary leaves were mixed distilled water or ethanol solution for 1, 2, and 4 h at 25 ± 2°C to extract phenolic compounds.	It was recovered from samples of about 80% of the total phenolic compounds. The method demonstrated to be a promising alternative regarding the time of the extraction and the absence of potentially toxic solvents. Furthermore, it was demonstrated the feasible extraction of oil and added-value products in a short time.	Ferreira et al. (2020)
Microwave hydrodiffusion and gravity	To compare the essential oil of rosemary extracted by using MHDG to those extracted by conventional HD and MAHD.	The experiment was carried out using 100 g of fresh plant material (rosemary leaves and steams) sliced into 1–2 cm. The innovative equipment of MHDG consisted of a stirring system able to work at low pressures. The treatment leads to the separation of intracellular water and essential oils.	The essential oil yields obtained were similar to those obtained by traditional methods but significantly shorter: from approximately 10–105 min extraction time for MAHD and 150 min extraction for HD, respectively.	Calinescu et al. (2017)
Assisted extraction	To evaluate the use of two solvents, i.e., water and ethanol are used to extract polar compounds from rosemary leaves. Different pretreatments were evaluated as well (deoiled and milled, deoiled and fresh plant).	Solvent extraction: Biomass samples were preheated in a water bath (40°C / 15 min); the samples were exposed to preheated solvent and rotated at 50 rpm. Microwave-assisted extraction: Samples were mixed with the solvent and irradiated with microwaves (250 W/30 s). For ultrasounds assisted extraction, it was maintained a 1:6 w/w plant to solvent ratio.	The efficiency was better in the extraction when the samples were treated with low energy intake for a short time (7 min). In addition, a higher antioxidant concentration was obtained in the samples subjected to extraction with benign solvents (water or ethanol) compared to other methods, i.e., microwave-assisted and ultrasound-assisted extraction. It was obtained a total phenolic content of between 110 and 180 mg gallic acid equivalents/g dried extract. The rosmarinic and carnosic acids concentrations were 50–140, and 80 mg/g dried extract, respectively.	Rodríguez-Rojo et al. (2012)

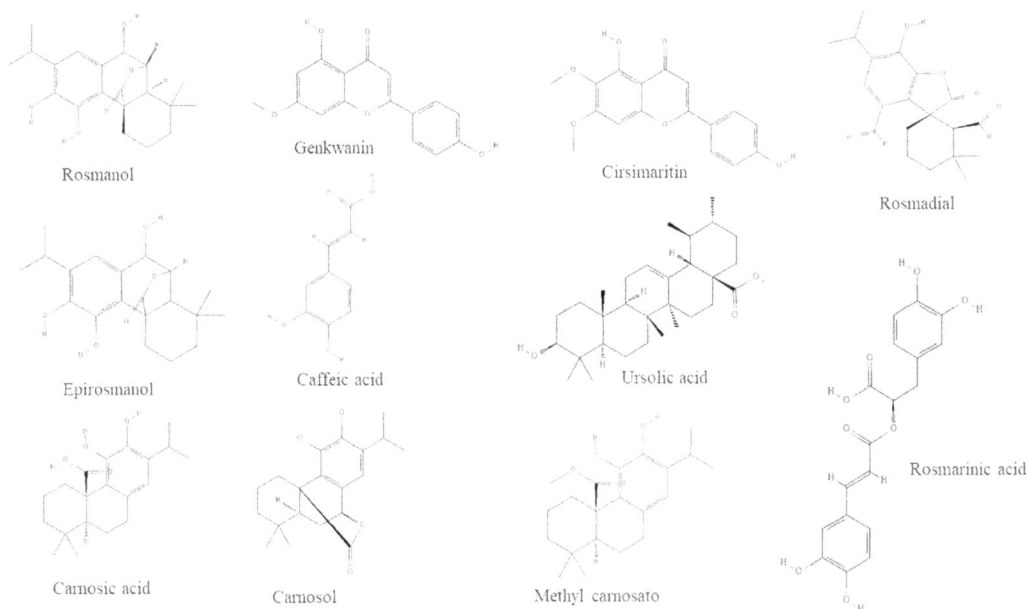

FIGURE 12.2 Main compounds found in the oleoresins of *S. rosmarinus*.

Source: https://pubchem.ncbi.nlm.nih.gov/.

12.4 PHARMACOLOGY EFFECTS OF ROSEMARY ESSENTIAL OIL AND OLEORESINS

Pharmacological actions are commonly related to essential oil and antioxidant phenolic compounds; these compounds are also the reason for antimicrobial, anti-inflammatory, antiulcerogenic, and antimutagenic activity (Alonso 2004). Studies based on the medicinal properties of rosemary have gradually increased, according to Andrade et al. (2018). The use of alcoholic extracts of rosemary leaves and flowers has been documented to treat gastric disorders, pain, and inflammation, antibacterial activities, and as an analgesic in muscles and joints (Andrade et al., 2018) in traditional medicine, additionally the essential oil of rosemary where bioactivity can be attributed to several molecules, mainly monoterpenes (limonene, camphor, 1,8-cineole, borneol, pinene, camphene, myrcene) (Borges et al., 2019a; Borges, Lima et al., 2018). Rosemary essential oil is commonly used to treat nonserious wounds, skin rashes, headaches, dyspepsia, spasmodic gastrointestinal disorders, circulatory problems, muscle and joint pain, and inflammation, and acts as an expectorant, diuretic, and antispasmodic in renal colic (Andrade et al., 2018; Rašković et al., 2014).

The studies concerning the pharmacological activity of the components of rosemary that are currently being carried out are directed mainly toward diterpenes (especially rosmanol) because of the great interest that their antioxidant properties have; They have been shown to prevent low-density lipoprotein (LDL) oxidation and skin aging (Petiwala and Johnson 2015; Rubió, Motilva, and Romero 2013). In addition, some studies have documented that carnosol promotes the synthesis of a neuronal growth factor essential for the growth and maintenance of nervous tissue (Satoh et al., 2008; Kosaka and Yokoi 2003). Furthermore, rosmarinic acid exhibits anti-inflammatory activity in carrageenan-induced plantar edema models in rats. Experimentally, it was shown that this acid acts on the formation of prostaglandins (PGE2) similarly to nonsteroidal anti-inflammatory drugs, causing inhibition of complement factor C3, a mediator of the inflammatory process, which does not involve the cyclooxygenase pathway or activity of prostacyclin synthetase. It was also shown to reduce leukotriene B4 production in human polymorphonuclear leukocytes.

On the other hand, rosmarinic acid demonstrated antioxidant activity in chemiluminescence inhibition tests and hydrogenated peroxides formed from human granulocytes. Studies carried out on pregnant rats indicate that the administration of rosemary extracts during the pre-implantation period interferes with the normal implantation of the egg, based on alterations in embryonic development observed after the autopsy of the animals. Consuming rosemary essential oil is contraindicated in epileptic patients (because of the risk of neurotoxicity), people with diabetes, children, and infants.

12.5 ANTIOXIDANT ACTIVITY AND MECHANISM OF ACTION OF ROSEMARY OLEORESIN

Antioxidants have been widely reported as compounds capable of delaying the oxidation of lipid compounds present in food (Martinello and Pramparo 2005). The antioxidants present in rosemary essential oil and other extracts are polyphenolic compounds commonly found in herbs, spices, and other plant-based materials. Compounds with antioxidant activity are obtained by hydrodistillation from plant extracts and are generically called "essential oils," highly aromatic. To minimize the aromas of the extracts while maintaining beneficial characteristics such as antioxidant power, solvent extraction (ethanol, methanol, acetone, hexane, etc.) is used to obtain extracts called "oleoresins" (Martinello and Pramparo 2005). The compounds present in the extracts of various origins isolated from plants are polyphenols; these compounds are bioactive substances that act as radical scavengers or metal chelators or stabilize lipid oxidation when they are in the natural stage in plants (Gad and Sayd 2015; Song et al., 2020; Farhat et al., 2009). In the particular case of *S. rosmarinus*, compounds such as phenolic acids, flavonoids, natural pigments (capsaicin and curcumin), and terpenes have been studied (Cuvelier, Richard, and Berset 1996; Ávila-Sosa et al., 2012). The polyphenolic profile of these plants is characterized by carnosic acid, carnosol, rosmarinic acid, and hesperidin (Tai et al., 2012).

It has been documented that extracts of rosemary (*S. rosmarinus*) have potential effects on health because of their anti-inflammatory and anticancer properties and at the same time that they have antioxidative stress properties (Žegura et al., 2011). Another reports hepatoprotective potential, the therapeutic potential for Alzheimer's disease, and its anti-angiogenic effect are also reported (Nieto et al., 2018). The bioactivity of rosemary extracts is derived from the mixture of compounds, such as oxygenated monoterpenes (linalol, verbenone, isobornyl acetate), and diterpenes, such as carnosol, methylcarnosate, carnosic acid, ursolic acid, rosmarinic acid, and caffeic acid (Rašković et al., 2014; Martinello and Pramparo 2005), although some studies focus on the antioxidant activity in the presence of carnosic acid, carnosol, and rosmarinic acid (Žegura et al., 2011; Cuvelier, Richard, and Berset 1996). Carnosic acid and carnosol inhibit lipid peroxidation in liposomal and microsomal systems; both are good scavengers of peroxyl radicals, reduce cytochrome C, and capture hydroxyl radicals; in a particular form, carnosol has been described as a molecule with the ability to interfere with tumor cell metastasis, chemotaxis, and inhibition of invasion by targeting metalloproteinase mediated cellular events (Song et al., 2020).

Other reported compounds, such as caffeic and rosmarinic acids, have double functions as antioxidants and stimulants. When caffeic acid derivatives react with the metallic ions present, chelates are formed; consequently, they react with peroxide radicals and thus stabilize these free radicals (Nieto, Ros, and Castillo 2018). Other antioxidative diterpenes, such as epirosmanol, isorosmanol, rosmaridiphenol, and rosmariquinone, have also been reported to contribute to the antioxidant activity of rosemary extracts (Hopia et al., 1996). Both oleoresin and rosemary essential oil have various uses in the food industry, especially for preventing oxidation and contamination of foods, rosemary for reaching higher sensory scores and lowering lipid oxidation in various foods (Georgantelis et al., 2007). RO has been reported to contain several components up to four times as effective as BHA and equal to BHT as an antioxidant (Gad and Sayd 2015). In addition, some of the compounds in rosemary extracts possess antibacterial properties (Georgantelis et al., 2007; Djenane et al., 2002). In the pharmaceutical industry, the properties of rosemary oil are used in the anti-aging of cosmetics and the development of drugs (Djenane et al., 2002).

12.6 ANTIMICROBIAL ACTIVITY OLEORESIN AND EXTRACTS IN ROSEMARY

The two significant phenotypic strategies for deciding the susceptibility of a microbial separate from an antimicrobial extract are agar disk diffusion and minimal inhibitory concentration (MIC) testing (Tenover 2019). The agar disk diffusion method consists of setting paper circles saturated with the antimicrobial substance on the surface of an agar medium with a standardized inoculum of one microorganism. Generally, an antimicrobial agent can diffuse into the agar and can inhibit growth. The zone of inhibition is determined by halos surrounding the paper disks (Tenover 2019; Balouiri, Sadiki, and Ibnsouda 2016). MIC testing can be achieved with different techniques as agar dilution, broth microdilution, or agar gradient dilution. MIC testing aims to determine a quantitative amount of antimicrobial agent as mg mL^{-1} (Tenover 2019).

Evaluation of the microbial activity of oleoresin in rosemary against different pathogenic microorganisms is done using the agar well diffusion method. Different concentrations of RO or extract are measured to calculate the minimal concentration MIC (Monisha et al., 2019). In another study, the oleoresin was assessed using broth dilution with bacterial culture in microtubes. The MIC was determined as the minor substance concentration, creating no bacterial pellet (inhibited growth) (Rodríguez-Calleja et al., 2014). Table 12.3 summarizes some rosemary extracts and oleoresin inhibition against different pathogen microorganisms.

Moreno et al. (2006) found that antibacterial activity on *Staphylococcus aureus* using methanolic extract and carnosic acid had a more significant effect than *Escherichia coli*. Methanolic and acetone extracts had modest inhibition on *Pseudomonas mirabilis*,

TABLE 12.3 Antimicrobial Activities Using Extracts and Oleoresin of *Salvia rosmarinus* for Food and Human Pathogens

Microorganism Used	Concentration	Effect	Reference
Listeria monocytogenes, Staphylococcus aureus, and *Bacillus cereus*	1250 ppm	In this assay, two of three bacteria showed MIC values for Gram (+)bacteria evaluated.	(Dussault, Vu, and Lacroix 2014)
Escherichia coli, Pseudomonas aeruginosa, S. aureus, B. cereus, and *C. albicans*	0.062–2.0 mg.mL^{-1}	Rosemary extracts demonstrated antimicrobial response against Gram (+) and Gram (−) bacteria. In addition, the extract was more effective with increasing extraction time for *S. aureus*. Inhibition of *C. albicans* needs more than 1 hour.	Genena et al. (2008)
Gram (+) bacteria *(Staphylococcus aureus, Bacillus megaterium, Bacillus subtilis, Enterococcus faecalis)* **Gram (−) bacteria** *(Escherichia coli, Klebsiella pneumoniae, Pseudomonas mirabilis, Xanthomonas campestris)* **Yeast** *(Saccharomyces cerevisiae, Candida albicans, Pichia pastoris)*	2–15 mg.mL^{-1} 2–125 mg.mL^{-1} 4–8 mg.mL^{-1}	Methanolic and acetone extracts of rosemary were most efficient in Gram (+) than Gram (−) bacteria. Also, carnosic acid was very effective.	Moreno et al. (2006)
Listeria monocytogenes, Escherichia coli, Pseudomonas fluorescens, and *Lactobacillus sake*	5–80 mg.mL^{-1}	Rosemary extracts had inhibition against all bacteria. Nevertheless, *L. monocytogenes* (Gram (+)) were the most susceptible.	(Zhang, Wu, and Guo 2016)
Staphylococcus aureus, Bacillus cereus, Escherichia coli, and *Pseudomonas fluorescens*	1.8–25 mg.mL^{-1}	The lowest concentration used was 1.8 mg/mL of rosemary oleoresin against Gram (+) bacteria *B. cereus*	Rodríguez-Calleja et al. (2014)
Escherichia coli O157:H7, Salmonella typhimurium, Listeria monocytogenes, and *Aeromonas hydrophila*	1%	Oleoresin of rosemary had more inhibition for *E. coli* strain O157:H7 later 9 days, also against *S. typhimurium* and most minor effect against *L. monocytogenes*. There was no inhibition effect for *A. hydrophila*	(Ahn, Grün, and Mustapha 2007)
Methicillin-resistant *Staphylococcus aureus* **(MRSA)**	25–100 µL	*S. rosmarinus* oleoresin showed inhibition against MRSA. The halo of inhibition was 18–28 mm.	Monisha et al. (2019)
Escherichia coli, Pseudomonas, Streptococcus mutans, and *Enterococcus*	2%–10%	Rosemary oleoresin showed antibacterial activity against all bacteria. However, the inhibition zone was higher against *Pseudomonas*.	(Mathew, Roy, and Geetha 2020)
Enterococcus faecalis	20–100 µL	The application of rosemary oleoresin was efficient against these bacteria with an inhibition halo in all concentrations.	Nivetha et al. (2019)

(Continued)

TABLE 12.3 *(Continued)*   Antimicrobial Activities Using Extracts and Oleoresin of Salvia rosmarinus for Food and Human Pathogens

Microorganism Used	Concentration	Effect	Reference
Staphylococcus aureus, Streptococcus mutans, **and** *Pseudomonas* sp.	20–100 µL	Rosemary oleoresin-mediated AgNPs showed antibacterial activity in three oral pathogens. The highest zone of inhibition was against *Pseudomonas* sp.	(Kandhan, Roy, and Rajeshkumar 2019)
Bacillus subtilis	0%–30%	Some structures, such as cyclic glucans, were applied to enhance the solubility of carnosic acid.	(Park, Rho, and Kim 2019)

Klebsiella pneumoniae, and *E. coli,* with MIC rates in the 60–125 mg/mL range. In addition, carnosic acid purified, as well as methanol and acetone extracts, turned up. In yeast, MIC values were minimal comparing with Gram (−) bacteria. Recently, Park, Rho, and Kim (2019) studied some complexing structures such as cycloamylose, branched dextrin, and β-cyclodextrin to enhance the dissolvability of carnosic acid; all of the complexes had an improved inhibitory effect against *Bacillus subtilis* contrasted to carnosic acid (Park, Rho, and Kim 2019).

Genena et al. (2008) evaluated antimicrobial activity utilizing the SFE method with the highest antioxidant ability. MIC rates were characterized as the most reduced concentration of the oil, which inhibited growth. In Gram (+) bacteria, the extracts improved time for *S. aureus,* and the opposite was observed for *Bacillus cereus.* Similarly, extracts showed inhibition for Gram (−) bacteria but notwithstanding extraction time. For fungi, the extraction had inhibition activity after 60 minutes. Similarly, Santoyo et al. (2005) investigated antimicrobial activity using disc diffusion and broth dilution methods against *B. subtilis, S. aureus, Pseudomonas aeruginosa, E. coli, Candida albicans,* and *Aspergillus niger.* They found that all parts obtained showed antimicrobial action against all the microorganisms tested.

Dussault, Vu, and Lacroix (2014) investigated the effect of RO and essential oils on various food pathogens. Whereas oleoresin of rosemary was only effective against Gram (+) bacteria. In contrast, Rosemary essential oil was also discovered that rosemary essential oil has antimicrobial properties against Gram (+) bacteria but not against Gram (−) bacteria (Ait-Ouazzou et al., 2011).

The findings of the antibacterial studies using the suitable diffusion method showed an elevated activity against the tested strains of Gram (−) bacteria, such as *E. coli* and *Pseudomonas,* and Gram (+) bacteria, such as *Streptococcus mutans* and *Enterococcus* zone of inhibition was shown by RO (Mathew, Roy, and Geetha 2020). Also, this oleoresin showed inhibition against *Enterococcus.* For example, the application of 25 µL showed a halo of 22 mm, whereas 50 and 100 µL showed 25 and 26 mm, respectively, and 24 mm for chlorhexidine (control) (Nivetha et al., 2019). In other studies, RO showed a dose-dependent zone in methicillin-resistant *S. aureus* 25 µL showed a halo of 18 mm, whereas 50 and 100 µL showed 20 and 28 mm, respectively. Chlorhexidine was used as a control and showed inhibition of 27 mm (Monisha et al., 2019).

Ahn, Grün, and Mustapha (2004) found that oleoresin rosemary (1%) can decrease the populations of *E. coli* O157:H7, *Salmonella typhimurium*, and *Listeria monocytogenes* in ground meat following 9 days of refrigerated stockpiling (Ahn et al., 2004). Different concentrations of RO were tested in *S. aureus*, *B. cereus*, *E. coli*, and *P. fluorescens*. The best effect was evidenced for the Gram (+) bacteria *B. cereus*. However, only a minor inhibition concentration (MIC) (1.8 mg/mL) was used for this Gram (+) bacteria. In contrast, this oleoresin not affected Gram (+)bacteria (Rodríguez-Calleja et al., 2014).

A pattern was observed for oleoresin than for essential oil when contrasted the antimicrobial movement agreeing with the Gram stain. Gram (+) microorganisms were more sensitive to oleoresin than Gram (−) bacteria by testing the broth dilution and disk agar diffusion. (Rodríguez-Calleja et al., 2014). A possible explanation is because Gram (−) bacteria have an outer cell membrane helping to be more resistant to the antimicrobial agent (Ceylan and Fung 2004). Another is that phenolic compounds can modify the membrane function and, in some instances, its structure, causing swelling and increased permeability. An increase in permeability results in loss of the cellular pH gradient, decreased ATP levels, proton motive force, and ends in cell death (Zhang, Wu, and Guo 2016).

12.7 ANTI-INFLAMMATORY ACTIVITY

The term "inflammation" derives from the Latin "inflammare," which means light a fire. On medicine is named with the suffix itis. It is a fundamental pathophysiological response whose objective is to eliminate any noxious stimulus introduced into the host and repair damaged tissue or organ. These noxious stimuli include causative agents external (microorganisms, physical agents, chemical agents) and causal agents internal (immune disorders and vascular disorders) (Borges et al., 2019a). Among the diseases that occur in the world population, those that involve inflammatory processes represent an important group. Although most infections that occur involve inflammatory processes as a natural response to physical trauma and allergies, which in many cases incapacitate those who suffer from it, particularly major infectious diseases, the inflammatory response may cause further damage than the offending agent. In traditional medicine in various places globally, herbal extracts have been used as the origin of medicines. Currently, there is a tendency to value natural compounds concerning their use instead of artificially synthetic compounds.

Inflammation is a regulated series of immunological, physiological, and behavioral processes orchestrated by soluble immune-signaling molecules called "cytokines" (Chereshnev and Gusev 2014). These inflammatory stimuli are first detected by host cells through transmembrane receptors called pattern (PRR) (innate and adaptive). PRR are receptors encoded in the germinal line responsible for detecting the presence of infectious microorganisms, as well as the occurrence of any cellular damage (Ramírez, Dranguet and Morales 2020). The first step in this series of reactions is the recognition of infection or damage. This is typically accomplished by detecting pathogen-associated molecular patterns (PAMPs), targeting general motifs of molecules expressed by pathogens, and damage-associated molecular patterns (DAMPs), which are endogenous molecules capable of signaling damage or necrosis, and they are also recognized by the innate immune system. During acute inflammation, these cells produce pro-inflammatory prostaglandins; induced by the enzyme cyclooxygenase-2 (COX-2) and regulated by phospholipase A2 (PLA2), which catalyzes the hydrolysis of membrane phospholipids, allowing the formation of free fatty acids (arachidonic acid (AA) and lysophospholipids. Both phospholipid metabolites act as precursors to inflammatory mediators such as eicosanoids) and leukotrienes, but rapidly switch to lipoxins, which further block neutrophil recruitment and instead promote enhanced infiltration of monocytes necessary for wound healing (Muñoz-Velázquez et al., 2012; Ramírez, Dranguet, and Morales 2020) anti-inflammatory activity of rosemary oil is due to its major components, mainly the pharmacological activity of 1,8-cineole, camphor, and α-pinene (Mekonnen et al., 2016; Machado et al., 2013; de Faria et al., 2011) and limonene and myrcene (Rufino et al., 2015). Some experimental studies have reported the anti-inflammatory activity of essential oils and biologically active terpenes, such as carnosic acid, carnosol, ursolic acid, and betulinic acid, as well as rosmarinic acid, rosmanol, and oleanolic acid, the activity of rosemary depends on a synergistic mechanism between its components (Kompelly et al., 2019). Rosemary essential oil was found to inhibit leukocyte migration *in vivo*. This reduced the number of leukocytes at the site of inflammation. Regarding *in vitro* studies, the anti-inflammatory studies were based on evaluating the inflammatory cytokines, COX-1/COX-2, iOS, and evaluation of nitric oxide production in macrophages cells (Kompelly et al., 2019; Andrade et al., 2018).

12.8 INVESTIGATIONS IN TRADITIONAL AND MODERN MEDICINAL USES OF ROSEMARY OLEORESINS

Plants have been of interest for medical use in humans and animals from prehistoric times to the present. Natural cures and herbal medicines have long been used to heal the sick by people worldwide, and this knowledge has been passed down through centuries. In recent decades, researchers, mostly from developing nations, have recognized the abundance of knowledge preserved in traditional medicine systems, focusing on herbs toward the discovery and characterization of active principles and the generation of new drugs with fewer side effects and fewer complications than conventional ones. In addition, growing drug resistance has rendered several antibiotics and other life-saving drugs useless. According to this improving demand, medicinal and pharmacological studies have been increasing worldwide and the emergence of novel markets based on herb exploitation. As a result, plant-based drugs, health goods, pharmaceuticals, food additives, and cosmetics are now vital contributors to the sector's global growth, as well as a way for people living in rural regions to build economic value chains.

Alternatively, "bioprospecting"—the search of indigenous sources for new drugs—has led to other phenomena that will need further awareness, such as the plundering of freely available resources and others. Beyond natural resource sustainability, combining traditional and modern medicine faces many issues stemming from fundamental differences in how each is practiced, evaluated, and managed, such as evidence documentation, intellectual property management, and adherence to efficacy and safety standards.

As reviewed above, *S. rosmarinus* L. has a wide range of medicinal uses because of its bioactive molecules (phytocompounds), mainly producing antioxidant and anti-inflammatory effects. These phytocompounds can be extracted from essential oils and extracts, and their concentration varies based on the plant specimen's characteristics (Council of Europe 2005). Caffeic acid, carnosic acid, chlorogenic acid, monomeric acid, oleanolic acid, rosmarinic acid, ursolic acid, alpha-pinene, camphor, carnosol, eucalyptol, rosmadial, rosmanol, rosmaquinones A and B, secohinokio, and eugenol and luteolin derivatives are some of them (de Oliveira, Afonso, and Dias 2019). As a result of the interaction of rosemary molecules with organic systems, distinct pharmacological effects result, leading to the therapeutic use of rosemary for pathological and nonpathological conditions, such as inflammatory diseases, skin cancer, wound healing, and mycoses, or alopecia, cellulite, ultraviolet damage, and aging (de Macedo et al., 2020).

The Natural Standard Research Collaboration published a comprehensive, evidence-based systematic review of rosemary that included written and statistical analysis of scientific literature, expert's opinion, history, pharmacology, interactions, kinetics and dynamics toxicology, adverse effects, and dosing (Ulbricht et al., 2010). Furthermore, a large body of evidence for *in vivo* and *in vitro* investigations on rosemary's therapeutic and preventative effects on several physiological illnesses caused by biochemical, chemical, or biological agents was compiled (de Oliveira, Afonso, and Dias 2019).

Rosemary extracts have been pharmacologically validated, recently documenting antibacterial, antiviral, antifungal, antidiabetic, anticancer, antinociceptive, anti-inflammatory, antioxidant, antiulcerogenic, antithrombotic, antidiuretic, antidepressant, and hepatoprotective effects (Habtemariam 2016). Other notable uses of rosemary include perfume and food industries, where essential oils are used as natural perfumes and additives. In the latter situation, rosemary extracts are frequently used to extend the shelf life of perishable goods, and the European Union recognizes them as natural antioxidants for food preservation.

Despite the growing importance and interest in the main constituents of rosemary for medicinal purposes, such as phenolic acid derivatives (i.e., rosmarinic acid) and polyphenolic compounds (i.e., flavonoids), polyphenolic diterpenes are a remarkable class of secondary metabolites that have recently received significant attention. Several types of diterpenes isolated from rosemary have been widely characterized by their therapeutic potential for tackling different targets of Alzheimer's disease (Habtemariam 2016). Furthermore, by examining the effects of rosemary compounds *in vitro* and *in vivo* models, a holistic overview of the chemistry and pharmacology of these compounds has been developed for applications to dementia (Habtemariam 2018). Beyond the well-known anti-inflammatory and antioxidant processes, significant pharmacological effects on amyloid, beta, and tau protein disorders, as well as potential neuronal loss recovery from stem cells, have been demonstrated. All of this evidence requires more investigation, specifically clinical trials that confirm the efficacy of rosmarinic acid in treating dementia caused by Alzheimer's disease or cerebrovascular diseases.

Substantial attempts have also been made to investigate rosemary's anti-(retro) viral activity, as well as the anti-(retro) viral activity of other Lamiaceae species. The antiviral impact is often strong and dose-dependent, with the most likely mode of action directly resulting in exterior structures (mainly the viral envelope), preventing viral adherence to target cells. Several other studies have yielded promising results; nonetheless, clinical trials should provide definitive judgments on antiviral activity and prospective patient applicability (Bekut et al., 2018).

A significant amount of pharmacological studies have demonstrated that rosemary extract and its phenolic components can drastically enhance metabolic conditions such as diabetes mellitus by modulating lipid metabolism, glucose metabolism, and anti-inflammatory and antioxidant activities, indicating that these compounds exhibit a higher research relevance. In this frame of reference, Bao et al. (2020) condensed the pharmacological mechanisms and effects reported for treating diabetes with rosemary, from 2000 and up to 2020, highlighting the scientific data and studies supporting its clinical application as an alternative to currently available antidiabetic drugs, which have efficacy and safety limitations (hypoglycemia, gastrointestinal problems, or weight gain).

Distinct cancer-fighting pharmaceuticals, such as paclitaxel, etoposide, and docetaxel, have been found by screening natural compounds from plants. Rosemary extracts and polyphenols have also been studied and discovered to exhibit anticancer properties (González-Vallinas, Reglero, and Ramírez De Molina 2015; Petiwala and Johnson 2015). A comprehensive review summarizes all studies on rosemary effects on many forms of cancer. To show how the research has progressed and what knowledge is accessible, *in vitro* and *in vivo* studies were classified by experimental treatment, cancer cell type, and study model in chronological order. The mechanistic information gathered and presented by these investigations was given specific attention to future research efforts (Moore, Yousef, and Tsiani 2016).

The data obtained from plant material research are often scattered, and the existing compendiums are usually out of date. This situation makes it difficult for decision-makers to design policies to regulate and integrate the traditional use of botanical products in health systems; hence, a suitable alternative solution may be the creation of quantitative and qualitative data sources based on the literature published worldwide. Geck et al. (2020) used 28 survey articles to analyze from the quantitative perspective, focused on the Mesoamerican use of botanical compounds, including rosemary, in the "Mesoamerican Medicinal Plants Database"; this database records the results of preclinical research of the *in vitro* and *in vivo* assays as an indicator of medical efficacy in humans.

However, despite the increasing evidence around rosemary medicinal properties, several challenges remain to make traditional medicine mainstream and introduce it into modern practices. Human clinical studies using technological advances are still lacking in investigating rosemary and its therapeutic applications. Nevertheless, some studies with documented effects show some promise in improving the mental status and as a treatment for alopecia. In addition to the study of the mechanisms of pharmacological action, there are several other fields of knowledge that require attention for future research and development activities: formulation types and dosages, routes of administration (i.e., topical), properties improvement of bioactive molecules, targeting and delivering vehicles (i.e., by the use of nanoparticles), innovative metabolite extraction methods, suitable preclinical and clinical models of study, among others (de Macedo et al., 2020; Kandhan, Roy, and Rajeshkumar 2019; Andrade et al., 2018).

The World Health Organization and some other relevant entities are aware of the critical place of traditional medicine in many societies and recognize the valuable contribution of traditional medicine to the provision of essential care. These organizations estimate that traditional medicine, rather than a modern one, is the primary contributor to health, benefiting around 80% of the world's population, using herbs for treatment, rehabilitation, and healthcare.

12.9 CONCLUDING REMARK

Plants are essential to discover new compounds with a broad spectrum of possible applications. Extraction methods play a crucial role in separating and characterizing different phytochemical compounds and screening plant extracts for novel leads. For example, the oleoresin and essential oil extracted from *S. Rosmarinus* (rosemary) have demonstrated high active bio compounds like rosmaniric acid, methylcarnosate, and carnosol carnosic acid, caffeic acid, and ursolic acid. Also, antimicrobial potential against a broad spectrum of human pathogens, i.e., *B. cereus*, *E. coli*, *S. aureus*, *Salmonella*, and *L. monocytogenes*. In addition, RO has different anti-inflammatory properties and antioxidants, and much traditional medicine uses polyphenolic compounds.

REFERENCES

Abuashwashi, M. 2017 Estudio Analítico y de La Actividad Antioxidante de *"Rosmarinus Officinalis"* L. de La Península Ibérica, Universidad Complutense de Madrid.

Abuashwashi, M., Palomino, O., and Gómez-Serranillos, P. 2014 Variability in the polyphenolic composition and antioxidant ability of wild, *Rosmarinus Officinalis L. Collected in Spain. In* Planta Medica, 80: 1. Georg Thieme Verlag KG.

Ahn, J., Grün, I.U., and Mustapha, A. 2004 Antimicrobial and antioxidant activities of natural extracts in vitro and in ground beef, *Journal of Food Protection*, 67(1): 148–55.

Ahn, J., Grün, I. U., and Mustapha, A. 2007 Effects of plant extracts on microbial growth, color change, and lipid oxidation in cooked beef, *Food Microbiology*, 24(1): 7–14.

Ait-Ouazzou, A., Lorán, S., Bakkali, M., Laglaoui, A., Rota, C., Herrera, A., Pagán, R., and Conchello, P. 2011 Chemical composition and antimicrobial activity of essential oils of *Thymus Algeriensis, Eucalyptus Globulus* and *Rosmarinus Officinalis* from Morocco, *Journal of the Science of Food and Agriculture*, 91(14): 2643–51.

Andrade, J.M., Faustino, C., Garcia, C., Ladeiras, D., Reis, C.P., and Rijo, P. 2018 *Rosmarinus Officinalis* L.: An update review of its phytochemistry and biological activity, *Future Science*, 4(4): 1–18.

Ávila-Sosa, R., Navarro-Cruz, A.R., Vera-López, O., Dávila-Márquez, R.M., Melgoza-Palma, N., and Meza, R. 2012. Romero (*Rosmarinus Officinalis* L.): Una Revisión de Sus Usos No Culinarios, *Ciencia y Mar*, 43: 23–36.

Azmir, J., Zaidul, I.S.M., Rahman, M.M., Sharif, K.M., Mohamed, A., Sahena, F., Jahurul, M.H.A., Ghafoor, K., Norulaini, N.A.N., and Omar, A.K.M. 2013 Techniques for extraction of bioactive compounds from plant materials: A review, *Journal of Food Engineering*, 117 (4): 426–36.

Balouiri, M., Sadiki, M., and Ibnsouda, S.K. 2016 Methods for in vitro evaluating antimicrobial activity: A review, *Journal of Pharmaceutical Analysis*, 6(2): 71–79.

Bekut, M., Brkić, S., Kladar, N., Dragović, G., Gavarić, N. and Božin, B. 2018 Potential of selected lamiaceae plants in anti(Retro)viral therapy, *Pharmacological Research*, 133 (2018): 301–14.

Borges, R.S., Keita, H., Ortiz, B.L.S., Santos Sampaio, T.I. dos, Ferreira, I.M., Lima, E.S., da Silva, M. de, Fernandes, C.P., Faria Mota Oliveira, A.E., de, Conceição, E.C., da, Rodrigues, A.B.L.,

Filho, A.C.M.P., Castro, A.N., and Carvalho, J.C.T. 2018 Anti-Inflammatory Activity of Nanoemulsions of Essential Oil from *Rosmarinus Officinalis* L.: In Vitro and in Zebrafish Studies, *Inflammopharmacology*, 26(4): 1057–80.

Borges, R.S., Lima, E.S., Keita, H., Ferreira, I.M., Fernandes, C.P., Cruz, R.A.S., Duarte, J.L., Velázquez-Moyado, J., Ortiz, B.L.S., Castro, A.N., Ferreira, J.V., Silva Hage-Melim, L.I, da, and Carvalho, J.C.T. 2018 Anti-inflammatory and antialgic actions of a nanoemulsion of *Rosmarinus Officinalis* L. essential oil and a molecular docking study of its major chemical constituents, *Inflammopharmacology*, 26(1): 183–95.

Borges, R.S., Ortiz, B.L.S., Pereira, A.C.M., Keita, H., and Carvalho, J.C.T. 2019 *Rosmarinus Officinalis* essential oil: A review of its phytochemistry, anti-inflammatory activity, and mechanisms of action involved, *Journal of Ethnopharmacology*, 229(30): 29–45.

Boutekedjiret, C., Bentahar, F., Belabbes, R., and Bessiere, J.M. 2003 Extraction of rosemary essential oil by steam distillation and hydrodistillation, *Flavour and Fragrance Journal*, 18(6): 481–84.

Calinescu, I., Asofiei, I., Gavrila, A.I., Trifan, A., Ighigeanu, D., Martin, D., Matei, C., and Buleandra, M. 2017 Integrating microwave-assisted extraction of essential oils and polyphenols from rosemary and thyme leaves, *Chemical Engineering Communications*, 204(8): 965–73.

Ceylan, E., and Fung, D.Y.C. 2004 Antimicrobial activity of spices, *Journal of Rapid Methods and Automation in Microbiology*, 12(1): 1–55.

Chemat, F., Fabiano-Tixier, A.S., Vian, M.A., Allaf, T., and Vorobiev, E. 2015 Solvent-free extraction of food and natural products, *TrAC - Trends in Analytical Chemistry*, 71(September): 157–68.

Chereshnev, V.A., and Gusev, E.Y. 2014 Immunological and pathophysiological mechanism of systemic inflammation, *Medical Immunology (Russia)*, 14(1–2): 9.

Conde-Hernández, L.A., Espinosa-Victoria, J.R., Trejo, A., and Guerrero-Beltrán, J. 2017 CO_2-supercritical extraction, hydrodistillation and steam distillation of essential oil of rosemary (*Rosmarinus Officinalis*), *Journal of Food Engineering*, 200(2016): 81–86.

Council of Europe 2005 *European Pharmacopoeia*. 5th ed. Vienna: EDQM. https://www.amazon.com/-/es/Council-Europe/dp/9287152810.

Cuvelier, M.E., Richard, H., and Berset, C. 1996 Antioxidative activity and phenolic composition of pilot-plant and commercial extracts of sage and rosemary, *JAOCS, Journal of the American Oil Chemists' Society*, 73(5): 645–52.

Djenane, D., Sánchez-Escalante, A., Beltrán, J.A., and Roncalés, P. 2002 Ability of α-tocopherol, taurine and rosemary, in combination with vitamin c, to increase the oxidative stability of beef steaks packaged in modified atmosphere, *Food Chemistry*, 76(4): 407–15.

Drew, B., González-Gallegos, J.G., Xiang, C.-L., Kriebel, R., Drummond, C., Walker, J., and Sytsma, K. 2017 Salvia united: The greatest good for the greatest number, *Taxon*, 66(1): 133–45.

Dussault, D., Vu, K.D., and Lacroix, M. 2014 In vitro evaluation of antimicrobial activities of various commercial essential oils, oleoresin and pure compounds against food pathogens and application in ham, *Meat Science*, 96(1): 514–20.

Farhat, M. Ben, Jordán, M.J., Chaouech-Hamada, R., Landoulsi, A., and Sotomayor, J.A. 2009 Variations in essential oil, phenolic compounds, and antioxidant activity of tunisian cultivated salvia officinalis L, *Journal of Agricultural and Food Chemistry*, 57(21): 10349–56.

Faria, L. de, Silva Lima, C., Ferreira Perazzo, F., and Tavares Carvalho, J. 2011. Anti-Inflammatory and Antinociceptive Activities Lf the Essential Oil from *Rosmarinus Officinalis* L. (Lamiaceae)Hydroalcoholic Extract of *Rosmarinus Officinalis*. *International Journal of Pharmaceutical Sciences Review and Research* 7 (2): 1–8. www.globalresearchonline.net.

Ferreira, D.F., Lucas, B.N., Voss, M., Santos, D., Mello, P.A., Wagner, R., Cravotto, G., and Barin, J.S. 2020 Solvent-free simultaneous extraction of volatile and non-volatile antioxidants from rosemary (*Rosmarinus Officinalis* L.) by microwave hydrodiffusion and gravity, *Industrial Crops and Products*, 145(112094): 1–8.

Filly, A., Fernandez, X., Minuti, M., Visinoni, F., Cravotto, G., and Chemat, F. 2014 Solvent-free microwave extraction of essential oil from aromatic herbs: from laboratory to pilot and industrial scale, *Food Chemistry*, 150 (May): 193–98.

Gad, A.S., and Sayd, A.F. 2015 Antioxidant properties of rosemary and its potential uses as natural antioxidant in dairy products—A review, *Food and Nutrition Sciences*, 06(01): 179–93.

Genena, A.K., Hense, H., Smânia, A., and Souza, S.M. De 2008 Rosemary (*Rosmarinus Officinalis*) - a study of the composition, antioxidant and antimicrobial activities of extracts obtained with supercritical carbon dioxide, *Ciencia e Tecnologia de Alimentos*, 28(2): 463–69.

Georgantelis, D., Ambrosiadis, I., Katikou, P., Blekas, G., and Georgakis, S.A. 2007. Effect of rosemary extract, chitosan and α-tocopherol on microbiological parameters and lipid oxidation of fresh pork sausages stored at 4°C, *Meat Science*, 76(1): 172–81.

González-Vallinas, M., Reglero, G., and Ramírez De Molina, A. 2015 Rosemary (*Rosmarinus Officinalis* L.) extract as a potential complementary agent in anticancer therapy, *Nutrition and Cancer*, 67(8): 1223–31.

Habtemariam, S. 2016 The therapeutic potential of rosemary (*rosmarinus officinalis*) diterpenes for alzheimer's disease, *Evidence-Based Complementary and Alternative Medicine*, 2016 (2680409): 1–14.

Habtemariam, S. 2018 Molecular pharmacology of rosmarinic and salvianolic acids: potential seeds for alzheimer's and vascular dementia drugs, *International Journal of Molecular Sciences*, 19 (2): 1–25.

Haraguchi, H., Saito, T., Okamura, N., and Yagi, A. 2007 Inhibition of lipid peroxidation and superoxide generation by diterpenoids from *Rosmarinus Officinalis*, *Planta Medica*, 61(4): 333–36.

Hopia, A.I., Shu-Wen, H., Schwarz, K., German, J.B., and Frankel, E. 1996 Effect of different lipid systems on antioxidant activity of rosemary constituents carnosol and carnosic acid with and without α-tocopherol, *Journal of Agricultural and Food Chemistry*, 44(8): 2030–36.

Jaimand, K., Rezaee, M.B., and Homami, S. 2018 Comparison extraction methods of essential oils of *Rosmarinus Officinalis* L. in Iran by microwave assisted water distillation; water distillation and steam distillation, *Journal of Medicinal Plants and By-Products*, 1(1): 9–14.

Kandhan, T.S., Roy, A., and Rajeshkumar, S. 2019 Green synthesis of rosemary oleoresin mediated silver nanoparticles and its effect on oral pathogens, *Research Journal Pharm. and Technology*, 12(11): 5379–82.

Karadağ, A.E., Demirci, B., Çaşkurlu, A., Demirci, F., Okur, M.E., Orak, D., Sipahi, H., and Başer, K.H.C. 2019. In vitro antibacterial, antioxidant, anti-inflammatory and analgesic evaluation of *Rosmarinus Officinalis* L. flower extract fractions, *South African Journal of Botany*, 125(September): 214–20.

Karakaya, S., El, S.N., Karagozlu, N., Sahin, S., Sumnu, G., and Bayramoglu, B. 2014 Microwave-assisted hydrodistillation of essential oil from rosemary, *Journal of Food Science and Technology*, 51(6): 1056–65.

Kompelly, A., Kompelly, S., Vasudha, B., and Narender, B. 2019 *Rosmarinus Officinalis* L.: An update review of its phytochemistry and biological activity, *Journal of Drug Delivery and Therapeutics*, 9(1): 323–30.

Kusuma, H.S., Putra, A.F.P., and Mahfud, M. 2016 Comparison of two isolation methods for essential oils from orange peel (*Citrus Auranticum* L) as a growth promoter for fish: Microwave steam distillation and conventional steam distillation, *Journal of Aquaculture Research and Developentment*, 7(2): 1–5.

Labib, R.M., Ayoub, I.M., Michel, H.E., Mehanny, M., Kamil, V., Hany, M., Magdy, M., Moataz, A., Maged, B., and Mohamed, A. 2019 Appraisal on the wound healing potential of melaleuca alternifolia and *Rosmarinus Officinalis* L. Essential oil-loaded chitosan topical preparations, *PLoS ONE* 14(9): 1–17.

Lesellier, E., Lefebvre, T., and Destandau, E. 2021 Recent developments for the analysis and the extraction of bioactive compounds from *Rosmarinus Officinalis* and medicinal plants of the lamiaceae family, *TrAC - Trends in Analytical Chemistry*, 135(116158): 1–14.

Lorenzo-Leal, A.C., Palou, E., López-Malo, A., and Bach, H. 2019 Antimicrobial, cytotoxic, and anti-inflammatory activities of pimenta dioica and *Rosmarinus Officinalis* essential oils. *BioMed Research International*, 2019(1639726): 1–8.

Macedo, L.M. de, Santos, É.M. Dos, Militão, L., Tundisi, L.L., Ataide, J.A., Souto, E.B., and Mazzola, P.G. 2020 Rosemary (*Rosmarinus Officinalis* L., Syn Salvia Rosmarinus Spenn.) and its topical applications: A Review, *Plants*, 9(5): 1–12.

Machado, D.G., Cunha, M.P., Neis, V.B., Balen, G.O., Colla, A., Bettio, L.E.B., Oliveira, Á., Pazini, F.L., Dalmarco, J.B., Simionatto, E.L., Pizzolatti, M.G., and Rodrigues, A.L.S. 2013 Antidepressant-like effects of fractions, essential oil, carnosol and betulinic acid isolated from *Rosmarinus Officinalis* L, *Food Chemistry*, 136(2): 999–1005.

Martinello, M.A., and Pramparo, M. 2005 Antioxidant potential of rosemary extracts concentrated by molecular distillation, *Información Tecnológica*, 16(5): 17–20.

Mathew, L.M., Roy, A., and Geetha, R. V. 2020 Antibacterial activity of nutmeg oleoresin, rosemary oleoresin, and ginger oleoresin-an in vitro study, *Drug Invention Today*, 14: 292–95. https://jprsolutions.info/files/final-file-5e7e0bf186f364.11803539.pdf.

Mejri, J., Aydi, A., Abderrabba, M., and Mejri, M. 2018 Emerging extraction processes of essential oils: A Review, *Asian Journal of Green Chemistry*, 2(3): 246–67. https://dx.doi.org/10.22034/ajgc.2018.61443.

Mekonnen, A., Yitayew, B., Tesema, A., and Taddese, S. 2016 In vitro antimicrobial activity of essential oil of *thymus schimperi, matricaria chamomilla, eucalyptus globulus*, and *rosmarinus officinalis*, *International Journal of Microbiology*, 2016(9545693): 1–8.

Monisha, K., Roy, A., Geetha, R. V., and Lakshmi, T. 2019 In vitro evaluation of antibacterial property of rosemary oleoresin against methicillin-resistant staphylococcus aureus, *Drug Invention Today*, 11(5): 1103–5. https://jprsolutions.info/files/final-file-5cda833c596cb5.39388546.pdf.

Moore, J., Yousef, M., and Tsiani, E. 2016 Anticancer effects of rosemary (*Rosmarinus Officinalis* L.) extract and rosemary extract polyphenols, *Nutrients*, 8(731): 1–32.

Moradi, S., Fazlali, A., and Hamedi, H. 2018 Microwave-assisted hydro-distillation of essential oil from rosemary: comparison with traditional distillation, *Avicenna Journal of Medical Biotechnology*, 10(1): 22–28. https://www.ncbi.nlm.nih.gov/pmc/articles/PMC5742650/.

Moreno, S., Scheyer, T., Romano, C.S., and Vojnov, A.A. 2006 Antioxidant and antimicrobial activities of rosemary extracts linked to their polyphenol composition, *Free Radical Research*, 40(-2): 223–31.

Muñoz-Velázquez, E.E., Rivas-Díaz, K., Loarca-Piña, M.G.F., Mendoza-Díaz, S., Reynoso-Camacho, R., and Ramos-Gómez, M. 2012 Comparación del contenido fenólico, capacidad antioxidante y actividad antiinflamatoria de infusiones herbales comerciales, *Revista Mexicana de Ciencias Agrícolas*, 3(3): 481–95. http://www.scielo.org.mx/scielo.php?script=sci_arttext&pid=S2007-09342012000300006&lng=es&nrm=iso&tlng=es.

Naz, S., Hanif, M.A., Bhatti, H.N., and Ansari, T.M. 2017 Impact of supercritical fluid extraction and traditional distillation on the isolation of aromatic compounds from cannabis indica and cannabis sativa, *Journal of Essential Oil-Bearing Plants*, 20(1): 175–84.

Neves, J.A., Neves, J.A., and Oliveira, R. de C.M. 2018 Pharmacological and biotechnological advances with *Rosmarinus Officinalis* L, *Expert Opinion on Therapeutic Patents*, 28(5): 399–413.

Nieto, G., Ros, G., and Castillo, J. 2018 Antioxidant and antimicrobial properties of rosemary (*Rosmarinus Officinalis*, L.): A Review, *Medicines*, 5(3): 1–13.

Nivetha, G.., Roy, A., Geetha, R.V.., and Lakshmi, T. 2019 Antibacterial activity of rosemary oleoresin against *Enterococcus Faecalis* – An in vitro study, *Drug Invention Today*, 11(5): 1201–3. https://jprsolutions.info/files/final-file-5cdec4f0473269.95315053.pdf.

Oliveira, J.R., Afonso Camargo, S.E., and Dias De Oliveira, L. 2019 *Rosmarinus Officinalis* L. (Rosemary) as therapeutic and prophylactic agent, *Journal of Biomedical Science*, 26(1): 1–22.

Oliveira, M.R. de, Custódio de Souza, I., and Fürstenau, C.R. 2017 Carnosic acid induces anti-inflammatory effects in paraquat-treated SH-SY5Y cells through a mechanism involving a crosstalk between the Nrf2/HO-1 Axis and NF-KB, *Molecular Neurobiology*, 55(1): 890–97.

Ozel, M.Z., and Kaymaz, H. 2004 Superheated water extraction, steam distillation and soxhlet extraction of essential oils of origanum onites, *Analytical and Bioanalytical Chemistry*, 379 (7–8): 1127–33.

Pagano, I., Sánchez-Camargo, A. del P., Mendiola, J.A., Campone, L., Cifuentes, A., Rastrelli, L., and Ibañez, E. 2018 Selective extraction of high-value phenolic compounds from distillation wastewater of basil (ocimum basilicum l.) by pressurized liquid extraction, *Electrophoresis*, 39(15): 1884–91.

Park, J., Rho, S.-J., and Kim, Y.-R. 2019 Enhancing antioxidant and antimicrobial activity of carnosic acid in rosemary (*Rosmarinus Officinalis* L.) extract by complexation with cyclic glucans, *Food Chemistry*, 299(125119): 1–10.

Petiwala, S.M., and Johnson, J.J. 2015 Diterpenes from rosemary (*Rosmarinus Officinalis*): defining their potential for anti-cancer activity, *Cancer Letters*, 367(2): 93–102.

Presti, M. Lo, Ragusa, S., Trozzi, A., Dugo, P., Visinoni, F., Fazio, A., Dugo, G., and Mondello, L. 2005 A comparison between different techniques for the isolation of rosemary essential oil, *Journal of Separation Science*, 28(3): 273–80.

Rahbardar, M.G., Amin, B., Mehri, S., Mirnajafi-Zadeh, S.J., and Hosseinzadeh, H. 2018 Rosmarinic acid attenuates development and existing pain in a rat model of neuropathic pain: An evidence of anti-oxidative and anti-inflammatory effects, *Phytomedicine*, 40(February): 59–67.

Ramírez, M.I., Dranguet, D., and Morales, J. 2020 Actividad antiinflamatoria de plantas medicinales, *Revista Granmense de Desarrollo Local*, 16: 320–32. http://redel.udg.co.cu.

Rašković, A., Milanović, I., Pavlović, N., Ćebović, T., Vukmirović, S. and Mikov, M. 2014 Antioxidant activity of rosemary (*Rosmarinus Officinalis* L.) essential oil and its hepatoprotective potential, *BMC Complementary and Alternative Medicine*, 14(1): 1–9.

Reverchon, E., and Senatore, F. 1992 Isolation of rosemary oil: Comparison between hydrodistillation and supercritical CO2 extraction, *Flavour and Fragrance Journal*, 7(4): 227–30.

Risaliti, L., Kehagia, A., Daoultzi, E., Lazari, D., Bergonzi, M.C., Vergkizi-Nikolakaki, S., Hadjipavlou-Litina, D., and Bilia, A.R. 2019 Liposomes loaded with salvia triloba and *Rosmarinus Officinalis* essential oils: In vitro assessment of antioxidant, antiinflammatory and antibacterial activities, *Journal of Drug Delivery Science and Technology*, 51(6): 493–98.

Rocha, J., Eduardo-Figueira, M., Barateiro, A., Fernandes, A., Brites, D., Bronze, R., Duarte, C.M., Serra, A.T., Pinto, R., Freitas, M., Fernandes, E., Silva-Lima, B., Mota-Filipe, H., and Sepodes, B. 2015 Anti-inflammatory effect of rosmarinic acid and an extract of *Rosmarinus Officinalis* in rat models of local and systemic inflammation, *Basic & Clinical Pharmacology & Toxicology*, 116(5): 398–413.

Rodríguez-Calleja, J.M., Cruz-Romero, M.C., Rodríguez-Calleja, J.M., Cruz-Romero, M.C., García-López, M.L., and Kerry, J.P. 2014 Antimicrobial and antioxidant activities of commercially available essential oils and their oleoresins, *Research & Reviews: Journal of Herbal Science*, 3(3): 1–11.

Rodríguez-Rojo, S., Visentin, A., Maestri, D., and Cocero, M.J. 2012 Assisted extraction of rosemary antioxidants with green solvents, *Journal of Food Engineering*, 109(1): 98–103.

Rufino, A.T., Ribeiro, M., Sousa, C., Judas, F., Salgueiro, L., Cavaleiro, C., and Mendes, A.F. 2015 Evaluation of the anti-inflammatory, anti-catabolic and pro-anabolic effects of e-caryophyllene, myrcene and limonene in a cell model of osteoarthritis, *European Journal of Pharmacology*, 750(5): 141–50.

Santoyo, S., Cavero, S., Jaime, L., Ibañez, E., Señoráns, F.J., and Reglero, G. 2005 Chemical composition and antimicrobial activity of *Rosmarinus Officinalis* L. Essential oil obtained via supercritical fluid extraction, *Journal of Food Protection*, 68(4): 790–95.

Senanayake, N. 2018 Rosemary extract as a natural source of bioactive compounds, *Journal Food Bioactives*, 2(2): 51–57.

Song, X.C., Canellas, E., Wrona, M., Becerril, R., and Nerin, C. 2020 Comparison of two antioxidant packaging based on rosemary oleoresin and green tea extract coated on polyethylene terephthalate for extending the shelf life of minced pork meat, *Food Packaging and Shelf Life*, 26: 1–9.

Tai, J., Cheung, S., Wu, M., and Hasman, D. 2012 Antiproliferation effect of rosemary (*Rosmarinus Officinalis*) on human ovarian cancer cells in vitro, *Phytomedicine*, 19(5): 436–43.

Tenover, F.C. 2019 Antimicrobial susceptibility testing. In *Encyclopedia of Microbiology*, edited by T. Schmidt, 166–75. Amsterdam: Elsevier.

Ulbricht, C., Abrams, T.R., Brigham, A., Ceurvels, J., Clubb, J., Curtiss, W., Kirkwood, C.D., Giese, N., Hoehn, K., Iovin, R., Isaac, R., Rusie, E., Serrano, J.M.G., Varghese, M., Weissner, W., and Windsor, R.C. 2010 An evidence-based systematic review of rosemary (*Rosmarinus Officinalis*) by the natural standard research collaboration, *Journal of Dietary Supplements*, 7(4): 351–413.

Wang, Y.Z., Fu, S.G., Wang, S.Y., Yang, D.J., Wu, Y.H.S., and Chen, Y.C. 2018 Effects of a natural antioxidant, polyphenol-rich rosemary (*Rosmarinus Officinalis* L.) extract, on lipid stability of plant-derived omega-3 fatty-acid rich oil, *LWT - Food Science and Technology*, 89(March): 210–16.

Yeo, I.J., Park, J.H., Jang, J.S., Lee, D.Y., Park, J.E., Choi, Y.E., Joo, J.H., Song, J.K., Jeon, H.O., and Hong, J.T. 2018 Inhibitory effect of carnosol on UVB-induced inflammation via inhibition of STAT3, *Archives of Pharmacal Research*, 42(3): 274–83.

Žegura, B., Dobnik, D., Niderl, M.H., and Filipič, M. 2011 Antioxidant and antigenotoxic effects of rosemary (*Rosmarinus Officinalis* L.) extracts in salmonella typhimurium TA98 and HepG2 cells, *Environmental Toxicology and Pharmacology*, 32(2): 296–305.

Zermane, A., Larkeche, O., Meniai, A.H., Crampon, C., and Badens, E. 2016 Optimization of algerian rosemary essential oil extraction yield by supercritical CO2 using response surface methodology, *Comptes Rendus Chimie*, 19(4): 538–43.

Zhang, H., Wu, J., and Guo, X. 2016 Effects of antimicrobial and antioxidant activities of spice extracts on raw chicken meat quality, *Food Science and Human Wellness*, 5(1): 39–48.

CHAPTER 13

Characterization of Lemongrass Oleoresins

Shafeeqa Irfan
University of Management & Technology (UMT)

Syeda Mahvish Zahra
Allama Iqbal Open University
University of Sargodha

Mian Anjum Murtaza
University of Sargodha

Saadia Zainab
Khwaja Fareed University of Engineering and Information Technology

Bakhtawar Shafique
University of Sargodha

Rabia Kanwal and Ume Roobab
South China University of Technology

Muhammad Modassar Ali Nawaz Ranjha
University of Sargodha

CONTENTS

DOI: 10.1201/9781003186205-13

13.1 INTRODUCTION

Since time immemorial, medicinal plants have exhibited great importance to the health of communities and individuals as folk medicine. Medicinal plants possess chemical/medicinal/bioactive constituents that influence the human body producing a definite physiological action, including phenolic compounds, flavonoids, tannins, and alkaloids (Nadeem et al., 2021; Ranjha et al., 2020a, b; Bonjar et al., 2004; Hill, 1952). The bioactive constituents have shown positive impact on human health, such as antimicrobial, antiinflammatory, antioxidant activity, anticarcinogenic potential, anti-mutagenic effects, digestive stimulation action, and hypolipidemic (Ranjha et al., 2021; Krishnaiah et al., 2007). The natural chemical profiles of plants, herbs, and spices make them the best alternative to fight against a number of different ailments (Irfan et al., 2019a, b; Sabtain et al., 2021; Shehzadi et al., 2020).

Lemongrass is a medicinal and aromatic plant that belongs to the family Poaceae and the genus Cymbopogon. Cymbopogon is a Greek word, where kymbe means "boat" and pogon means "beard," referring to species' flower spike arrangement, having about 180 species (including varieties, sub-varieties, and subspecies) (Shah et al. 2011). It's a tall C4 (subtropical and tropical) (Tovar et al., 2010) monocotyledonous perennial grass having sharp, slender, and pointed apex leaves (Ernst, 2008).Lemongrass shoots contain essential oils having a typical lemon-like odor, because of which it was named lemongrass (Skaria et al., 2006). India produces three species of lemongrass: *Cymbopogon pendulus* has limited production in the Jammu region and contains high citral content, *Cymbopogon citratus* contains less citral and is cultivated in the West Indian States, *Cymbopogon flexuosus* is well-known for its essential oil and is cultivated in the East Indian States (Tovar et al., 2010). It has different local names in different languages, such as Gawati Chah, Nimmagaddi, Nibugrass, Vasanapullu, Bhustarah, and Puthigandaetc (Farooqi and Sreeramu, 2001; Tovar et al., 2010).

C. citratus herb has broad utilization in tropical countries (particularly in Southeast Asia). *C. citratus* oil (amber or yellow) is utilized in aromatherapy and is composed of 75%–85% of aldehydes: citral (chiefly), neral, and geranial. Reportedly, essential oil also comprises phytochemicals, such as terpinol methylheptenone, myrecene, citral α, citral β, geranyl acetate, terpinolene, citronellal, and nerol geraniol (Shah et al., 2011; Vazquez-Briones et al., 2015). Additionally, the extract of *C. citratus* contains many different compounds, such as citral (about 65%–85%), geraniol, monoterpene olefins, and geranylacetate (Fair and Kormas, 2008). Moreover, researchers have isolated flavones (luteolin and its 6-C-glucoside), cymbopogonol, cymbopogone and triterpenoids from *C. citratus* leaves (Becker et al., 2004).

Studies indicates that lemongrass possesses phytochemicals, such as phenolic compounds (esters, aldehyde, ketones, terpenes, and alcohols), apigenin, kaempferol, quercetin, isoorientin 2'-O-rhamnoside, luteolin, and flavonoids (Shah et al., 2011). Reportedly, lemongrass exhibits certain pharmacological properties and other effects in humans, such as antioxidant, antibacterial, anticarcinogenic, antiseptic, antidiabetic, insecticidal, mosquito repellent, and antifungal activities. Similarly, it shows antimutagenic properties in some *Salmonella typhimurium* strains against chemical-induced mutation (Tiwari et al., 2010). Commonly, lemongrass is used in Asian cooking because of its aromatic (lemon fragrant) property and its leaves as traditional remedies. Furthermore, *C. citratus* has many industrial applications, such as in cosmetics, food flavoring, medicine, and perfume industries, based on its essential oil (Sah et al., 2012).

13.2 ORIGIN, DISTRIBUTION, AND PRODUCTION

Origin of lemongrass cultivation can be tracked from India. Today, it's widely distributed in many parts of the world, including tropics and subtropics, and grown in North America, South America, Europe, and Australia. In the worldwide trade, commercial lemongrass oil is also called as Cochin oil, as more than 90% of the oil is exported through Cochin port. India is the major producer of lemongrass by cultivating around 250 tons per 4000 ha annually. India's Kerala state is known as monopoly in producing and exporting lemongrass oil. Worldwide, lemongrass oil is produced at around 1000 tons per 16,000 ha annually (Skaria et al., 2006). *C. citratus* or *C. flexuosus* make the major share of oil produced in the world (Skaria et al., 2012). However, the leading traders of lemongrass are Guatemala and Russia, with an annual production of around 250,000 and 70,000 kg, respectively (Anonymous, 2012). Additionally, the cultivation of lemongrass provides about 300 USD net profit annually to low-income growers as a profitable source of earning (Singh and Jha, 2008). Lemongrass helps in soil and water conservation because of its well-ramified root system. Therefore, it is extensively grown along live mulch bunds and in waste, marginal, and poor lands (Skaria et al., 2006).

13.3 ECONOMIC IMPORTANCE

The lemongrass oil is steam distilled from flowering tops and leaves of the plants. Lemongrass oil is a mixture of two geometric isomers of citral. A high percentage of citral (above 75%) in lemongrass essential oil develops a strong lemon-like fragrance and a citrus-like flavor. Therefore, lemongrass oil is believed to be one of the most important essential oils that is broadly used to isolate citral by fractional distillation. Citral was later on utilized as a starter material in industries for producing a number of important products.

Citral is used as a starting material to prepare two types of ionones: α-ionone and β-ionone. α-Ionone is further utilized in making perfumes, cosmetics, and flavors, whereas β-ionone is used in producing vitamin A. On the other hand, citral b, which is the other main constituent of lemongrass oil, possesses the ability to inhibit β-glucuronidase (Balz, 1999; Saikia et al., 1999). Lemongrass oil is also used to extract fragrance and flavoring substances, such as citronellol, linalool, and geraniol (acyclic terpene alcohols). Pinene plays an important role as a starter material in fragrance and flavoring industries. Citronellol is added in citrus compositions for the purpose of bouquet-ting. Nerol is also used in citrus flavors as bouquet-ting. On the contrary, small quantities of geraniol are used in flavor compositions to emphasize citrus notes (Joy et al., 2006).

Lemongrass oil is also known for many other uses, such as medicine, insect repellent, and bactericide. It shows important repellent activities, such as larvicidal and antifeedant against *Helicoverpa armigera* (Rao et al., 2000). It's also effective against repelling mosquitos for 2–3 hours (Oyedele et al., 2002) and against storage pests (Rajapakse and Emden, 1997). Studies revealed that lemongrass oil is potentially anticarcinogenic (Vinitketkumnuen et al., 2003) and acts as fungicidal against human and plant pathogens (Dubey et al., 2000; Cimanga et al., 2002). *C. citratus* essential oil has been tested against P388 leukemia cells for its cytotoxic activity (Dubey et al., 1997). Various researches have revealed that lemongrass oil possesses antioxidative properties as compared to butylated hydroxyl toluene and α-tocopherol (Baratta et al., 1998; Lean and Mohammad, 1999). Z-asarone, a compound of *C. pendulus* oil, has antiallergic properties and is used as such, whereas the oil itself has been utilized in preparing trimethoxyprim (antibacterial) drug (Skaria et al., 2006).

Lemongrass oil is used to increase the storage life of butter cakes by retarding mold growth in them (Yadav and Bhargava, 2002). It is also used in developing desired odor for special designer blends of oils and beverages (Skaria et al., 2006). *C. citratus* oil has shown potential results in the inhibition of egg hatch (Yadav and Bhargava, 2002). It's antidiabetic, antiinflammatory, carminative, febrifuge, antiseptic, and a stimulant as well as it regulates vascular expansion and nervous system, promotes digestion, stimulates appetite, useful against rickets, and strengthens the stomach (Skaria et al., 2006).

Lemongrass leaves have applications in paper and cardboard manufacturing as a cellulose source. *C. flexuosus* leaves have shown a potential decrease in root-knot nematode disease in soil amended with them. Lemongrass leaves are used as a poultice externally to relieve arthritis and pain. Primarily, lemongrass is considered as a herb that reduces fever in the Caribbean; the leaves' paste is smeared on ringworm patches in India (Chevallier, 2001).

13.4 CHEMISTRY AND PROPERTIES

C. citratus is a medicinal plant, belonging to the family Poaceae, that possesses bioactive compounds having the capability to control pathogens and pathogenic diseases by rising herbal resistance. Its chief components are myrecene and citral monoterpene aldehyde. Citral (2,3-dimethyl 2,6-octadienal) basically occurs in two geometric isomeric mixtures, geranial, which is citral A, and neral, which is citral B, and both have medicinal importance along with antibacterial activities as illustrated in Figure 13.1. Antimicrobial and antifungal characteristics of citral monoterpenes lead to its applications in the agronomy. This aromatic grass is cultivated for business purposes, such as extracting essential oils

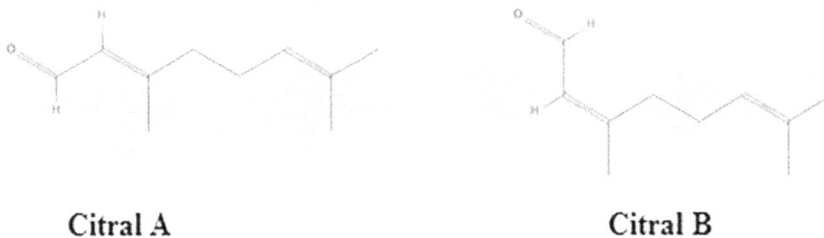

Citral A   **Citral B**

FIGURE 13.1   Chemical structure of citral A and citral B.

and production of perfumes. It has different applications in the pharmaceutical industry, owing to suitable aroma, such as in preparing soaps, deodorants, and colognes (de Almeida Costa et al., 2011).

13.5 CHEMICAL COMPOSITION

13.5.1 Oleoresins

Oleoresin (total extracts of the natural spice or herb) represents volatile and nonvolatile compounds, which develop distinguishing aroma and flavor, as they principally comprise resin and oil. Generally, small quantities of extracted spice oleoresins give improved availability and release of active principles in comparison to raw spices. However, the availability of essential oils is the source of attributed flavor of the oleoresins (Mathulla et al., 1996). Sterilization by manufacturing process, good economy, processed food standardized flavor and aroma, and instant flavor are the some advantages of extracted oleoresins (Mariwala, 2001). Oleoresins are extracted from the herb by using an appropriate solvent or combination of solvents; end products contain <25–30 ppm solvent residues. Oleoresins have better storage character, as compared to oil, as it's a concentrated wholesome product (Skaria et al., 2012).

Joy et al. (2009a) reported in their study that leaves and inflorescence of East Indian lemongrass comprise 17.3% and 15.6% oleoresins, respectively. Similarly, Joy et al. (2009b), in another study, reported that lemongrass stem (11.33%) and inflorescence (15.64%) contain less oleoresin than other parts, such as leaf lamina and leaf sheath, which contain 17.29% and 17.28% oleoresins, respectively, as mentioned in Table 13.1. They also tested eight solvents out of which methanol was found to be the best for extracting oleoresins.

The oleoresin of lemongrass is a dark green viscous liquid having a distinguished green flavor and lemongrass aroma. The volatile oil content of oleoresins is adjusted in the range of 5%–10% by diluting with sunflower seed oil.

13.5.2 Essential Oil

Lemongrass leaves are the chief source of essential oil, which make up 12% of the dry matter (Skaria et al., 2012). Plant accumulates the essential oil in certain parenchyma tissues oil cells (Ganjewala and Luthra, 2010). Lemongrass essential oil has a specific lemon-like odor, a pungent taste, and a sherry color, which makes it different from other essential oils. Chemical composition of lemongrass essential oil has been widely studied with the help

TABLE 13.1 Oleoresins Content in Different Parts of Lemongrass Plant

Plant Part	Oleoresins Content (% w/w)		
	Fresh	Dry Weight Basis	Dried
Culm	8.3360	16.6720	11.3300
Inflorescence	11.6650	23.3300	15.6430
Leaf lamina	8.0230	25.0720	17.2880
Leaf sheath	6.6180	22.0610	17.2780

Source: Adapted from Joy et al. (2016).

of GC and GC/MS methods, which varies broadly depending on the extraction methods, genetic differences, harvest period, photoperiod, plant age, farming practices, environment's geobotanical conditions, and geographical origin (Majewska et al., 2019). Table 13.2, shows the chemical compositions of different lemongrass essential oils.

13.6 EXTRACTION AND CHARACTERIZATION OF LEMONGRASS OLEORESINS

Different extraction methods, such as solvent extraction (SE), hydrodistillation (HD), microwave-assisted HD, steam distillation (SD), and supercritical fluid extraction (SFE), are used to extract lemongrass essential oil (Desai and Parikh, 2015). These different extraction methods are employed to obtain an appreciable yield of good quality oil, but extraction time and cost of production may vary (Khan and Dwivedi, 2018). Studies have reported that essential oil's quality based on its own constituent and its yield is directly influenced by the methods of extraction (Wu et al., 2019). However, it is important to note that thermal extraction methods can induce hydrolysis or degradation of instable constituents (Majewska et al., 2019) (Figure 13.2).

13.6.1 Solvent Extraction

Essential oil is dissolved from the plant material with the addition of hydrocarbon solvent usually *n*-hexane. A distillation process is employed to filter the solution and concentrate it, which results in resinoid (resin-containing substance) or a combination of substances (mixture of essential oil and wax). SE has applications in the processing of biodiesel, vegetable oil, or perfume. Usually, this method is followed to produce essential oil in high amount at lower cut in delicate plants (Chrissie et al., 1996). Relatively, it's a simple method requiring a higher solvent amount and sometimes resulting in unsatisfactory reproducibility. During the evaporation process, volatiles might be evaporated along with the

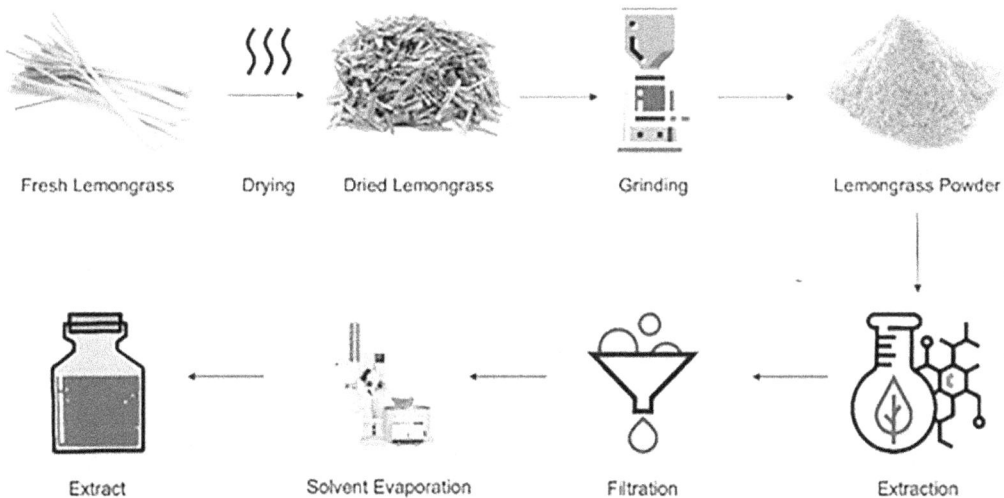

Fresh Lemongrass   Drying   Dried Lemongrass   Grinding   Lemongrass Powder

Extract   Solvent Evaporation   Filtration   Extraction

FIGURE 13.2   Extraction of oleoresins from lemongrass.

TABLE 13.2   Chemical Compositions of *C. citratus* Oil, *C. pendulus* Oil, and *C. flexuosus* Oil

Components	*C. citratus* Oil (%)	*C. pendulus* Oil (%)	*C. flexuosus* Oil (%)
1,8 Cineole	NR	NR	-
Camphene	NR	0.01	NR
Car-3-ene	NR	0.04	NR
Caryophyllene	NR	NR	0.32
Citral a	41.82	43.29	51.19
Citral b	0.18	32.27	26.21
Citronellal	0.73	0.49	0.37
Citronellol	NR	NR	0.44
Citronellyl acetate	0.96	0.72	NR
Delta-3-catrene	0.16	NR	NR
Dipentene	0.23	0.35	NR
Elemol	1.2	2.29	NR
Geraniol	1.85	2.6	5.00
Geraniol acetate	NR	3.58	NR
Geranyl acetate	3.00	NR	1.95
Limonene	NR	NR	2.42
Linalool	1.85	3.07	1.34
Linalyl acetate	NR	NR	-
Methyl heptanene	2.62	NR	NR
Methyl heptanone	NR	1.05	1.50
Myrcene	12.75	0.04	0.46
Nerol	NR	NR	2.20
P-Cymene	NR	0.36	NR
Phellandrene	NR	0.3	NR
Pinene	NR	0.19	NR
Terpinolene	NR	NR	0.05
α-Pinene	0.13	NR	0.24
α-Terpineol	NR	NR	0.24
β-Caryophyllene	0.18	2.15	NR
β-Caryophyllene Oxide	0.61	1.56	NR
β-Cymene	0.2	NR	NR
β-Elemene	1.33	0.7	NR
β-Ocimene	NR	NR	0.06
β-Phellandrene	0.07	NR	NR
β-Pinene	-	0.16	NR
β-Thujene	NR	NR	0.03
cis-β-Ocimene	NR	NR	0.06
trans-β-Ocimene	NR	NR	0.07
δ-3-Catrene	0.16	NR	NR
β-Phellandrene	0.07	NR	NR
Source: Adapted from	Saleem et al. (2003a, b)	Shahi et al. (1997); Sharma et al. (2002)	Weiss (1997); Ranade (2004)

NR, not reported.

concentration of the sample following extraction. Besides, there are chances of essential oil contamination with solvent residues (Majewska et al., 2019).

In recent years, this method has shown satisfactory results for extracting lemongrass essential oil from dry and fresh lemongrass leaves (Schaneberg and Khan, 2002). The Soxhlet apparatus is sometimes used for SE of lemongrass essential oil (Alhassan et al., 2018). Suryawanshi et al. (2016) and Alhassan et al. (2018) conducted a study on lemongrass leaves using *n*-hexane as solvent. Suryawanshi and his coworkers obtained 1.85% oil yield, while, Alhassan and his coworker obtained 4.5% oil yield. Moreover, Schaneberg and Khan (2002) in their study reported that extraction of lemongrass essential oil with sonication-assisted *n*-hexane extraction yielded similar oils having main compounds to SD.

Soxhlet extraction results higher extraction efficiency as plant materials are in continuous contact with refluxing liquid phase. However, in comparison to other conventional extraction method, Soxhlet extraction has a significant drawback of heating at high temperature, usually around solvent's boiling point, for a longer period that results in thermal degradation of fragile compounds of plant material. The choice of the correct solvent is very important for both Soxhlet extraction and maceration extraction in order to prevent volatile's loss and achieve high yield of extraction (Majewska et al., 2019).

13.6.2 Hydrodistillation

HD is among the most employed traditional extraction methods which sometimes can be used in place of SD. It works on the principle of isotropic distillation (Rassem et al., 2016). In this method, plant material is fully submerged into water in a container, which is direct heated and essential oil distills along with water molecules. When cooled, oil gathers on the top of the hydrosol, which is then collected. This process has been employed to extract essential oil from various plants and different parts of the plants. The yield of essential oil depends on a number of parameters, such as nature, size, weight of raw material, and volume of water (Parish et al., 2011).

Generally, citral from lemongrass is isolated by using the HD method, which is then utilized in prepare lemongrass tea. It has been reported that maximum extract yield is obtained from wet lemongrass (Diwan et al., 2014). Marongiu et al. (2006) and Desai and Parikh (2015) reported that HD yields essential oil in a range of 0.43% and 1.80%, respectively. In 2016, Ajayi and coworkers conducted a study on lemongrass leaves using neutral, basic, and weakly acidic medium and adopting HD and microwave-assisted HD (MAHD) methods. They reported that the composition of essential oil was significantly affected by mediums of isolation. Subsequently, HD showed 0.73%, MAHD showed 0.64%, base-distillation showed 0.45%, and acid-distillation resulted in a 0.7% total yield of volatile fractions. Moreover, HD resulted in 72.6%, MAHD 44.7%, base-distillation 78.61%, and acid-distillation 30.07% citral content as the main component in obtained essential oil. They also observed significant differences in geranial, neral, and myrcene contents. In acidic distillation, essential oil showed a low concentration of citral because of the chemical transformation of citral in an acidic solution (Ajayi et al., 2016). However, basic medium provides the suitable conditions to extract the high citral content of lemongrass essential oil.

The advantages of HD are relatively easy method and cost-effective setup. However, this is a slow process involving heat exposure, which may cause the degradation of sensitive constituents during polymerization reactions or hydrolysis (Majewska et al., 2019).

13.6.3 Microwave-Assisted Extraction Hydrodistillation (MAHD)

Recently, extraction of essential oils using MAHD has grabbed the attention of researchers. But a drawback is associated with the use of MAHD that samples may deteriorate because of the external exposure of microwaves to a sample (Golmakani et al., 2008). MAHD works on the principle that based on dipole rotation and ionic conduction the polarity of solvents is influenced by irradiations, which occurs simultaneously in most cases (Letellier et al., 1999).

Basically, MAHD and traditional HD have same working, but the only difference is MAHD involves the use of microwaves to heat the solvent instead of direct heating. The flask is filled with plant material and water (as solvent) and put inside the microwave oven working at 2.45 GHz frequency. Desai and Parikh (2015) verified MAHD as a potential and powerful technique for the extraction of lemongrass essential oil as compared to conventional extraction techniques. There is no substantial difference in the chemical composition of essential oil extracted by MAHD and traditional HD. However, there may be significant differences in geranial, neral, and myrcene contents of essential oils (Desai and Parikh, 2015). In another study, Tran et al. (2019) reported the yield of essential oil with citral content obtained using HD and MAHD. HD reported 0.2% essential oil yield having an 83.85% citral content, while MAHD yielded 0.35% essential oil having a 93.28% citral content.

In comparison to conventional methods, the use of microwaves offers advantages: accelerates oil extraction, significant extraction yield, less time consumption, environment friendly, fast transfer of energy, and effective heating, which makes it attractive to both laboratories and industries (Majewska et al., 2019).

13.6.4 Steam Distillation

Mostly, SD is employed for heat-sensitive materials, water insoluble and that may decay at their boiling point, such as hydrocarbons, resins, oils, etc. Furthermore, it's employed for the extraction of other essential oils (Fernandes et al., 2019).

In this method, the temperature of steam is maintained high enough to vaporize the essential oil and keeping in view to avoid the burn to essential oil or damage to the plant material. Fresh or dried plant material is exposed to steam that softens the plant materials' cells and releases essential oil in the form of vapors along with molecules of steam that are then cooled in a condenser and collected. This method has an advantage of carrying out extraction process below boiling point(s) of the individual component(s) of essential oils as they possess compounds having 200°C above boiling points (Berk, 2013). However, steam assists in the extraction of such substances near to 100°C at atmospheric pressure.

Still, SD is a well-known and leading method for extracting lemongrass essential oil. Lemongrass can be exposed to distillation both fresh and wilted, but wilted herbage has an advantage, as it possesses less moisture content and a high-yield oil before distillation (Skaria et al., 2012). Previous studies have reported a wide range of yields of essential oil extracted through this method: 0.71% (Kpoviessi et al., 2014), 0.6% (Boukhatem et al., 2014a), 0.3% (Santin et al., 2009), and 0.24% (Anggraeni et al., 2018).

The advantages of SD include simple method, low-cost apparatus, unchanged properties of essential oil, no decomposition of essential oil's constituents, and can be used under pressure (Majewska et al., 2019).

13.6.5 Supercritical Fluid Extraction (SFE)

SFE, one of the most ecofriendly techniques, has been developed to isolate the essential oil and meet the demand of high-quality natural products over the last decades. Haloui and Meniai (2017) reported that SFE has a great advantage over the SE as it can extract various compounds from natural solid matrices without any solvent trace. It produces better quality essential oils as compared to HD, SD, and SE (Al-Marzouqi et al., 2007). SFE properties can be modified, which allow the selective extraction by influencing the density of solvent by adjusting the critical pressure and temperature, and play a significant role in food and pharmaceutical systems. Carbon dioxide has low critical temperature (23°C–50°C) and pressure (8–12 MPa), suitable physical and chemical properties because of which it is used as the supercritical fluid in most cases (Carlson et al., 2001). It is an inexpensive, non-ammable, non-corrosive, and non-toxic gas as a natural constituent of many foods and also has been generally recognized as safe (21 CFR § 184.1240, 2019). Carbon dioxide with SFE at 30°C can be performed to preserve the properties and composition of original oil.

In the literature, only a few studies have reported on the extraction of lemongrass essential oil by employing supercritical carbon dioxide, which were designed to optimize the pressure and temperature of the extraction process of essential oil. In 2001, Carlson and his coworkers conducted a study on fresh lemongrass leaves under different pressure and temperature conditions of supercritical carbon dioxide extraction. They unveiled that changes in parameters of pressure and temperature significantly influence the composition of essential oil. The parameters of 9 MPa & 23°C and 12 MPa & 40°C resulted in maximum extraction yields of 1.7% and 1.51% of essential oil, respectively. Under all the pressure and temperature conditions, neral (26.7%–31.9%) and geranial (44.6%–53.0%) were recorded as the maximum quantities in the essential oil (Carlson et al., 2001). In 2006, Marongiu and his fellow researchers carried out a research to extract lemongrass essential oil with maximum citral content and followed the supercritical extraction with a series of experiments at different pressures, such as 9, 10, 11, and 12 MPa, at 50°C for 360 minutes based on maximizing citral content in obtained oil. They compared the composition of obtained extract with HD- and SD-isolated essential oil. They found that 9 MPa essential oil extraction condition achieved the highest 0.65% process yield and the highest 68% citral content in the essential oil, on the other hand, HD resulted in 0.43% process yield and the highest 73% citral content. Because of the high molecular mass during the compound's extraction, the appearance changed from a characteristic yellow oil to a yellowish semi-solid product at higher solvent density (Marongiu et al., 2006). In 2019, Wu and co-researchers adopted the response surface methodology for predicting optimum supercritical CO_2 extraction's operational parameters to extract essential oil from *Cymbopogon citronella* (lemongrass). They determined that at 25 MPa, 35°C, CO_2 flow rate 18 L/hour, for 120 minutes parameter of SFE extraction yielded 4.4% essential oil as compared to that obtained employing HD. SFE-extracted essential oil showed contents of 20.02% geranial, 10.22% geraniol, and 15.11% neral as the main components, whereas, in comparison, HD showed 15.12% geranial, 25.45% geraniol, and 11.15% neral content. It was concluded that SFE doesn't change the main components of essential oil of lemongrass (Wu et al., 2019).

SFE is an innovative and ecofriendly method of extraction for essential oils. However, the major concern associated with SFE is the cost of the equipment, which has restricted its applications in extremely sensitive industrial systems where the major priority is high-quality and pure final products (Majewska et al., 2019).

13.7 PHYTOCHEMISTRY AND PHARMACOLOGY APPLICATIONS

Medicinal plants are used as an edge to compete the inclined interest in consumption of "natural and vegan," especially regarding market of food, nutraceuticals, and pharmaceuticals, perfumes, toiletries, and cosmetics industries (Rocha et al., 2011). Variety and geographic location of growing *C. citratus* has a great impact on the composition of its essential oils. Aldehydes, fatty acids, esters, ketones, alcohols, and hydrocarbon terpenes have been constantly found and registered with progress in extraction techniques. Myrcene is a bioactive component of lemongrass; it has properties of pain relieving and inhibition of bacterial infestation; and other bioactive contents include geraniol, citral, citronellal, and citronellol. Citral contributes specific lemon flavor: it's basically a mixture of two stereoisomeric monoterpene aldehydes, the cis isomer neral (25%–38%) dominated by the trans isomer geranial (40%–62%) and is specifically utilized to make perfumes, soaps, and vitamin A (Shah et al., 2011).

13.7.1 Antimicrobial Activity

Ethanol-assisted extracts of lemongrass have an inhibitory impact on the growth of *Staphylococcus aureus*, which is associated with flavonoids and tannins (Danlami et al., 2011). The antioxidant potential of lemongrass is active as antibacterial in wound infections as well as against respiratory, urinary, or digestive tract infections (Mickiene et al., 2011).

13.7.2 Antifungal Activity

Candida albicans is an extremely active pathogen regarding infections in humans as compared to other fungal species. A study proved the antifungal effects of lemongrass specific to the active compound citral, which is often associated with limiting the growth of species *Candida* (Silva et al., 2008). Essential oils of lemongrass can be used for internal or external fungal infestation because of its antifungal potential (Handique and Singh, 1990; Alam et al., 1994; Mehmood et al., 1997). Essential oils of lemongrass act efficiently to limit

C. albicans infection if utilized in vapor phase (Tyagi and Malik, 2010a, 2010b), and these repressed the activity of *Aspergillus flavus* at 750 ppm (Singh et al., 2010).

13.7.3 Antiprotozoan Activity

Protozoans belonging to the Trypanosomatidae family cause serious infections in humans, plants, and animals. *Crithidia*, *Blastocrithidia*, *Herpetomonas*, and monoxenous protozoans that are commonly found in insect hosts, are also members of this family. The lemongrass essential oils possess antiprotozoan activity against *Crithidia deanei* (Pedroso et al., 2006).

13.7.4 Antioxidant Activity

Flavonoids and phenolic acid have been investigated as free radical scavengers and natural antioxidants because of their pharmacological activity. Plant-based phenolic acids represent the antioxidant potential (Garg et al., 2012). Studies by Tiwari et al. (2010) publicized antioxidative, anti-inflammation, and cell-protecting properties of *C. citratus* after intervening as supplement, also represented good potential against inflammatory and detrimental lung diseases.

13.7.5 Antidiarrheal Activity

It is a common trial and tested practice in traditional medicine to use the decoction of lemongrass leaf and whole stalk as a relief to diarrheal patients, as citral in stalk is a potent bioactive component, which has antidiarrheal properties (Tangpu and Yadav, 2006).

13.7.6 Antimutagenic Activity

Lemongrass extracts with ethanol were found to be anti-mutative when investigated against mutations caused by chemicals in TA 100 and TA 98 strains of *S. typhimurium* (Vinitketkumnuen et al., 1994).

13.7.7 Antiinflammatory Activity

Leaf infusion of *C. citratus* yielded results of inhibiting inflammatory stress with special regard to gastrointestinal tract (Figueirinha et al., 2010). Francisco et al. (2011) extrapolated *C. citratus* leaf extracts as a safe drug against inflammation in traditional medicines by associating its unique polyphenol profile, especially flavonoid "luteolin glycosides."

13.7.8 Antimalarial Activity

Antimalarial potential of lemongrass essential oils was exhibited by an animal model with *Plasmodium berghei* infestation (Tchoumbougnang et al., 2005).

13.7.9 Antinociceptive Activity

Essential oil of *C. citrates* retains a noteworthy anti-nociceptive action, paralleling the consequences of three experimental methods of nociception, namely acetic acid-induced writhing in mice, hot-plate, and formalin test, essential oils impact at the peripheral and central levels, both (Viana et al., 2000).

13.7.10 Antihepatotoxic Activity

Cisplatin toxicity increases the risks of hepatopathies, while lemongrass extracts act as an elixir in managing the hepatic health by improving hepatic health and limiting the action of cisplatin (Arhoghro et al., 2012).

13.7.11 Diuretic

In certain infections, it is necessary to consume diuretic substances, yet lemongrass causes frequent urination and also increases urine concentration, which helps in the excretion of causative agents (Carbajal et al., 1989).

13.7.12 Nervine

Blanco et al. (2009) reported that lemon grass oil can be helpful in curing different nervous disorders like lack of reflexes, sluggishness, convulsions, vertigo, nervousness, shivering of hands and limbs, etc. It may be used by people suffering from Parkinson's and Alzheimer's diseases.

13.7.13 Sedative

Blanco et al. (2009) studied curative effects of essential oils from lemongrass, especially relieving insomnia due to sedative action, soothing and mind-calming effects. It relieves anxiety, and soothes inflammation and skin itches.

13.7.14 Tonic

Lemongrass strengthens all body systems, i.e., nervous, digestive, respirators, and excretory, for smooth functioning, and its action on enhancement of nutrient absorption into body tissues facilitates immune system activity and improvement (Skaria et al., 2012).

13.7.15 Analgesic

Lemongrass essential oils are miraculously analgesic for joints and muscle pains, and also relieve headaches caused by viral infestations in body, such as chicken pox, fever, cough, and common influenza; these oils are effective in minimizing lethargy and help manage toothaches (Lorenzetti et al., 1991).

13.7.16 Antidepressant

Lemongrass essential oils maintain mental stress, confine confidence and self-esteem, hope, and mitigate depression (Costa et al., 2011).

13.7.17 Antipyretic

The antipyretic effects of essential oils from lemongrass increase when lemongrass is used as a hot decoction in tea, mainly because of the antiviral perspiration-causing properties (Skaria et al., 2012).

13.8 INDUSTRIAL APPLICATIONS

13.8.1 Cosmetics and Perfumes

The lemony misty fragrance of essential oils of *C. citratus* is well associated to citral in it that freshens up the mood, and for this activity, it is used by perfume, grooming product, soap, and deodorant-making industries and is also used in mopping and cleaning detergents. Lemongrass essential oils are immensely used in aroma therapies and massage applications because of the ameliorative actions on pain caused by rheumatoid, nerve issues, also for headaches. Lemongrass essential oils are benefiting in foot bath. Its stimulating fragrance reverts drowsiness and revitalizes the mind and soul, which is why it is being added to candle waxes. The essential oils of lemongrass can be used in massage applications by mixing with essential oils of lavender, jasmine, tea tree, basil, and cedar wood (Skaria et al., 2012).

The bioactive properties of lemongrass leaves and stalk extracts, be it ethanol extracts or essential oils, are not limited just to food or medicinal industries but also hold havoc for cosmetology. Citral is known as a precursor to produce rose aroma yielding compound beta-ionone in just a little amount, and is economic to perfume production business. *Cymbopogon* genus essential oils have extensive use in palmarosa oil, a basic component of perfume and soap production (Davis et al., 1983). Several blends of glycerol and lemon balm are well-known patents of cosmetic products (Yongtian et al., 2015). A unique patent has ensemble, release of pleasing aroma from pods of lemon grass, with the action of bacteria (Yuhua et al., 2014). Mosquera established the antibacterial potential of lemongrass against gram negative and positive bacteria and marked exclamatory use in soaps (Mosquera, 2016; Naik et al., 2010); similar activity was investigated by a team of researchers extrapolating it against pathogens causing skin acne and irritation (Lertsatitthanakorn et al., 2006; Melo et al., 2015), and it prevents skin disease by managing oxidative stress. The exotic smell of lemongrass makes it to be used as insect-repelling agent finalizing it to be suitable for using as a lotion during excursion trips and tours (Lima et al., 2009). The antioxidant property of this oil is very significant for cosmetic industries as this activity can be used to prevent several dermal diseases that result from oxidative stress (Pereira et al., 2009), which is the main cause of skin aging (Saraí et al., 2006).

13.8.2 Food Preservation

Oleoresins in lemongrass are healthy flavoring components, which are being used for flavor enhancement in drinks, bakery items, and also being consumed as flavored tea (Joy et al., 2009a). Lemongrass essential oils have proven their antibacterial actions to limit the growth of at least 12 food spoilage and disease-causing strains (de Silveira et al. 2012). Moreover, lemongrass possesses effective antifungal (Mishra and Dubey 1994; Paranagama et al., 2003) and antibacterial properties against *Salmonella enteritidis* and *E. coli* (Raybaudi-Massilia et al., 2006; Moore-Neibel et al., 2012). Lemongrass has proved itself against the pathogens *Cladosporium herbarum*, *Colletotrichum coccodes*, *Botrytis cinerea*, and *Rhizopus stolonifer*, which are a threat of food spoilage and cause post-harvest losses to fresh and processed commodities, if got germinated in suitable storage conditions

(Tzortzakis and Economakis, 2007). Lemongrass enacts as shelf-life increaser for guava, cucumber, and also fruit juices (Murmu and Mishra, 2018; Omoba and Onyekwere, 2016; Tyagi et al., 2014). Essential oils of lemon grass serve as extravaganza preservative in processed cheese, yogurt, non-fermentative dairy products, cake, bread, and bakery (Abd-El Fattah et al., 2010; Belewu et al., 2012; Abd-El Fattah et al., 2010; Guynot et al., 2003; Suhr and Nielsen, 2003). Lemongrass has promising research-based results of becoming a superb preservative, yet it can be extremely toxic if used at high dose and exposed directly to olfactory organs (Smith et al., 2005) as supported by Ekpenyong and research team (Ekpenyong et al., 2015; Ekpenyong and Akpan, 2017).

13.9 QUALITY ISSUES

13.9.1 Oleoresin

Generally, there are two ways to evaluate the oleoresin quality: (a) impartation of aroma by components of essential oil or volatile and (b) impartation of bite from resin portion, which is a mixture of pigments, gums, alkaloids, etc. Moreover, quality parameters of oleoresin as flavor ingredients include consistency of blending, dispersibility, pourability, viscosity, color, and flavor (Skaria et al., 2012).

13.9.2 Essential Oil

13.9.2.1 Citral Estimation

The main component of lemongrass essential oil is citral content, which is the important quality characteristic, is estimated using sulfite or bisulfite method that also helps to determine a part of methyl heptanone and other aldehydes achieving higher results (Guenther, 1948). Generally, this method is followed to evaluate the oil quality in trade because of insignificant error. However, gas chromatography can be used to precisely estimate the citral.

13.9.2.2 Organic Lemongrass Oil

The organic production standards of lemongrass oil start from growing, processing, packaging to shipping, which have been setup by many countries. Generally, lemongrass oil is believed to be "organic" as its production mainly doesn't involve any chemical fertilizers and pesticides. Every country has its own set of procedures and regulations for any product believed to be "organic," which must be observed. Before labeling product as organic, the process of certification must be fulfilled (Skaria et al., 2012).

13.9.3 Adulteration of Oil

Lemongrass oils must be solely extracted from specific *Cymbopogon* species to achieve its 100% purity. Adulteration of pure lemongrass oil is carried out by the conscious addition of cheap synthetics, alternative oils, isolates, byproducts, oil fractions, etc. Rarely, marketed lemongrass oil has been reported to have several contaminants because of defective practices of production and processing. Moreover, its adulteration can be done by consciously adding synthetic odorants and citral but those have some concerns such as imparting irritancy and/or toxicity, and altering beneficial properties of lemongrass oil. The detection of adulterants in lemongrass oil can be achieved by variation in phys-icochemical characteristics, uncharacteristic or poor odor profile, and using advanced analytical techniques (HPLC–MS, GC–13C NMR, GC–FTIR, and GC–MS), however, thin-layer chromatography (TLC) is the best method to opt as it is more appropriate and practical (Skaria et al., 2012).

13.10 SAFETY AND TOXICITY

In 1996, Leung and Foster reported that lemongrass oil has not shown any adverse effects on protein, kidney function, liver function, blood, and metabolism of lipid and carbohy-drate of rats. Moreover, studies have not reported any toxicological or mutagenic reactions in humans (Leung and Foster, 1996).

13.11 CONCLUSION

In literature, few studies have been reported on lemongrass oleoresin; therefore, there is a huge gap in studying the potential of lemongrass oleoresins in future. Lemongrass is an abundant source of oleoresins, which has the enormous potential to be utilized as a flavor-ing ingredient. Lemongrass oil has great applications in some toiletries and cosmetics as a low-cost fragrance material. Its oil is also a significant source of citral, which is utilized to synthesize vitamin A, β-ionone, and as a starter material to manufacture several com-pounds. Oil is also used in some confectionary, baked goods, and several beverages.

REFERENCES

21CFR184.1240, 2019. https://www.accessdata.fda.gov/scripts/cdrh/cfdocs/cfcfr/CFRSearch.cfm?fr=184.1240

Abd-El Fattah, S. M., Yahia Hassan, A., Bayoum, H. M. and Eissa, H. A. 2010. The use of lemon-grass extracts as antimicrobial and food additive potential in yoghurt. *The Journal of American Science*, 6: 582–594.

Ajayi, E. O., Sadimenko, A. P. and Afolayan, A. J. 2016. GC–MS evaluation of *Cymbopogon citratus* (DC) Stapf oil obtained using modified hydro distillation and microwave extraction methods. *Food Chemistry*, 209: 262–266.

Alam, K., Agua, T., Maven, H., Taie, R., Rao, K. S., Burrows, I., et al. 1994. Preliminary screening of seaweeds, seagrass and lemongrass oil from Papua New Guinea for antimicrobial and antifun-gal activity. *International Journal of Pharmacognosy*, 32(4): 396–399.

Alhassan, M., Lawal, A., Nasiru, Y., Suleiman, M., Safiya, A. M. and Bello, N. 2018. Extraction and formulation of perfume from locally available lemon grass leaves. *ChemSearch Journal*, 9(2):40–44. Al-Marzouqi, A. H., Rao, M. V. and Jobe, B. 2007. Comparative evaluation of SFE and steam distillation methods on the yield and composition of essential oil extracted from spearmint (*Mentha spicata*). *Journal of Liquid Chromatography & Related Technologies*, 30(4): 463–475.

Anggraeni, N. I., Hidayat, I. W., Rachman, S. D., and Ersanda. 2018. Bioactivity of essential oil from lemongrass (*Cymbopogon citratus* Stapf) as antioxidant agent. In *AIP Conference Proceedings*. AIP Publishing LLC. Melville, NY, USA. https://doi.org/10.1063/1.5021200.

Anonymous. 2012. *Lemongrass Production: in Essential Oil Crops, Production Guidelines for Lemongrass*. Pretoria, South Africa: A Publication of the Department of Agriculture, Forestry and Fisheries; Directorate Communication Services, Department of Agriculture, Forestry and Fisheries Pretoria, pp. 1–26. https://www.nda.agric.za/docs/brochures/proguilemongrass.pdf.

Arhoghro, E. M., Kpomah, D. E. and Uwakwe, A. A. 2012. Curative potential of aqueous extract of lemon Grass (*Cymbopogon citratus*) on cisplatin induced hepatotoxicity in Albino Wistar rats. *Journal of Physiology and Pharmacology Advances*, 2(8): 282–294.

Balz, R. 1999. *The Healing Power of Essential Oils*. Delhi: Motilal Banarsidass Publishers Pvt Ltd.

Baratta, M. T., Dorman, H. D., Deans, S. G., Figueiredo, A. C., Barroso, J. G. and Ruberto, G. 1998. Antimicrobial and antioxidant properties of some commercial essential oils. *Flavour and Fragrance Journal*, 13(4): 235–244.

Becker, E. M., Nissen, L. R. and Skibsted, L. H. 2004. Antioxidant evaluation protocols: food quality or health effects. *European Food Research and Technology*, 219(6): 561–571.

Belewu, M. A., El-Imam, A. A., Adeyemi, K. D. and Oladunjoye, S. A. 2012. Eucalyptus oil and lemon grass oil: effect on chemical composition and shelf-life of soft cheese. *Environment and Natural Resources Research*, 2(1): 114.

Berk, Z. (2013). Distillation. In *Food Process Engineering and Technology*, ed. Z. Berk. Elsevier Inc, USA. pp. 329–352.

Blanco, M. M., Costa, C. A. R. A., Freire, A. O., Santos Jr, J. G. and Costa, M. 2009. Neurobehavioral effect of essential oil of *Cymbopogon citratus* in mice. *Phytomedicine*, 16(2–3): 265–270.

Bonjar, G. S. and Farrokhi, P. R. 2004. Anti-bacillus activity of some plants used in traditional medicine of Iran. *Nigerian Journal of Natural Products and Medicine*, 8: 34–39.

Boukhatem, M. N., Ferhat, M. A., Kameli, A., Saidi, F. and Kebir, H. T. 2014a. Lemongrass (*Cymbopogon citratus*) essential oil as a potent anti-inflammatory and antifungal drugs. *Libyan Journal of Medicine*, 9(1): 25431.

Carbajal, D., Casaco, A., Arruzazabala, L., Gonzalez, R. and Tolon, Z. 1989. Pharmacological study of *Cymbopogon citratus* leaves. *Journal of Ethnopharmacology*, 25(1): 103–107.

Carlson, L. H. C., Machado, R. A. F., Spricigo, C. B., Pereira, L. K. and Bolzan, A. 2001. Extraction of lemongrass essential oil with dense carbon dioxide. *The Journal of Supercritical Fluids*, 21(1): 33–39.

Chevallier, A. 2001. *Encyclopedia of Medicinal Plants*. Great Britain: Dorling Kindersley Ltd.

Chrissie, W. 1996. *The Encyclopedia of Aromatherapy*. Vermont: Healing Arts Press.

Cimanga, K., Apers, S., de Bruyne, T., Van Miert, S., Hermans, N., Totté, J. et al. 2002. Chemical composition and antifungal activity of essential oils of some aromatic medicinal plants growing in the Democratic Republic of Congo. *Journal of Essential Oil Research*, 14(5): 382–387.

Danlami, U., Rebecca, A., Machan, D. B. and Asuquo, T. S. 2011. Comparative study on the antimicrobial activities of the ethanolic extracts of lemon grass and *Polyalthia longifolia*. *Journal of Applied Pharmaceutical Science*, 1(9): 174.

Davis, J. B., Kay, D. E. and Clark, V. 1983. *Plants Tolerant of Arid, or Semi-Arid, Conditions with Non-Food Constituents of Potential Use*. London: Tropical Development and Research Institute.

de Almeida Costa, C. A. R., Kohn, D. O., de Lima, V. M., Gargano, A. C., Flório, J. C. and Costa, M. 2011. The GABAergic system contributes to the anxiolytic-like effect of essential oil from *Cymbopogon citratus* (lemongrass). *Journal of Ethnopharmacology*, 137(1): 828–836.

del Carmen Vázquez-Briones, M., Hernández, L. R. and Guerrero-Beltrán, J. Á. 2015. Physicochemical and antioxidant properties of *Cymbopogon citratus* essential oil. *Journal of Food Research*, 4(3): 36–45.

Desai, M.A. and Parikh, J. 2015. Extraction of essential oil from leaves of lemongrass using microwave radiation: optimization, comparative, kinetic, and biological studies. *ACS Sustainable Chemistry and Engineering*, 3(3): 421–431.

Dubey, N. K., Kishore, N., Jaya, V. and Lee, S. 1997. Cytotoxicity of the essential oils of *Cymbopogon citratus* and *Ocimum gratissimum*. *Indian Journal of Pharmaceutical Sciences*, 59(5):263–264.

Dubey, N. K., Pramila, T. and Singh, H. B. 2000. Prospects of some essential oils as antifungal agents. *Journal of Medicinal and Aromatic Plant Sciences*, 22(1B):350–354.

Ekpenyong, C. E., Akpan, E. and Nyoh, A. 2015. Ethnopharmacology, phytochemistry, and biological activities of *Cymbopogon citratus* (DC.) Stapf extracts. *Chinese Journal of Natural Medicines*, 13(5): 321–337.

Ekpenyong, C. E. and Akpan, E. E. 2017. Use of *Cymbopogon citratus* essential oil in food preservation: recent advances and future perspectives. *Critical Reviews in Food Science and Nutrition*, 57(12):2541–2559.

Ernst, E. 2008. Chiropractic: a critical evaluation. *Journal of Pain and Symptom Management*, 35(5): 544–562.

Fair, J. D. and Kormos, C. M. 2008. Flash column chromatograms estimated from thin-layer chromatography data. *Journal of Chromatography A*, 1211(1–2): 49–54.

Farooqi, A. A. and Sreeramu, B. S. 2001. *Cultivation of Aromatic and Medicinal Crop.* Hyderabad: Universities Press (India) Pvt. Ltd.

Fernandes, S. S., Tonato, D., Mazutti, M. A., de Abreu, B. R., da Costa Cabrera, D., D'Oca, C. D. R. M. et al. 2019. Yield and quality of chia oil extracted via different methods. *Journal of Food Engineering*, 262: 200–208.

Figueirinha, A., Cruz, M. T., Francisco, V., Lopes, M. C. and Batista, M. T. 2010. Anti-inflammatory activity of *Cymbopogon citratus* leaf infusion in lipopolysaccharide-stimulated dendritic cells: contribution of the polyphenols. *Journal of Medicinal Food*, 13(3): 681–690.

Francisco, V., Figueirinha, A., Neves, B. M., García-Rodríguez, C., Lopes, M. C., Cruz, M. T. and Batista, M. T. 2011. *Cymbopogon citratus* as source of new and safe anti-inflammatory drugs: bioguided assay using lipopolysaccharide-stimulated macrophages. *Journal of Ethnopharmacology*, 133(2): 818–827.

Ganjewala, D. and Luthra, R. 2010. Essential oil biosynthesis and regulation in the genus *Cymbopogon*. *Natural Product Communications*, 5(1): 163–172.

Garg, D., Muley, A., Khare, N. and Marar, T. 2012. Comparative analysis of phytochemical profile and antioxidant activity of some Indian culinary herbs. *Research Journal of Pharmaceutical, Biological and Chemical Sciences*, 3(3): 845–854.

Golmakani, M. T., and Rezaei, K. 2008. Microwave-assisted hydrodistillation of essential oil from *Zataria multiflora* Boiss. *European Journal of Lipid Science and Technology*, 110(5):448–454.

Guenther, E. and Althausen, D. 1948. *The Essential Oils.* New York: Van Nostrand Company Inc.

Guynot, M. E., Ramos, A. J., Seto, L., Purroy, P., Sanchis, V. and Marin, S. 2003. Antifungal activity of volatile compounds generated by essential oils against fungi commonly causing deterioration of bakery products. *Journal of Applied Microbiology*, 94(5):893–899.

Haloui, I. and Meniai, A.H. 2017. Supercritical CO2 extraction of essential oil from Algerian Argan (Argania spinosa L.) seeds and yield optimization. *International Journal of Hydrogen Energy*, 42(17): 12912–12919.

Handique, A. K. and Singh, H. B. 1990. Antifungal action of lemongrass oil on some soil-borne plant pathogens. *Indian Perfumer*, 34(3):232–234.

Hill A. F. 1952. *Economic Botany.* New York: McGarw-Hill Book Company Inc.

Irfan, S., Ranjha, M. M. A. N., Mahmood, S., Mueen-ud-Din, G., Rehman, S., Saeed, W., Alam, M. Q., Zahra, S. M., Ramzan, I., Rafique, A. and Masood, A. B. 2019b. A critical review on pharmaceutical and medicinal importance of ginger. *Acta Scientific Nutritional Health*, 3:78–82.

Irfan, S., Ranjha, M. M. A. N., Mahmood, S., Saeed, W. and Alam, M. Q. 2019a. Lemon peel: a natural medicine. *International Journal of Biotechnology and Allied Fields*. 7(10): 185–194.

Joy, P. P., Skaria, B. P., Mathew, S., Mathew, G. and Joseph, A. 2009a. Standardization of oleoresin extraction in lemongrass (*Cymbopogon flexuosus*), In *Proceedings of National Workshop on Spices and Aromatic Plants, Ludhiana*, India.

Joy, P. P., Skaria, B. P., Mathew, S., Mathew, G. and Joseph, A. 2009b. Evaluation of lemongrass for oleoresin, In *Abstracts of CIMAP Golden Jubilee Symposium on Medicinal and Aromatic Plants, Bangalore*, India.

Joy, P. P., Skaria, B. P., Mathew, S., Mathew, G. and Joseph, A. 2006. Lemongrass: the fame of Cochin. *Indian Journal of Arecanut, Spices and Medicinal Plants*, 8(2): 55–64.

Joy, P. P., Skaria, B. P., Mathew, S., Mathew, G. and Joseph, A. 2016. Standardisation of oleoresin extraction in lemongrass (*Cymbopogon flexuosus*). In *Conference: National Seminar, Navasari*, India. 1–13.

Khan, M. F. and Dwivedi, A. K. 2018. A review on techniques available for the extraction of essential oils from various plants. *International Research Journal of Engineering and Technology*, 5(5): 5–8.

Kpoviessi, S., Bero, J., Agbani, P., Gbaguidi, F., Kpadonou-Kpoviessi, B., Sinsin, B., Accrombessi, G., Frederich, M., Mou-dachirou, M. and Quetin-Leclercq, J. 2014. Chemical composition, cytotoxicity and in vitro antitrypanosomal and antiplasmodial activity of the essential oils of four *Cymbopogon* species from Benin. *Journal of Ethnopharmacology*, 151(1): 652–659.

Krishnaiah, D., Sarbatly, R. and Bono, A. 2007. Phytochemical antioxidants for health and medicine a move towards nature. *Biotechnology and Molecular Biology Reviews*, 2(4): 97–104.

Lean, L. P. and Mohamed, S. 1999. Antioxidative and antimycotic effects of turmeric, lemon-grass, betel leaves, clove, black pepper leaves and Garcinia atriviridis on butter cakes. *Journal of the Science of Food and Agriculture*, 79(13): 1817–1822.

Lertsatitthanakorn, P., Taweechaisupapong, S., Aromdee, C. and Khunkitti, W. 2006. In vitro bioactivities of essential oils used for acne control. *International Journal of Aromatherapy*, 16(1): 43–49.

Letellier, M., Budzinski, H., Charrier, L., Capes, S. and Dorthe, A. M. 1999. Optimization by factorial design of focused microwave assisted extraction of polycyclic aromatic hydrocarbons from marine sediment. *Fresenius' Journal of Analytical Chemistry*, 364(3): 228–237.

Leung A. Y. and Foster S. 1996. *Encyclopedia of Common Natural Ingredients Used in Food, Drugs and Cosmetics*. Toronto, Canada: John Wiley & Sons, Inc.

Lima, R., das Graças Cardoso, M., Moraes, J., Vieira, S., Melo, B. and Filgueiras, C. 2009. Composition of essential oils of *Illicium verum* L. and lemongrass *Cymbopogon citratus* (DC.) Stapf: evaluation of the repellent effect on *Brevicoryne brassicae* (L.) (Hemiptera: Aphididae). *BioAssay*, 3: 1–6.

Lorenzetti, B. B., Souza, G. E., Sarti, S. J., Santos Filho, D. and Ferreira, S. H. 1991. Myrcene mimics the peripheral analgesic activity of lemon grass tea. *Journal of Ethnopharmacology*. 34(1): 43–48.

Majewska, E., Kozlowska, M., Gruszczynska-Sekowska, E., Kowalska, D. and Tarnowska, K. 2019. Lemongrass (*Cymbopogon citratus*) essential oil: extraction, composition, bioactivity and uses for food preservation-a review. *Polish Journal of Food and Nutrition Sciences*, 69(4): 327–341.

Mariwala, S. 2001. Spice oils and oleoresins, *FAFAI*, 3(4): 23–24.

Marongiu, B., Piras, A., Porcedda, S. and Tuveri, E. 2006. Comparative analysis of the oil and supercritical CO_2 extract of *Cymbopogon citratus* Stapf. *Natural Product Research*, 20(5): 455–459.

Mathulla, T., Issac, A., Roy, N. C. and Mathew, A. G. 1996. Spice oleoresins. *PAFAI Journal*, 18:9–14.

Mehmood, Z., Ahmad, S. and Mohammad, F. 1997. Antifungal activity of some essential oils and their major constituents, *Indian Journal of Natural Products*, 13:10–13.

Melo, G. E. M., López, K. F., and Méndez, G, L. 2015. Microencapsulation of thyme (*Thymus vulgaris*) essential oil in polymeric matrices of modified yam (Dioscorea rotundata) starch. *Colombian Journal of Chemical-Pharmaceutical Sciences*, 44 (2): 189–207.

Mickiene, R., Bakutis, B. and Baliukoniene, V. 2011. Antimicrobial activity of two essential oils. *Annals of Agricultural and Environmental Medicine*, 18(1): 139–144.

Mishra, A. K. and Dubey, N. 1994. Evaluation of some essential oils for their toxicity against fungi causing deterioration of stored food commodities. *Applied and Environmental Microbiology*, 60(4): 1101–1105.

Moore-Neibel, K., Gerber, C., Patel, J., Friedman, M. and Ravishankar, S. (2012). Antimicrobial activity of lemongrass oil against *Salmonella enterica* on organic leafy greens. *Journal of Applied Microbiology*, 112(3): 485–492.

Mosquera, T., Noriega, P., Cornejo, J. and Pardo, M. L. 2016. Biological activity of *Cymbopogon citratus* (DC) Stapf and its potential cosmetic activities. *International Journal of Phytocosmetics and Natural Ingredients*, 3(1): 1–7.

Murmu, S. B. and Mishra, H. N. 2018. The effect of edible coating based on Arabic gum, sodium caseinate and essential oil of cinnamon and lemon grass on guava. *Food Chemistry*, 245:820–828.

Nadeem, H. R., Akhtar, S., Ismail, T., Sestili, P., Lorenzo, J. M., Ranjha, M. M. A. N., Jooste, L., Hano, C. and Aadil, R. M. 2021. Heterocyclic aromatic amines in meat: formation, isolation, risk assessment, and inhibitory effect of plant extracts. *Foods*, 10(7): 1466.

Naik, M. I., Fomda, B. A., Jaykumar, E. and Bhat, J. A. 2010. Antibacterial activity of lemongrass (*Cymbopogon citratus*) oil against some selected pathogenic bacterias. *Asian Pacific Journal of Tropical Medicine*, 3(7): 535–538.

Omoba, O. S. and Onyekwere, U. 2016. Postharvest physicochemical properties of cucumber fruits (*Cucumber sativus* L) treated with chitosan-lemon grass extracts under different storage durations. *African Journal of Biotechnology*, 15(50): 2758–2766.

Oyedele, A. O., Gbolade, A. A., Sosan, M. B., Adewoyin, F. B., Soyelu, O. L. and Orafidiya, O. O. 2002. Formulation of an effective mosquito-repellent topical product from lemongrass oil. *Phytomedicine*, 9(3): 259–262.

Paranagama, P. A., Abeysekera, K. H. T., Abeywickrama, K. and Nugaliyadde, L. 2003. Fungicidal and anti-aflatoxigenic effects of the essential oil of *Cymbopogon citratus* (DC.) Stapf. (lemon grass) against *Aspergillus flavus* Link. isolated from stored rice. *Letters in Applied Microbiology*, 37(1): 86–90.

Parikh, J. K. and Desai, M. A. 2011. Hydrodistillation of essential oil from *Cymbopogon flexuosus*. *International Journal of Food Engineering*, 7(1).

Pedroso, R. B., Ueda-Nakamura, T., Filho, B. P. D., Cortez, D. A. G., Cortez, L. E. R., Morgado-Diaz, J. A. and Nakamura, C. V. 2007. Biological activities of essential oil obtained from *Cymbopogon citratus* on *Crithidia deanei*. *Acta Protozoologica*, 45(3):231.

Pereira, R. P., Fachinetto, R., de Souza Prestes, A., Puntel, R. L., Da Silva, G. N. S., Heinzmann, B. M., et al. 2009. Antioxidant effects of different extracts from *Melissa officinalis*, *Matricaria recutita* and *Cymbopogon citratus*. *Neurochemical Research*, 34(5):973–983.

Rajapakse, R. and Van Emden, H. F. 1997. Potential of four vegetable oils and ten botanical powders for reducing infestation of cowpeas by *Callosobruchus maculatus*, *C. chinesis* and *C. rhodesianus*. *Journal of Stored Products Research*, 33(1):59–68.

Ranade, G. S. 2004. Essential oil (lemongrass oil). *FAFAI Journal*, 6(3): 89.

Ranjha, M. M. A. N., Amjad, S., Ashraf, S., Khawar, L., Safdar, M. N., Jabbar, S., Nadeem, M., Mahmood, S. and Murtaza, M. A. 2020b. Extraction of polyphenols from apple and pomegranate peels employing different extraction techniques for the development of functional date bars. *International Journal of Fruit Science*, 20 (sup 3): S1201–S1221.

Ranjha, M. M. A. N., Irfan, S., Nadeem, M. and Mahmood, S. 2020a. A comprehensive review on nutritional value, medicinal uses, and processing of Banana. *Food Reviews International*, 38: 1–27.

Ranjha, M. M. A. N., Shafique, B., Wang, L., Irfan, S., Safdar, M. N., Murtaza, M. A., Nadeem, M., Mahmood, S., Mueen-ud-Din, G. and Nadeem, H. R. 2021. A comprehensive review on phytochemistry, bioactivity and medicinal value of bioactive compounds of pomegranate (*Punica granatum*). *Advances in Traditional Medicine*. 1–21.

Rao, M. S., Pratibha, G. and Korwar, G. R. 2000. Evaluation of aromatic oils against *Helicoverpa armigera*. *Annals of Plant Protection Sciences*, 8(2): 236–238.

Rassem, H. H., Nour, A. H. and Yunus, R. M. 2016. Techniques for extraction of essential oils from plants: a review. *Australian Journal of Basic and Applied Sciences*, 10(16): 117–127.

Raybaudi-Massilia, R. M., Mosqueda-Melgar, J. and Martin-Belloso, O. 2006. Antimicrobial activity of essential oils on *Salmonella enteritidis*, *Escherichia coli*, and *Listeria innocua* in fruit juices. *Journal of Food Protection*, 69(7):1579–1586.

Rocha, R. P., Melo, E. D. C., Demuner, A. J., Radünz, L. L. and Corbín, J. B. 2011. Influence of drying air velocity on the chemical composition of essential oil from lemon grass. *African Journal of Food Science and Technology*, 2(6): 132–139.

Sabtain, B., Farooq, R., Shafique, B., Ranjha, M. M. A. N., Mahmood, S., Mueen-Ud-Din, G., and Ishfaq, M. A. 2021. Narrative review on the phytochemistry, nutritional profile and properties of prickly pear fruit. *Open Access Journal of Biogeneric Science and Research*, 7(2): 1–12.

Sah, S. Y., Sia, C. M., Chang, S. K., Ang, Y. K. and Yim, H. S. 2012. Antioxidant capacity and total phenolic content of lemon grass (*Cymbopogon citratus*) leave. *Annals Food Science and Technology*, 13(2): 150–155.

Saikia, D., Kumar, T. R. S., Kahol, A. P. and Khanuja, S. P. S. 1999. Comparative bioevaluation of essential oil of three species of *Cymbopogon* for their antimicrobial activities. *Journal of Medicinal and Aromatic Plant Sciences*, 21: 24.

Saleem, M., Afza, N., Anwar, M. A., Hai, S. M. A. and Ali, M. S. 2003. A comparative study of essential oils of *Cymbopogon citratus* and some members of the genus Citrus. *Natural Product Research*, 17(5): 369–373.

Saleem, M., Afza, N., Anwar, M. A., Hai, S. M. A., Ali, M. S., Shujaat, S. and Atta-Ur-Rahman. 2003. Chemistry and biological significance of essential oils of *Cymbopogon citratus* from Pakistan. *Natural Product Research*, 17(3): 159–163.

Santin, M.R., dos Santos, A.O., Nakamura, C.V., Dias, B.P., Ferreira, I.C.P. and Ueda-Nakamura, T. 2009. In vitro activity of the essential oil of *Cymbopogon citratus* and its major component (citral) on *Leishmania amazonensis*. *Parasitology Research*, 105(6): 1489–1496.

Saraí, B. P. A., Martha, S. R., Mirna, R. R., Retana-Ugalde, R. and Mendoza-Núñez, V. M. 2006. Is oxidative stress the cause of aging? *Bioquimia*, 31(SA): 113.

Schaneberg, B.T. and Khan, I.A. 2002. Comparison of extraction methods for marker compounds in the essential oil of lemon grass by GC. *Journal of Agricultural and Food Chemistry*, 50(6): 1345.

Shah, G., Shri, R., Panchal, V., Sharma, N., Singh, B. and Mann, A. S. 2011. Scientific basis for the therapeutic use of *Cymbopogon citratus*, Stapf (lemon grass). *Journal of Advanced Pharmaceutical Technology & Research*, 2(1): 3–8.

Shahi, A. K., Sharma, S. N. and Tava, A. 1997. Composition of *Cymbopogon pendulus* (Nees ex Steud) Wats, an elemicin-rich oil grass grown in Jammu region of India. *Journal of Essential Oil Research*, 9(5): 561–563.

Sharma, S. N. and Taneja, S. C. 2002. Growth studies on an elemicin containing grass: *Cymbopogon pendulus* (Nees ex. Steud) Wats in Jammu. *Indian Perfumer*, 46(2): 105–108.

Shehzadi, K., Rubab, Q., Asad, L., Ishfaq, M., Shafique, B., Ranjha, M. M. A. N. et al. 2020. A critical review on presence of polyphenols in commercial varieties of apple peel, their extraction and health benefits. *Open Access Journal of Biogeneric Science and Research*, 6(2): 1–8.

Silva, C. D. B. D., Guterres, S. S., Weisheimer, V. and Schapoval, E. E. 2008. Antifungal activity of the lemongrass oil and citral against *Candida* spp. *Brazilian Journal of Infectious Diseases*, 12(1): 63–66.

Silveira, S. M. D., Cunha Júnior, A., Scheuermann, G. N., Secchi, F. L. and Vieira, C. R. W. 2012. Chemical composition and antimicrobial activity of essential oils from selected herbs cultivated in the South of Brazil against food spoilage and foodborne pathogens. *Ciênciar Rural*, 42(7):1300–1306.

Singh, K. M. and Jha, A. 2008. Medicinal and aromatic plants cultivation in Bihar, India: economic potential and condition for adoption. https://mpra.ub.uni-muenchen.de/id/eprint/47091.

Singh, P., Shukla, R., Kumar, A., Prakash, B., Singh, S. and Dubey, N. K. 2010. Effect of *Citrus reticulata* and *Cymbopogon citratus* essential oils on *Aspergillus flavus* growth and aflatoxin production on *Asparagus racemosus*. *Mycopathologia*, 170(3): 195–202.

Skaria, B.P., Joy, P.P., Mathew, G., Mathew, S. and Joseph, A. 2012. Lemongrass. In *Handbook of Herbs and Spices*, ed. K.V. Peter. England: Woodhead Publishing Ltd, pp. 348–370

Smith, R. L., Cohen, S. M., Doull, J., Feron, V. J., Goodman, J. I., Marnett, L. J., et al. 2005. GRAS flavoring substances 22. *Food Technology*, 59: 24–62.

Suhr, K. I. and Nielsen, P. V. 2003. Antifungal activity of essential oils evaluated by two different application techniques against rye bread spoilage fungi. *Journal of Applied Microbiology*, 94(4): 665–674.

Suryawanshi, M.A., Mane, V.B. and Kumbhar, G.G. 2016. Methodology to extract essential oils from lemongrass: solvent ex- traction approach. *International Research Journal of Engineering and Technology*, 3(8): 1775–1780.

Tangpu, V. and Yadav, A. K. 2006. Antidiarrhoeal activity of *Cymbopogon citratus* and its main constituent, citral. *Pharmacology Online*, 2: 290–298.

Tapoja, M. D. and Desai, S. A. 2014. Studies on extraction of ingredient oil from lemongrass. *International Journal of Engineering Research and Technology*, 3: 509–512.

Tchoumbougnang, F., Zollo, P. A., Dagne, E. and Mekonnen, Y. 2005. In vivo antimalarial activity of essential oils from *Cymbopogon citratus* and *Ocimum gratissimum* on mice infected with *Plasmodium berghei*. *Planta Medica*, 71(01): 20–23.

Tiwari, M., Dwivedi, U. N. and Kakkar, P. 2010. Suppression of oxidative stress and pro-inflammatory mediators by *Cymbopogon citratus* D. Stapf extract in lipopolysaccharide stimulated murine alveolar macrophages. *Food and Chemical Toxicology*, 48(10): 2913–2919.

Tovar, L. P., Maciel, M. R. W., Pinto, G. M. F., Filho, R. M. and Gomes, D. R. 2010. Chemical engineering research and design. *Food Chemistry*, 88: 239–244.

Tran, T. H., Nguyen, D. C., Phu, T. N. N., Bach, L. G. and Nguyen, T. D. 2019. Research on lemongrass oil extraction technology (hydrodistillation, microwave-assisted hydrodistillation). *Indonesian Journal of Chemistry*, 19(4): 1000–1007.

Tyagi, A. K. and Malik, A. 2010a. Liquid and vapour-phase antifungal activities of selected essential oils against *Candida albicans*: microscopic observations and chemical characterization of *Cymbopogon citratus*. *BMC Complementary and Alternative Medicine*, 10(1): 1–11.

Tyagi, A. K. and Malik, A. 2010b. In situ SEM, TEM and AFM studies of the antimicrobial activity of lemon grass oil in liquid and vapour phase against *Candida albicans*. *Micron*, 41(7): 797–805.

Tyagi, A. K., Gottardi, D., Malik, A. and Guerzoni, M. E. 2014. Chemical composition, in vitro anti-yeast activity and fruit juice preservation potential of lemon grass oil. *LWT-Food Science and Technology*, 57(2): 731–737.

Tzortzakis, N. G. and Economakis, C. D. 2007. Antifungal activity of lemongrass (*Cympopogon citratus* L.) essential oil against key postharvest pathogens. *Innovative Food Science & Emerging Technologies*, 8(2): 253–258.

Viana, G. S. B., Vale, T. G., Pinho, R. S. N. and Matos, F. J. A. 2000. Antinociceptive effect of the essential oil from *Cymbopogon citratus* in mice. *Journal of Ethnopharmacology*, 70(3): 323–327.

Vinitketkumnuen, U., Lertprasertsuk, N. and Puatanachokchai, R. 2003. Isolation of chemopreventive agents against colon cancer from lemongrass. *Journal of National Research Council of Thailand*, 35(1): 61–94.

Vinitketkumnuen, U., Puatanachokchai, R., Kongtawelert, P., Lertprasertsuke, N. and Matsushima, T. 1994. Antimutagenicity of lemon grass (*Cymbopogon citratus* Stapf) to various known mutagens in salmonella mutation assay. *Mutation Research/Genetic Toxicology*, 341(1): 71–75.

Wu, H., Li, J., Jia, Y., Xiao, Z., Li, P., Xie, Y. et al. 2019. Essential oil extracted from *Cymbopogon citronella* leaves by supercritical carbon dioxide: antioxidant and antimicrobial activities. *Journal of Analytical Methods in Chemistry*, 2019: 1–10.

Yadav, J. P. and Bhargava, M. C. 2002. Efficacy of some plant products on the eggs of *Corcyra cephalonicastationa*. *Acta Ecologica*, 24(2): 141–144.

Yongtian, C., Mengyu, C. and Xiangyu, C. 2015. Preparation method of *Cymbopogon citratus* handmade soap. China Patent No. CN104862130A. https://patents.google.com/patent/CN104862130A/en.

Yuhua, Z., Xuanming, L., Hongdong, L. et al. 2014. *Cymbopogon citratus* fragrance producing endophytic bacterium. China Patent No. CN104195063A. https://patents.google.com/patent/CN104195063A/en.

CHAPTER 14

Health and Medicinal Properties of Turmeric Oleoresin

Muhammad Rizwan Tariq, Shinawar Waseem Ali, Sajid Ali, and Muhamad Shafiq

University of the Punjab

CONTENTS

DOI: 10.1201/9781003186205-14

14.1 INTRODUCTION

Spice oleoresins are a combination of oil and resins, which can be used as a substitute of whole spices in different food products, and non-food products as well, because they are similar in properties, such as taste, flavor, texture, and aroma. It cannot only be used if the appearance and the filler aspect of spices is necessary. Despite being advantageous in the aspects of standardization, consistency, and hygiene provision by oleoresins, it has a great beneficial impact for its use in new product development and value addition.

Their use has been enhanced because of its production quality, easy handling, easier preparation, and cost-saving benefits. There is a fast move from the use of traditional seasonings toward dispersed or encapsulated oleoresins and oils. There has been an accelerated demand for their use in the cheese and dairy products, bakery goods, dressings, confectionery, snacks, beverages, cosmetics, perfumes, hygienic products, and pharmaceuticals. Raw spices are cleaned and then grounded. The extraction is carried out by using a proper solvent. The dark-colored extract that is of high viscosity and contains about 10% of the total soluble solids (TSS), which is obtained, and then to remove the excess amount of the solvent, distillation is carried out under reduced pressure. The essential oil (EO) is procured by the process of steam distillation. Oleoresins are more advantageous than whole or ground spices as they are in concentrated form, which saves space and are easier to store; moreover, they are less heat sensitive and have a longer shelf life because of less amount of moisture content in them.

14.2 TYPES OF OLEORESINS

The species from which oleoresins can be extracted are ajowan seeds, black pepper, cardamom, capsicum, celery seeds, cassia bark, cinnamon bark, coriander seeds, cloves, curcumin, cumin seeds, fennel seeds, galangal, dates, ginger, juniper berries, nutmeg, olibanum resinoid, turmeric, parsley seeds, white pepper, paprika, mace, and *Zingiber*.

14.2.1 Paprika Oleoresin

It is basically a soluble extract of oil from the fruits of capsicum. Another name is Paprika Extract. The purpose for which it is used is flavoring and coloring in different food products. It mainly consists of a compound, namely, capsaicin, which is the key flavoring agent and provides pungency when used in relatively high concentrations. Among other carotenoids, first, capsanthin and, the second one, capsorubin, are the major coloring agents. The foods that are colored with the coloring agent of paprika oleoresin include different types of cheese, variety of sauces and sweets, orange juice, mixtures of spices, and processed meats, which are then emulsified. In the feed, which is used in poultry, the color of egg yolks is deepened by using it.

14.2.2 Turmeric Oleoresin

Its color is orange-red and consists of a layer of oil, which is the upper one, and a layer is crystalline that is the lower one. Coloring components are curcumin and curcuminoids. These are soluble in fat, alcohol, insoluble in cold water. To make it dispersible in water, dissolve curcumin in a solution of polysorbate-80 or -60, commercially. It is stable in heat but unstable in light. There are changes in color with the change in pH, that is:

- Green colored in pH range, which is acidic

- Orange yellowish in the neutral pH range

- Stable in acidic pH

It is being used in several pickles, bakery products, confectionery items, puddings, gelatin, jellies, yogurt, and many flavors of popcorn and finger foods as well.

14.2.3 Black Pepper Oleoresin

Its color is basically yellowish brown, and it is a viscous type of liquid with a slightly biting and pungent aroma of black pepper. Almost 5–10 kg of the Oleoresin can replace 100 kg of the black pepper (dried). Most importantly it should be kept in fully airtight containers and should be placed in a controlled atmosphere and should be protected from direct heat and any light sources.

14.2.4 Rosemary Oleoresin

It is also known as rosemary oleoresin extract (ROE). It does not have protective properties, basically, it has antioxidant properties, which slows down the process rancidity in oils. If these are being used to increase the shelf life of the oils (fixed), when oils are fresh ROE must be added into them, before the beginning of oxidation in the oils. It is the most effective if and only if it is completely dispersed in the oil.

Because of its viscosity, it is difficult to blend. It is preferred to eliminate a little part of the base oil, and blend it completely, and then re-establish it into the bulk amount of fixed oil. Rosemary oleoresin increases the shelf life of several sugar/salt scrubs and many balms and moisturizers as well, and it is usually added during the phase of cooling down or when there is addition of preservative in the formula.

14.2.5 Ginger Oleoresin

Ginger oleoresin manufacturing is being done on a large scale in different countries, and it has a dire need in the different food industries. The aroma of ginger is so spicy and pleasant, while the flavor is kind of pungent and marginally bitter because of the presence of pungent compounds or antiseptic in it that makes it valuable to the manufacturer of many food products, such as ginger breads, several confectionery items, ginger ale, different curry powders, many flavors of soft drinks, vegetables, meat and fish curries, cocktails of ginger, sauces containing ginger flavor, etc. The preserves of ginger and its candies are prepared from green or fresh ginger, which is the preference of a number of food industries and have a great demand as well. A number of alcoholic beverages are prepared from ginger in foreign countries, such as brandy, beer, and wine made from ginger, etc.

14.2.6 Cinnamon Bark Oleoresin

This type of oleoresin is basically dispersed on sugar and salt and is used for flavoring in various processed foods.

14.3 CHEMISTRY OF OLEORESINS

These are terpenoids, which are thought to be formed in the epithelial secretory cells that are specialized for its manufacturing. Terpenoids are basically the biggest class of secondary metabolites of plants, having at least 50,000 structural variants. There are various number of structurally different terpenoids of plants that are known and have some particular purposes that are associated with interactions of sessile plants with other organisms. Oleoresins chiefly consist of monoterpenes (C10) and diterpene resin acids (C20) as well as smaller amounts of sesquiterpene (C15) compounds, which constitute both volatile and non-volatile components. They can be solid or semi-liquid but are always insoluble in water. If the percentage of volatile component is high, the substance will be more of liquid and will be known as oleoresin or wood oil. Volatile terpenoids and the compounds relating to it, which occur with no non-volatile fractions, are termed essential (aromatic or volatile) oils.

There are various oleoresins that are obtained from different trees, such as Agarwood (*Aquilaria* spp.), Aguaribay (*Schinus molle* spp.), Dipterocarp (*Dipterocarpaceae* spp.), Pine Cinnamon (*Cinnamomum* spp.), and Copaiba (*Copaifera* spp.).

14.4 PROPERTIES

Turmeric contains resin, starch grains, Zingiberaceae (ginger family), and oils (volatile-5%–6%). A large quantity of curcumin is present in curcuminoids, which imparts a bright yellow color to turmeric. Some other constituents present in turmeric include *p-α-dimethyl benzyl alcohol*, *caprylic acid*, and *1-methyl-4-acetyl-1-cyclohexene*. Oleoresin is not soluble in water, which makes it difficult to be used in food matrices.

During distillation, the fraction that is soluble in ethanol is identified by its light green fluorescence and yellow color. When sulfuric acid is added to the extract, it gives a crimson red appearance.

Turmeric oleoresin, from *Curcuma longa* L., is an orange-brown oily liquid and is used to impart special flavor and color to the food. It is basically because of *curcumin*. It is a natural antioxidant; however, turmeric is sensitive to light, heat, and oxygen.

14.5 USES AND BENEFITS

Oleoresin is of great importance in our day-to-day life and has the following major uses:

14.5.1 Processed Meats

Traditional seasoning of fresh meat consists of pepper, capsicum, and herbs, etc. With an increase in the size of manufacturing and production plants, the use of oleoresin has remarkably increased. It is mostly because of lesser time and the ease of handling.

14.5.2 Fish and Vegetables Seasoning Mixes

Vegetables and fish, especially pickled/brined products, contain a diverse range of herbs and spices. Oleoresin, dispersed on a soluble base, provides an easier means of preparation. It greatly reduces the handling and cost of the product under consideration.

14.5.3 Soups, Sauces, Chutneys, and Dressings

A rapid switch from traditional toward conventional products greatly enhanced the use of oleoresins. Oleoresin—from different sources—is used in coexistence with oils of onion and garlic. Ginger sauce is readily used for barbeque, etc.

14.5.4 Cheeses and Dairy Products

Oleoresin as well as other spice oils are significantly used in cheese (processed) and savory, etc. It was used in Germany for the first time.

14.5.5 Baked Goods

Ginger, nutmeg, etc. are frequently used in the baking industry to impart taste and flavor. The simplicity in the manufacture and ease of handling oleoresin is a major cause of this taste shift toward conventional products.

14.5.6 Confectionery

The use of oleoresin in the confectionery industry is an uncommon approach; however, the use of it and other such ingredients such as oil extracted from cardamom, etc. have proven it to be an important and pleasing step and would give a new taste to the market.

14.5.7 Snacks

Because of the leading increasing demand for quality snacks in the market, it is required that flavors are applied over the surface of the snack, by either dusting or spraying to increase the efficiency and reduce the time of application. Oleoresin is widely used because they stay over the surface, if applied efficiently. Turmeric and chili flakes are also used to impart color.

14.5.8 Beverages

Special juices are made by adding spice oil. Ginger beer contains a special ingredient, ginger oil, to impart a unique taste to the product.

14.5.9 Cosmetics

Spice oils are generally used in the making of creams, soaps, etc. It is widely used because of the recent trend of herbal products and lesser side effects recorded.

14.5.10 Perfumes

A wide range of organic oils, including oleoresins, are being used in perfume making. EOs give off a nice, pleasant smell.

14.5.11 Hygiene Products

A wide variety of mouthwash, toothpaste, etc., contain oleoresins. Their antiseptic role—as in the case of dental products—is well known. The offensive odor of some house cleaning materials is eradicated by the addition of organic oils into them.

14.5.12 Aerosols

All the perfumes and related products get their smell because of enough quantity of natural oils. Oleoresin plays an important role in such cases.

14.5.13 Pharmaceuticals

Various medicines, including skin creams and cold remedies, efficiently use oleoresin to play its role in improving the sensory properties of otherwise difficult-to-accept medicines. The functionality of the immune system is increased. Enough oleoresins are used to repel the endoparasites. The anthelmintic role of it helps in the proper digestion of food.

14.5.14 Coloring Agent

Oleoresin, and especially *turmeric oleoresin*, is used as a coloring agent for food, medicines, and various cleaning products.

14.5.15 Cold and Cough Treatment

A small amount of turmeric mixed with milk proves to be a wonder against colds and coughs.

14.6 BIOSYNTHETIC PATHWAY OF OLEORESINS

The exact biosynthesis pathway of producing oleoresins is still unknown, but as a model, conifers are used to study the mechanism by which they produce resins and synthesize terpenoids. The biosynthesis of oleoresins produces all other terpenoids by the formation of isopentenyl diphosphate (IPP) through mevalonic acid pathway or methylerythritol phosphate pathway. Building blocks of terpenoids, that is, IPP and isomer of IPP dimethylallyl diphosphate (DMAPP), undergo consecutive condensation to farnesyl diphosphate (FPP), geranyl diphosphate (GPP) and geranyl GPP (GGPP). These intermediate molecules are precursor molecules of sesquiterpenes, monoterpenoids, and diterpenes, respectively, and many other large products. The first step involved in the synthesis of pathways of MEP and MEV occurs in plastids and endoplasmic reticulum, respectively. The production of TPS and DT enzymes involved in central terpenoids pathway also starts in cytosol and in plastids. Monoterpenoids and diterpenoids are formed in plastids, which are guiders from MEP pathway while sesquiterpenoids are preferably made in the cytosol by using guider from pathway of MEV. P_{450} enzyme involved in the modification of sesqui, mono, and diterpenoids are linked with endoplasmic reticulum; after this step, enzymes that are involved in catalysis of condensation of IPP and DMAPP to FPP, GPP, and GGPP are assigned to join as small chain isoprenyl diphosphate synthases (IDSs), which is member of a huge enzyme class known as prenyltransfrase. IDS is mostly studied because it is used in many branches of terpenoid biosynthesis and that is why it controls product distribution. FPP, GPP, and GGPP are each formed by a specific small chain IDS, as GPP synthase condenses DMAPP with one molecule of IPP, FPP synthase combines DMAPP with two IPP molecules, and GGPP synthase condenses DMAPP with three IPP molecules. During these reactions intermediate prenyl diphosphates are bound and not released by any enzyme. The paIDS1 protein is believed to act like a GGPP synthase, but it eliminates major portion of GPP, which is formed as intermediate. The left over GPP is converted directly to GGPP without elimination of FPP.

α-Pinene and β-pinene are produced by principal wound-inducible monoterpenes cyclase of resinous tree stem in a fixed ration of 2:3 from geranyl pyrophosphate by cationic intermediates. The principal abietic acid is produced from corresponding C_{20} isoprenoid precursor GGP to abietic-diene, which comes after sequential oxidation of a-methyl of olefin to carboxyl function, which have two cytochromes: P450-dependent hydroxylases and aldehyde dehydrogenase. Most of the common resin acids possess double bond position isomer of abiotic acid and most probably they are originated from changes in the biogenetic theme. Already allocated step of resin acid biosynthesis is catalyzed abietadiene synthase. This inducible diterpenes cyclase is a soluble enzyme. Enzymatic cyclization sequence from geranylgeranyl pyrophosphate to abietic-diene surely involves the production of pimaradiene and copalyl pyrophosphate as intermediate.

Agarwood contains a large variety of fragrant sesquiterpenes, and the study of *Aquilaria*-cultured cells shows that production of α-humulene, sesquiterpene, and δ-guaiene, which are produced by treatment of methyl jasmonate. Guaiane type is thought to be produced by two cyclization reactions.

14.7 MANUFACTURING PROCESS

Very first, raw spices are cleaned followed by grinding to very small size. The extraction is taken with the help of a suitable solvent. Hexane, acetone, ethylene dichloride, and alcohol are the mostly used solvents for extraction. Extraction is taken by infiltration of the solvents at ambient temperature through ground spices, which are packed in the stainless-steel percolator. The dark, thick extract obtained must have at least 10% of TSS, which are drawn off and then distilled under less pressure to eliminate the excess of solvent. The EO is extracted by distillation using steam.

14.7.1 Paprika Oleoresins

Extraction process is carried out by infiltration with different varieties of solvents, mostly hexane, which is separated prior to utilization. Foods that are colored with paprika oleoresins comprise orange, cheese, spice mixtures, juice, sauces, sweets, and emulsified processed meats. It is necessary in poultry feed to darken the color of egg yolks. In the United States, paprika oleoresin is considered as a color additive and categorized as a natural color. Paprika oleoresin and capsanthin and capsorubin are marked by E160c in Europe.

14.7.2 Turmeric Oleoresin

It is obtained by *C. longa* L., which is a member of the ginger family. It is extracted by solvent extraction of the finely grounded spice and contains volatile oil, coloring matter, fatty oil.

14.7.3 Black Pepper Oleoresin

It is extracted by using the solvent extraction technique of black pepper, and the solvent traces are eliminated by distilling it in vacuum at controllable temperature.

14.7.4 Ginger Oleoresin

On steam distillation, cracked, dried, and comminuted ginger gives 1.0%–3.0% of dark yellow viscid oil. This is extracted by abstraction of crushed dried ginger with appropriate solvents, e.g., acetone and alcohol. Concentration of the acetone extract with vacuum and on completely removal of the solvent used yields the so-called ginger oleoresin.

14.7.5 Cinnamon Bark Oleoresin

This is obtained from the bark of cinnamon using organic solvent. Yield of oleoresin differs from 10% to 12%. The oleoresin can spread on salt and sugar, and utilized to flavor processed foods.

14.8 FENNEL AND ITS OLEORESIN

Oleoresins are hugely homegrown just as fare markets. These are devoured by an expansive range of producers, such as drinks, soup powders, noodles, curry powders, desserts, sauces, canned meats, and poultry items. The greater part of the end-use enterprises are developing consistently and bound to increment with increment inclination of value items. The utilization of zest is quickly replaced with oleoresins and the crude flavors brings about significant impact.

14.9 TOXICOLOGY

Oleoresin capsicum (OC) is a synthetic antimicrobial that can be used in a variety of plants. Products containing capsaicin, active ingredient in OC, cause irritation and aggravation in the immediate area. In humans, prolonged or rehashed openness to OC may cause antagonistic nasal and aspiratory problems.

14.9.1 Toxicity of Inhalation

Capsaicin fumes inhaled inwardly can cause massive pneumonic initiation and delayed hacking. The effect of different concentrations of 0.6–19.8 g/m^3 on bringing in healthy people was investigated. Also in subjects with mild asthma, OC at these fixations induced a portion subordinate hack reaction without genuine pneumonic contribution. Extra research has shown that when humans are exposed to vaporized arrangements of 2%–10% capsaicin, hacking starts rapidly but fades away quickly until the exposure is over.

To assess the effect of ongoing openness of laborers to OC in the bean stew pepper industry, Blanc et al. estimated three respiratory lists, extensiveness of respiratory manifestations, improvement in lung work, and an expansion in the hack edge. Strong bronchial compressions were also measured *in vitro* with "10-M (3.0 g/m^3)" capsaicin in refined bronchial tissue. Regardless, no significant negative effects on lung function or respiratory rates were observed in these individuals. In other human studies, eight standard subjects inhaled "nebulized capsaicin (lC7 M, 0.03 g/m^3)" to investigate its effects on the example of calming. Capsaicin increased mean inspiratory path by faster but not shallower relaxing as compared to the diluent alone.

The effect of inhaled capsaicin on aviation path conductance, or the ease with which air passes through the respiratory tract, has also been considered in humans. Breathing in 2.4× ward drops in overt aviation path conductance that peaked within 20 seconds of opening and remained at least for 60 seconds.

Philip et al. investigated a variety of capsaicin-induced strong secretory effects in the nose of humans. After a challenge with capsaicin, the absolute protein content of the nasal lavage liquid increased dramatically. In comparison to respiratory effects, a capsicum challenge at regular intervals resulted in a reduction in complete protein emission and lactoferrin discharge, both of which are indicators of tactile nerve inactivation in the nose.

14.9.2 Toxicity of the Dermal Route

The dermal course of OC is considered tolerably toxic, with a dermal LD50 >512 mg/kg in the mouse. People with open skin to OC experience disturbance, erythema or redness, and consuming anguish. The main component for the subsequent agony following dermal openness gives off the impression of being the arrival of "substance."

Furthermore, when OC is applied to the skin or mouth, it induces a localized, consistent desensitization. As a result, although the primary reaction is torment, a long-term desensitization to consuming and torment by various professionals is often administered at the site of transparency. As a result, OC has been discovered to be effective as a pain reliever when applied to over-the-counter salves. Furthermore, Simone et al. discovered that 0.1 pg was the least amount of capsaicin that could induce pain when delivered intradermally, under trial conditions designed to obtain managed improvements and overcome the skin's dissemination hindrance. The torment could last anywhere from 2 to 17 minutes, depending on the section.

14.9.3 Toxicity of Eye

In studies looking into the toxicity of OC to the skin, 0.1 mL of fluid from a research shower of a 5% OC arrangement was injected into the conjunctival sac of the left eyes of four bunnies. After instillation, the treated eyes were momentarily closed and not cleaned. Eyes that had not been handled served as sensors. At 24, 48, and 72 hours, net indications of eye aggravation and fundamental poisonousness were reported. Following instillation, the usual poisonous effects of flickering, trimming, and noisy uneasiness were noted. Within the first 24 hours, three out of four bunnies developed mild conjunctival erythema. In three of the eyes, the redness was completely gone after 48 hours, and in the fourth eye, it was gone after 72 hours; 50 pg/day capsaicin ingested into rats caused clear torment and uncontrollable squinting in various studies. Furthermore, the rodents' conjunctiva veins and tops were found to be exceptionally porous.

A few manufacturers of OC protection products have focused on the effects of OC on bunny paws. The effects of distilled water on hares with delayed and rehashed eye openness to capsaicin were compared to the effects of distilled water on hares with delayed and rehashed eye openness to capsaicin. In the OC-exposed bunnies, eye station was slightly higher than in the refined water bunnies. Furthermore, the discomfort was restricted to the conjunctiva, with mild to average erythema of the tops and vascularization of the layers. The most severe aggravation was noticed almost straight away after the use, and by 94–96 hours, it had mostly subsided.

14.9.4 Toxicity of Oral Route

Consumption of OC in food has long been recorded in humans. Ingestion can result in severe stinging of the lips, tongue, and oral mucosa, as well as retching and loose bowels. The guinea pig appears to be the animal most susceptible to the dangers of oral capsaicin openness, with an extreme oral LD50 of 1.10 mg/kg, while the intense oral LD50 in mice was discovered to be >190 mg/kg.

Respiratory loss of motion is the cause of death after poisonous oral openness. Oral transparency contemplates were guided by guiding 50 mg/kg glasslike capsaicinoids through a stomach tube on a sub-constant (now) and ongoing (long-term) basis. Food and water intake, growth, rectal temperature, blood and pee science, and posthumous gross assessment of various organs and their relative loads were all subjected to extensive estimations.

14.9.5 Toxicity in Reproduction and Carcinogen Studies

IARC, NTP, and ACGIH have not classified this substance as a carcinogen. Furthermore, the lack of epidemiological proof of any unfavorable effects from consuming stew peppers containing capsaicin, as well as hundreds of years of culinary use as a topping, suggests that capsaicin as a food-fixing agent poses no health risks.

14.10 EXPOSURE TO HUMAN BEINGS

Over 900 individuals were either given great numbers directly in the face or placed in kept within bands, parts and subject to OC arrangements ranging from 1% to 10% OCiIn harmony with a written statement by the Federal Bureau of Investigation of the United States Department of being just, between July 1987 and July 1989. Eye irritancy, which ranged from severe uncontrollable blinking to forced closing of the eyes, was one of the physiological effects observed in these individuals; respiratory annoyance with symptoms ranging from coughing and windedness to gasping for air and a choking feeling in the throat; and dermal discomfort with symptoms ranging from a consuming sensation to an extreme eating sensation and skin redness. After disinfecting, respiratory functions and visual acuity returned to normal within 2–5 minutes. Similarly, varying degrees of transient lack of motion of the larynx and eventual powerlessness to speak were observed, but restored until OC openness was interrupted, depending on the breathing rates of the participants and the measure of openness duration. Since being exposed to OC, none of the participants observed any long-term negative effects.

Midgren et al. studied capsaicin's hack response in solid human subjects. The participants were able to breathe in rehashed breaths of a 5% capsaicin vaporized for 60 seconds without difficulty, including frequent hacking. Hacking started almost immediately after taking an internal breath and was usually outstanding for the first 30 seconds. When the capsaicin transparency was stopped, the hack reaction came to an end almost instantly.

There was no evidence of excessive touchiness after transparency in examinations of mild asthmatics, and there have been no reported cases of occupationally induced asthma because of OC. Furthermore, OC has been used as a skin pain reliever in ludicrous balms and therapies with no known antagonistic effects.

In studies sponsored by the International Association of Chiefs of Police, data on in-care deaths where pepper splash was used in the capture method were analyzed. These tests were carried out to see whether there was a chance that OC was a factor in the in-care passing. The inquiry concluded that OC was not considered as a cause or sponsor of the deaths in any of these circumstances.

14.11 CONCERNS ABOUT THE ENVIRONMENT

Unlike other plastic aggravations, OC particles scatter from a person's clothing in a moderately short timeframe. As a result, sterilization of people merely entails excluding them from contact with the outside world. To get rid of the consuming feeling, you may need to wash and rinse your eyes with water. The encased region is ventilated by opening entryways or windows during territory disinfection. Since OC does not persist lib CS or CN, cross ventilation is unnecessary.

14.12 MARKET OVERVIEW

The worldwide oleoresin market is estimated to enlist a CAGR of 5.6%, during the figure time frame (2020–2025).

Oleoresins are famous in the drinks business since they can be an extraordinary base flavor or some portion of an intricate flavor profile. These can likewise be utilized to add normal tone to drinks, further expanding their ease of use in this industry. The developing refreshment industry straightforwardly drives the market development for oleoresins. The wide assortment of oleoresins gives them various prospects to figure out new or improved regular food varieties and flavorings. Manufacturers of food and drink, drugs, and different ventures lean toward using it, as oleoresins are a practical alternative, with simpler quality control and furthermore require lesser extra room. In difference to fundamental oils, oleoresins are a lot more non-volatile. This reality makes them more intriguing in the flavor and food industry.

A portion of the unmistakable oleoresins incorporate paprika, capsicum, turmeric, vanilla, dark pepper, cardamom, and cinnamon, among others. Every one of them have their own utilities and part in each industry such as food and drink (refreshment, bread kitchen, flavors, and fixings, meat and fish items, and different items), aroma industry, and drugs and nutraceuticals. The market is ready for various nations under every field.

14.13 KEY MARKET TRENDS

14.13.1 Increasing Demand from Food Manufacturers

Ethnic food varieties are acquiring prevalence around the world. Indian, Thai, and Mexican food sources are the absolute most well-known worldwide flavors. Oleoresins from flavors are intriguing elements for food producers to make such ethnic food sources. Particularly makers of meat items, such as hotdogs, regularly apply oleoresins as fixings. Rather than utilizing marinades from seasoning producers, some of them set up their own marinades from oleoresins and different types of flavors (for instance, dried flavors). A few makers of mayonnaise, sauces, marinades, and pickles additionally apply oleoresins as fixings, rather than utilizing items from enhancing makers. Oleoresins are additionally heat-steady and simple to store. They are not defenseless to microbiological pollution and have a longer lapse period than new or even dried flavors. Food and seasoning makers are continually searching for extraordinary flavors to grow new items. They are especially keen on new kinds of oleoresins that are practical and can give extraordinary outcomes with restricted use.

14.13.2 Europe Holds a Significant Market Share

The United Kingdom, Germany, and Spain are unmistakable clients of oleoresins in the locale, with the biggest food and drink ventures. The district imports the vast majority of its oleoresins from Asian regions, especially India. The ports in Belgium and the Netherlands are significant places of passage for imports to Northwestern Europe. The rising fame of ethnic cooking styles, such as Indian, Mexican, and Thai, has prodded the interest in oleoresins obtained from flavors among food makers, for example, pepper oleoresin, to imitate new pepper flavor. The locale offers colossal potential for oleoresin makers, inferable from expanding request and changes in the crude material inventory inside the district. For example, oleoresin extractions for cardamom occur in nations, such as India and Sri Lanka; so they have sent out promising circumstances in the locale, given that they agree with the European guidelines and principles for oleoresins. For instance, the European enactment has allowed the utilization of just not many extraction solvents, in particular, propane, butane, ethyl acetic acid derivation, ethanol, carbon dioxide ($CH_3)_2CO$), and nitrous oxide.

14.14 ABTS°+ FREE RADICAL SCAVENGING ACTIVITY OF GINGER OLEORESIN

The radical cation decolorization assay was used to determine antioxidant activity. The absorbance of the free radical cation from (ABTS) (2,2'-azinobis-(3-ethylbenzothiazoline-6-sulfonic acid) diammonium salt is inhibited by antioxidants in this assay. To generate the free radical cation, ABTS was incubated with potassium persulfate. In a nutshell, ABTS was dissolved in deionized water to create a concentration solution of 7 mmol/L. ABTS°+ was a form of ABTS.

The blend was permitted to place in the darkness at room temperature for 12–16 hours prior to utilization, and it was made by mixing ABTS stock solution with 2.45 mmol/L potassium persulfate (final concentration). The ABTS°+ solution was diluted with PBS, pH 7.4, to achieve an absorbance of 0.70 at 734 nm in our experiment. The absorbance reading was taken exactly 6 minutes after adding 2 mL of diluted ABTS°+ to 20 mL of ginger oleoresin or EO in PBS. Each assay included a PBS blank. The positive regulation was ascorbic acid. Many of the experiments were done in triplicate. The percentage of inhibition was used to measure radical scavenging activity.

14.15 EXTRACTION METHODS

Hydro-distillation is one of the most popular methods used for the purpose of extraction of EOs. The extracted EO should be placed in the glass vials, which are sealed airtight, enclosed with aluminum foil, and is held at 4°C till more process is completed. The Soxhlet apparatus method is used to extract oleoresin compounds from dry ginger powder. Briefly, 10 g samples were wrapped in filter paper, bound, and dipped in methanol for 4–8 hours at 70°C. To obtain the oleoresin, the methanol extract was fully vaporized using a rotary evaporator. Each dry oleoresin sample should be weighed and reconstituted in 10 mL methanol before being placed in the dark at 4°C until checked.

14.16 PACKAGING

The impact of modified atmosphere packaging on spoilage fungus was extensively carried out. *Endomyces fibuliger*, *Penicillium roqueforti*, *Penicillium commune*, and *Aspergillus flavus* were capable to grow up at oxygen saturation as low as 0.03%, whereas the chalk mold *E. fibuliger* was able to grow yet in the presence of an oxygen absorber. Carbon dioxide levels were high enough to slow development, but not absolutely. Active packaging employing oleoresins (OL) and volatile EOs from herbs and spices were checked alongside a variety of fungus typically present on bread as an alternative to MAP. A filter paper was put in the lid of a Petri dish inoculated with one of the test fungi and EO or OL concentrations of 1, 10, or 100 mL were applied. To prevent the exchange of gases, the Petri dish was hermetically sealed. The EO of mustard had the most powerful influence. Oregano oleoresin only had a minor effect on development while garlic, cinnamon, and clove all had a lot of activity. Vanilla had no repressing effect on the microorganisms measured at the concentrations used. *P. roqueforti* was the most vulnerable while flavus was the most resistant of the bacteria. The basic oil of mustard was studied. For same species, as well as three additional molds and one yeast, the minimum inhibitory concentration (MIC) for the active ingredient, allyl isothiocyanate (AITC) was calculated. MIC values in the gas phase ranged from 1.8 to 3.5 mg/mL. The results revealed that whether AITC was fungistatic or fungicidal was dependent on its concentration as well as the spore concentration. AITC was fungicidal to all tested fungi when the gas phase contained at least 3.5 mg/mL. According to the results of the sensory test, hot-dog bread was more susceptible to AITC than rye bread. For rye bread, the minimum detectable concentration of AITC was 2.4 mg/mL gas phase, and for hot-dog bread, it was between 1.8 and 3.5 mg/mL gas phase. These findings demonstrated that active packaging with AITC could provide the necessary shelf life for rye bread. However, to prevent off-flavor formation, active packaging of hot-dog bread can require the addition of other preserving factors. While modified atmosphere packaging can offer necessary further shelf life. Laboratory's findings showed that in several cases, particularly when chalk molds are involved, adequate defense cannot be achieved. The deep draw method, which also included sensory evaluation of bread, produces the best results. It requires an evacuation of the package until it is flushed with the desired gas, but it has a much lower throughput than flow pack. Level in the final box, as it is simply blowing the package gas sealed off, pushing out the air surrounding the product.

The use of volatile antimicrobial substances derived from herbs and spices has been shown to be effective in preventing fungal damage caused by common spoilage fungi. When isothiocyanates against postharvest were applied at 1 µL per 250 mL culture flask, mustard oil, which contains AITC, had a potent effect in stopping all fungi for more than 14 days. For showing fungal growth, garlic oil and cinnamon oil need a slightly higher concentration.

14.17 CONCLUSION

Oleoresins are of much importance, as these are being extracted from spices, thus having aroma and flavor of the spice. Oleoresins consist of various high-strength active compounds that enables their utilization in small quantities. Oleoresins and spice oils can be utilized advantageously over the spices that are excessively being used nowadays, rather in the cases where filler requirements can be necessary for the products. Usage of spice oleoresins leads toward a constant state in taste and consistency in flavor.

REFERENCES

Anubhuti, P., S., Rahul, and K. C. Kant. 2011. Standardization of fennel (*Foeniculum vulgare*), its oleoresin and marketed Ayurvedic dosage forms. International Journal of Pharmaceutical Sciences and Drug Research 3: 265–269.

Archuleta, M. 1995. Oleoresin Capsicum: toxicology evaluation and hazard review. Albuquerque, NM: Sandia report SAN 95-2129.

Bannan, M. W. 1936. Vertical resin ducts in the secondary wood of the Abietineae. *New Phytologist* 35: 11–46.

Bellik, Y. 2014. Total antioxidant activity and antimicrobial potency of the essential oil and oleoresin of *Zingiber officinale* Roscoe. *Asian Pacific Journal of Tropical Disease* 4: 40–44.

Blanc, P., D. Liu, C. Juarez, and H. A Boushey. 1991. Cough in hot pepper workers. *Chest* 99: 27–32.

Busker, R. W., and H. P. M. Van Helde. 1998. Toxicologic evaluation of pepper spray as a possible weapon for the Dutch police force: risk assessment and efficacy. *The American Journal of Forensic Medicine and Pathology* 19: 309–316.

Carpenter, S. E., B. Lynn. 1981. Vascular and sensory responses of human skin to mild injury after topical treatment with capsaicin. *British Journal of Pharmacology* 73: 755–758.

Collier, J. G., and R. W. Fuller. 1984. Capsaicin inhalation in man and the effects of sodium cromoglycate. *British Journal of Pharmacology* 81: 113–117.

Fonger, G. C. 1995. Hazardous substances data bank (HSDB) as a source of environmental fate information on chemicals. *Toxicology* 103: 137–145.

Fuller, R. W., C. M. Dixon., and P. J. Barnes. 1985. Bronchoconstrictor response to inhaled capsaicin in humans. *Journal of Applied Physiology* 58: 1080–1084.

Gershenzon, J. and N. Dudareva. 2007. The function of terpene natural products in the natural world. *Nature Chemical Biology* 3: 408–414.

Glinsukon, T., V. Stitmunnaithum, C. Toskulkao, T. Buranawuti, and V. Tangkrisanavinont, 1980. Acute toxicity of capsaicin in several animal species. *Toxicon* 18: 215–220.

Granfield, J. P., J. Onnen, and C. S. Petty. 1994. Pepper spray and in-custody deaths. *The American Journal of Forensic Medicine and Pathology* 16: 185–192.

Kulp, K. 2016. *Batters and Breadings in Food Processing*. Academic Press. USA.

Leandro, L. M., F. de Sousa Vargas., P. C. S. Barbosa., J. K. O. Neves, J. A. Da Silva, D. Veiga-Junior, and V. Florêncio. 2012. Chemistry and biological activities of terpenoids from copaiba (*Copaifera* spp.) oleoresins. *Molecules* 17: 3866–3889.

Maxwell, D. L., R. W. Fuller., and C. M. S. Dixon. 1987. Ventilatory effects of inhaled capsaicin in man. *European Journal of Clinical Pharmacology* 31: 715–717.

McCaskill, D. and R. Croteau. 1997. Prospects for the bioengineering of isoprenoid biosynthesis. *Biotechnology of Aroma Compounds* 55: 107–146.

Midgren, B., L. Hansson., J. A. Karlsson, B. O. G. Simonsson, and C. G. Persson. 1992. Capsaicin-induced cough in humans. *American Review of Respiratory Disease* 146: 347–351.

Morabito, E. V., and W. G. Doerner. 1997. Police use of less-than-lethal force: *Oleoresin capsicum* (OC) spray. *Policing: An International Journal of Police Strategies & Management*.

National Law Enforcement and Corrections Technology Center (NLECTC), and United States of America. 1994. *Oleoresin Capsicum: Pepper Spray as a Force Alternative*.

Parimal, K., A. Khale., and K. Pramod. 2011. Resins from herbal origin and a focus on their applications. *International Journal of Pharmaceutical Sciences and Research* 2: 1077.

Philip, G., F. M. Baroody., D. Proud, R. M. Naclerio, and A. G. Togias. 1994. The human nasal response to capsaicin. *Journal of Allergy and Clinical Immunology* 94: 1035–1045.

Rumsfield, J. A., and D. P. West. 1991. Topical capsaicin in dermatologic and peripheral pain disorders. *The Dalian Institute of Chemical Physics* 25: 381–387.

Sachetti, C. G., M. L. Fascineli, J. A. Sampaio, O. A. Lameira, and E. D. Caldas. 2009. Avaliação da toxicidade aguda e potencial neurotóxico do óleo-resina de copaíba (*Copaifera reticulata* Ducke, Fabaceae). *Revista Brasileira de Farmacognosia* 19: 937–941.

Simone, D. A., T. K. Baumann., and R. H. LaMotte. 1989. Dose-dependent pain and mechanical hyperalgesia in humans after intradermal injection of capsaicin. *Pain* 38: 99–107.

Weaver, W., and M. B. Jett. 1989. Oleoresin capsicum training and use. *Firearms Training Unit*, FBI Academy, Quantico, VA.

CHAPTER 15

Onion Oleoresin

Extraction, Characterization, and Application

Shafiya Rafiq
Lovely Professional University

Bababode Adesegun Kehinde
University of Kentucky

Priyanka Suthar
Dr Y.S. Parmar University of Horticulture & Forestry

Suheela Bhat
Sant Longowal Institute of Engineering and Technology

Gulzar Ahmad Nayik
Government Degree College, Shopian

Yash D. Jagdale
MIT ADT University

CONTENTS

DOI: 10.1201/9781003186205-15

15.1 INTRODUCTION

The history of onion cultivation, though somewhat uncertain, bears some traces with eastern and western Asia, though domestic cultivation has a higher origin-likelihood from central or southwest Asian regions, precisely from Pakistan or Iran. Around 5000 BC, during the Bronze Age, onions were dietetically applied in China for their flavors and stability during carriage and storage (Ansari, 2007). Early Egyptians venerated onion, based on the concentric arrangement and spherical shape of its bulb, spurring them to use it for burial occasions. In ancient Europe, the Romans in ancient Italy used onion as a traditional remedy for diverse bodily ailments, such as digestive disorders, eye ailments, sleep deprivation, muscular ailments, and even oral injuries.

Over 718 cultivars of onion (*Allium cepa*) have been reported with prominent ones, including *A. cepa* var. viviparum, *A. cepa* var. solaninum, *A. cepa* var. proliferum, *A. cepa* var. multiplicans, *A. cepa* var. cepa, *A. cepa* var. bulbiferum, and *A. cepa* var. aggregatum. These cultivars and varieties differ based on their respective flavor (ranging from strongly sweet to mildly sweet), color (green, white, red, and yellow), with approximate nutrient compositions of about 1.5% fat, 2.6% protein, 14.7% carbohydrate, and above 82% moisture content (Arshad et al., 2017). The flavonoid constituency of fleshy and dry onion scales offers their specific appearance characteristics and also has considerable effects on their antioxidant profiles (Kehinde et al., 2019; Sharma et al., 2019; Majid et al., 2015). The red appearance of some onion varieties is sometimes associated with softer flavors by some consumers, though scientific evidence for this has not been fully established (McCallum, 2007). Tri-, di-, and monoglucoside quercetins are naturally available in virtually all the colored onions, but the oxidation metabolites and conjugates of these constituents promote their dry-scale colors, though red onions have a predominant presence of malonylglucoside and cyanidin3-glucoside anthocyanins (Ly et al., 2005). Carbohydrates present in onions have been reported to influence their culinary and storage attributes and they include the fructans (neoketose and ketose), fructooligosaccharides, sucrose, fructose, and glucose, while the organosulfur compounds that constitute their medicinal and aroma characteristics include propyl- and methyl-cysteine sulfoxides, and larger amounts of 1-propenyl cysteine sulfoxide, though substantial amounts of gamma-glutamyl sulfoxides may also be present (McCallum, 2007).

The global cultivation of onion spans across over 170 countries with a recent estimate of 78.31 million tons and India ranking as the largest producer of about 15.88 million tons, and a cultivation capacity of 22.46 million tons places China as the second, as of 2015 (Teshika et al., 2018). The global cultivation however has been strongly affected by pest and disease infestation issues over the years. These biological agents negatively affect the cultivation yield, nutritional quality, physiological appearance, shelf life, and overall usage. Diseases such as white rot (caused by the soil-borne fungus *Sclerotium cepivorum*), splitting and neck rot affect the bulbs, slimy shanking of the leaves, and white tip, rust and smut, and mildew affect the foliage. Prominent pests include onion eelworm (*Ditylenchus dipsaci*), onion fly (*Delia antiqua*), and leek moth (*Acrolepiopsis assectella*).

Several scientific studies in recent years have investigated the biological functionalities of onions and its derivatives and reported them to possess neuroprotective, antioxidant, antimicrobial, anticancer, and hepatoprotective properties, among several others, thus making onion consumption an optimal dietetic selection for patients of metabolic syndrome diseases (Galavi et al., 2021; Kehinde et al., 2021). These health functionalities are usually experimentally examined beginning with an extraction procedure using solvents or other solvent-free methodologies, a further purification and identification of one or more desirable constituents, followed by an *in vivo* and/or *in vitro* evaluation of the purified bioactive component(s) (Kaur et al., 2020; Kehinde et al., 2020).

15.2 CHEMISTRY, CHARACTERIZATION, AND PROPERTIES

Phytochemicals have the potential to promote health benefits in humans and offer protection from a variety of diseases, including cancer. Onion oleoresins are a potential source of many drugs produced from onions. Chemically these are terpenoids thought to be produced using biosynthesis in specialized secondary cells. Normally, plants use these compounds as a defense mechanism to prevent themselves from insect and herbivorous attacks (Shahzadi et al., 2017). Terpenoids are a broader group of chemical compounds that are complex in function and structure. Onion oleoresins consist mainly of monoterpenes (C10) and diterpene resin acids (C20). Many plant oleoresins may also consist of a small amount of sesquiterpenes (C15). Normally onion oleoresins consist of both volatile and non-volatile components. Different phytochemical studies performed on *A. cepa* oleoresin revealed that a large number of compounds were responsible for its peculiar flavor and pharmacological properties.

Among these phytochemicals, phenolic components received much attention because of the role in biological and medicinal properties. A simultaneous determination of 4-vinylphenol, rutin, syringic acid, catechin, chlorogenic acid, naringenin, vanillic acid, quercetin, and caffenic acid were most prominent in *A. cepa* oleoresins. Albishi et al. (2013) also reported the presence of quercetin 3,4'-diglucoside, quercetin, and kaempferol as predominant phenolics in all onion extracts tested using high-performance liquid chromatography (HPLC)-MS. HPLC of different varieties of *A. cepa* oleoresins revealed the presence of a significant amount of phenolic components such as gallic acid (9.3–354 µg/mL), ferulic acid (13.5–116 µg/mL), protocatechuic acid (3.1–138 µg/mL), and kaempferol (3.2–481 µg/mL). Many minor phenolic compounds were also found in trace amounts (Prakash et al., 2007).

Another class of predominant phytochemicals in *A. cepa* oleoresins responsible for its distinguished pigment are flavonoids. *A. cepa* is very rich in flavonoids, and three diverse and most valuable groups of phytochemicals are present in it in perfect proportion: flavonoids, fructans, and organo-sulfur compounds. More than 25 different flavonoids have been identified and characterized in *A. cepa* oleoresins. Their glycosyl moieties are almost exclusively glucose, which is mainly attached to the 4', 3, and/or 7-positions of the aglycones. Quercetin 4'-glucoside and quercetin 3,4'-diglucoside are in most cases reported as the main flavonols in recent literature. Analogous derivatives of kaempferol and isorhamnetin have been identified as minor pigments (Slimestad et al., 2007). Moreover, quercetin 3-glycoside, delphinidin 3,5-diglycosides, quercetin 3,7,4 tri-glycoside, quercetin 7,4 diglucoside, quercetin 3,4 diglucoside, isorhamnetin 3,4 diglucoside, and many more were reported in *A. cepa* oleoresins (Zhang et al., 2016). Some of the *A. cepa* pigments facilitate unique structural features, such as 4′-glycosylation and unusual substitution patterns of sugar moieties.

Another class of phytochemicals in *A. cepa* oleoresins is anthocyanins. Altogether at least 25 different anthocyanins have been reported, including two novel 5-carboxypyranocyanidin-derivatives. The quantitative content of anthocyanins in different varieties of onion oleoresins contribute to nearly 10% of the total flavonoid content. The dihydroflavonol taxifolin and its 3-, 7-, and 4′-glucosides are also present in *A. cepa*. Although the structural diversity of different dihydroflavonols characterized is restricted compared with a wide structural assortment of flavonols and anthocyanins identified, they may occur at high concentrations in some cultivars.

Several studies have revealed the presence of cyanidine 3-O-(3″-O-β-gluco phyranosyl-6″-O-malonyl-β-glucophyranoside), cyanidin 7-O-(3″-O-β-glucophyranosyl-6″-O-malonyl-β-glucophyranoside), cyanidin 3–4 di-O-β-glucophyranosyl, and cyanidin 4-O glucoside. The most important types of anthocynins present in *A. cepa* oleoresins were dipropyl disulfide and dipropyl trisulfide. Moreover, the most active classes of organo sulfuric compounds, such as S-alk(en)yl-L-cystein sulfoxides, were present. Alliin and γ-glutamylcysteine were found to be dominant in such sulfoxides. The taste of *A. cepa* oleoresins was found to be associated with the presence of allicin, methiin, propiin, iso-alliin, and lipid-soluble components, such as diallyl sulfide and diallyl disulfide (Griffiths et al., 2002). Apart from compounds such as sulfur and flavonoids, many more constituents, e.g., lectins, prostaglandins, fructan, pectin, adenosine, vitamins B1, B2, B6, C, and E, biotin, nicotinic acid, fatty acids, glycolipids, phospholipids, and essential amino acids, have been studied for their biological effects over several decades.

15.3 EXTRACTION OF ONION OLEORESIN

Onion is one of the most abundantly used spice in various food products. Presently, various onion-based products are available in market in different forms, such as onion powder, dehydrated onion pieces, onion juice, toasted dehydrated onions, onion flavoring, encapsulated flavor, canned, frozen and packaged onion, oleoresins, onion salt, pickled onion, and essential oil. The flavor of onion is mostly incorporated into the food by adding raw material or onion powder. However, in few cases, onion oil or solvent-extracted oleoresins are also used to enhance the flavor of foodstuffs. According to Heath (1981), onion oleoresin is a concentrated juice of onion, which is further subjected to vacuum evaporated in stirrer pan to yield 80%–85% dry solid content and further heating resulting into non-enzymatic browning to get dark brown, soft, and stable cooked onion characteristics of the end product. In one of the recent studies by Liu et al. (2016), Lingling red onions were used for the extraction of oleoresins to evaluate the effect of reaction time, various solvents, solid–liquid ratio, extraction time, and temperature. It was reported that the optimal extraction conditions include utilization of petroleum ether as an extraction solvent with reaction time 100 minutes, reaction temperature 47°C with 1:8 solid–liquid ratio with two times extraction. Under above conduction, the extraction rate was observed to reach at 0.6384% from 50 g of Lingline red onion. The study also reviled the presence of 18 different volatile compounds, which is 97.81% of total extractions. In volatile compounds, 24.47% were acids, sulfur-containing compounds were 3.83%, alcohols were 17.06%, ketones were 2.71%, aldehydes were 0.36, and esters were 10.81%. The reported volatile compounds were 2-methyl-2-pentanol, dimethyl disulfide, gadoleyl alcohol, octadecadienoic acid, 1,3-dithiane, 3-hydroxy-2-butanone, octadecenoate, 5,7-dimethylchromone-3-carboxalde hyde, dioctyl phthalate, palmitic acid, and hexanol. In a study by Wang et al. (2018), a total of 42 compounds were reported in onion oil. The study showed that the sulfur compounds such as esters, alkanes, sulfides, alcohols, and alkenes are major constituents in onion oil. Also, sulfide compounds such as dipropyl trisulfide, diallyl disulfide, allyl propyl disulfide, allyl methyl disulfide, 2,4-dimethyl thiophene, dipropyl disulfide, and dimethyl trisulfide are main onion's odor contributing compounds. In a study by Shi et al. (2009), oleoresin was extracted from Welsh-onion stalk powder by using ethanol as a solvent. According to the authors, the final results reported that, 70°C temperature with 20 time solvent volume as much as the sample powder of Welsh onions and extraction time 5 hours was optimized conditions for extraction. The extracted oleoresin was subjected to emulsification, centrifugation and then spray drying by using wall materials like dextrin and gum arabic.

Another extraction technology, i.e., steam distillation, is most commonly used for the extraction of essential oils from aromatic plants or herbs. Steam distillation usually follows liquid-liquid extraction with different types of solvents (Figure 15.1). The application of high temperature (100°C) to the starting plant sample in order to generate steam usually leads to degradation of the flavor oil components as they are generally thermolabile. Along with this, water can also exert hydrolytic effects and result in modification in chemical changes in aromatic oils. Therefore, most of the studies are reported with the utilization of green technologies such as supercritical fluid extraction (SFE) for the extraction of oleo-resins from onions. Recently, a study by Devani et al. (2020) used dried rotten onions and extracted oleoresins of high quality by using SFE. The optimized condition for extraction of oleoresin from onion was reported as 60 minutes dynamic time, pressure of 400 bar, extraction temperature 80°C with 0.53 mm particle size. Under optimized conditions, oleoresin extraction from supercritical fluid yielded 1.012% oleoresin along with 10.41 µmol pyruvate/g fresh weight of onion and 31 g sulfur content/kg of oleoresin. Earlier, Sass-Kiss et al. (1998) used carbon dioxide as a supercritical fluid to produce oleoresins extracts from the onion at pilot scale. The results showed that the temperature and pressure during extraction process are the main influencing factors of onion oleoresin yield as well as sulfur content concentration. The authors discussed that increased temperature to 65°C from 45°C at 300 bar pressure led to an increase in both sulfur concentration and total extraction yield. However, at 45°C temperature and 300 bar, pressure yield is higher than at 100 bar, whereas sulfur concentration in oleoresin got reduced at higher pressure (300 bar) than at lower pressure (100 bar). The authors compared various extraction techniques with respect to extraction yield and concluded that supercritical carbon dioxide extraction yields 22 times higher when compared to the steam distillation; however, the yield is 14 times lower than that of alcohol extraction at 25°C shaking or 39 times lower yields than soxhlet apparatus. The sulfur content in onion oleoresin extraction from dried onion was also previously studied by Simándi et al. (2000). In this study, the authors evaluated

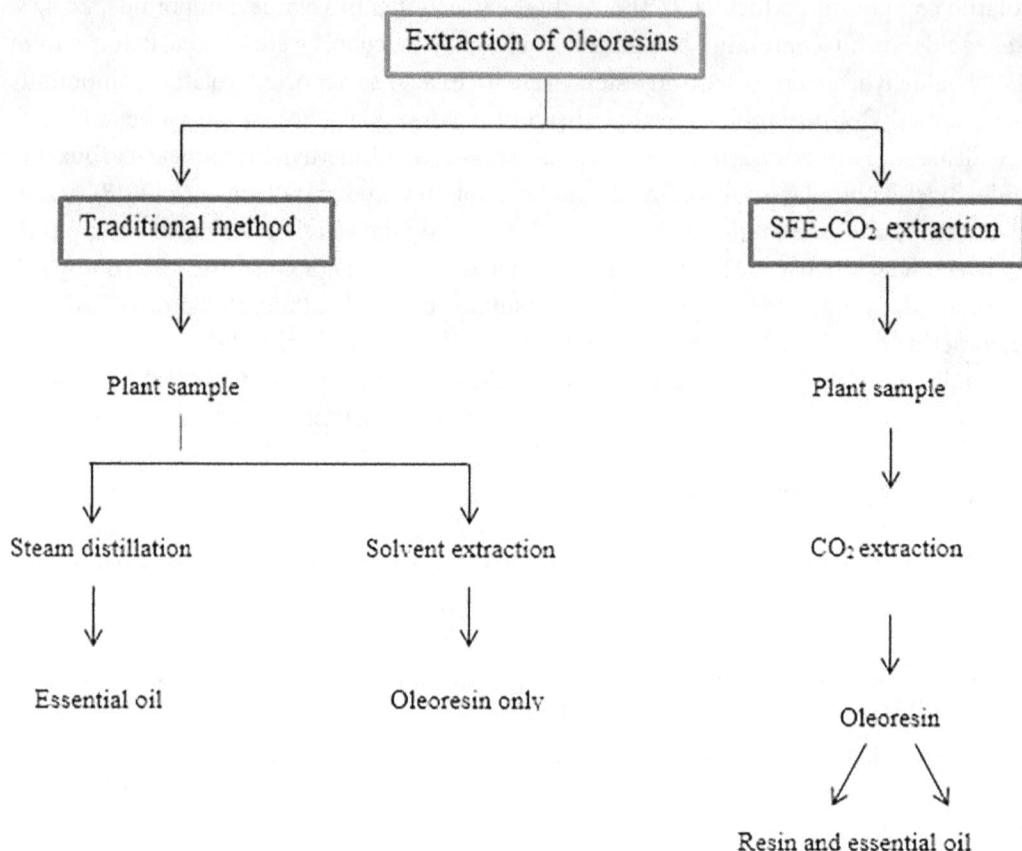

FIGURE 15.1 Flowchart showing different extraction processes.

the sulfur content and distilled oil showed highest and followed SFE and hexane. The sulfur content in these extractions was one tenth of distilled oil. However, the lowest sulfur concentration for alcoholic solvents was because of the highest recovery of other oleoresin components. The authors also concluded that supercritical carbon dioxide extraction can be used for the production of excellent quality onion oleoresin.

The flavors in onions are majorly attributed to primary and secondary products of enzymatic breakdown of S-alk(en)yl cysteine sulfoxide (ACSO), which is a common flavor precursor compound. The enzyme alliinase is released from plant cell vacuoles and further acts on ACSOs during chopping or crushing of onion bulbs, which is present in the cytoplasm and leads to the formation of characteristic aroma and flavor (Bhat et al., 2010). In 1997, Dron et al. (1997) extracted onion oil by using supercritical carbon dioxide with extraction condition as 3600 psi or 24.5 MPa, 37°C temperature with 0.89 g/cm^3 CO_2 density, and CO_2 flow rate was 0.5 L/minute to give maximum extraction yield. The brown amber liquid was yielded as 0.002%–0.03% by distillation of minced onions, which was kept a side to stand for few hours before distillation. Authors also reported the sulfur volatile compounds present in extracted oil. The compounds found in various supercritical extracts (SFE-CO_2 without entrainer, SFE-CO_2, C with ethanol and SFE-CO_2 with octane were 3-ethenyl-l, 2-dithi-5-ene, 3-ethenyl-l, 2-dithi4-ene, 3,4-dihydro-3-vinyl-1,2-dithi in, diallyl thiosulfinate (or its isomer), and diallyl trisulfide. Sinha et al. (1992) studied the supercritical carbon dioxide extract for over a storage period of 3 months to evaluate whether the presence of diallyl thiosulfinate or its isomers was still there or not. The result showed the presence of diallyl thiosulfide and dithiin derivatives even after 3 months in onion extract. The analysis suggests that the above volatile compound was detected in very low quantity even after the first week of extraction (peak area 0.075%) and found absent after the storage of 3 months, which was kept at 20°C–22°C temperature. However, the presence of dithiin and diallyl thiosulfinate derivatives supports that the SFE-CO_2 process is useful in the extraction of significant quantity of diallyl thiosulfinate. In 2005, the study by Guyer et al. reported that when onion oil was loaded on XAD-16, an adsorbent before supercritical extraction with carbon dioxide and desorption at 20.7 MPa pressure was observed; 37°C temperature and a flow rate of 1 L/minute showed an increased yield in onion oil (gravimetric yield). However, great volumes of onion juices loaded on the adsorbent led to a reduced gravimetric yield of onion oil. In conclusion, the authors suggest that the adsorption of onion juice on the adsorbent before the supercritical CO_2 desorption may be helpful in improving the supercritical CO_2 extraction of onion juice as it increases the gravimetric yield as per CO_2 volume used.

15.4 APPLICATIONS OF ONION OLEORESIN

Storage of onion bulbs has become a serious problem in tropical countries like India. The onion aroma concentrate (oleoresin) is finding favor in the food industry. It can be used for flavoring many food products, especially those of smooth texture, in dairy products, such as flavored cream cheese, sour cream, or in meat products, such as sausage, processed hams, cold meats, meat cans, and pickles. It is used in alcoholic and soft drinks and for the treatment of cold and infection and for blood cleansing (Devani et al., 2020).

15.5 SAFETY, TOXICITY, AND FUTURE SCOPE

Vegetable foods (including onions), their processed forms, and by-products have had their global production and consumption increase over the years. This is associated with their concomitant bioactive components, their natural availability, their affordability, and general acceptance as food materials (Sosalagere, Kehinde, and Sharma, 2022). Furthermore, the increasing socio-religious sentiments against consumption and general usage of animals and animal products is increasing on a global scale. However, high moisture content, nutritional constituencies, and natural matrices of plant foods like onions qualify them as suitable carriers for physical, chemical, microbial, and allergenic hazards. These hazards obtain their influxes into food materials from virtually every point of the food supply chain: from farm to fork, or even sea to spoon. Vegetative materials such as onions usually begin their exposure to hazards from the farms where they are cultivated. The cultivating soils, irrigation water, agrochemicals, farming equipment, and farm personnel are some prominent entry points for hazardous materials. Modern and urban agriculture has been observed to be constrained by toxic trace elements found in the produce cultivated and even the soil on which they are cultivated (Adjuik et al., 2020). These elements could accumulate on onion produce through various means, such as anthropogenic activities, dust, fossil fuel combustion initiating atmospheric deposits, metallurgical industries, metalliferous mining and smelting, and urban waste and sewage sludge dumping (Alfaro et al., 2017; Weber et al., 2019). Uptake of elements, such as zinc, copper, chromium, lead, and arsenic, has been observed in onion, and though some of them might be beneficial to health in trace quantities, they can be imbibed to toxic concentrations by the plant (Weber et al., 2019). Atamaleki et al. (2019) performed a meta-analytical systematic review of potentially toxic elements in cultivated onions irrigated by wastewater. The edible part of the plant was observed to contain larger concentrations of the elements, which include iron, zinc, copper, chromium, lead, nickel, and cadmium. Jha, Nayak, and Sharma (2009) studied the concentration of fluoride uptake in different parts of onion grown in contaminated soils. The study reported a fluoride (F) concentration in the root, bulb, and shoot to range between 18.6 and 151.6, 15.8 and 54.3, and 16.3 and 109.1 mg F/kg, respectively.

Agrochemicals, such as fungicides, insecticides, and herbicides, applied in excess dosages or without following regulatory guidelines can be deposited on onions and serve as potential hazards. Pesticides such as Fluopyram plus Tebuconazole, Propiconazole, Spinosad, Spinetoram, Propiconazole, and Thiacloprid are prominent types used for onions. Contaminated irrigation water has also been studied to infect onions with mold, *Salmonella* spp., *Escherichia coli*, and *Listeria monocytogenes* (Zhao et al., 2021).

Strict compliance and adherence to regulatory guidelines on the use of agrochemicals by local and international agencies by farmers would doubtlessly aid the reduction of hazards in onion foods. Furthermore, proper hygiene and sanitary practices, and safety management procedures and policies are effective tools for checking diverse hazards at different points of the onion food supply chain (Kehinde et al., 2020). In addition, the use of emerging technologies, biofunctional polymers, and food agents that are Generally Recognized as Safe (GRAS) would further assist in the control of these hazards (Kehinde and Sharma, 2018; Sharma et al., 2020).

15.6 CONCLUSION

Onions have been used since ancient times for dietetic and nutritional purposes based on their flavors and other organoleptic characteristics they impart for such applications. Furthermore, they have been known to be beneficial as traditional agents to remedy bodily disorders in several parts of the body, such as skin, eyes, and mouth, among others, though these require more extensive scientific studies. However, numerous investigations have shown that onion oleoresin is an exceptional bioactive component of food and has health benefits. They are conventionally extracted through the usage of suitable solvents, but there has been an emerging adoption of SFE using carbon dioxide. Onion oleoresin contains several phytochemicals that can function as nutraceuticals for the management of diverse metabolic syndrome disorders. In addition, they have been found to be highly beneficial as flavorings in various food-processing industries, such as beverages, sauces, seasoning, and pickles. It is a potential food agent for more uses as safe, natural, and plant-originated additives of general acceptability and significant safety with more research and industrial focus imparted for its continuous improvement.

REFERENCES

Adjuik, T., Rodjom, A. M., Miller, K. E., Reza, M. T. M., and Davis, S. C. 2020. Application of hydrochar, digestate, and synthetic fertilizer to a miscanthus X giganteus crop: implications for biomass and greenhouse gas emissions. *Applied Sciences* 10(24): 8953.

Albishi, T., John, J. A., Al-Khalifa, A. S., and Shahidi, F. 2013. Antioxidative phenolic constituents of skins of onion varieties and their activities. *Journal of Functional Foods* 5(3):1191–1203.

Alemzadeh Ansari, N. 2007. Onion cultivation and production in Iran. *Middle Eastern and Russian Journal of Plant Science and Biotechnology* 1(2):26–38.

Alfaro, M. R., Do Nascimento, C. W. A., Ugarte, O. M., Álvarez, A. M., de Aguiar Accioly, A. M., Martín, B. C. et al. 2017. First national-wide survey of trace elements in Cuban urban agriculture. *Agronomy for Sustainable Development* 37(4): 1–7.

Arshad, M. S., Sohaib, M., Nadeem, M., Saeed, F., Imran, A., Javed, A., Zaid Amjad, Batool, S. M. 2017. Status and trends of nutraceuticals from onion and onion by-products: a critical review. *Cogent Food and Agriculture* 3(1). doi:10.1080/23311932.2017.1280254.

Atamaleki, A., Yazdanbakhsh, A., Fakhri, Y., Mahdipour, F., Khodakarim, S., and Khaneghah, A. M. 2019. The concentration of potentially toxic elements (PTEs) in the onion and tomato irrigated by wastewater: a systematic review; meta-analysis and health risk assessment. *Food Research International* 108518. doi:10.1016/j.foodres.2019.1085

Bhat, N. R., Desai, B. B., and Suleiman, M. K. 2010. Flavors in onion: characterization and commercial applications. In: *Handbook of Fruit and Vegetable Flavors*, eds. Y. H. Hui, 849–872, John Wiley & Sons, New Jersey, USA.

Devani, B. M., Jani, B. L., Balani, P. C., and Akbari, S. H. 2020. Optimization of supercritical CO$_2$ extraction process for oleoresin from rotten onion waste. *Food and Bioproducts Processing* 119:287–295.

Dron, A., Guyeru, D. E., Gage, D. A., and Lira, C. T. 1997. Yield and quality of onion flavor oil obtained by supercritical fluid extraction and other methods. *Journal of Food Process Engineering* 20(2):107–124.

Galavi, A., Hosseinzadeh, H., and Razavi, B. M. 2021. The effects of *Allium cepa* L. (onion) and its active constituents on metabolic syndrome: a review. *Iranian Journal of Basic Medical Sciences* 24(1): 3.

Griffiths, G., Trueman, L., Crowther, T., Thomas, B., and Smith, B. 2002. Onions—a global benefits to health. *Phytotherapy Research* 16:603–615

Guyer, D. E., Saengcharoenrat, C., and Lira, C. T. 2005. Onion flavor recovery in the process of adsorption and supercritical carbon dioxide desorption. *Journal of Food Process Engineering* 28(3):205–218.

Heath, H. B. 1981. *Source Book of Flavors: (AVI Sourcebook and Handbook Series)* (Vol. 2). Springer Science and Business Media.

Jha, S. K., Nayak, A. K., and Sharma, Y. K. 2009. Fluoride toxicity effects in onion (*Allium cepa* L.) grown in contaminated soils. *Chemosphere* 76(3): 353–356.

Kaur A., Kehinde, B. A, Sharma, P., Sharma, D., Kaur, S. 2020. Recently isolated food-derived ACE inhibitory hydrolysates and peptides: a review. *Food Chemistry* 346: 128719. doi:10.1016/j.foodchem.2020.128719.

Kehinde, B. A., Chhikara, N., Sharma, P., Garg, M., and Panghal, A. 2021. Application of polymer nanocomposites in food and bioprocessing industries. *Handbook of Polymer Nanocomposites for Industrial Applications*. doi:10.1016/B978-0-12-821497-8.00006-X.

Kehinde, B. A., Panghal, A., Garg, M. K., Sharma, P., Chhikara, N. 2020. Vegetable milk as probiotic and prebiotic food. *Advances in Food and Nutrition*. doi:10.1016/bs.afnr.2020.06.003.

Kehinde, B. A, Sharma, P., Kaur, S. 2020. Recent nano-, micro- and macrotechnological applications of ultrasonication in food-based systems. *Critical Reviews in Food Science and Nutrition* 61(4):599–621. doi:10.1080/10408398.2020.1740646.

Kehinde, B. A., Sharma, P., Kaur S., and Panghal, P. 2019. Effects of drying temperature on the drying kinetics, engineering, microstructural and phytochemical profile of cassava. *Think India Journal* 636–664.

Liu, X., Pan, J., Chen, X., Quan, Q., Ao, Y., Hu, S. et al. 2016. Study on the extraction and analysis of red onion oleoresin. *Acta Agriculturae Zhejiangensis* 28(8):1401–1407.

Ly, T. N., Hazama, C., Shimoyamada, M., Ando, H., Kato, K., and Yamauchi, R. 2005. Antioxidative compounds from the outer scales of onion. *Journal of Agricultural and Food Chemistry* 53(21):8183–8189.

Majid, I., Dhatt, A.S., Sharma, S., Nayik, G.A. and Nanda, V. 2015. Effect of sprouting on physicochemical, antioxidant and flavonoid profile of onion varieties. *International Journal of Food Science & Technology* 51(2):317–324.

McCallum, J. (2007). Onion. *Genome Mapping and Molecular Breeding in Plants.* Springer, Berlin, Heidelberg, pp. 331–347. doi:10.1007/978-3-540-34536-7_11.

Prakash, D., Singh, B. N., and Upadhyay, G. 2007. Antioxidant and free radical scavenging activities of phenols from onion (*Allium cepa*). *Food Chemistry* 102(4):1389–1393.

Sass-Kiss, A., Simandi, B., Gao, Y., Boross, F., and Vamos-Falusi, Z. 1998. Study on the pilot-scale extraction of onion oleoresin using supercritical CO_2. *Journal of the Science of Food and Agriculture* 76(3):320–326.

Shahzadi, I., Nadeem, R., Hanif, M. A., Mumtaz, S., Jilani, M. I., and Nisar, S. 2017. Chemistry and biosynthesis pathways of plant oleoresins: important drug sources. *International Journal of Chemical & Biochemical Sciences* 12:18–52.

Sharma, P., Kaur, G., Kehinde, B. A., Chhikara, N., Panghal, A., and Kaur, H. 2019. Pharmacological and biomedical uses of extracts of pumpkin and its relatives and applications in the food industry: a review. *International Journal of Vegetable Science* 26(1): 79–95.

Sharma, P., Kaur, H., Kehinde, B. A, Chhikara, N., Sharma, D., and Panghal, A. 2020. Food-derived anticancer peptides: a review. *International Journal of Peptide Research and Therapeutics* 27:55–70. doi:10.1007/s10989-020-10063-1.

Shi, X., Zhang, W., Qian, J., and Zhang, Y. 2009. Extraction and microencapsulating process of the oleoresin from welsh-onion stalk the residue of the green onion in Xinghua. *China Condiment* 3: 54–58.

Simándi, B., Sass-Kiss, Á., Czukor, B., Deák, A., Prechl, A., Csordás, A., and Sawinsky, J. 2000. Pilot-scale extraction and fractional separation of onion oleoresin using supercritical carbon dioxide. *Journal of Food Engineering* 46(3): 183–188.

Sinha, N. K., Guyer, D. E., Gage, D. A., and Lira, C. T. 1992. Supercritical carbon dioxide extraction of onion flavors and their analysis by gas chromatography-mass spectrometry. *Journal of Agricultural and Food Chemistry* 40(5):842–845.

Slimestad, R, Fossen, T., and Vagen, I. M. 2007. Onions: a source of unique dietary flavonoids. *Journal of Agricultural and Food Chemistry* 25(55):1067–1080.

Sosalagere, C., Kehinde, B. A, Sharma, P. 2022. Isolation and functionalities of bioactive peptides from fruits and vegetables: a review. *Food Chemistry* 366: 130494

Teshika, J. D., Zakariyyah, A. M., Toorabally, Z., Zengin, G., Rengasamy, K. R., Pandian, S. K., and Mahomoodally, F. M. 2018. Traditional and modern uses of onion bulb (*Allium cepa* L.): a systematic review. *Critical Reviews in Food Science and Nutrition* 1–75. doi:10.1080/10408398.2018.1499074.

Wang, Z. D., Li, L. H., Xia, H., Wang, F., Yang, L. G., Wang, S. K., and Sun, G. J. 2018. Optimisation of steam distillation extraction oil from onion by response surface methodology and its chemical composition. *Natural Product Research* 32(1):112–115.

Weber, A. M., Mawodza, T., Sarkar, B., and Menon, M. 2019. Assessment of potentially toxic trace element contamination in urban allotment soils and their uptake by onions: a preliminary case study from Sheffield, England. *Ecotoxicology and Environmental Safety* 170:156–165.

Zhang, S-L., D. Peng, Y-C Xu, S-W Lu, and J-J Wang. 2016. Quantification and analysis of anthocyanin and flavonoids compositions, and antioxidant activities in onions with three different colors. *Journal of Integrative Agriculture* 15 (9):2175–2181.

Zhao, X. X., Lin, F. J., Li, H., Li, H. B., Wu, D. T., Geng, F., et al. 2021. Recent advances in bioactive compounds, health functions, and safety concerns of onion (*Allium cepa* L.). *Frontiers in Nutrition* 8:669805. doi:10.3389/fnut.2021.669805.

CHAPTER 16

Production, Characterization, and Health Benefits of Cardamom Oleoresins

Jasmeet Kour
Government P.G. College for Women, Jammu

Renu Sharma
Akal Degree College

Sangeeta
Guru Nanak College

Vikas Bansal
Jaipur National University

Monika Hans
Government P.G. College for Women, Jammu

Ashwani Kumar Khajuria
Government Degree College for Women, Kathua

CONTENTS

DOI: 10.1201/9781003186205-16

16.1 INTRODUCTION

The history of cardamom popularly called as "queen of spices" owing to its distinctive taste as well as aroma dates back to human race (Pearley Jesylne et al., 2016). Humans have been utilizing it as one of the ancient spices (Mal and Gharde, 2019). India holds its paramount position with respect to area and production of prominent spices across the globe such as black pepper, large cardamom, ginger, chili, and turmeric (Sasikumar and Sharma, 2001). Across the globe, the major cultivating areas of cardamom include tropical regions, such as South-Western parts of the Indian Peninsula, Sri Lanka, Thailand, Vietnam, Mexico and Tanzania. The application of cardamom has been as a medicinal herb in the 4th century in India mainly for trade purpose by Romans and Greeks (Asghar et al., 2017). The botanical names of large cardamom and small cardamom are *Amomum subulatum Roxburg* and *Elettaria cardamomum Maton* (Mal and Gharde, 2019).

The plant of cardamom comprises thick clump consisting of 20 leafy shoots and can attain a height between 2 and 6 m approximately (Pearley Jesylne et al., 2016). The oil of this spice is used as a valuable ingredient in culinary world, perfumery, and the beverage world (Kapoor et al., 2008). A perennial herb capable of growing up to 10 feet high with blade-shaped leaves bears small yellow flowers with purple tips, followed by ovoid fruit (Pearley Jesylne et al., 2016). Cardamom (*Elettaria cardamomum*) is a perennial herbaceous plant pertaining to order Zingiberaceae used to prohibit several infections (Asghar et al., 2017).

Cardamom is one of the most significant species of plant world hailing from the Zingiberaceae family from India and Southeast Asia (Kapoor et al., 2008). The usage of cardamom finds in the field of diseases, such as asthma, heart-related disorders, rectal diseases, and congestive jaundice (Jamal et al., 2005; Savan and Kucukbay, 2013). Cardamom finds its cultivation in the form of two species: small and large cardamom.

There is a dearth in literature highlighting the chemistry and activity of the cardamom essential oil and its oleoresins. Processed foods involving the incorporation of cardamom flavor is incorporated in the form of cardamom essential oil or the cardamom oleoresins obtained by solvent extraction process. It is the total extracts or oleoresins in various spices that are indicative parameters of the flavor quality in comparison with the distilled volatile oil (Savitha Krishnan et al., 2005).

In one of the pivotal works, compounds detected in cardamom oleoresin were 1,8-cineole and α-terpinyl acetate (Lewis et al., 1966). The oleoresins obtained by extraction with various solvents were reported to contain 5-(hydroxymethyl)-2-furaldehyde (16.2%), 1,8-cineole (19.7%), 1,8-cineole (9.2%), β-sitosterol (7.0%), α-terpineol (5.1%), 1,8-cineole (16.2%), and α-terpineol (4.1%) in methanol, acetone, carbon tetrachloride, and isooctane, respectively (Kapoor et al., 2008). Oleoresins have to be protected against various environmental factors such as moisture, oxygen, and light, which leads to its deterioration (Savitha Krishnan et al., 2005).

Earlier, the antioxidative evaluation of essential oil and oleoresins of mustard oil was carried out using various antioxidant parameters. Few studies can act as a starting point to acknowledge cardamom essential oil and oleoresins as food preservatives of natural origin (Kapoor et al., 2008). One of the most pivotal techniques to encapsulate spice oils and oleoresins is the spray-drying technique (Raghavan et al., 1990). However, there are no data reporting the encapsulation of oleoresins derived from cardamom (Krishnan et al., 2005).

16.2 DISTRIBUTION, PRODUCTION, AND ECONOMIC IMPORTANCE OF CARDAMOM OLEORESIN

Spices constitute an important category of ingredients utilized mostly in food products. Among various species, India leads the world in terms of producing chili, turmeric, black pepper, ginger, and large cardamom (Sasikumar and Sharma, 2001). Cardamom (*E. cardamomum*), a perennial herb of family *Zingiberaceae*, is also recognized as the "Queen of Spices" (Mathai, 1985). These are broadly classified as large cardamom (*Aframomum* and *Amomum* species) and small cardamom (*E. cardamomum Maton*) (Ravindran & Madhusoodanan, 2002.). Since ancient times, cardamom is well-known for imparting characteristic flavor and aroma to food products. The pleasant aroma of this spice is credited to either its essential oil or the solvent-extracted oleoresin.

For most of the known spices, the oleoresin is credited for reflecting flavor quality (Govindarajan et al., 1982). The flavor-imparting quality of oleoresin might be because of the essential volatile oil (52%–58%) contained in cardamom oleoresin. This volatile oil is also known for having analgesic, antispasmodic, antifungal (Utta-'Ur et al., 2000; Al-Zuhair et al., 1996), and anti-inflammatory activities (Nirmala, 2000). Cardamom oleoresin, due to the mellower and lesser harsh flavoring properties of cardamom (Krishnan, 1981; Sankarikutty et al., 1988), is used as a flavoring agent in various food products (Krishnan et al., 2005).

Cardamom is expanded to tropical regions, such as Sri Lanka, Tanzania, and a few Central American nations, from its native evergreen rainforests of southern India's Western Ghats. In India, the cardamom-developing tract lying between 75–70′ E longitude and 8°30′–14°30′ N latitude extends over 2000 km from north to south, including Sirsi (Karnataka) to Tirunelveli (Tamil Nadu). In the east–west direction, it is expanded over the Western Ghats as a narrow land belt (Madhusoodanan et al., 1994). Nelliampathy, Wayanad, and Idukki (Kerala); Shimoga, Uttar Kannada, Chickmagalur, and Hassan (Karnataka); and the southern and northern foothills of Tirunelveli, Salem, Dindigul,

Theni, and Nilgiris (Tamil Nadu) are reported to be major cultivation areas of cardamom (Parthasarathy and Prasath, 2012).

Cardamom has been considered as a significant spice commodity of International importance since ancient periods. The production of cardamom varies from 2900 metric tons to 10,075 metric tons during 1987–1988 and 2009–2010. The increased productivity during this period might be owing to the usage of high-yield-providing varieties as well as better agro-techniques. However, during the same time period, the demand for exported cardamom was extremely low. The decline in traded cardamom can be due to enhanced domestic consumption as well as competition among other cardamom-producing nations (Joseph, 2010). Currently, Guatemala exports about 90% of cardamom in the world.

Till 1979–1980, India was the prominent International spice exporter. But in the past few years, Guatemala has replaced Indian cardamom export with an annual production of 13,000 metric tons. Because of lower yields and lesser productivity, the cost of cardamom production in India is relatively more in comparison to Guatemala. Poor varieties, monsoon overdependence, land tenure issues, prolonged drought, defective postharvest procedures, and inadequate consideration to production management practices are some of the main causes for the lesser production. India and Guatemala are the chief producers in the cardamom world economy, while countries such as Tanzania, Sri Lanka, Thailand, and Vietnam are known to be small producers of cardamom. Despite negligible local demand for cardamom in Guatemala, all quantity produced is exported. The share of Guatemala in cardamom production has amplified by 30%–90% in the world market (Nair, 2006).

Oleoresins obtained from spices exhibit similar characteristics as that of spices. Besides providing aroma to the food products, these oleoresins are known to have antimicrobial, antifungal, preservative, antiviral, antioxidant, and insect repellent properties (Gautam et al., 2017; Su and Horvat, 1981). Cardamom oleoresin is mainly produced in India and other spice-producing western countries. Because of the similar application of oleoresin and the volatile oil in flavor quality, the commercial production of cardamom oleoresin is usually poor (Govindarajan et al., 1982). Both of these components undergo some chemical changes during prolonged storage as well as on exposure to air, which ultimately affects their organoleptic properties. These are mainly used in food products with short shelf life, such as meat and sausages (Nair, 2006). Several researchers reported the use of various oleoresin-extracting techniques. About 10% oleoresin is obtained from solvent extraction technique. The yield obtained depends upon the raw material and the solvents employed. It is also seen that oleoresin is usually dispersed in salt, flour, rusk, or dextrose before using.

16.3 EXTRACTION TECHNIQUES

Plants are well-known sources for several valuable biocomponents. A number of methods, such as steam distillation, high hydrostatic pressure extraction, pulse electric field process, high-pressure process, maceration using organic solvents, Soxhlet extraction techniques, have been reported for extracting oleoresins. These traditional extraction methods employed to obtain oleoresin are usually two-step processes involving use of organic solvents, such as alcohols, ethyl acetate, hexane, and acetone in the first step and then followed by removal of solvent in the second step (Steele et al., 1995; Gautam et al., 2017; Lee et al., 2020).

Oleoresins are concentrated spice extracts and possess similar profile as that of spice from which they are attained. These are composed of volatile essential oils and non-volatile resins. Various sensory differences have been observed among essential oil and resin parts of cardamom. The blending of these two fractions provides flavoring effect to spice. Steam or hydro-distillation processes are meant for essential volatile extraction, while resin is obtained with solvent extraction method. Later on, supercritical fluid extraction (SFE) technique was also implemented. Like other oleoresins, the lesser demand for cardamom oleoresin limits its production. Appropriate raw material, optimum particle size of raw material, solvent type, extraction process, and blending are the major considerations for oleoresin preparation (Nair, 2006). For extracting oleoresin, either Soxhlet process (Goldman, 1949) or batch countercurrent extraction process is industrially adopted (Nambudiri et al., 1970). The various techniques of cardamom oleoresin are briefly discussed below:

16.3.1 Solvent Extraction

In the solvent extraction process, a powdered sample of cardamom seed having particle size 500–700μm is extracted with suitable solvent. The various solvents, such as acetone, methanol, ethyl acetate, ethyl methyl ketone individually or a combination, can be employed for extraction process. A proper selection of solvent is an important step for oleoresin extraction process, and it should be standardized in laboratory before attempting commercial production. In this process, the coarse powdered spice extracted with solvent is laden into the extractor (also termed as percolator). The solvent is then permitted to the feedstock by keeping the drain valve opened for air circulation. After soaking the whole raw feedstock, drain valve is bolted and adequate time is provided for leaching of solvent into the solute. Afterwards, the extract, termed miscella, is obtained. The finished product is recovered by distillation of miscella. About 90%–95% solvent is recovered by normal atmospheric distillation. The distillation processes should be handled with care as heat might destruct the product.

After solvent stripping, the hot product is discharged and stored in containers. The spent meal, discharged from the extractor, is utilized in animal feed composition because of the presence of starch, fiber, carbohydrate, and protein. It can also be used as manure for many crops as well as broiler feed. Cardamom spent meal has find its application in fabrication of fragrant sticks, locally termed as "Agarbathi" (Suresh, 1987). The final yield and quality of cardamom oleoresin is significantly affected by the nature of solvent, the kind of raw material, and the method of extraction. Oleoresin containing 10%–20% fixed oil has been obtained with hydrocarbon solvents, whereas oil-free product is obtained with alcohol (Naves, 1974). Literature studies revealed the presence of oleic acid (62.6%), linoleic acid (10.5%), caproic and caprylic acids (0.3%), palmitic acid (8.4%), and stearic acid (18.3%) in fixed oil.

16.3.2 Supercritical Extraction of Cardamom Oleoresin

SFE is considered to be one of the most important techniques for extraction of oleoresins. The chief motivational factor in the use of SFE process in oleoresin is the introduction of the green chemistry principles in early 1990s. The 12 green chemistry principles assist as the strategies for maximizing efficiency and minimizing the adverse influences of chemicals on human health and environment. The above goals can only be attained with eco-friendly, highly efficient SFE process. Out of the various super-critical fluids (SCFs), supercritical CO_2 is generally preferred for oleoresin extractions. The wide utilization of SC-CO_2 is owing to its lower critical temperature and pressure (31.1°C, 7.39 MPa) and higher purity grade at relatively lower price. Also, SC-CO_2 is eco-friendly, inflammable, non-corrosive, cheap, abundantly available, and safer solvent. The extraction conditions, such as pressure, temperature, time, flow rate of carbon dioxide (CO_2), and the co-solvent addition, can be altered during the SFE process to allow for variations in viscosity and density, thereby altering the solvation power of CO_2 in order to attain a selective extraction process. Higher selectivity, lesser extraction time, high yield of oleoresin, and easy gas recovery at the end indicates the high efficacy of the process (Lee et al., 2020).

Literature revealed the destruction of several volatile oil constituents of cardamom oleoresin on exposure to high temperature. The terpenoids present in cardamom volatile oil are found to be highly unstable in the presence of acid, light, oxygen, and heat and develop petroleum-like smell due to rise in p-cymene (terpenoid) levels. Hence, the protection of oleoresin against these detrimental factors is required. This problem can be overcome by microencapsulation, a widely accepted technique in food industry that involves packing of core material particles surrounded by an incessant polymer film, which is meant for discharging its contents in expected mode under predefined circumstances (Beristain et al., 2001; Parthasarathy and Prasath, 2012). Microencapsulation using hydrolyzed and emulsifying starches and gums (especially gum acacia) serve as the most commonly employed carrier material (Krishnan et al., 2005).

Krishnan et al. (2005) reported the preparation of encapsulated cardamom oleoresin by using a mixture of gum acacia/emulsifying starch solution with spray drying. They presented that stabilization of oleoresins in the presence of damaging factors, such as light, oxygen, and heat, can be attained by integrating oleoresin in sugar environment. These cardamom co-crystallized sugar cubes offer their application in beverages and several other food products. Thus, co-crystallization method can be favorable for formulating cardamom oleoresin-flavored sugar cubes for utilization in ready-to-drink beverages (Sarder et al., 2013).

16.4 CHARACTERIZATION OF CARDAMOM OLEORESINS

Cardamom oleoresin, also known as Cardomomi, a yellow-colored concentrated viscous liquid or semi-solid material with a sweet-spicy, non-irritant, and warming fragrance, is used as a domestic spice and fragrance component of various processed food dishes. The mellower and less harsh flavor of cardamom oleoresin has become the reason behind the increase of its popularity day by day (Sankarikutty et al., 1982).

The process of obtaining cardamom oleoresin consists of solvent extraction of either finely crushed fresh cardamom powder or essential oil-free cardamom powder, and contains a wholesome character of spice in concentrated form; therefore, it can be used in small dosages with reduced storage space and easy transport; moreover, it has many micro-biological advantages. In addition, cardamom oleoresin has the advantage of its capability of processing at a higher temperature in comparison to direct steam distillate volatile oil (Eiserle and Rogers, 1972).

Cardamom oleoresin consists of two major portions of essential volatile oil (60%) and non-volatile oil (40%). The essential volatile oil contains isoprenoids and benzenoids while fixed oils, alkaloids, carotenoids, and anthocyanins are part of non-volatiles (Boelens and Boelens, 2000).

Oleoresins do not lose their quality easily and, therefore, are stable during their storage with a shelf life of a minimum of 1 year. The significant components of cardamom oleoresin are 1,8-cineole, α-terpineol, trans-nerolidol, terpinene-4-ol, and spathulenol. These components are present in different proportions in different oleoresins (Kapoor et al., 2008):

- Methanol oleoresin contains 5-(hydroxymethyl)-2-furaldehyde (16.2%), α-terpineol (6.1%), 1,8-cineole (5.4%), 2,3-dihydrobenzofuran (coumaran) (2.1%), and terpinen-4-ol (1.4%).

- Acetone oleoresin contains 1,8-cineole (19.7%), eugenol (12.5%), α-terpineol (8.1%), 5-(hydroxymethyl)-2-furaldehyde (3.7%), and trans-nerolidol (3.6%).

- Isooctane oleoresin contains 1,8-cineole (16.2%), α-terpineol (4.1%), n-heptacosane (4.2%), and n-nonacosane (4.0%).

- Carbon tetrachloride oleoresin contains 1,8-cineole (16.2%), α-terpineol (5.1%), and β-sitosterol (7.0%).

Various researchers, Nigam and Purohit (1960), Lawrence (1970), Hussain et al. (1988), Patra et al. (198), and Gurudutt et al. (1982), have confirmed the presence of 1,8-cineole as significant component along with sabinene, terpinen-4-ol, α-terpineol, α-and β-pinene by analyzing the GC-MS graphs closely. However, factors such as environmental, developmental, genetic, the nature of the solvent used for extraction, and some other factors affect the proportion of these components in oleoresin (Blair et al., 2001).

Another major constituent of cardamom oleoresin, i.e., α-terpineol, when exposed to light, heat, oxygen, or acid, undergoes polymerization, hydrolysis, rearrangement, and oxidation reactions and affects the flavor of the oleoresin due to increase in the quantity of p-cymene (responsible for petroleum-like fragrance) (Brennand and Heinz, 1970). The occurrence of these reactions can be reduced or prevented by following the process of encapsulation and ultimately retaining the true flavor of cardamom oleoresin for a longer period. The encapsulation process makes the oleoresin non-volatile, dry, and free-flowing, which provides a uniform flavor to the various food mixes.

Cardamom oleoresin also contains some non-aromatic fats, resinoids, colors, and waxes along with the aforesaid flavoring constituents. These non-aromatic constituents act as a preservative for the volatiles and this characteristic has a very important application in bakery and confectionary processing industry (Farell, 1985).

16.5 CHEMISTRY AND PROPERTIES

16.5.1 Chemistry

Oleoresin mainly comprises two major components: one is the volatile part, i.e., oil (gives aroma), and the other is the non-volatile part, i.e., resin, which is composed of fat, color, wax, pungent constituents, etc. The volatile oil and resin give the total flavor effect of spice only in combined form, i.e., after blending (Parthasarathy and Prasath, 2012; Peter, 2012). Steam/hydro-distillation and solvent extraction methods are used for the production of volatile oil and resin, respectively (Sankarikutty et al., 1982). Cardamom oleoresin is a darkish brown liquid with viscous consistency, warming fragrance, rich in aroma, and has sweet-spicy flavor (Govindarajan et al., 1982).

Cardamom oleoresin has many components and major constituents, which according to importance are 1,8-cineole; α-terpineol; 2, 3-dihydrobenzofuran (coumaran); 5-(hydroxymethyl)-2-furaldehyde; eugenol; β-sitosterol; terpinen-4-ol; *n*-heptacosane; trans-nerolidol; *n*-nonacosane; and *n*-heptacosane (Gautam et al., 2016). The components present in volatile oil of cardamom were reported in literature by Guenther (1975) and their analysis reported in detail for the first time by Nigam et al. (1965). The volatile components in cardamom are dominated by oxygenated compounds having potential aroma properties and have few hydrocarbons (mono- or sesquiterpenic). However, cardamom has many common constituents (esters, alcohols, and aldehydes) as found in the oils of many spices, but the presence of 1,8-cineole (ether) and acetates of linalyl and terpinyl (ester) dominates and makes a unique combination in the volatiles of cardamom (Lewis et al., 1966; Salzer, 1975).

The composition of oleoresin and its quality depends on the variety, part of cardamom, rate, extraction process, and time of distillation (Khajeh et al., 2004; Marongiu et al., 2004; Kaskoos et al., 2006; Lucchesi et al., 2007). The difference in aroma of cardamom from different sources is reported mainly due to the presence and amount of components 1,8-cineole (ether) and esters (Gautam et al., 2016).

Method of extraction significantly affects the composition of oleoresin and volatile part as reported in various studies. The monoterpenes (87.6%) were reported to be higher in the steam-distilled portion of cardamom having 1,8-cineole (35.6%) as the main monoterpene ether, and then acetates of α-terpenyl (27.1%), α-terpineol (4.9%), and thujyl alcohol comes in terms of importance (Kaskoos et al., 2006). However, the composition of cardamom seeds extract obtained by supercritical CO_2 extraction also vary and the main components reported were 42.3% α-terpinyl acetate, 21.4% 1,8-cineole, 8.2% linalyl acetate, 5.6% limonene, and 5.4% linalool. The strong compositional differences were observed in the extract obtained by using hexane as the solvent, and important components reported were 36.4% limonene; 23.5% 1,8-cineole; 8.6% terpinolene; and 6.6% myrcene (Marongiu et al., 2004). Recently, solvent-free microwave extraction (SFME) has also been successfully employed (Lucchesi et al., 2007) and six major components have been identified. All the compounds were oxygenated and their order as per importance is 1,8-cineole, α-terpinyl acetate, linalool, linalyl acetate, α-terpineol, and terpin-4-ol.

Variation in the amount of oxygenated components and yields of the two major aromatic compounds (1,8-cineole and α-terpinyl acetate) were reported when SFME and hydro-distillation were compared (Lucchesi et al., 2007). The distinct cardamom flavor is mainly because of compounds 1,8-cineole, terpinyl acetate, linalyl acetate, and linalool (Kapoor et al., 2008). Different components of oleoresins and volatile oil have different characteristics such as higher amount of cineole contributes pungency, while pleasant aroma is because of terpenyl acetate (Chempakam and Sindhu, 2008, Gautam et al., 2016). Seeds of cardamom were reported to have various components, such as cardamonin (2,4-dihydroxy-6-methoxyalcone) and alpinetin (7-hydroxy-5-methoxyflavanone) and glycosides (petunidin 3,5-diglucoside, leucocyanidin-3-O-β-D-glucopyranoside), and a new aurone glycoside subulin (6,3,4,5-tetrahydroxy-4-methoxyaurone-6-O-α-L-rhamno pyranosyl (1–4)-β-D glucopyranoside) (Gopal et al., 2012). Various non-volatile pigments were reported in large cardamom part from aforementioned components, which make its chemistry unique on its own (Naik et al., 2004). As explained above, Kapoor et al. (2008) and Gautam et al. (2016) also reported that the percent recovery of oleoresin and its chemical composition is affected by the cardamom variety, conditions of production, and type of solvent used for extraction. The yield and recovery of different components was found to be different, when different solvents (methanol, acetone, isooctane, and CCl4) were used for extraction of oleoresins using steam distillation (Soxhlet apparatus) as the extraction method. The viscous oleoresins were produced by removal of solvent using distillation, and the oleoresins were stored under cold condition until further use (Kapoor et al., 2008).

16.5.2 Properties of Cardamom Oleoresins

Oleoresins (concentrated form of spice) are characterized by high efficiency of active compounds, which enable them to be used in small dosages. Cardamom oleoresin, containing all the volatile as well as non-volatile components of spices, represents closely the whole flavor of the fresh spice in a highly concentrated form. Therefore, oleoresins are preferred spice extracts used for flavoring purposes, and its demand in the snacks and fast food industry is increasing sharply because of producing a standardized effect on taste (Gautam et al., 2016).

Cardamom oleoresins possess various health beneficial properties, i.e., antioxidant, antimicrobial properties, antispasmodic, anticancer, and many more. Because of their aromatic and medicinal properties, oleoresins of different cardamom are widely used in aromatherapy, food, and pharmaceutical industries, and are considered as luxurious items. A wide range of pharmacological and physiological properties have been reported in the extract of large cardamom (Bisht et al., 2011). Some of the important properties as reported in literature are discussed in this section.

16.5.2.1 Anti-Inflammatory Properties

Alam et al. (2011) reported that the ethanolic extract (100 mg/mL) and aqueous extract (200 mg/mL) of cardamom (large) showed anti-inflammatory activity. Cardamom is used for the treatment of various infections related to teeth and gums, inflammation of eyelids, throat troubles, lung congestion, digestive disorders, etc. (Chempakam and Sindhu, 2008).

16.5.2.2 Antimicrobial Properties

Cardamom oleoresins are used as a preservative for orange juice and have a significant effect on shelf life because of their antimicrobial properties, and superior (safe and effective) than synthetic preservatives (Singh et al., 2009). Various studies have reported that cardamom extract in various solvents exhibits antimicrobial properties against various bacteria and fungus. The extract of large cardamom in petroleum ether has an antimicrobial effect against *Staphylococcus aureus, Escherichia coli, Pseudomonas aeruginosa,* and *Bacillus cereus* (Kumar et al., 2010; Satyal et al., 2012). The acetonic, ethanolic, and methanolic extracts were reported to exhibit antimicrobial activity against *Streptococcus mutans* and *S. aureus* (bacteria causing dental caries) (Hussain et al., 2011); and an antifungal effect against *Candida albicans* and *Saccharomyces cerevisiae* (Aneja and Joshi, 2009). Gautam et al. (2016) reported that cardamom extracts have much broader antifungal spectrum and not only limited to various dermophytic and keratinophilic fungi. Hence, it is necessary to explore the "broad spectrum fungal inhibition" attribute of compounds present in cardamom extract (oleoresins and essential oils) by active research and study in future.

16.5.2.3 Antioxidant and Scavenging Activity

Cardamom extract has a high level of phenolic compounds and is reported to have notable activities in antioxidant assays (Gautam et al., 2016). Yadav and Bhatnagar (2007) reported that these polyphenols are superoxide radical scavenging compounds and found to have strong inhibitory attributes against lipid peroxidation in rat liver homogenate. As per data reported in literature, the main components present in extract of cardamom seeds exhibiting antioxidant property against lipid peroxidation and potential health benefits are 1,8-cineole, protocatechualdehyde, alphaterpineol, and protocatechuic acid (Kikuzaki et al., 2001; Jessie and Krishnakantha, 2005). Various active components of cardamom seed extracts have been reported for their antioxidant effect in cardiac and hepatic antioxidant enzymes, and also activate other antioxidant enzymes (Verma et al., 2010).

16.5.2.4 Other Activities

In addition to the properties discussed above, cardamom extracts (oleoresins and volatile oil) have been reported to have various other health beneficial properties. Jafri et al. (2001) reported the anti-ulcer activity of crude methanolic extract of cardamom in albino rats. Similarly, various fractions (methanolic, ethyl acetate soluble, and petrol soluble) of cardamom have been reported for their notable effect in opposition to ethanol induced ulcer, lower aspirin-induced gastric ulcer (60%), etc. (Parmar et al., 2009; Verma et al., 2010). Large cardamom extract has been found to be effective in the treatment of ischemic heart disease (IHD) (Bisht et al., 2011). Shukla et al. (2010) reported the remarkable analgesic effect of cardamom seeds extract at higher dose in various solvents. Cardamom oleoresin and oils are widely used as spice in food, in medicines (mainly in Ayurveda medicines), as antioxidants, and are non-toxic in nature. Cardamom oleoresins have also been reported for their antispasmodic, anticancer property (neutralizes adverse effects of chemotherapy), metabolism maintaining property (stimulant; anti-depression, anti-fatigue, etc.), anti-septic (disinfects oral cavity, drinking water), flavoring as well as antimicrobial action in various food stuffs, warming effect, detoxification property, and aphrodisiac property, etc. (Gautam et al., 2016).

16.6 APPLICATIONS (HEALTH AND MEDICINE)

Two genera correspond to two types of cardamom: large cardamom (*Amommum cardamomum*) and true cardamom, i.e., green cardamom or small cardamom (*E. cardamom*) (Bhide, 2010). Small cardamom (green cardamom) has long been used around the world in cooking and also has medicinal values. This spice is used not only as flavoring and spicy ingredient in a variety of food products, but it is also used as folk remedy to treat teeth and gum infections, lungs and pulmonary tuberculosis, and digestive and kidney disorders (Saeed et al., 2014). The oleoresins of cardamom seeds and other high value gastroprotective have characteristic aroma and have involvement as functional foods. They also have wide range of medicinal and pharmaceutical applications (Hamzaa and Osman, 2012).

Oleoresin consists of volatile oil and resin. The flavor consists of volatile oil, while the resin is a mixture of non-volatile compounds, such as color, fat, odor, waxes, and so on. Just after the oils and resins have been mixed, the flavor of spices become totally apparent. Volatile oil is obtained using hydro or steam distillation, while the resin extraction is done by using solvent extraction. Cardamom oleoresin demand is gradually increasing, owing to its tentful and less palatable flavor characteristics (Sankarikutty et al., 1982). Because of their applications in aromatherapy, food and pharmaceutical industries, essential oils and oleoresins of spices are considered luxurious items. They are also effective antioxidants and antimicrobials.

The presence of phenolics, 1,8-cineole, limonene, linalool, terpinolene, myrcene, and volatile oils and resins (Oleoresin) and other bioactives as such contribute to the pharmaceutical uses of this spice (Kurt, 2011). Some of the health properties are shown by cardamom extract such as antioxidant, antihypertensive, antidiabetic, gastroprotective, laxative, antispasmodic, antibacterial, antiplatelet aggregation, and anticancer properties (Padmakumari et al., 2010). Pain and swelling, especially on mucous membrane, mouth, and throat can be helped by cardamom oil and resins. The dry seeds of cardamom and its oil are utilized for the treatment of stomach and other gastrointestinal diseases (Jamal et al., 2006). The dry seeds of cardamom and its oil are utilized for the treatment of stomach and other gastrointestinal diseases (Jamal et al., 2006). In the same manner, phytonutrients, vitamins, and essential oil of cardamom act as antioxidants, helping to remove free radicals and prevent cell ageing (Saeed et al., 2014).

Moreover, cardamom and its essential extracts are known for improving poor sexual responses and impotence (Lwasa and Bwowe, 2007). Knowing that Arabian countries' consumption is in the highest proportion (Ravindran and Madhusoodanan, 2002), the preference or aspiration of multiple marriages among men can be associated with wide-ranging consumption of a popular hot drink (Gahwa) containing an important ingredient, cardamom extract. The essential oil along with resins of cardamom is used in aromatherapy as a massage oil to relieve digestive and throat infections and has revitalizing properties.

The antibacterial, antispasmodic, analgesic, and anti-inflammatory qualities of essential cardamom oil have proved to be effective in delaying the proliferation of viruses, bacteria, and molds (Al-Zuhair et al., 1996). Cardamom essential oils are renowned for their soft nervous system tonic to alleviate headaches. Furthermore, cardamom essential oil and resins combined with ginger, fennel and some oils can alleviate colic indications in children's. This essential oil has a dramatic influence on the respiratory system, encouraging clear breathing health due to its high level of 1,8 cineole and terpinyl acetate (Ravindran and Madhusoodanan, 2002; Davis, 2005).

Green cardamom was chewed by the ancient Egyptians to keep their teeth clean and a healthy digestion (Lwasa and Bwowe, 2007). Cardamom fruit/pudding, extract and essential oil can be utilized as a natural antioxidant and food preservatives because of the presence of phenolic and antibacterial compounds (Martins et al., 2001). The development of poisonous histamine in mast vells has been demonstrated to be greatly inhibited and can therefore be restricted to lessen histamine food toxicity as a natural remedy. The oil has the ability to operate as wheat protective by contact and fumigation action (Huang et al., 2000) to target *Tribolium castaneum* and *Sitophilus zeamais* acting as a preservative. Natural antioxidants present in the resins of cardamom are proven to be safer and have a variety of potential health benefits (Saeed et al., 2014). Cardamom pods and their extracts contain high levels of antioxidants, phenolics, and flavonoids (quercetin, kaempferol, luteolins, and pelargonidin) and are a natural antioxidant ingredient in the food industry (Nair et al., 1998). The important extract and volatile compounds can be combined with vegetable oils such as from coconut to make valuable lotions and ointments that promote healthy skin cell function. Cardamom essential oil and oleoresin compounds can be combined with lemon extract which can be used as a natural wood preservative and polish as it has good cleansing, purifying and insect repellent properties. The essential compound, which is primarily used to flavor processed foods, can also be found in products such as beverages and fruit drinks, alcoholic preparations, and liquors. At present, the perfume and cosmetics industries use essential oils as well as fruit extracts from many herbs and plant species, including cardamom, to mixing with other volatile oil and vegetables. In the processed food sector, cardamom essential oil and oleoresin are utilized for aroma as a soluble spice (Ravindran and Madhusoodanan, 2002).

16.7 SAFETY, TOXICITY, AND FUTURE GROWTH

In line with the new development of natural and unique products, a range of marketable cardamom products have now been launched. Cardamom odor has been developed in new ways so that the commercial use of cardamom for the manufacture of unique products is more diversified and improved. The encapsulated spice resins are characterized by uniformity in flavor, quick release and dispersal of the flavor, flexibility of flow, and ease of usage. Some of researcher's unique processed goods are cardamom coffee and tea with an additional immediate cardamom flavor. It is vital to undertake further development programs in order to diversify the various uses of this rare plant, which led to the production of new cardamom flavors or beverages (Ravindran and Madhusoodanan, 2002).

16.8 CONCLUSION

Over the years, a spike in the production of meat products and ready-to-eat meals at industrial levels has led to an upsurge in the utilization of seasoning extracts as a substitute for natural seasonings. One of the best sources of natural antioxidants and antimicrobials have been plant extracts in foods. Oleoresins have proven to have high antioxidative values than synthetic ones such as butylated hydroxytoulene (BHT). These are promising in showing a broad spectrum of antifungal activity against fungal isolates, which makes the essential oil and oleoresin of cardamom to be used as natural food preservatives.

REFERENCES

Alam, K., Pathak, D., and Ansari, S.H. 2011. Evaluation of anti-inflammatory activity of *Ammomum subulatum* fruit extract. *International Journal of Pharmaceutical Sciences and Drug Research* 3(1): 35–37.

Al-Zuhair, H., El-sayeh, B., Ameen, H.A., and Al-Shoora, H. 1996. Pharmacological studies of cardamom oil in animals. *Pharmacological Research* 34(1–2): 79–82.

Aneja, K.R., and Joshi, R. 2009. Antimicrobial activity of *Amomum subulatum* and *Elettaria cardamomum* against dental caries causing microorganisms. *Ethnobotanical Leaflets* 13: 840–849.

Asghar, A., Butt, M.S., Shahid, M., and Huang, Q. 2017. Evaluating the antimicrobial potential of green cardamom essential oil focusing on quorum sensing inhibition of *Chromobacterium violaceum*. *Journal of Food Science and Technology* 54(8): 2306–2315.

Bhide, M. 2010. Queen of spices. *Saveur.* http://www.saveur.com/article/Kitchen/Queen-of-Spices (Retrieved 4.12.14.).

Beristain, C. I., Garcıa, H. S., and Vernon-Carter, E. J. 2001. Spray-dried encapsulation of cardamom (Elettariacardamomum) essential oil with mesquite (Prosopisjuliflora) gum. *LWT-Food Science and Technology* 34(6): 398–401.

Bisht, V.K., Negi, J.S., Bhandari, A.K., and Sundriyal, R.C. 2011. *Amomum subulatum* Roxb: traditional, phytochemical and biological activities-an overview. *African Journal of Agricultural Research* 6(24): 5386–5390.

Blair, J., Aichinger, T., Hackal, G., Hueber, K., and Dachler, M. 2001. Essential oil content and composition in commercially available dill cultivars in comparison to caraway. *Industrial Crops and Products Journal* 14: 229–239

Boelens, M., and Boelens, H. 2000. The chemical and sensory evaluation of edible oleoresins. *Perfumer and Flavourist* 25(4): 10–23.

Brennand, C.P., and Heinz, D.E. 1970. Effects of pH and temperature on volatile constituents of cardamom. *Journal of Food Science* 35: 533–537.

Chempakam, B., and Sindhu, S. 2008. Small cardamom. In V.A. Parthasarathy, B. Chempakam, T.J. Zachariah *Chemistry of Spices*, CABI, UK, pp. 41–58.

Eiserle, R.J., and Rogers, J.A. 1972. The composition of volatiles derived from oleoresins. *Journal of the American Oil Chemists Society* 49: 573–577.

Farell, K.T. (1985) *Spices, Condiments, and Seasonings.* The AVI Publishing Company, USA.

Gautam, N., Bhattarai, R.R., Khanal, B.K.S., and Oli, P. 2016. Technology, chemistry and bioactive properties of large cardamom (*Amomum subulatum* Roxb.): an overview. *International Journal of Applied Sciences and Biotechnology* 4(2): 139–149.

Gautam, D., Loach, N., Yadav, S. K., Srivastava, C. N., and Mohan, L. 2017. Bioefficacy evaluation of certain oleoresins against the larvae of Rhipicephalusmicroplus (Acari: Ixodidae). *Advances in Bioresearch* 8(5). 188–194.

Goldman, A. 1949. How spice oleoresins are made. *American perfume fragrance and Essential Oil Review* 53: 320–323.

Gopal, K., Baby, C., and Mohammed, A. 2012. *Amomum subulatum* Roxb: an overview in all aspects. *International Research Journal of Pharmacy* 3(7): 96–99.

Govindarajan, V.S., Narasimhan, S., Raghuveer, K.G., Lewis, Y.S., and Stahl, W.H. 1982. Cardamom—production, technology, chemistry, and quality. *Critical Reviews in Food Science & Nutrition* 16(3): 229–326.

Guenther, E. 1975. Cardamom. In *The Essential Oils*, Vol. 5. Van Nostrand, New York, p. 85.

Gurudutt, K.N., Naik, J.P., Srinivas, P., and Ravindranath, B. 1996. Volatile constituents of large Cardamon (*Amomum subulatum* Roxb). *Flavor and Fragnance Journal* 11: 7–9.

Hamzaa, R., and Osman, N. 2012. Using of coffee and cardamom mixture to ameliorate oxidative stress induced in γ-irradiated rats. *Biochemistry and Analytical Biochemistry* 1: 113–119.

Huang, Y., Lam, S.L., and Ho, S.H. 2000. Bioactivities of essential oil from *Elletaria cardamomum* (L.) Maton to *Sitophilus zeamais* Motschulsky and *Tribolium castaneum* (Herbst). *Journal of Stored Products Research* 36: 107–117.

Hussain, A., Virmani, O.P., Sharma, A., Kumar, A., and Misra, L.N. 1988. *Major Essential Oil-Bearing Plants of India*. Central Institute of Medicinal and Aromatic Plants, Lucknow, India.

Hussain, T., Arshad, M., Khan, S., Hamid, S., and Qureshi, M.S. 2011. In vitro screening of methanol plant extracts for their antibacterial activity. *Pakistan Journal of Botany* 43(1): 531–538.

Jafri, M.A., Javed, K., and Singh, S. 2001. Evaluation of the gastric antiulcerogenic effect of large cardamom (fruits of *Amomum subulatum* Roxb). *Journal of Ethnopharmacology* 75(2–3): 89–94.

Jamal, A., Javed, K., Aslam, M., and Jafri, M.A. 2006. Gastroprotective effect of cardamom, *Elettaria cardamomum* Maton fruits in rats. *Journal of Ethnopharmacology* 103: 149–153.

Jamal, A., Siddiqui, A., Aslam, M., Javed, K., and Jafri, M. 2005. Antiulcerogenic activity of *Elettaria cardamomum* Maton and *Amomum subulatum* Roxb seeds. *Indian Journal of Traditional Knowledge* 4: 298–302.

Jessie, S.W., and Krishnakantha, T.P. 2005. Inhibition of human platelet aggregation and membrane lipid peroxidation by food spice, saffron. *Molecular and Cellular Biochemistry* 278(1): 59–63.

Jesylne, P., Soundarajan, S., Murthykumar, K., and Meenakshi, M. 2016. The role of cardamom oil in oral health: a short review. *Research Journal of Pharmacy and Technology* 9(3):272–274.

Joesph, R. 2010. Cardamom industry scaling new heights. *Spice India* 23(7): 11–14.

Kapoor, I.P.S., Singh, B., Singh, G., Isidorov, V., and Szczepaniak, L. 2008. Chemistry, antifungal and antioxidant activities of cardamom (*Amomum subulatum*) essential oil and oleoresins. *International Journal of Essential Oil Therapeutics* 2(1): 29–40.

Kaskoos, R.A., Ali, M., Kapoor, R., Akhtar, M.M.S., and Mir, S.R. 2006. Essential oil composition of the fruits of *Eletteria cardamomum*. *Journal of Essential Oil Bearing Plants* 9(1): 81–84.

Khajeh, M., Yamini, Y., Sefidkon, F., and Bahramifar, N. 2004. Comparison of essential oil composition of *Carum copticum* obtained by supercritical carbon dioxide extraction and hydrodistillation methods. *Food Chemistry* 86(4): 587–591.

Kikuzaki, H., Kawai, Y., and Nakatani, N. 2001. 1, 1-Diphenyl-2-picrylhydrazyl radical-scavenging active compounds from greater cardamom (*Amomum subulatum* Roxb.). *Journal of Nutritional Science and Vitaminology* 47(2): 167–171.

Krishnan, S. 1981. Natural flavouring ingredients. 33. In *Proceedings of seminar on spices, oleoresins and flavours*. Bombay: AFSTI (Bombay chapter) 48–51.

Krishnan, S., Bhosale, R., and Singhal, R.S. 2005. Microencapsulation of cardamom oleoresin: evaluation of blends of gum Arabic, maltodextrin and a modified starch as wall materials. *Carbohydrate Polymers* 61(1): 95–102.

Kumar, U., Kumar, B., Bhandari, A., and Kumar, Y. 2010. Phytochemical investigation and comparison of antimicrobial screening of clove and cardamom. *International Journal of Pharmaceutical Sciences and Research* 1(12): 138–147.

Kurt, S. 2011. The healing intelligence of essential oils: the science of advanced aromatherapy paperback. http://www.goodreads.com/book/show/11631089-the-healing-intelligence-of-essential-oils (Retrieved 3.01.15.).

Lawrence, B.M. 1970. Terpenes in two *Amomum* species. *Phytochemicals* 9: 665.

Lee, W. J., Suleiman, N., Hadzir, N. H. N., and Chong, G. H. 2020. Supercritical fluids for the extraction of oleoresins and plant phenolics. In *Green Sustainable Process for Chemical and Environmental Engineering and Science* Ed(1), Inamuddin; Bodulla, R and Asiri, A.M, Elsevier Inc, MA, USA (pp. 279–328).

Lewis, Y.S., Nambudiri, E.S., and Philip, T. 1966. Composition of cardamom oils. *Perfumery and Essential Oil Records* 57: 623–628.

Lucchesi, M.E., Smadja, J., Bradshaw, S., Louw, W., and Chemat, F. 2007. Solvent free microwave extraction of *Elletaria cardamomum* L.: a multivariate study of a new technique for the extraction of essential oil. *Journal of Food Engineering* 79(3): 1079–1086.

Lwasa, S., and Bwowe, F. 2007. Exploring the economic potential of cardamom (*Elettaria cardamomum*) as an alternative and promising income source for Uganda's smallholder farmers. *ACSS Science Conference Proceedings* 8: 1317–1321.

Mal D. and Gharde S. K. (2019). Medicinal uses of Cardamom: A review. *Journal of Emerging Technologies and Innovative Research (JETIR)* 6 (1): 877–980.

Marongiu, B., Piras, A., and Porcedda, S. 2004. Comparative analysis of the oil and supercritical CO_2 extract of *Elettaria cardamomum* (L.) Maton. *Journal of Agricultural and Food Chemistry* 52(20): 6278–6282.

Martins, A.P., Salgueiro, L., and Goncalves, M.J. 2001. Essential oil composition and antimicrobial activity of three Zingiberaceae from S. Tome e Principe. *Planta Medica* 67 (6): 580–584.

Mathai, C. K. 1985. Quality evaluation of the 'agmark' grades of cardamom Elettaria cardamomum. *Journal of the Science of Food and Agriculture* 36(6): 450–452.

Naik, J.P., Jagan Mohan Rao, L., Mohan Kumar, T.M., and Sampathu, S.R. 2004. Chemical composition of the volatile oil from the pericarp (husk) of large cardamom (*Amomum subulatum* Roxb.). *Flavour and Fragrance Journal* 19(5): 441–444.

Nair, S., Nagar, R., and Gupta, R. 1998. Antioxidant phenolics and flavonoids in common Indian foods. *Journal of the Association of Physicians of India* 46 (8): 708–710.

Nair, K. P. 2006. The agronomy and economy of Cardamom (Elettaria cardamomum M.): the "queen of spices". *Advances in agronomy* 91: 179–471.

Nambudiri, E. S., Lewis, Y. S., Krishnamurthy, N., and Mathew, A. G. 1970. Oleoresin pepper. *Flavour Indus.* 1:97–99.

Naves, Y.R. 1974. Technologie et chimie des parfums Naturess Paris. Masson & Cie.

Nigam, M.C., Nigam, I.C., Handa, K.L., and Levi, L. 1965. Essential oils and their constituents XXVIII. Examination of oil of cardamom by gas chromatography. *Journal of Pharmaceutical Sciences* 54(5): 799–801.

Nigam, S.S., and Purohit, R.M. 1960. Chemical examination of essential oil driven from the seed of *Amomum subulatum* Roxb. *Journal of Essential Oil Research* 51: 12–123.

Nirmala Menon, A. 2000. Studies on the volatiles of cardamom (Elleteria cardamomum). *Journal of Food Science and Technology* 37(4): 406–408.

Padmakumari, A.K.P., Rani, M.P., and Sasidharan, I., et al. 2010. Chemical composition, flavonoid-phenolic contents and radical scavenging activity of four major varieties of cardamom. *International Journal of Biological and Medical Research* 1: 20–24.

Parmar, M.Y., Shah, P., Thakkar, V., and Gandhi, T.R. 2009. Hepatoprotective activity of *Amomum subulatum* Roxb against ethanol-induced liver damage. *International Journal of Green Pharmacy (IJGP)* 3(3): 250–254.

Parthasarathy, V.A., and Prasath, D. 2012. Cardamom. In *Handbook of Herbs and Spices*. Woodhead Publishing Limited, Cambridge, UK.

Patra, N.K., Siddiqui, M.M., Akhila, A., Nigam, M.C., and Naqvi, A. 1982. Gas chromatography examination of the oil from fruit of *Amomum subulatum* growing wild in Darjeeling, *Perfumes and Flavours Association of India Journal* 4(4): 29–31.

Ravindran, P.N., & Madhusoodanan, K.J. (Eds.). (2002). Cardamom: The Genus Elettaria (1st ed.). CRC Press, London, UK. https://doi.org/10.1201/9780203216637.

Peter, K.V. 2012. *Biodiversity, Conservation and Utilization of Spices, Medicinal and Aromatic Plants*. Woodhead Publishing Limited, Cambridge, UK.

Raghavan, B., Abraham, K.O., and Shankaranarayana, M.L. 1990. Encapsulation of spice and other flavour materials. *Indian Perfumer* 34(1): 75–85.

Ravindran, P.N., Johny, A.K., and Nirmal, B.K. 2002. Spices in our daily life. *Satabdi Smaranika* 2: 102–105.

Ravindran, P.N., and Madhusoodanan, K.J. 2002. *Cardamom: The Genus Elettaria (Medicinal and Aromatic Plants Industrial Series)*. pp. 269–283. CRC Press, Taylor and Francis Group, London.

Saeed, A., Sultana, B., Anwar, F., Mushtaq, M., Alkharfy, K.M., and Gilani, A.H. 2014. Antioxidant and antimutagenic potential of seeds and pods of Green cardamom (*Elettaria cardamomum*). *International Journal of Pharmaceutics* 10(8): 461–469.

Salzer, U.J. 1975. Analytical evaluation of seasoning extracts (oleoresins) and essential oils from seasonings. *International Flavours Food Additives* 6(3): 151–157.

Sankarikutty, B., Narayanan, C.S., Rajamani, K., Sumanthikutty, M.A., Omanakutty, M., and Mathew, A.G. 1982. Oil and oleoresin from major spices. *Journal of Plantation Crops* 10(1): 1–20.

Sankarikutty, B., Sreekumar, M. M., Narayanan, C. S., and Mathew, A. G. 1988. Studies on microencapsulation of cardamom oil by spray drying technique. *Journal of food science and technology* 25(6): 352–356.

Sarder, B. R., Tarade, K. M., and Singhal, R. S. 2013. Stability of active components of cardamom oleoresin in co-crystallized sugar cube during storage. *Journal of Food Engineering* 117(4): 530–537.

Sasikumar, B., and Sharma, Y.R. 2001. Role of spices in national economy. *FAFAI*, 21–23.

Satyal, P., Dosoky, N.S., Kincer, B.L., and Setzer, W.N. 2012. Chemical compositions and biological activities of *Amomum subulatum* essential oils from Nepal. *Natural Product Communications* 7(9): 1233–1236.

Savan, E.K., and Kucukbay, F.Z. 2013. Essential oil composition of *Elettaria cardamomum* Maton. *Journal of Applied Biological Sciences* 7: 42–45.

Shukla, S.H., Mistry, H.A., Patel, V.G., and Jogi, B.V. 2010. Pharmacognostical, preliminary phytochemical studies and analgesic activity of *Amomum subulatum* Roxb. *Pharma Science Monitor* 1(1): 90–102.

Singh, G., Kapoor, I.P.S., and Singh, B. 2009. Essential oil and oleoresins of cardamom (*Amomum subulatum* Roxb.) as natural food preservatives for sweet orange (*Citrus sinensis*) juice. *Journal of Food Process Engineering* 34: 1101–1113.

Steele, C. L., Lewinsohn, E., and Croteau, R. 1995. Induced oleoresin biosynthesis in grand fir as a defense against bark beetles. *Proceedings of the National Academy of Sciences* 92 (10): 4164–4168.

Su, H. C. and Horvat, R. 1981. Isolation, identification, and insecticidal properties of Piper nigrum amides. *Journal of Agricultural and Food Chemistry* 29(1): 115–118.

Suresh, M. P. 1987. Value added products: better scope with cardamom. *Cardamom* 20(1): 8–11.

Utta-'Ur, R., Choudhary, M. I., Ahmed, A., Iqbal, M. Z., Demirci, B., Demirci, F., and Baser, K.H.C. 2000. Antifungal activity and essential oil constituent of some spices from Pakistan. *Journal of Chemical Society Pakistan* 22: 60–65.

Verma, S.K., Rajeevan, V., Bordia, A., and Jain, V. 2010. Greater cardamom (*Amomum subulatum* Roxb.)–a cardio-adaptogen against physical stress. *Journal of Herbal Medicine and Toxicology* 4(2): 55–58.

Yadav, A.S., and Bhatnagar, D. 2007. Modulatory effect of spice extracts on iron-induced lipid peroxidation in rat liver. *Biofactors* 29: 147–157.

CHAPTER 17

Chemistry and Characterization of Clove Oleoresin

Gurpreet Kaur, Kamalpreet Kaur, and Preeti Kukkar

Mata Gujri College

Navneet Kaur Panag

Baba Banda Singh Bahadur Engineering College

Jashanpreet Kaur

Mata Gujri College

CONTENTS

DOI: 10.1201/9781003186205-17

329

17.1 INTRODUCTION

Currently, usage of medicinal herbs is becoming more in demand as a safe and effective measure for controlling various fatal diseases. Plants are often favoured because they are safe, economical, and do not exhibit adverse effects (Dhinahar and Lakshmi, 2011). A massive number of people (75%–80%) in growing regions are based on herbals for the maintenance of their health (Ekor, 2014). Plants show several medicinal values like antiviral, antibacterial, fungicidal, microbicidal, and anti-inflammatory. Various pharmacological applications of medicinal plants might be attributed to their phytochemicals, such as flavonoids, alkaloids, terpenes, tannins, glycosides, and saponins (Batiha et al., 2018; Beshbishy et al., 2019). These phytoconstituents may serve as an ideal agent in the exploration of effective and novel drugs.

Syzygium aromaticum or *Eugenia cariophylata* belongs to the Myrtaceae family and is often called a clove. It is an 8–12 m average-sized tree indigenous to the Moluccas in the eastern part of Indonesia. The discovery of this valuable spice and the marketing of clove enhanced the economic status of the Asiatic zone (Kamatou et al., 2012). Clove oil is secreted by plants by secondary metabolic pathways (Atanasova-Pancevska et al., 2017) and isolated from leaves, buds, and flower (Riyanto et al., 2016; Uddin et al., 2017) through distillation (Sahraoui and Boutekedjiret, 2015; Rassem et al., 2016; Nam et al., 2017). Essential oil derivatives such as oleoresin (Kamatou et al., 2012; Gaspar et al., 2018) are commercially significant in the food, health, and cosmetics industries (Nejad et al., 2017), as food preservatives, and pesticides (Kamatou et al., 2012; Xu et al., 2016). Cloves are employed as a warming agent and stimulator in Chinese and Indian traditional medicine (Batiha et al., 2019). Clove has been found valuable for centuries in the cure of intestinal gas, hepatic complications, nausea and neurological and gastric diseases. Moreover, in tropical Asia, it has been shown protective potential against various pathogenic diseases such as malaria, cholera, and tuberculosis. Clove has been traditionally used in the cure of several fatal infections in America (Bhowmik et al., 2012). The protective efficacy of clove against various fatal infections is due to the presence of several phytoconstituents in greater amounts with antioxidant potential (Hu and Willett, 2002; Astuti et al., 2019). Clove oil is being valued for the main component eugenol, which possesses antiviral, antiseptic, antioxidant, anticancer, antibacterial, and immunomodulatory properties (Riyanto et al., 2016; Kasai et al., 2016; Mohamed and Badri, 2017; Rathinam dan Viswanathan, 2018; Rahman et al., 2018), and majorly employed in the cure of teeth and gums traditionally (Pulikottil and Nath, 2015). Eugenol can cross the dental pulp tissue easily and enter the blood flow. Other major constituents of clove oil are trans-caryophyllene, rhamnetin, eugenol acetate, kaempferol, 4-Hydroxy-3-methoxybenzaldehyde, oleanolic acid, Maslinic acid, bicornin, methyl ester of salicylic acid, gallotannic acid, eugenitin, campesterol, and stigmasterol (Mittal et al., 2014; Issac et al., 2015). The clove is reaped mainly from the unopened flower buds, which are dehydrated to secrete the familiar spice, i.e., whole clove buds. In addition, other derivatives of clove are volatile oils, produced from clove buds, ground cloves, and oleoresins (Nurdjannah and Bermawie, 2012). Clove oil, buds, and clove oleoresins (CORs) are sanctioned by US-FDA (Food and Drug Administration) as safe food additives (FEMA, 1978).

17.2 DISTRIBUTION, PRODUCTION, AND ECONOMIC IMPORTANCE

Clove is an aromatic spice tree. The clove name is taken from the French word "clou," which means "nail." The major manufacturers of clove are Indonesia, India, Tanzania, Malaysia, Madagascar, and Sri Lanka (Kamatou et al., 2012). In Brazil, 8000 ha of clove are cultivated in the Camamu, Itubera, Taperoa, Valenca, and Nilo Pecanha in the state of Bahia and producing around 2500 tonnes per year (Oliveira et al., 2007, 2009). Moreover, few countries like Malaysia, Kenya, China, and Grenada produce less amount of clove. The main producer is Indonesia, which exports more than 75%–80% of clove to its domestic market, followed by Madagascar, while the United Arab Emirates and Indonesia are the principal importers. After Indonesia, India became the second major consumer of clove. In India, clove is limited to Tamil Nadu, Karnataka, and Kerala. The chief clove-growing regions in Tamil Nadu are Tirunelveli, Nilgiris, Ramanathapuram, Kanyakumari, and Nagercoil. Major clove production in Kerala is found in Kollam (Kottayam), Kozhikode, and Thiruvananthapuram and in the South Kanara district of Karnataka (Board, 2010). The world annual clove output in the standard international trade is higher than 160,000 tonnes (Figure 17.1). The monetary value of cloves in the world accounts for 500 million dollars per year, which accounts for about 4% of the international spice trade. Generally, every continent of the globe is a consumer of clove up to some extent, but Asia is the largest consumer.

The import and export of the clove in the world mainly transit through two hubs: the UAE and Singapore. Apart from it, there is also a direct flow of clove between the producing and the consumer countries, e.g., Brazil exports directly to South American Countries, Madagascar to European countries, and Asian countries. On the other hand, Indonesia imports both directly and indirectly from the producing countries as well as through the transit hubs (Figure 17.2).

Clove is a conical myrtle, a medium-sized tree with a straight trunk with a height of 10–13 m. The greyish branches of clove are semi-erect and dense. Leaves are large oblong to elliptic, simple obovate opposite, glabrous, and possess plenty of essential oil secretory

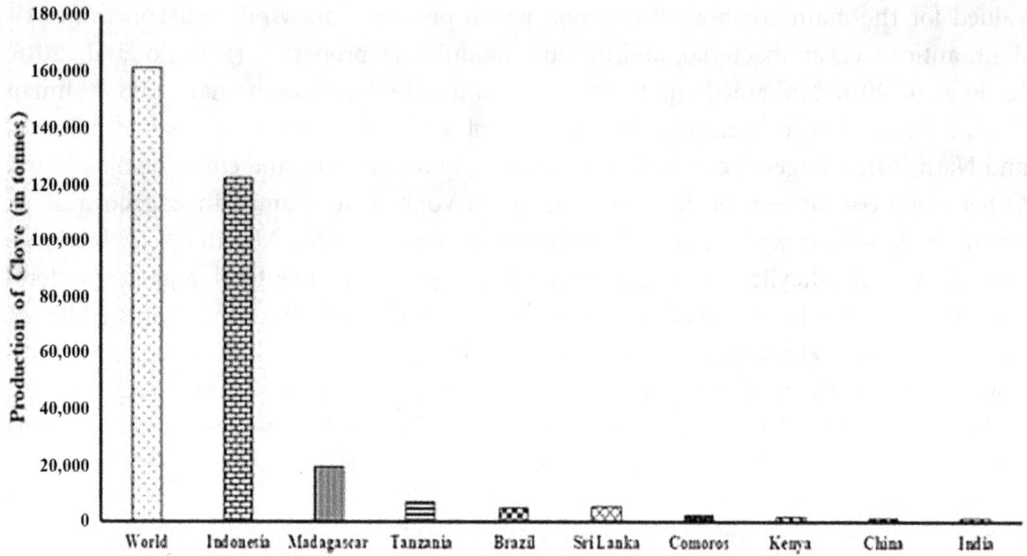

FIGURE 17.1   Clove production in the world (adapted from Danthu et al., 2020).

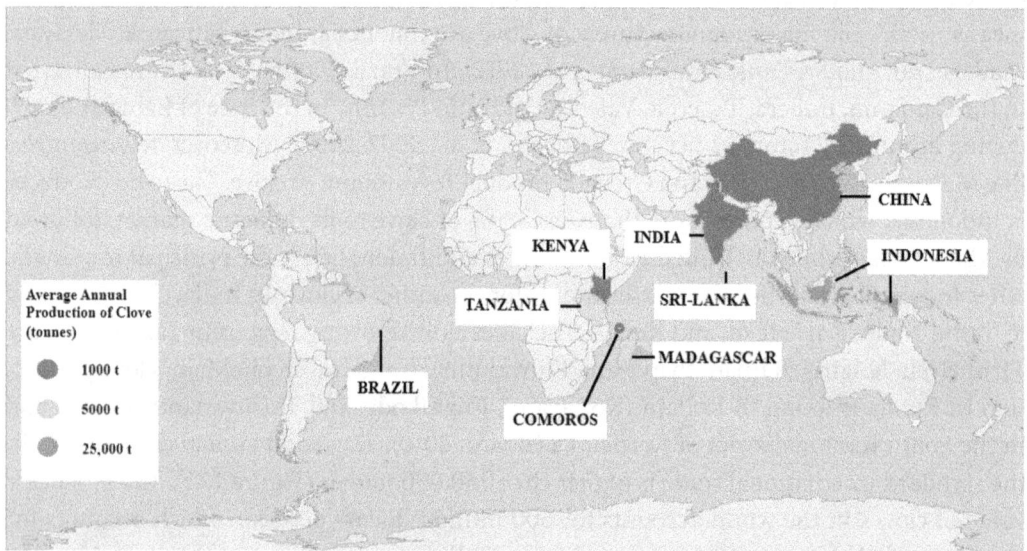

FIGURE 17.2   Distribution and production of the clove worldwide (adapted from Danthu et al., 2020).

glands on the bottom surface (Kamatou et al., 2012; Cortés-Rojas et al., 2014). Cloves have gained extraordinary attention because they are present all the time in several countries because of varied reaping periods. Various species of clove trees vary in the uppermost spreading branchy layer from pyramidal to cylindrical. It starts flowering in about 6–7 years and cannot tolerate a waterlogged environment. The life span of clove is up to a hundred years and prefers to grow in well-drained soil with sufficient soil moisture. Clove trees require heavy sunlight with high atmospheric temperature (25°C–35°C), well-distributed rainfall above 150 cm, and high humidity above 70% (Danthu et al., 2014). In India, this crop prefers deep black loamy soil or red soil and humid tropical environments for growth and to flourish well in Kerala, the Western Ghats in Tamil Nadu, and Karnataka (Byng et al., 2016). The clove tree is commonly planted in marshy regions at 200 m altitude above sea level. The flower buds begin after 4 years of sowing and are assembled in the ripening stage prior to flowering (Filho et al., 2013). Cloves are cultivated by small farmers in Indonesia, and they generate major income from it (Blakeney and Mengistie, 2012; Danthu et al., 2014). More than 31,000 farmers in Madagascar are dependent upon the farming of clove which has been combined into their agro-systems (Arimalala et al., 2019). Similarly, most of the people live from clove farming in Brazil. Clove is the reservoir of clove essential oil (CEO), extracted by various methods of extraction from the different components of the tree, such as leaves, cloves, and stems. The major portions of CEO are produced by Indonesia and Madagascar (Kraus, 2015).

Clove products and vanilla are considered to be the second-largest segment of Madagascar's agricultural exports. The export of cloves in Indonesia is employed in the secretion of the local cigarettes called Kretek. They use a mixture of clove and tobacco in a ratio of 1:2 for the formation of these cigarettes. The essence of the oil of clove is based on the quantity of a bioactive component eugenol in several commercial regions, such as pharmaceuticals, costumery, and the food industry (Danthu et al., 2014). Cloves have significant importance from culinary to medicine. Cloves in dried form are the main flavour enhancers in tea. Cloves also act as a flavouring agent in cookies, meat products, chewing gums, chocolates, spiced fruits, pastries, pickles, sandwiches, and candies. It is a beneficial spice in the kitchen that is employed for studding onions, salads, and herbal tea. This spice is employed in the cuisines of Russia, India, Greece, Scandinavia, and China. Usage of volatile clove oil provides fragrance to toothpaste, perfumes, soaps, and pharmaceuticals. Clove exhibits bactericidal activity and is employed in various dental creams, throat sprays, and mouthwashes to kill pathogens. It finds application in reducing the pain of sore gums. In the filling of dental cavities, eugenol (a huge active component of clove) and zinc oxide in combination is used transiently (Cai and Wu, 1996). The presence of flavonoids imparts anti-inflammatory activities in clove oil. Pure clove oil showed significant activity against arthritis and rheumatism. The mixture of clove and honey is employed to cure dermatological problems. Clove paste also enhances the healing of bites and cuts or injuries. The use of clove is recommended to cure several digestive complications such as loose motion, nausea, flatulence, and dyspepsia. It improves the immune system of the body and assists to resist invading pathogens. Clove is also known to treat Athlete's foot disease and Onychomycosis. CEO assists in relaxing several respiratory problems, such as cold, cough, sinusitis, asthma, and bronchiolitis. They exhibit protective efficacy against lung and skin carcinoma. Clove is used to lower the blood glucose level and hinders the development of blood clots. Topical application of clove can reduce muscular pain. It also hampers the disruption in the retina, which decreases the deterioration of muscles as well as enhances eyesight in aged people. Inhalation of clove fragrance lowers headache, drowsiness, and anxiety. It causes improvement in cognitive development by enhancing memory and reducing mental fog, tension, nervousness, and desperation. Clove oil is used as a repellent against mosquitoes (Trongtokit et al., 2005). Clove has more antioxidant activity as compared to other medicinal herbs. Clove oil has shown 400 times more potency in comparison to blueberries. Clove oil has a good remedy to treat inflammation of the ear in cats and dogs. These are used in herbal formulations to treat animals. Clove tea supplemented with peppermint, and ginger is used for the cure of puking in dogs. It is given thrice times daily according to the size of the animal (Hussain et al., 2017).

17.3 EXTRACTION, ISOLATION, CHARACTERIZATION, AND CHEMICAL COMPOSITION OF CLOVE OLEORESIN

The various chemical compounds isolated from clove include flavonoids, hydroxybenzoic acid, hydroxyphenyl propens, hydroxycinnamic acid, and phenolic acid (Hussain et al., 2017). The major flavonoid compound isolated from CEO and CRO includes eugenol, which constitutes nearly 72%–90% of the extracted chemical compounds. In addition to eugenol, the CEO also comprises eugenol acetate (~15%) and trans caryophyllene (~5%–12%) as other flavonoid compounds (Sebaaly et al., 2015). The other important compounds constituting the CEO include α-humulene (~2.1%), and numerous other volatile organic compounds (VOCs) (e.g., β-pinene, benzaldehyde, farnesol, and 2-heptanone) in traces (Aguilar and Malo, 2013) (Table 17.1). The daily safe limit for CEO consumption has been standardized as less than 2.5 mg/kg b.w.t. by the World Health Organization (WHO) (Nagababu and Lakshmaiah, 1992).

Eugenol with intensive analgesic, anti-inflammatory, anaesthetic, and antioxidant activities is approved by the US-FDA (Yogalakshmi et al., 2010). It constitutes between 9.38 and 14.65 g/100g of flower buds (Marchese et al., 2017). Chemically, eugenol is 2-methoxy-4-(2-propenyl) phenol with a yellowish appearance, having the chemical formula of $C_{10}H_{12}O_2$ (Pramod et al., 2010). Eugenol exhibits appreciable solubility in water and ethanol and accounts for the aromatic flavour of cloves (Table 17.2).

Extraction performs a crucial role in the chemical analysis and the retrieval of biologically active components from plant tissue. Various conventional methods of extraction like maceration, percolation, and Soxhlet are simple and easy techniques for the extraction of bioactive components from clove. With the advancements in technology, high purity extracts can be prepared, which can be used in the treatment of diseases and for improving health conditions (Belwal et al., 2018). Traditionally, clove oils are extracted by the solvent extraction method, steam distillation, or hydrodistillation (HD). These conventional processes of extraction have the advantage of being inexpensive, but suffer from serious disadvantages such as being time consuming, higher solvent volume requirements, inducing hydrolysis, possible thermal degradation, and water solubilization and hydrolysis of various fragrant components. The distinctive fragrance of plant materials is generally the consequence of complicated interactions that take place among the various components. The task of a precise reproduction of the normal fragrance in a concentrated extract is a difficult task. The most common hindrances in the reproduction of natural fragrances of plant materials are the existence of thermally unstable compounds, the likelihood of hydrolysis, and the solubility in water of a few fragrant compounds (Jeyaratnam et al., 2016). In addition, these conventional methods of extraction are associated with a few parameters that can be adjusted or controlled. It results in the extraction of less pure essential oils. The presence of organic solvents in essential oils is objectionable and is dangerous for both mankind and the environment. Currently, stringent legislative restrictions are enacted to remove solvent residues in cosmetic, pharmaceutical, and food

TABLE 17.1   Important Phytoconstituents of Clove Oleoresin

Oleanolic acid

2-Methoxy-4-(prop-2-en-1-yl)phenol

(Eugenol)

Gallic acid

Ellagic acid

2-methyl-5-propan-2-ylphenol

(Carvacrol)

3,5,7-Trihydroxy-2-(4-hydroxyphenyl)-
4H-chromen-4-one

(Kaempferol)

4-Hydroxy 3 methoxybenzaldehyde

(Vanillin)

(Continued)

TABLE 17.1 (*Continued*)   Important Phytoconstituents of Clove Oleoresin

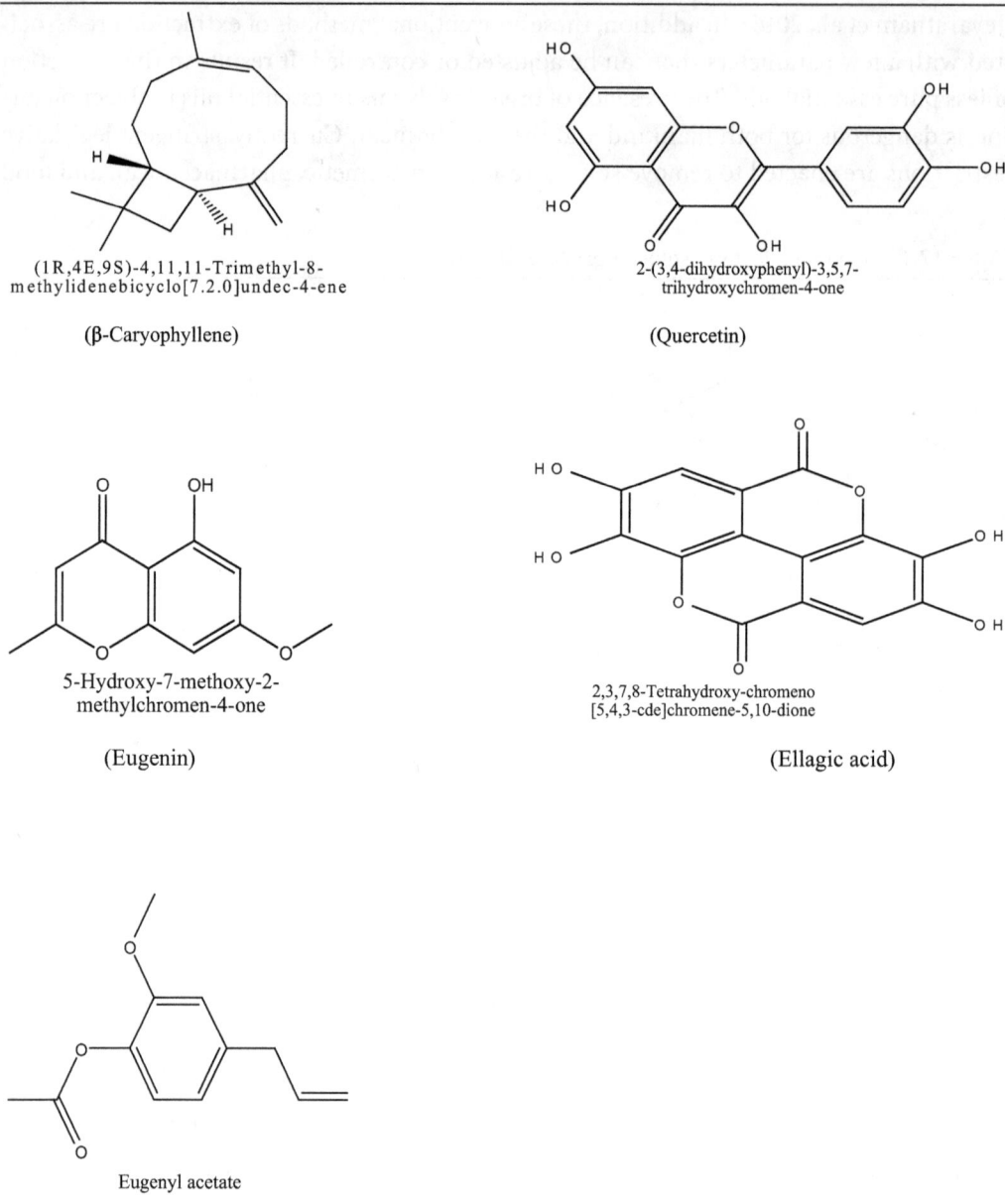

(1R,4E,9S)-4,11,11-Trimethyl-8-
methylidenebicyclo[7.2.0]undec-4-ene

(β-Caryophyllene)

2-(3,4-dihydroxyphenyl)-3,5,7-
trihydroxychromen-4-one

(Quercetin)

5-Hydroxy-7-methoxy-2-
methylchromen-4-one

(Eugenin)

2,3,7,8-Tetrahydroxy-chromeno
[5,4,3-cde]chromene-5,10-dione

(Ellagic acid)

Eugenyl acetate

industries. Various experimental modifications are performed to overcome these limitations. Nonconventional extraction methods like microwave-assisted extraction (MWAE),
high-pressure liquid extraction, supercritical CO_2-assisted extraction, ultrasound-assisted
extraction, and enzyme-assisted extraction methods are more selective approaches of
extraction. Recently, the use of green solvents in lab-scale extraction has resulted in the
production of first-class quality plant extracts with economical profits (Belwal et al., 2020).
Over the past many years, numerous researchers have attempted the extraction and chemical analysis of CEO owing to its myriad of medicinal properties. Herein, we review some

TABLE 17.2   Chemical Composition and Pharmacological Potential of the Clove

Phytoconstituents	Part of the Plant	Biological Activity	References
Volatile Constituents (Pino et al., 2001)			
Eugenol (73%–79%)	Clove bud oil	Antioxidant	Saeed et al. (2021)
Eugenyl acetate (15%)		Antimicrobial	Pino et al. (2001)
β-Caryophyllene		Anti-inflammatory	Uddin et al. (2017)
Methyl salicylate		Neuroprotective	Francomano et al. (2019)
β-Humulene		Antitumour	Cai and Wu (1996)
Benzaldehyde		Anti-apoptotic	Xin et al. (2014)
Chavicol		Anti-arthritis	Deans and Svoboda (1989)
		Anti-inflammatory	Ramos-Nino et al. (1996)
		Antibacterial	Ohigashi and Koshimizu
		Antilisterial	(1976)
		Larvicidal	
Eugenol (76.4%–84.8%)	Stem oil	Antioxidant, Anticancer,	Kamatou et al. (2012)
Eugenyl acetate (1.5%–8.0%)	Leaf oil	Anthelmintic, Antiulcer,	Gopalakrishnan et al. (1988)
β-Caryophyllene		Anti-inflammatory,	Francomano et al. (2019)
α-Humulene		Anti-depressant,	Fernandes et al. (2007)
		Neuroprotective	
		Anticancer	
		Anti-inflammatory	
Eugenol (50%–55%)	Fruit oil	Antimicrobial	Kamatou et al. (2012)
		Analgesic	
		Antioxidant	
Polar Constituents			
Flavonoids (Nassar, 2006)	Seeds	Antioxidant	Bhuiyan et al. (2010)
Isobiflorin	Flower buds	Anticancer	Vasconcellos et al. (2011)
Biflorin		Antibacterial	Zhang et al. (2011)
Apigenin		Antioxidant	Imran et al. (2020)
Gossypetin 7-O		Antibacterial	Ghai et al. (2014)
rhamnopyranoside		Anticancer	Ming et al. (2005)
Triterpenes	Buds of clove	Anti-diabetic	Castellano et al. (2013)
Oleanolic acid		Antitumour	Sánchez-Tena et al. (2013)
Maslinic acid			
Tannins	Leaves of clove	Antioxidant	Wang et al. (2016)
Eugenol glucoside gallate		Anticancer	Tanaka et al. (1993)
Syzyginin A		Anti-inflammatory	Gupta et al. (2014)
Syzyginin B		Hepatoprotective	
		Antioxidant	

of the studies published in the past decade that exhibit the extraction and purification of CEO. Various significant conventional/nonconventional modes of extraction of bioactive constituents from the clove are briefly described herein:

17.3.1 Solvent Extraction

It is a commonly employed technique for obtaining COR. Therefore, several solvents like ethanol, hexane, and petroleum ether can be exploited for obtaining eugenol from different parts of the clove plant. The solvent extraction process is associated with some limitations like the addition of other soluble products, disagreeable flavour variations in the food items, etc. (Guan et al., 2007). Despite the limitations, the solvent extraction method finds extensive applications in the extraction process of COR. Clove buds are first ground to a fine powder, which is then wrapped in filter paper. The filter paper is then put into the extraction thimble and transferred into a refluxing flask of suitable capacity. Then a suitable solvent is used to extract eugenol oil using a Soxhlet apparatus. The product obtained is concentrated by heating it at 50°C temperature using a rotary vacuum evaporator. This conventional method of solvent extraction can be modified in various ways to increase efficiency, like the batch extraction process, can act as an interesting substitute for the Soxhlet extraction process. El-Refai et al. (2020) collected organic and aqueous extracts of clove buds in 95% ethanol and distilled water, sieved and then ethanol was evaporated in a rotary evaporator and yielded dry product under controlled conditions of temperature (600°C) and reduced pressure. Comparison of ethanolic and aqueous extracts was done for the presence of total phenols and flavonols. The Folin–Ciocalteu procedure (2016) was employed for the estimation of total phenolic compounds, which were expressed in terms of (GAE)/g, i.e., milligram gallic acid equivalent. Total flavonoids were monitored by using the method given by Li et al. (2007) and were expressed as QE/g extract, i.e., mg of quercetin equivalent.

It was found that ethanolic extract of clove buds contained a large quantity of TPC (372.21 mg GAE/g of extract) and the highest total flavonoid compound, i.e., (177.15 mg QE/g of extract) (Figure 17.3). El-Maati et al. (2016) also obtained comparable results. So, the ethanol/water system was a superior solvent system for obtaining phenolic compounds, and water behaved as the most superior solvent for obtaining flavonoids. Moreover, Mohammed et al. (2016) characterized the chemical composition of ethanolic extract of clove for monitoring the content of sulphur, nitrogen, ketones, aldehydes, phenolics, and anthraquinones. The chief constituents of the extract were found to be anthraquinones and ketones as validated using Ultraviolet and Fourier Transform Infrared (FTIR) analysis data.

17.3.2 Hydrodistillation

Hydrodistillation (HD) is the most commonly used conventional inexpensive extraction technique for extracting essential oils, and it uses modified Clevenger apparatus for the extraction process. Volatile essential oils are first converted into vapours and are then converted into liquids by the process of condensation. COR is extracted using the HD process extensively by many research groups. To extract eugenol from clove oil (Jeyaratnam et al., 2016; Khalil et al., 2017), a finely powdered sample of dehydrated and ground clove buds was initially submerged into water and then was subjected to the HD process for a period of 4–6 hours. The volatile distillate accumulated in a clean flask was saturated with sodium chloride. A suitable organic solvent such as petroleum ether was then used to extract COR from the distillate. The two separate layers of water-soluble and ether soluble components were separated. The organic layer was dehydrated using a suitable dehydrating agent such as anhydrous sodium sulphate. The extract was concentrated by distilling the sample in a water bath. The product was obtained in 11.5% yield with 50.5%–53.5% concentration of eugenol. The product yield showed an indirect relationship with the particle size of pulverized buds of clove. Uddin et al. (2017) extracted clove oil from ground clove buds by the HD method using Clevenger apparatus consisting of a double glass boiler

Phenolic compounds (mg GAE/g)

(a)

■ Ethanolic Extract whole   ▫ Ethanolic Extract powder   ▣ Aqueous Extract whole
⊞ Aqueous Extract powder   ▯ Essential Oil Extract whole

Flavonoid compounds (mg QE/g)

(b)

■ Ethanolic Extract whole   ▫ Ethanolic Extract powder   ▣ Aqueous Extract whole
⊞ Aqueous Extract powder   ▥ Essential Oil Extract whole

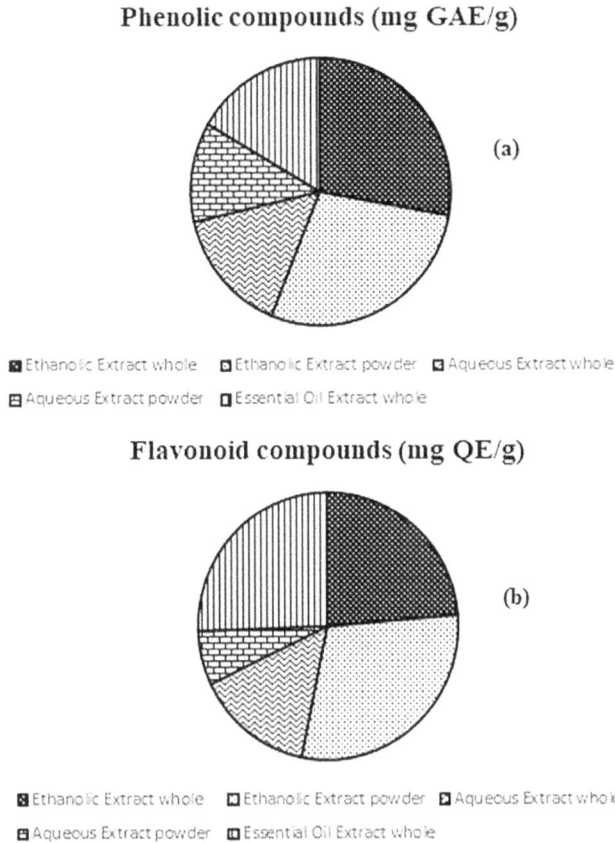

FIGURE 17.3   (a) Total phenolic and (b) flavonoid compounds of clove extracts (adapted from El-Refai et al., 2020).

having many valves, and the volatile distillate was collected. The extract so collected was dried by using anhydrous sodium sulphate. The chemical composition of the COR was monitored by Gas chromatography–mass spectrometry (GC-MS) analysis, which indicated the existence of 13 unique constituents in it. The major compounds present in clove oil were (a) eugenol acetate; (b) 2-pentanone, 4-hydroxy-4-methyl; (c) caryophyllene; and (d) 3-allyl-6-methoxyphenol, while the components present in minor amounts were (a) 1,4,7-cycloundecatriene; (b) copaene; (c) 2-pentanone-3-methylene; (d) 2,4,4,6-tetram ethyl-4,5-dihydro-1,3-oxazine; (e) 1,5,9,9-tetramethyl-Z,Z,Z-toluene; (f) alpha-farnesene; (g) meta dioxan-4-ol; (h) 6-diethyl-5-methylacetate; and (i) 2,6-diethyl-5-methyl acetate as indicated in Table 17.3. Similarly, Santos et al. (2009) characterized the oil from clove buds using gas chromatography and differential scanning calorimetry. It was found that oil of clove bud contains the maximum amount (90%) of eugenol.

17.3.3 Steam HD

Ratri et al. (2020) used the steam HD method for extracting clove oil from dried clove buds. For this, 25 g of dried clove buds were taken in a steam distillation flask. The steam

TABLE 17.3   Chemical Composition of the COR Extracted from the Buds of *Eugenia caryophyllum*

Component	Concentration (%)
Toluene	1.873
Tetramethyl-dihydro-1,3-oxazine	0.15
2-Pentanone, 4-hydroxy-4-methyl	7.785
3-Allyl-6-methoxyphenol	69.436
Copaene	0.219
Alpha-farnesene	0.163
Caryophyllene	6.803
Caryophyllene oxide	0.048
Eugenol acetate	10.798
2-Pentanone-3-methylene	0.286

Adapted from Uddin et al. (2017).

HD was performed for several hours, namely 3, 4, 5, and 6 hours. The distillation so collected was extracted with n-hexane as solvent with the help of a separatory funnel. The essential oil was obtained by evaporating the solvent. Moreover, enhancing the extraction time also boosts the yield of extracted products. The maximum yield of clove oil (7.04%) was collected when extraction time was lengthened from 2 to 6 hours. The main constituents obtained from clove oil were eugenol and eugenol acetate. Clove bud waste was utilized for making eco-friendly packaging, such as cardboards.

The composition of COR was evaluated using FTIR and GC-MS studies, and the findings were compared with commercial clove oil (100% purity). ATR-FTIR studies were also carried out to find the functional groups present in the compounds. Besides this, GC-MS utilizing the electrospray ionization method was employed to quantify clove oil contents based on their mass-to-charge (m/z). The extracted COR and commercially available clove oil samples show similarity in IR peaks, indicating that extracted COR had similar components as present in commercially available oil. GC-MS spectra of extracted clove oil indicated two major components, viz. eugenol and eugenyl acetate, in 85.01% and 13.06% compositions, respectively (Table 17.4).

17.3.4 Two-Phase Extraction Method

Aqueous two-phase extraction systems (e.g., water and inorganic salts) provide a benign substitute for the conventional organic solvent–water systems used for purification of CEO. Consequently, the aqueous two-phase extraction acts as a more feasible approach for the purification of labile bioactive materials susceptible to degradation in the organic solvents. Likewise, microencapsulation of CEOs can substantially increase their shelf life by reducing their evaporation and slower release rate. Considering the benefits of aqueous two-phase extraction and microencapsulation technologies, Xiong et al. (2018) combined these two approaches for the separation and purification of CEO by utilizing sodium sulphate and β-cyclodextrin. The various VOCs present in the CEO were characterized using nuclear magnetic resonance (NMR) spectroscopy. The two-phase extraction cum

TABLE 17.4 Phytoconstituents of Extracted Oil of Clove and Commercial Clove Oil

Compound	Extracted Oil of Clove		Commercial Pure Clove Oil	
	Retention Time (RT)	% Area	Retention Time (RT)	% Area
Methyl salicylate	14.33	0.06	14.29	0.05
Chavicol	16.00	0.19	15.98	0.04
Eugenol	18.99	85.01	18.98	81.35
α-Ylangene	20.27	0.04	20.23	0.11
Caryophyllene	21.55	1.14	21.52	5.05
Humulene	22.61	0.18	22.58	0.76
Eugenyl acetate	23.93	13.06	23.90	12.50
Caryophyllene oxide	26.88	0.32	26.83	0.14

Adapted from Ratri et al. (2020).

microencapsulation method yielded two major components as eugenol acetate (9.23%) and eugenol (90.77%) (Xiong et al., 2018). On a comparative note, the authors noted the presence of multiple components, including eugenol (70.42%), eugenol acetate (15.50%), and trans-caryophyllene (14.08%) in crude olive oil extracted using the steam distillation method. The authors concluded that cyclodextrin encapsulation of CEO offered excellent separation of the major component of CEO relative to the steam distillation method. Further, FTIR analysis of the encapsulated samples indicated the presence of characteristic peaks of β-cyclodextrin. These observations confirmed the consistency of the β-cyclodextrin structure before and after the encapsulation of CEO (Xiong et al., 2018). Overall, this study exemplified the applicability of the encapsulation method for the separation and purification of CEO.

17.3.5 Low-Temperature Extraction of COR by Liquid Gases

Many reports are available in literature where essential oils are extracted by using liquefied gases like air, carbon dioxide, Freon, etc. The extracted products have the advantage of being harmless and thus find extensive application in the cosmetic, medicine, food, and flavour industries (Reverchon and Senatore, 1994; Reverchon et al., 1995; Belwal et al., 2020). Stoyanova et al. (1998) employed 1,1,1,2-tetrafluoroethane to obtain extracts of clove oil (*S. aromaticum*) and thus determined its antimicrobial and antioxidant properties. Clove buds having a humidity level of 10% were crushed to a size of 0.15–0.25 mm in an attrition mill. 1 dm^3 volume of $C_2H_2F_4$ was used to obtain the extract under conditions of continuous flow and subsequent evaporation of the solvent for 60 minutes at 0.5 MPa pressure and 18°C–20°C temperature. A dark yellow oily product was obtained in 8%–12% yield (v/w) having an intense characteristic smell of raw clove. The clove oil extract in $C_2H_2F_4$ was analysed using GC/MS analysis. When compared with other extracts obtained with 1,1,1,2-tetrafluoroethane, it was noticed that the clove extract exhibited remarkable antioxidant properties against commonly spread infective and spoilage bacteria and excellent antioxidant properties in contrast to other extracts

TABLE 17.5   Chemical Composition of Extracted Clove Oil

Components	wt%
Myrcene	0.31
α-Humulene	1.08
β-Caryophyllene	9.28
α-Copaene	0.81
Methyl eugenol	0.14
δ-Cardinene	0.18
Eugenol	69.72
Eugenyl acetate	13.42
Caryophyllene oxide	1.32

Adapted from Atanasova et al. (2013).

obtained by using the low-temperature extraction technique. The chief components of the clove extract are indicated in Table 17.5.

17.3.6 Supercritical Fluid Extraction

Extraction of essential oils/flavouring materials through liquid and supercritical CO_2 has been a fascinating technique of extraction for the last many decades. There are many reasons for using this extraction technique like the ability of carbon dioxide to serve as an appropriate solvent under prevailing conditions of high-pressure and subcritical /supercritical conditions of temperature (Della Porta et al., 1998). The supercritical carbon dioxide extraction technique acts as a good substitute to overcome the limitations associated with conventional extraction methods utilizing HD and solvent extraction. The natural aroma of essential oils is not affected by heat, water, and the presence of solvent residues. Gopalakrishanan et al. (1990) found that chlorophyll content in extracted clove oil increased as pressure was increased from 100 to 500 bar, temperature being fixed at 40°C. The supercritical CO_2 extraction (supercritical fluid extraction (SFE)) has the advantage that it can be executed at ambient temperature and a relatively lower pressure. At the end of the extraction method, CO_2 is removed from the reaction mixture (Reverchon and Senatore, 1994; Reverchon et al., 1995). Also, supercritical CO_2 behaves like a lipophilic solvent, so its solvent power and/or selective nature can be modified by alteration in temperature and pressure conditions. But the choice of the correct extraction conditions is required to prevent the co-extraction of other high molecular weight components. Moreover, many research groups have reported the efficient extraction of CEO by employing supercritical extraction techniques (Moyler, 1986; Huston and Ji, 1991). CO_2 acts as the most suitable solvent in SFE because of the following reasons: (a) it is comparatively cheaper; (b) simpler to use; (c) has strong affinity for lipophilic compounds; (d) non-toxic in nature; and (e) adjustable solvent ability in comparison to other solvents, which can be adjusted for values extending from gas-like to liquid-like (Della Porta et al., 1998).

Della Porta et al. (1998) isolated volatile oils from the buds of clove and star anise by performing SFE-CO_2 extraction. The conditions of temperature and pressure for the extraction and fractionation of volatile essential oils were optimized. They evaluated the influence of extraction time and pressure (200–300 bar) on the composition of extracted oil. GC-MS analysis was performed on the various fractions retrieved after varying the extraction times and pressure. The optimum conditions of pressure and temperature were investigated not only for procuring an ample amount of terpene compounds accountable for the strong fragrance but also to circumvent the extraction of undesirable products such as fatty acids, anthocyanins, polymethoxyflavones, methyl esters, and other colouring materials. Diverse solvent pressures extending from 80 to 200 bar and various temperatures varying from 40°C to 50°C were studied to establish the best suited conditions for extraction. The best results were attained at pressure of 90 bar and temperature being set at 50°C (Reverchon, 1992).

17.3.7 Modified Supercritical Fluid Extraction (SFE)

The selectivity as well as the solubility of the extraction of COR can be enhanced by optimizing the SFE process by adding a fixed amount of co-solvent or entrainer to the SC-CO_2 flow (Della Porta et al. 1998). If any effort is made to evaporate the co-solvent from the extract, it is generally accompanied by the loss of desirable and valuable volatile components. Efficiency can be further increased by either using a blend of two distinct plant materials or adding essential oil of one pure plant to the other. Oszagyan et al. (1994) obtained extracts of essential oils from a blend of thyme/rosemary (T/R) and thyme/lavender systems to prevent loss of required volatile components obtained from pure plants of rosemary and lavender. The same components were present in the extracts obtained from one-to-one mixtures of T/R or T/L as extracted from the individual plants but in totally different concentrations. It was also suggested and proved that essential oil obtained from another plant when mixed with thyme could be used as a potential agent and it does not need to be removed from the desired end product. There was a blending of the biological activities of different plants and a few reports proved that the effect was synergistic.

Ivanovic et al. (2011) carried out simultaneous analysis of kinetics and mass transfer phenomenon of extraction of CEO employing SFE from the blend of two plants (clove/thyme and clove/oregano) by varying their initial compositions. The extraction of essential oils from pure clove buds (C), thyme leaves (T), and oregano leaves (O) was performed, and the results were compared with the products obtained from clove/oregano (C/O) and clove/thyme (C/T) mixtures by taking various compositions using the supercritical CO_2 extraction process under conditions of 10 MPa pressure and 40°C temperature. Clove, thyme, and oregano were selected for the present studies owing to the existence of high levels of antimicrobials such as eugenol in clove, and thymol and carvacrol in oregano and thyme. Studies on the chemical composition in addition to kinetic survey of SFE of COR from clove buds under varied conditions of pressure (10–30 MPa) and temperature (25–55°C) are available in the literature (Clifford et al., 1999; Yazdani et al., 2005; Guan et al., 2007; Martínez et al., 2007; Hatami et al., 2010). The chemical compositions and kinetics of supercritical CO_2 extraction of essential oils from oregano (Menaker et al., 2004; Cavero et al., 2006; Ocana-Fuentes et al., 2010) and thyme (Zeković et al. 2000; Díaz-Maroto et al., 2005; Grosso et al., 2010; Babovic et al., 2010) at a pressure ranging from 8 to 40 MPa and temperature varying from 20°C to 100°C have already been notified by various research groups.

The existence of lighter compounds at the commencement of the supercritical CO_2 extraction process from oregano or thyme leaves (C/T-84:16% weight/weight and C/O-90:10%, weight/weight) intensified the rate of extraction of compounds from clove buds with negligible effect on total extraction yields as extracted from pure clove buds was detected. The experimental data were also simulated by mathematical modelling, which demonstrated increased solubility of the extracted products accompanied by increased mass transfer rate of extracted compounds in solid-state when extracted from a mixture of C/O (90:10, w/w) and C/T (84:16, w/w). The extracts obtained from this chemical composition have only bits of compounds existing in thyme or oregano (like thymoquinone, thymol, and carvacrol). Also, an insignificant enhancement in extraction rate was detected when the proportion of oregano in the clove/oregano mixture was increased. This decrease in the extraction time for obtaining extraction product in desirable yield was accompanied by lesser consumption (app. 70%) of SC-CO_2 in SFE of the clove buds, which can find extensive utility in industrial-scale application. Notably, the occurrence of even trace amounts of oregano and thyme in the starting mixture with clove buds facilitated a significant enhancement in extraction rates. However, the presence of a small amount of either oregano or thyme to clove buds had an insignificant effect on extraction yields in comparison to the extraction from pure clove. Both oregano and thyme contained few components that are primarily soluble in supercritical CO_2 in the pre-treatment step. Comparatively lighter compounds procured from the pre-treatment of oregano or thyme solubilize in CO_2 and behave as modifiers or co-solvents and thus alter the solubility potential of SC-CO_2. This increased the solubility of comparatively less soluble and heavier components prevailing in clove buds (like eugenol acetate, eugenol, and trans-caryophyllene). The products extracted from a mixture of C/O (90:10, w/w):C/T (84:16, w/w) by employing SFE comprising insignificant amounts of compounds present in oregano or thyme (thymol, thymoquinone, and carvacrol). In contrast, an inconsiderable increase in extraction rate was observed in the presence of excess amounts of oregano present in the clove/oregano mixture (C/O:<50:50%, w/w).

17.3.8 Microwave-Assisted Extraction of COR

The MWAE is considered the best green extraction process that could produce essential clove oil without compromising the quality of the product. This method requires many microwave-absorbing solvents for the extraction. In comparison to conventional extraction methods, COR is produced cost-effectively along with the decreased time required for the extraction process. Solvent-free extraction (Périno-Issartier et al., 2011) essential oils are also possible with MWAE and it is another advantage of the MWAE technique over other methods (Chemat et al., 2019). In this green extraction approach, plant material is dipped in a non-absorbing fluid and microwave radiations are irradiated on the plant material. Huge pressure, higher than the expansion capability, is developed inside the oil glands because of high thermal current and localized strong pressure, causing the bursting of oil glands and releasing essential oil at rates faster than that in conventional methods. The MWAE technique makes use of various configurations such as microwave-assisted HD (MWHD), coaxial MWHD (coaxial MWHD), microwave steam distillation (MWSD), and microwave-assisted hydro-diffusion and gravity (MWHG) method (Khalil et al., 2017). Out of these green methods, coaxial MWHD is more beneficial because of (a) lesser energy consumption (30%); (b) more energy savings vis-à-vis heating time (400%); (c) cost-effective; (d) safe; and (e) easier scale-up configurations. Gonzalez-Rivera et al. (2016) investigated that coaxial MWHD had the potential for the extraction of various oils such as rosemary, clove, fennel, and lavender. Extraction through coaxial MWHD technique showed that essential products such as eugenol exhibited high thermal stability accompanied by lesser extraction time as compared to traditional extraction methods. At the same time, MWAE techniques can be used for industrial level scale-up. MWHD method makes use of HD using water as a solvent in presence of microwave heating and has the potential to replace conventional methods of extraction.

Haqqyana et al. (2020) used the MWHD for the extraction of COR from the dried stem of the clove. Kinetic mechanisms and appropriate kinetic models were evaluated by them for microwave-assisted HD of clove oil. From kinetic mechanism studies and modelling, the extraction behaviour of essential oils can be predicted and can be utilized for scaling up the extraction processes. To check the effect of irradiating power of the microwave as the heating source on parameters of the kinetic model, heating of the sample was performed at different settings of power (300, 450, 600, and 800 W), with a total extraction time of 120 minutes, which was done at an interval of 10 minutes. In their studies on the extraction of oils from solid material, two-parametric kinetic models were used based on four models: Hyperbolic model, Weibull's exponential equation, Elovich's equation, and Power-law model were evaluated. The yield of extracted clove oil was calculated in different power settings and was then fitted in the parameters of the kinetic model. It was found that the experimental data obtained and all the four kinetic models applied were in good agreement with each other, but Weibull's exponential equation gave the best results. There was a direct relationship between microwave power and extraction yield.

Kapadiya et al. (2018) applied the MWAE method for the isolation of CEO from clove buds. The extraction process was optimized by varying various experimental parameters (e.g., plant material (30 g), quantity of water used (200 mL), microwave power (600 W), and extraction time (30 minutes) by using the Taguchi method). Under the optimized conditions, the maximum yields of CEO, eugenol content, and bacterial inhibition (zone of inhibition) were estimated to be 13.11% (w/w), 11.93% (w/w), and 24.80 mm, respectively (Kapadiya et al., 2018). Of late, a green technique of *in situ* microwave-assisted extraction (IMWAE) was utilized for isolation and chemical analysis of CEO from dried buds of clove (Gonzalez-Rivera et al., 2021). These authors also compared the performance of IMWAE and HD methods towards the quantification of byproducts including residual condensed water and solid residues. The IMWAE was performed at 150 W for 10 minutes for the extraction of the CEO. In a parallel experiment, the HD process was carried out in a Clevenger extractor operating at 250 W of power. The quantitative chemical analysis of the extracted CEO from both techniques was performed using headspace GC-MS methods (Gonzalez-Rivera et al., 2021). The GC-MS analysis of the extracted CEO displayed the occurrence of eugenol (48.9%±2.5%), trans-caryophyllene (42.8%±2.1%), alpha-caryophyllene (3.7%±0.2%), alpha-cubebene (2.3%±0.1%), and copaene (2.2%±0.1%),

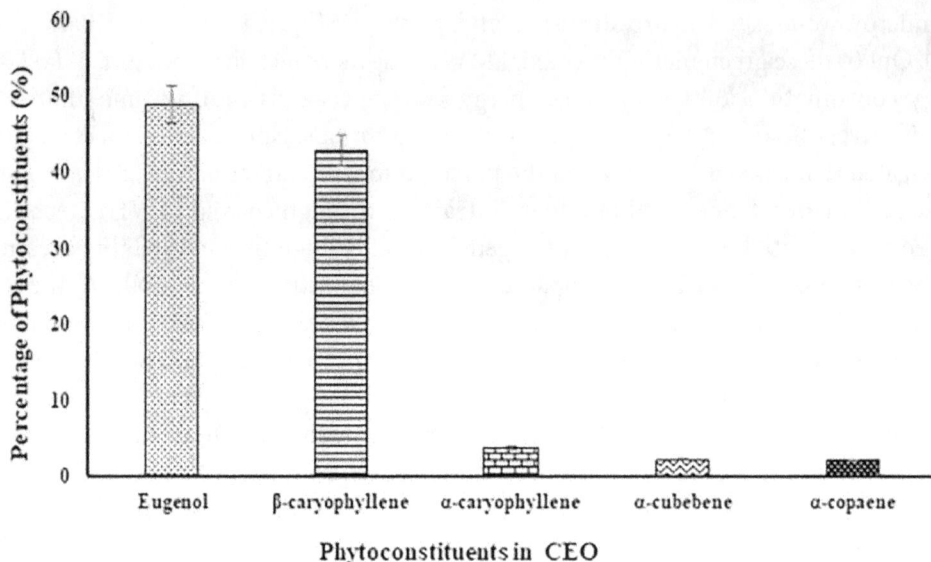

FIGURE 17.4   GC-MS analysis of extracted CEO (adapted from Gonzalez-Rivera et al., 2021).

respectively (Figure 17.4). However, the chemical composition of the CEO derived from both the methods was indistinguishable to compare their performance. Nevertheless, the high-pressure liquid chromatography (HPLC-DAD-FD) analysis of IMWAE yielded water residues, containing 1/3 of eugenol content relative to that derived from HD. The relatively lower content of eugenol in water residues suggested more efficient extraction and separation performance of IMWAE in comparison to the HD approach. Further, the CEO yield using IMWAE and HD methods was 16%±1.5% and 7.8%±0.8%, respectively. Moreover, thermo-gravimetric and FTIR spectroscopy proved the excess of hemicellulose, lignin, and cellulose in IMWAE-derived residues in contrast to that procured from the HD. These observations indicated the higher efficiency of microwave radiation towards the removal of lignin/ phenolic compounds oligomers relative to the HD process (Gonzalez-Rivera et al., 2021).

17.3.9 Ultrasound-Assisted Extraction

Ultrasound-assisted extraction (UAE) is a budding vivid green technology used for extraction of clove oil where ultrasonic waves after interaction with plant material change the physical as well as chemical properties and release the extracted product because of the rupturing of cell walls. Using UAE, extraction is completed within minutes, whereas the conventional methods require hours for the extraction process (Chemat and Khan, 2011). It has several advantages over other conventional as well as nonconventional methods like (a) smaller volumes of solvents used; (b) faster extraction rates; (c) high reproducibility; (d) simple workup; (e) simple and faster method of extraction; (f) elimination of post-treatment of wastewater; (g) high purity of extracted essential oils; (h) lesser consumption of energy; (i) economical; and (j) non-degradation of extracted products.

Wei et al. (2016) made use of ultrasound-assisted supercritical carbon dioxide (UASC–CO_2) extraction method. The performance of UASC–CO_2 extraction was compared with the conventional techniques. Clove oils and other bioactive components were obtained in excellent yields without producing any chemical waste. USC–CO_2 extraction caused higher yield of COR (23.2%) in small extraction time with excellent quality and more volumes of eugenol acetate (14.2%) and eugenol (71.4%) fractions. Temperature and pressure conditions played a major role in the extraction. The solubility of eugenol and clove oil in SC-CO_2 under a wide range of temperature (32°C–50°C) and pressure (9.0–28.5 MPa) was studied for the first time. Noteworthy differences in the yield of extracted oil (COR) were detected. Best results were attained at 50°C temperature and 28.5 MPa pressure with a fixed extraction duration of 10–15 minutes and 0.35 g/minute flow rate of CO_2 when operated at an ultrasonic frequency of 40 kHz, power 185 W, and ultrasound cycle of 75%.

In other findings, Alexandru et al. (2013) carried out UAE of COR using batch and flow ultrasonic reactors from dry clove buds. The results were then compared with the conventional maceration in view of yield, biological activity, and total phenols. The phytoconstituents of the extracted crude oil and the efficiency of the process were found to be dependent on (a) extraction conditions, (b) technique used, and (c) type of reactor. The constituent components were studied using headspace gas chromatographic method coupled with mass spectrometry (HS-GC/MS). The continuous flow UAE method employs a novel multiprobe reactor consisting of titanium horns. Various flow rates (450, 900, and 1350 mL/minute) were carried out during three independent cycles. At higher flow rates, flow UAE was found to give maximum yield, whereas maceration gave the lowest yields. At low flow rates, batch reactor UAE was observed to be more effective than the other methods. The antioxidant potential and total phenols (191–215 mg gallic acid equivalents/L of extract) was maximum under flow UAE, which was done at 1350 mL/minute in contrast to other methods. Likewise, Tekin et al. (2015) employed UAE of oils of clove using a central composite design (CCD). These authors studied the effect of three extraction parameters, namely extraction temperatures (32°C–52°C), plant concentrations (wt/ethanol volume) (3%–7%), and extraction times (30–60 minutes). The ultrasound frequency was kept constant at 53 kHz while varying the rest of the parameters mentioned above. The outcomes of the research indicated that yield of extraction was greatly affected by temperature. The highest yield was achieved under the temperature of extraction, duration of extraction, and clove extract concentration values of 60°C, 45 minutes, and 5%, respectively, with a satisfactory correlation coefficient (r^2) of 0.94 (Tekin et al., 2015). The gas chromatography-mass spectroscopy (GC-MS) of CEO demonstrated that it consisted of eugenol (64%), methoxy-4-(2-propenyl) phenol acetate, alpha-caryophyllene, and caryophyllene oxide. Considering the well-established antibacterial properties of the CEO, the authors also studied its bacteriostatic effects. The CEO was observed to substantially inhibit the multiplication of *Escherichia coli* and *Staphylococcus aureus* with an inhibitory concentration of 800 and 1600 mg/L, respectively (Tekin et al., 2015). These studies established that the UAE is a powerful method for the setup of commercial applications in many fields.

17.3.10 Polymeric Membrane-Assisted Purification of Clove Oil

In the literature, many studies are available where extraction of the bioactive components is carried out with the assistance of membranes (Peev et al., 2011; Kim et al., 2016). Polymer-based membranes result in the selective separation of essential oils under milder processing conditions. The usage of polymeric membrane for the purification of COR was described by Nasution et al. (2013). A polymeric cellulose chitosan membrane was used for the purification of COR and gave clove oil permeate with the more eugenol content of approximately 58%. Kusworo et al. (2020) devised a novel method where nanohybrid cellulose acetate (CA) nano-TiO_2/crosslinked polyvinyl alcohol (PVA)-coated membrane was used for the purification of COR. GC-MS analysis confirmed the main components present in crude clove oil (without using membrane) were eugenol (69.51%), caryophyllene (25.19%), and hexadecanoic acid ethanediyl ester (1.58%) along with alpha-Cubebene and alpha-Humulene as indicated in Table 17.5. Performance of the membrane was significantly affected by membrane selectivity, which is decided by membrane potential to discard impurities present in the COR. It was detected that as the amount of eugenol in permeate increased, selectivity of the membrane also improved. Eugenol content in each permeate collected from the fabricated membranes was determined using GC-MS analysis as given in Table 17.6. The wt% of eugenol in clove oil is 74.25; similar results were obtained using the gravimetric method. The permeate contains a small amount of residual solvent hexane in it, which was not suggested by the GC-MS analysis of crude clove oil feed. The presence of a small amount of alpha-copaene was because of the difficulty of GC-MS analysis in differentiating between alpha-copaene and alpha-cubebene, isomers with the same molecular formula $C_{15}H_{24}$. The amount of trans-caryophyllene declined from 25% to 22%. No esters of hexadecanoic acid were detected in the permeate owing to the rejection of fatty acids by the membrane. The effect of the variables such as CA polymer concentration, concentration of TiO_2 nanoparticles, and PVA concentration used for designing the hybrid CA membrane on the permeate flux in the isolation of clove oil was investigated. It was found that the total flux decreased on increasing both CA and PVA concentrations. On increasing the concentration of coating material PVA, a thicker layer develops, which increases

TABLE 17.6 Comparison of Chemical Components in Crude Clove Leaf Oil and Membrane-Assisted Extracted Permeate (MAEP)

Component	Crude Clove Leaf Oil (wt%)	MAEP (wt%)
Phenol,-methoxy-4-(2-propenyl)-(Eugenol)	70	74.24
Beta-caryophyllene	25.19	22.06
Hexadecanoic acid	1.58	–
Alpha-copaene	–	0.8
Alpha-humulene	2.79	2.41
Alpha-cubebene	0.93	–
Hexane	–	0.49

Adapted from Kusworo et al. (2020).

membrane hydrophilicity and which in turn increases the resistance of eugenol to penetrate the membrane. The highest eugenol amount in permeate on using CA membrane (20 wt% concentration) was found to be 87.5%. In general, CA membranes can be used as potential candidates for clove oil purification. PVA coating increased hydrophilicity of the membrane and increased separation efficiency but was not able to offer a non-porous, dense layer to the membrane.

17.3.11 Miscellaneous

In addition to the methods explained above, COR extraction and characterization are also done by many more methods. In another study, Xu et al. (2016) attempted extraction of CEO from *Syringa yunnanensis*. The chemical constituents of the extracted CEO were analysed using the GC-MS method with helium as the carrier gas. The authors were able to isolate the CEO with a yield of 12.8% (v/w). Screening of the CEO using gas chromatography-flame ionization detector revealed the presence of 22 components (Table 17.7). The chief constituents in the extract included eugenol, trans-caryophyllene, caryophyllene oxide, and eugenyl acetate (Xu et al., 2016). The CEO demonstrated outstanding inhibition of *S. aureus*. The diameter of inhibition zone (DIZ) values for eugenol- and β-caryophyllene-induced *S. aureus* inhibition were estimated in the range of 21.2 and 15.8 mm, respectively. The inhibitory concentrations were calculated to be 0.625 and 1.25 mg/mL, respectively. The kill time analysis and cell-permeability assays established the rapid cell membrane permeation and disintegration properties of CEO, thereby leading to its high antibacterial efficacy. Overall, the potent antibacterial effect of CEO was ascribable to its molecular-level toxicity (Xu et al., 2016).

Recently, Fuentes and co-workers attempted a GC-MS analysis of the commercially procured *S. aromaticum* (Fuentes et al., 2020). The GC-MS was furnished with FID and a capillary column. The quantification of CEO was performed in 0.1% $CHCl_3$ using H_2 as a carrier gas over the temperature range of 50°C–250°C (Fuentes et al., 2020). The major components as identified included eugenol (79.47%), copaene (1.76%), α-humulene (2.65%),

TABLE 17.7 Chemical Composition of CEO as Identified from Gas Chromatography-Flame Ionization Detector

Phytocompounds	Peak Area (%)	Phytocompounds	Peak Area (%)
Pinene	0.02	Eugenol	76.23
(–)-b-Cadinene	0.12	Methyl salicylate	0.06
Eugenol acetate	2	Alpha-caryophyllene	0.64
α-Pinene	0.03	Trans-caryophyllene	11.54
Chavicol	0.1	Selinene	0.25
α-Selinene	0.16	4-Allylanisole	0.13
Jasmone	0.07	Cedrene	0.02
Globulol	0.04	Valencene	0.01
α-Copaene	0.05	Ledol	0.03

Adapted from Xu et al. (2016).
Peak area calculated by GC-FID.

and humulene (2.48%). The amount of eugenol quantified in this study by following earlier reported studies to confirm these observations.

The traditional extraction methods are more time consuming and use more solvent, which results in undesirable reproducibility. The extraction specialists aim at strengthening the extraction processes by increasing extraction efficiency, quality of the extracted essential oils and by lowering the extraction duration, unit operations, energy consumption, volume of the solvent produced, economic expenses, and amount of waste produced. In the last few decades because of enhancing interest in safety, economic, and environmental considerations, novel green substitutes have been greatly applied in cosmetic, food processing, and pharmacological industries and would be a novel initiative to meet the challenges of the 21st century, to safeguard both the environment and the users.

17.4 PHARMACOLOGICAL APPLICATIONS

17.4.1 Antimicrobial and Antibacterial Activity

Antibiotic resistance is an alarming scenario to public health, which encourages the use of medicines based on plant origin in place of chemotherapeutic medicines. The protective efficacy of water and alcohol extracts of clove as well as garlic were monitored against gram-positive MRSA (methicillin-resistant *S. aureus*, *Streptococcus* spp.) and gram-negative (*Pseudomonas aeruginosa*, *E. coli*, *Klebsiella pneumoniae*) bacteria. Alcoholic extract of clove revealed more antimicrobial potential followed by an aqueous extract of clove. However, the extracts of garlic showed moderate antibacterial activity. The highest zone of inhibition (20–26 mm) was induced by ethanolic extract of clove against MRSA and *K. pneumoniae* at 1.0 μg/mL concentration. The alcoholic and water extract of clove revealed 64–128 μg/mL minimum inhibitory concentration (MIC) against all pathogens (Liu et al., 2021). In another study, antimicrobial potential of water, alcoholic, and hydroethanolic extracts of clove was determined against *Salmonella typhimurium*, *E. coli*, *S. aureus*, *P. aeruginosa*, *Candida albicans*, *Shigella flexneri*, and their clinical counterparts. The aqueous extract decreased the 67% growth of tested germs, but the hydroethanolic and ethanolic extracts showed 100% protective efficacy in the killing of all the germs. The microbicidal potential of clove extracts might be related to the active phytochemicals present in the fruits of the plant. Eugenol is the active component present in cloves and is already well known for its antifungal and antibacterial potential, thus it can be a reason for antimicrobial potential (Tampieri et al., 2005; Afanyibo et al., 2018). The flavonols, alkaloids, saponins, and tannins in the plant have shown curative effects against many pathogens such as *E. coli*, *P. aeruginosa*, *C. albicans*, and *S. aureus* (Usman and Osuji, 2007; Jimoh et al., 2017). In addition, antimicrobial activity of clove oil was checked against multidrug-resistant strains *Enterococcus faecalis*, *P. aeruginosa*, *Acinetobacter baumannii*, and *S. aureus*. It showed minimum inhibitory concentrations ranging from 0.31% to 1.3% (v/v) against tested strains (Abdullah et al., 2015). Similarly, in another study, essential oil of clove demonstrated protective efficacy against *S. aureus* (Mishra and Sharma, 2014) and *Listeria monocytogenes* in pasteurized milk (Cava et al., 2007). Moreover, Zengin and Baysal (2015) found clove to be effective against *Carnobacterium divergens*, *Listeria innocua*, *S. aureus*, *S. typhimurium*, *E. coli*, *Shewanella putrefacians*, and *Serratia lique-faciens* using broth dilution method. This study revealed that CEO hampered the multi-plication of all bacteria, however *Shewanella* and *Listeria* were found to be resistant to oil. Likewise, Gupta et al. (2013) also demonstrated the protective potential of clove oil against food-borne bacteria (*S. aureus*, *P. aerugenosa*, *E. coli*, *S. chloeraesius*, *Yersinia enteroco-litica*, *Bacillus cereus*, *L. monocytogenes*, and *E. faecalis*). Various studies demonstrated that CEO revealed more microbicidal resistance against *Penicillium* sp., *Aspergillus flavus*, and *S. aureus* occur in fish (Matan, 2012). In another study, the antiseptic potential of etha-nolic extract of clove and clove oil was determined against food-borne pathogens. In this study, ten bacterial and seven fungal strains were checked by agar well diffusion technique. It displayed more microbicidal effects of clove oil as compared to extract and standard food preservative, sodium propionate. Moreover, antibacterial potential of clove and other spices (Garlic, mint, and ginger) was monitored against *Escherichia coli*, *B. cereus*, and *S. aureus*. It was observed that the clove showed maximum inhibitory activity at 1% concen-tration. Garlic exhibited maximum inhibition at 3% concentration. However, mint and ginger revealed very little inhibition at the same concentration (Sofia et al., 2007). In addi-tion, another study also reported that clove oil at low concentration hindered the growth of *L. monocytogenes*. Antibacterial and antimicrobial potential of clove oil was because of the existence of eugenol, gallic acid, isoeugenol, methyl salicylate, kaempferol, heptanone, and oleanolic acid (Mytle et al., 2006; Chaieb et al., 2007). The free –OH groups of eugenol bind to the proteins of bacteria and hinder the action of enzymes of bacterial cells. In another study, Devi et al. (2013) demonstrated the microbicidal potential of clove extracts might be attributed to high content of eugenol, which alters the penetrability of the cytoplasmic membrane and causes hindrance disruption in the distribution of ions, ATP transport, and apoptosis. Further, Das et al. (2016) demonstrated that the eugenol causes the upregu-lation in the levels of free radical species (ROS), which leads to a change in the permeability of cell membrane, the disintegration of DNA, and the ultimately cell death of *S. aureus*. More phenols in clove oil cause antimicrobial activity against various microbes through impairment in the flow of electrons and proton motive force leads to flocculation of cell content of bacterium (Elhoussine et al., 2010). All of these studies indicate the potential of clove extracts in the secretion of ideal microbicidal and antibacterial agents.

17.4.2 Antitumour Activity

S. aromaticum has been employed from ancient times in Ayurveda to cure the tumour. Other treatments like chemotherapeutics, surgery, radiation therapy, and transplanta-tion have been used to cure the tumour, but these therapies reveal several toxic effects on the human body (Reddy et al., 2003). Herbal extracts give a good alternative option in combating cancer cells to circumvent the adverse effects of chemotherapeutic drugs (Mbaveng et al., 2011). Several research investigations demonstrated that clove and its active compounds are an ideal anticancer agent. Various active components of *Syzygium* sp. like betulinic acids, oleanolic acids, and dimethyl cardamonins possess anticancer properties. The anticancer potential of clove extracts against HCT (human colon carci-noma) cell line was determined using MTT assay. The clove ethanolic extract exhibited the marked protective efficacy against HCT cell line and IC_{50} was found to be 2.53 mg/mL (Yassin et al., 2020). *S. aromaticum* extracts have a large number of tannins that display good antitumour potential (Batiha et al., 2020). Similarly, Tejasari et al. (2020) demonstrated that flavonoid compounds from clove oil exhibited robust cytotoxic activity against malignant liver cells, which indicated the potential of clove as good candidates for treatment of hepatic cancer. Moreover, nanoscale emulsion of the *S. aromaticum* was observed to be effective against the thyroid cancer cell line (HTH-7) and caused a marked reduction in tumour cells (Nirmala et al., 2019). Likewise, Kubatka et al. (2017) suggested anticancer potential of *S. aromaticum* against oestrogen-responsive and oestrogen-unresponsive breast cancer cell lines. It was found that clove extract suppressed the multiplication of tumour cells in time and dose-dependent means. Moreover, treatment with *S. aromaticum* hampered the growth of tumour cells by stimulating cell cycle arrest at the S phase. It was also observed that this extract enhanced the percentage of cells in the sub-Go/G1 phase after 72 hours of treatment, which depicts the efficacy of *S. aromaticum* in the stimulation of cell death. The cytotoxicity of clove extracts was verified by Kumar et al. (2014), which showed the significant toxic effect against MCF-7 breast cancer cell line. Likewise, various extracts of clove were tested against human breast cancer cells through MTT and brine shrimp lethality test assay. These extracts displayed strong cytotoxic activity and LD_{50} was found to be of 36–37 μg/mL against breast cancer cells (Kumar et al., 2014). Moreover, in another study, the cytotoxic activity of leaves, bark, and stem extract of clove was tested against MCF-7 cells. Among these extracts, stem extract was found to reveal the potent inhibitory activity in the cells. The extract activates the caspase 3/7 and leads to cell death in MCF-7 cells. The potent antitumour potential of clove extracts might be due to their phytocompounds like eugenol, which was already known to have anti-proliferative activity against oral squamous carcinoma, prostatic cancer cells, and malignant melanoma cell lines (Carrasco et al., 2008). In another study, *S. aromaticum* extract showed anticancer efficiency due to the existence of terpenoids and phenylpropanoids in the extract. This extract causes the induction of protein caspases, cell cycle arrest, and apoptosis in cancer cells. Clove extract seemed to induce the free radical's generation in cancer cells, regulation of hepatic detoxifying enzymes, as well as obliteration of angiogenesis (Lesgards et al., 2014; Liu et al., 2014). Likewise, anti-proliferative potential of aqueous, ethanolic, and clove oil extracts were checked against breast, cervical, prostate, and oesophageal cancer cell lines, along with normal blood lymphocytes. Out of these extracts, the oil extracts revealed more cell growth inhibition activity. Maximum cell death (80%) occurred in oesophageal cancer cells by clove oil at 300 μL/mL; however, prostate cancer cells revealed the least apoptosis. Moreover, a negligible cytotoxic effect was observed in human lymphocytes at a similar concentration (Dwivedi et al., 2011).

Further protective activity of *S. aromaticum* was checked in a mammary carcinoma rat model. Extract of *S. aromaticum* was injected to the rats for 1 week before the injection of N-nitroso-N-methylurea and continued to be given for 3 months. Treatment of clove extract leads to reduce the tumour frequency in the rats but average tumour volume and tumour latency were found to be ineffective. The anticancer function was achieved by the activation of caspase 3, caspase 7, Bax, ALDH1A1, H4K16ac, H4K20me3, and suppression

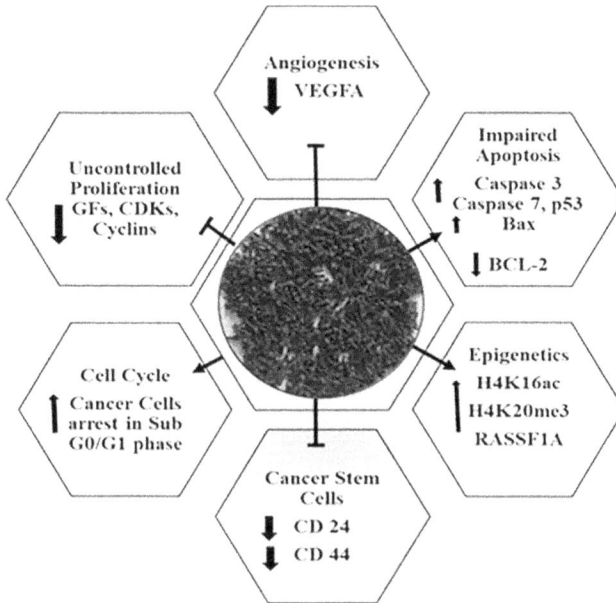

FIGURE 17.5 Anticancer activity of *Syzygium aromaticum*.

of levels of CD24, vascular endothelial growth factor A, BCL-2, CD44. Total RASSF1A promoter methylation (three CpG sites) was found to be enhanced in clove-treated animals (Kubatka et al., 2017). In another study, the *in vivo* activity of clove extract was checked in the murine model against colon cancer. Then mice were injected with clove extract for 5 days and it was observed that tumour growth reduced markedly in the extract-treated group than the untreated control group (Liu et al., 2014). Moreover, chemopreventive potential of water extract of clove was also determined on benzopyrene-stimulated lung carcinogenesis in mice. Treatment of aqueous extract of clove resulted in suppression of the hypergenesis, hypertrophy, and carcinoma in mice. It showed a remarkable reduction in the quantity of dividing cells and enhanced apoptotic bodies in lung lesions of benzopyrene-induced mice. The levels of caspase 3, Bax, and p53 were found to be increased in lung lesions of BP-induced mice. However, clove treatment in mice revealed a marked decrease in the concentration of anti-apoptotic and growth-promoting factors. These results elucidate the protective activity of clove in respect of its anti-proliferative and apoptogenic potential (Banerjee et al., 2006). It depicts that clove extracts can be used as natural anticarcinogenic agents (Figure 17.5).

17.4.3 Antiviral Activity

The antiviral potential of ethanol extract of the whole clove was examined against herpes simplex virus (HSV). It was observed that clove extract directly inactivated the growth of the HSV. In another study, the HSV viral load was found to be reduced after treatment with the clove extract (Tragoolpua and Jatisatienr, 2007). In addition, methanolic extracts of cloves revealed more than 90% HCV protease inhibition (Hussein et al., 2000).

Similarly, the antiviral activity of clove phyto-components particularly eugenol was determined against HSV-1 and HSV-2, and IC_{50} (inhibitory concentration 50%) was observed to be 26 and 16 µg/mL, respectively. Moreover, it was observed to be active against Ebola and influenza A virus (Benencia and Courreges, 2000; Dai et al., 2013). Other phytochemicals of clove-like eugeniin possess the anti-HSV property at a 5-µg/mL concentration. Eugeniin inhibits the DNA polymerases of the virus and thereby hampers the DNA replication of HSV (Kurokawa et al., 1998).

17.4.4 Clove in the Fight against COVID-19

Traditionally, clove has been employed for the cure of respiratory infections, and its various properties, such as anti-inflammatory, immunomodulatory, and cardioprotective, highlight its efficacy against the COVID-19 infection. Clove is one of the medicinal herbs presently used for the treatment of the SARS-CoV-2 infection, in combination with cinnamon, ginger, neem, basil, and other herbs enriched with the benefits of being economical and sufficiently obtainable around the globe. A method in the early stages of the infection was described by J. N. M. Kanyinda for the prevention and cure of COVID 19. In this method (decoction), first boil the cloves in water with other herbs for approximately 20 minutes. Then discharged volatile compounds are breathed by patients for 5 minutes. A similar procedure was also proposed for a decoction made with cloves and other medicinal herbs (Kanyinda, 2020). 92–98% of the surveyed Indian population presumed that spices are useful in bettering the SARS-CoV-2 infection and may assist in enhancing immune response. Cloves are also being used by herbalists in Morocco to control and cure coronavirus infection (Chaachouay et al., 2021). Various molecular computational researches suggested that phytochemicals present in cloves act as strong anti-COVID-19 agents, and among these phytochemicals, kaempferol displayed the ability to attach with the substrate-binding site of the proteinase of SARS-CoV-2, which depicts that natural component like clove flavonoids, can be ideal agents against this virus (Pandey et al., 2020; Joshi et al., 2020). In another study, molecular docking revealed that clove compounds like bicornin and biflorin showed high affinities for M[pro] recommending their potential inhibitory activity (Rehman et al., 2020).

17.4.5 Anti-Inflammatory Activity

S. aromaticum extract is a natural reservoir of phytochemicals and it assists to decrease inflammation in many diseases. The chief compound in clove is eugenol, which alters cell signalling and immunological responses (Rusmana et al., 2015). Clove oil showed protective efficacy in the reduction of proliferation and swelling of fibroblasts of skin (Han and Parker, 2017). Moreover, it also reduced the secretion of proinflammatory markers like collagen III and vascular cell adhesion molecule-1. Nikoui et al. (2017) described the antipyretic and inflammatory potential of clove oil in dogs. Treatment with clove oil showed a decline in neutrophils and white blood cells in comparison to control. However, no effect was seen on erythrocytes, and it ultimately led to a reduction in inflammation. Bachiega et al. (2012) suggested clove and eugenol exhibited anti-inflammatory activity on the production of cytokines using ELISA (enzyme-linked immunosorbent assay). *S. aromaticum* showed a remarkable decrease in the amount of IL-10, IL-1, and IL-6 and eugenol hampered the secretion of IL-10 and IL-6. CEO revealed protective efficacy for the cure of inflammatory diseases, such as arthritis and rheumatism in aromatherapy, and was found to be effective in animal models at a concentration of 0.05 and 0.20 mL/kg (Öztürk and Özbek, 2005). In another study, the ethanol extracts of clove buds were monitored for anti-inflammatory activity (50, 100, and 200 mg/kg) in animals. The lethal dose of clove extract was found to be 565.7 mg/kg, which revealed remarkable effects at all doses, validating the usage of the clove extract in inflammatory diseases (Tanko et al., 2008).

From a molecular context, clove buds consist of flavonoids, such as β-caryophyllene, kaempferol, and rhamnetin, which play an important role in anti-inflammatory effect of clove (García-Mediavilla et al., 2007; Rho et al., 2011; Jnawali et al., 2014; Novo Belchor et al., 2017). Eugenol (200 and 400 mg/kg) showed a decline in the number of pleural exudates in animal models and showed a negligible effect on the total leukocytes, which depicts the anti-inflammatory nature of this molecule (Daniel et al., 2009). Moreover, treatment with both whole clove aqueous extract and eugenol demonstrated a significant decrease in LPS (lipopolysaccharide)-induced lung inflammation. It was mediated through a decline in the levels of TNF-α (tumour necrosis factor-alpha) and impaired NF-κB signalling, which leads to recovery of lung injury (Magalhães et al., 2010; Chniguir et al., 2019). Interestingly, water extract of clove displayed cytoprotective effects against pyelonephritis (a kidney inflammation seen in COVID-19 patients) in the animal model. Clove oil showed anti-inflammatory properties through inhibition of the cyclo-oxygenase-2 and lipo-oxygenase enzymes (Nassan et al., 2015; Su et al., 2020).

17.4.6 Immunostimulatory Activity

One of the strategies to prevent and alleviate many diseases is the stimulation of the immune system. Many plants have been examined for the same and are used as immunomodulators. Clove is known to be the stimulator of the immune system and enhance disease resistance traditionally. It was observed that this herb increased the total leukocyte count and delayed-type hypersensitivity response in animal models. COR has restored the antibody and cell-mediated immunity in cyclophosphamide-immunosuppressed animal models in a concentration-dependent means (Carrasco et al., 2009; Bhowmik et al., 2012). Moreover, treatment of clove extract showed enhancement in the levels of lymphoblasts, lymphocytes, and microbicidal molecules of macrophages in infected BALB/c mice with *S. typhimurium* (Wael et al., 2018). Additionally, Bachiega et al. (2009) described that treatment with clove in mice did not affect the balance of Th1/Th2 cytokine.

17.4.7 Cardiovascular Activity

Intake of cloves can decrease the complications of heart disease, arteriosclerosis, and other vascular infections. Eugenol causes vasodilation and relaxation of smooth muscle in a dose-dependent manner (Damiani et al., 2003; Scalbert et al., 2005). Usage of clove is considered as an inducer for the cardiovascular system through improvement in blood supply to the brain and heart (Bahramsoltani and Rahimi, 2020). Moreover, clove oil was demonstrated to hinder the clustering of thrombocytes stimulated by the platelet-activating factor. *In vivo* studies conducted on rabbits revealed that essential oil of clove at 50–100 mg/kg concentration exhibited a protective effect against the platelet-activating factor and 70%–75% efficacy against arachidonic acid-induced shock because of pulmonary embolism (Mittal et al., 2014). Antithrombotic and antiplatelet aggregation effects were also studied on clove extracts by *ex vivo* methods measuring the inhibitory and fibrinolytic activity on thrombin-stimulated platelet assemblage. In another study, the clove extracts revealed marked fibrinolytic and inhibitory activity against platelet aggregation, suggesting the anti-atherosclerotic potential of the clove (Yang et al., 2011). Owing to the basis for the anti-thrombotic potential of clove could be because of the presence of platelet inhibitor components like eugenol, rhamnetin, kaempferol, gallic acid, myricetin, and β-caryophyllene, thus prohibiting blood clots (García-Mediavilla et al., 2007). Moreover, it also inhibits the synthesis of thromboxanes, prostaglandins, and arachidonic acid-stimulated platelet assemblage (Rasheed et al., 1984).

17.4.8 Antioxidant Activity

Clove oil and COR showed antioxidant activity as compared to synthetic antioxidant Tertiary Butyl HydroQuinone (TBHQ) and natural antioxidants (tocopherol and ascorbic acid). These plant products exhibited strong inhibition against lipid oxidation and extended the durability of cooked chicken and chevon meat for 3 weeks. Clove oil and COR are naturally strong antioxidants that can replace artificial antioxidants (Sultana et al., 2017). In another study, the COR in combination with capsicum oleoresin and kalonji seed extract showed efficient antioxidant activity. It also depicted the synergic activity of COR to be employed as an alternative for artificial antioxidants (Rege and Momin, 2018). Clove buds showed antioxidant activity and reduced the reactive oxygen species in our body. The high antioxidant potential shown by *S. aromaticum* oil was attributed to the existence of phenols like eugenol acetate, eugenol, and thymol (Yadav and Bhatnagar 2007; Gulcin et al., 2012; Dai et al. 2013; Nam and Kim, 2013).

17.4.9 Hepatoprotective Activity

The liver is a crucial organ that regulates the normal internal environment and also plays a key role in metabolic activities, inflammatory actions, and detoxification. Many studies are supporting the hepatoprotective properties of cloves. Hepatoprotective activity of aqueous extract of clove was determined at a concentration of 0.1 and 0.2 g/kg in paracetamol-intoxicated rats. It was found that paracetamol resulted in liver damage as it enhanced the concentration of various enzymes in the liver, i.e., SGOT, SGPT in the serum. It was found that clove extract ameliorated the hepatic damage by restoring the normal concentrations of enzymes in serum (Sallie et al., 1991; Milind and Deepa, 2011).

17.4.10 Other Therapeutic Effects

Clove is one of the richest sources of manganese and it is crucial for enzyme metabolism, enhances the strength of bone, and antioxidant value. It is high in fibre, omega-3, calcium, magnesium, and vitamins K and C. It has been found to assist in preventing diabetes by tripling insulin levels. In addition, it showed antifungal, larvicidal, analgesic, neuroprotective, and antipyretic activities (Mittal et al., 2014; Bhowmik et al., 2012).

17.5 SAFETY, TOXICITY, AND FUTURE SCOPE

Clove oil is not toxic to take at a concentration of less than 1500 ppm, and the admissible amount of cloves/day in humans is 2.5 mg/kg weight (Fischer and Dengler, 1990; Anderson et al., 1997). Moreover, a phenolic extract of clove displayed negligible toxicity in Wistar rats at a concentration of 1 g/kg b.wt./day. Additionally, it revealed the least genotoxic effects against *S. typhimurium* (Vijayasteltar et al., 2016). However, many studies suggested contradictory results from these herbs. Aqueous extract of *S. aromaticum* demonstrated a minimum percentage of lethality at a dose of <125 µg/mL. However, ethanolic extract of clove demonstrated toxic effects even at small doses, with a 100% mortality found at the dose of 250 µg/mL (Kumar et al., 2014). Moreover, the alcoholic as well as aqueous clove extracts did not reveal any toxicity against murine embryonic fibroblast T3 cells (Ling et al., 2010). Further, in *in vivo* studies, there was no acute chronic toxicity found in rats administered with alcoholic clove leaves extract (Manaharan et al., 2014). Similarly, Mollika et al. (2014) described that methanolic leaves extract of *Syzygium* sp. in albino Swiss mice was observed to be safe up to a concentration of 1 g/kg. In another study, the *S. jambos* leaf extract was cytotoxic against *Artemia franciscana*, and lethal concentration (LC_{50}) was found to be 388 ± 39 µg/mL (Mohanty and Cock, 2010). In another study, *Syzygium campanulatum* revealed no cytotoxicity against normal human fibroblasts and epithelial cells (Aisha et al., 2013).

The FDA has authenticated the safe profile of clove buds, oil of clove, oleoresins, and eugenol as a food additive; but there have been substantial reports in context to its cytotoxicity currently (Vijayasteltar et al., 2016). Cytotoxic potential of clove oil and eugenol have been examined *in vitro* against human endothelial cells and fibroblasts, and these are observed to be safe (Prashar et al., 2006). However, many researchers suggested that eugenol displayed allergic contact dermatitis, ulcers, necrosis, irritation of the skin, and anaphylaxis when used in dentistry (Sarrami et al., 2002; Anuj and Sanjay, 2010). Moreover, ingestion of clove oil is also reported to cause acute adverse effects like liver toxicity, seizures, and disseminated intravascular coagulopathy (Janes et al., 2005). In another study, clove oil showed a lethal dose (LD_{50}) of 18.2 ± 5.52 and 1.7 ± 0.8 mg/mL in zebrafish and guppy fish, respectively (Doleželová et al., 2011). It was observed that clove oil exhibited marked detoxification and maintained good heart health in humans by decreasing peroxidation of lipids and enhancing the concentration of redox enzymes (Gülçin et al., 2012). Further research is still imperative to know the extent of cytotoxicity of clove.

This review discussed several extraction methods, phytochemicals, and health benefits of clove. There is a demand for more investigations done on the natural death of clove trees. Current clove trees seem to fall off to a greater extent and there will be limited clove trees in Mkoani District in the next 10 years. The chief future prospective lies at detecting the novel biological properties of clove and employ it as an active therapeutic against several diseases with negligible toxicity. The treatment using herbal medicine will be economical and it will be present at a large level. Clove and its major phytochemical eugenol can be used as an adjuvant in many medications. Moreover, the protective efficacy of COR and their phytochemicals should be determined against COVID-19 infection. More molecular studies are required to monitor the specific clove phytochemical interactions with protein targets of SARS-CoV-2, which will help to develop the new drugs based on clove phytochemicals with optimized characteristics.

17.6 CONCLUSION

Based on the discussion in this chapter, it could be concluded that clove is an alluring plant with highly valued multifunctional phytoconstituents and has tremendous potential in the preservation of food. The proven protective effect of clove recommends the development of herbal medicines for the welfare of humans and validates the usage of this herb for centuries. Clove contains major phytoconstituents eugenol, carvacrol, thymol, and cinnamaldehyde. Out of these, eugenol is the most efficacious component of clove and the FDA authenticated it as a non-toxic compound. Moreover, clove and its active components showed numerous biological activities like antibacterial, antimicrobial, antioxidant, anti-inflammatory, immunomodulatory, antipyretic, antitumour, and antiviral. Moreover, they showed insecticidal, larvicidal, and mosquito repellent activities. Furthermore, given its multifaceted medicinal uses, there is plenty of scope for designing novel drugs of plant origin from COR.

REFERENCES

Abdullah, B. H., Hatem, S. F., and Jumaa, W. 2015. A comparative study of the antibacterial activity of clove and rosemary essential oils on multidrug resistant bacteria. *UK Journal of Pharmaceutical and Biosciences* 3, (1): 18–22.

Afanyibo, Y. G., Anani, K., Esseh, K., et al. 2018. Antimicrobial activities of *Syzygium aromaticum* (L.) Merr. & LM Perry (myrtaceae) fruit extracts on six standard microorganisms and their clinical counterpart. *Open Access Library Journal* 5, (12): 1. https://doi.org/10.4236/oalib.1104951.

Aisha, A. F., Ismail, Z., Abu-Salah, K. M., et al. 2013. *Syzygium campanulatum* korth methanolic extract inhibits angiogenesis and tumor growth in nude mice. *BMC Complementary and Alternative Medicine* 13, (1): 1–11.

Alexandru, L., Cravotto, G., Giordana, L., et al. 2013. Ultrasound-assisted extraction of clove buds using batch and flow-reactors: a comparative study on a pilot scale. *Innovative Food Science & Emerging Technologies* 20: 167–172.

Anderson, W. G., McKinley, R. S. and M. Colavecchia. 1997. The use of clove oil as an anesthetic for rainbow trout and its effects on swimming performance. *North American Journal of Fisheries Management* 17, (2): 301–307.

Anuj, G., and S. Sanjay. 2010. Eugenol: a potential phytochemical with multifaceted therapeutic activities. *Pharmacologyonline* 2, 108–120.

Arimalala, N., Penot, E., Michels, T., et al. 2019. Clove based cropping systems on the east coast of Madagascar: how history leaves its mark on the landscape. *Agroforestry Systems* 93, (4): 1577–1592.

Astuti, R. I., Listyowati, S., and W. T. Wahyuni. 2019. Life span extension of model yeast *Saccharomyces cerevisiae* upon ethanol derived-clover bud extract treatment. In *IOP Conference Series: Earth and Environmental Science* 299, (1): 012059.

Atanasova, T., Nenov, N., Gochev, V., et al. 2013. *Low Temperature Extraction of Essential Oil-Bearing Plants by Liquid Gases. 14 Clove (Syzygium aromaticum (L.) Merryl and Perry)*. In the Proceeding of International Scientific And Practical Conference On Development Of

Agricultural Sectors Of The Economy In The Conditions Of Globalization Materials, Russia, Voronezh, June 19-20, 2013, 978-5-7267-0676-4.

Atanasova-Pancevska, N., Bogdanov, J., and D. Kungulovski. 2017. *In vitro* antimicrobial activity and chemical composition of two essential oils and eugenol from flower buds of *Eugenia caryophyllata*. *Open Biological Sciences Journal*, 3, (1): 16–25.

Babovic, N., Djilas, S., Jadranin, M., et al. 2010. Supercritical carbon dioxide extraction of antioxidant fractions from selected Lamiaceae herbs and their antioxidant capacity. *Innovative Food Science & Emerging Technologies* 11, (1): 98–107.

Bachiega, T. F., de Sousa, J. P. B., Bastos, J. K., et al. 2012. Clove and eugenol in noncytotoxic concentrations exert immunomodulatory/anti-inflammatory action on cytokine production by murine macrophages. *Journal of Pharmacy and Pharmacology* 64, (4): 610–616.

Bachiega, T. F., Orsatti, C. L., Pagliarone, A. C., et al. 2009. Th1/Th2 cytokine production by clove-treated mice. *Natural Product Research* 23, (16): 1552–1558.

Bahramsoltani, R., and R. Rahimi. 2020. An evaluation of traditional Persian medicine for the management of SARS-CoV-2. *Frontiers in Pharmacology*, 11.

Banerjee, S., Panda, C. K., and S. Das. 2006. Clove (*Syzygium aromaticum* L.), a potential chemopreventive agent for lung cancer. *Carcinogenesis* 27, (8): 1645–1654.

Batiha, G. E. S., Beshbishy, A. M., Tayebwa, D. S., et al. 2018. Inhibitory effects of *Uncaria tomentosa* bark, *Myrtus communis* roots, *Origanum vulgare* leaves and *Cuminum cyminum* seeds extracts against the growth of *Babesia* and *Theileria in vitro*. *JPN. Veterinary Parasitology* 17, (1): 1–13.

Batiha, G. E. S., Beshbishy, A. M., Tayebwa, D. S., et al. 2019. Inhibitory effects of *Syzygium aromaticum* and *Camellia sinensis* methanolic extracts on the growth of *Babesia* and *Theileria* parasites. *Ticks and Tick-Borne Diseases* 10, (5): 949–958.

Belwal, T., Chemat, F., Venskutonis, P. R., et al. 2020. Recent advances in scaling-up of non-conventional extraction techniques: learning from successes and failures. *TrAC Trends in Analytical Chemistry*, 127: 1–25.

Belwal, T., Ezzat, S. M., Rastrelli, L., et al. 2018. A critical analysis of extraction techniques used for botanicals: trends, priorities, industrial uses and optimization strategies. *TrAC Trends in Analytical Chemistry* 100, 82–102.

Benencia, F., and M. C. Courreges. 2000. *In vitro* and *in vivo* activity of eugenol on human herpesvirus. *Phytotherapy Research: An International Journal Devoted to Pharmacological and Toxicological Evaluation of Natural Product Derivatives* 14, (7): 495–500.

Beshbishy, A. M., Batiha, G. E. S., Adeyemi, O. S., et al. 2019. Inhibitory effects of methanolic *Olea europaea* and acetonic *Acacia laeta* on growth of *Babesia* and *Theileria*. *Asian Pacific Journal of Tropical Medicine* 12, (9): 425.

Bhowmik, D., Kumar, K. S., Yadav, A., et al. 2012. Recent trends in Indian traditional herbs *Syzygium aromaticum* and its health benefits. *Journal of Pharmacognosy and Phytochemistry* 1, (1): 13–22.

Bhuiyan, M. N. I., Begum, J., and F. Akter. 2010. Constituents of the essential oil from leaves and buds of clove (*Syzigium caryophyllatum* (L.) Alston). *African Journal of Plant Science* 4, (11): 451–454.

Blakeney, M., and G. Mengistie. 2012. Zanzibar: cloves. In *Extending the Protection of Geographical Indications – Case Studies of Agricultural Products in Africa*, eds. M. Blakeney, T. Coulet, G. Mengistie, and M.T. Mahop, Taylor & Francis (Oxon, England: Earthscan from Routledge), 330–344. https://doi.org/10.4324/9780203133316.

Board, N. 2010. *Handbook on Spices*. Delhi: Asia Pacific Business Press Inc, 199–213.

Byng, J. W., Barthelat, F., Snow, N., and B. Bernardini. 2016. Revision of *Eugenia* and *Syzygium* (Myrtaceae) from the Comoros archipelago. *Phytotaxa* 252, (3): 163.

Cai, L., and C. D. Wu. 1996. Compounds from *Syzygium aromaticum* possessing growth inhibitory activity against oral pathogens. *Journal of Natural Products* 59, (10): 987–990.

Carrasco A, H., Espinoza C, L., Cardile, V., et al. 2008. Eugenol and its synthetic analogues inhibit cell growth of human cancer cells (Part I). *Journal of the Brazilian Chemical Society* 19, (3): 543–548.

Carrasco, F. R., Schmidt, G., Romero, A. L., et al. 2009. Immunomodulatory activity of *Zingiber officinale* Roscoe, *Salvia officinalis* L. and *Syzygium aromaticum* L. essential oils: evidence for humor-and cell-mediated responses. *Journal of Pharmacy and Pharmacology* 61, (7): 961–967.

Castellano, J. M., Guinda, A., Delgado, T., et al. 2013. Biochemical basis of the antidiabetic activity of oleanolic acid and related pentacyclic triterpenes. *Diabetes* 62, (6): 1791–1799.

Cava, R., Nowak, E., Taboada, A., et al. 2007. Antimicrobial activity of clove and cinnamon essential oils against *Listeria monocytogenes* in pasteurized milk. *Journal of Food Protection* 70, (12): 2757–2763.

Cavero, S., García-Risco, M. R., Marín, F. R., et al. 2006. Supercritical fluid extraction of antioxidant compounds from oregano: chemical and functional characterization via LC–MS and *in vitro* assays. *The Journal of Supercritical Fluids* 38, (1): 62–69.

Chaachouay, N., Douira, A., and L. Zidane. 2021. COVID-19, prevention and treatment with herbal medicine in the herbal markets of Salé Prefecture, North-Western Morocco. *European Journal of Integrative Medicine* 42, 101285.

Chaieb, K., Hajlaoui, H., Zmantar, T., et al. 2007. The chemical composition and biological activity of clove essential oil, *Eugenia caryophyllata* (*Syzygium aromaticum* L. Myrtaceae): a short review. *Phytotherapy Research: An International Journal Devoted to Pharmacological and Toxicological Evaluation of Natural Product Derivatives* 21, (6): 501–506.

Chemat, F., and M. K. Khan. 2011. Applications of ultrasound in food technology: processing, preservation and extraction. *Ultrasonics Sonochemistry* 18, (4): 813–835.

Chemat, F., Abert-Vian, M., Fabiano-Tixier, A. S., et al. 2019. Green extraction of natural products. Origins, status, and future challenges. *TrAC Trends in Analytical Chemistry* 118, 248–263.

Chniguir, A., Zioud, F., Marzaioli, V., et al. 2019. *Syzygium aromaticum* aqueous extract inhibits human neutrophils myeloperoxidase and protects mice from LPS-induced lung inflammation. *Pharmaceutical Biology* 57, (1): 55–63.

Clifford, A. A., Basile, A., and S. H. Al-Saidi. 1999. A comparison of the extraction of clove buds with supercritical carbon dioxide and superheated water. *Fresenius' Journal of Analytical Chemistry* 364, (7): 635–637.

Cortés-Rojas, D. F., de Souza, C. R. F., and W. P. Oliveira. 2014. Clove (*Syzygium aromaticum*): a precious spice. *Asian Pacific Journal of Tropical Biomedicine* 4, (2): 90–96.

Dai, J. P., Zhao, X. F., Zeng, J., et al. 2013. Drug screening for autophagy inhibitors based on the dissociation of Beclin1-Bcl2 complex using BiFC technique and mechanism of eugenol on anti-influenza A virus activity. *PLoS One* 8, (4): e61026.

Damiani, C. E. N., Rossoni, L. V., and D. V. Vassallo. 2003. Vasorelaxant effects of eugenol on rat thoracic aorta. *Vascular Pharmacology* 40, (1): 59–66.

Daniel, A. N., Sartoretto, S. M., Schmidt, G., et al. 2009. Anti-inflammatory and antinociceptive activities A of eugenol essential oil in experimental animal models. *Revista Brasileira de Farmacognosia* 19, (1B): 212–217.

Danthu, P., Penot, E., Ranoarisoa, K. M., et al. 2014. The clove tree of Madagascar: a success story with an unpredictable future. *Bois et forêts des tropiques* 320, (2): 83–96.

Danthu, P., Simanjuntak, R., Fawbush, F., et al. 2020. The clove tree and its products (clove bud, clove oil, eugenol): prosperous today but what of tomorrow's restrictions?. *International Journal of Tropical and Subtropical Horticulture* 161: 52–915.

Das, B., Mandal, D., Dash, S. K., et al. 2016. Eugenol provokes ROS-mediated membrane damage-associated antibacterial activity against clinically isolated multidrug-resistant *Staphylococcus aureus* strains. *Infectious Diseases: Research and Treatment* 9, S31741.

Deans, S. G., and K. P. Svoboda. 1989. Antibacterial activity of summer savory (*Satureja hortensis L*) essential oil and its constituents. *Journal of Horticultural Science* 64, (2): 205–210.

Della Porta, G., Taddeo, R., D'Urso, E., et al. 1998. Isolation of clove bud and star anise essential oil by supercritical CO_2 extraction. *LWT-Food Science and Technology* 31, (5): 454–460.

Devi, K. P., Sakthivel, R., Nisha, S. A., et al. 2013. Eugenol alters the integrity of cell membrane and acts against the nosocomial pathogen Proteus mirabilis. *Archives of Pharmacal Research* 36, (3): 282–292.

Dhinahar, S., and T. Lakshmi. 2011. Role of botanicals as antimicrobial agents in management of dental infections–a review. *International Journal of Pharma and Bio Sciences* 2, (4): 690–704.

Díaz-Maroto, M. C., Díaz-Maroto Hidalgo, I. J., Sánchez-Palomo, E., et al. 2005. Volatile components and key odorants of Fennel (*Foeniculum vulgare* Mill.) and Thyme (*Thymus vulgaris* L.) oil extracts obtained by simultaneous distillation– extraction and supercritical fluid extraction. *Journal of Agricultural and Food Chemistry* 53, (13): 5385–5389.

Doleželová, P., Mácová, S., Plhalová, L., et al. 2011. The acute toxicity of clove oil to fish *Danio rerio* and *Poecilia reticulata*. *Acta Veterinaria Brno* 80, (3): 305–308.

Dwivedi, V., Shrivastava, R., Hussain, S., et al. 2011. Comparative anticancer potential of clove (*Syzygium aromaticum*)—an Indian spice—against cancer cell lines of various anatomical origin. *Asian Pacific Journal of Cancer Prevention* 12, (8): 1989–1993.

Ekor, M. 2014. The growing use of herbal medicines: issues relating to adverse reactions and challenges in monitoring safety. *Frontiers in Pharmacology*. 4: 177.

Elhoussine, D., Zineb, B., and B. Abdellatif. 2010. GC/MS analysis and antibacterial activity of the essential oil of *Mentha pulegium* grown in Morocco. *Research Journal of Agriculture and Biological Sciences* 6, (3): 191–198.

El-Maati, M. F. A., Mahgoub, S. A., Labib, S. M., et al. 2016. Phenolic extracts of clove (*Syzygium aromaticum*) with novel antioxidant and antibacterial activities. *European Journal of Integrative Medicine* 8, (4): 494–504.

El-Refai, A. A., Sharaf, A. M., Azzaz, N. A. E., et al. 2020. Antioxidants and antibacterial activities of bioactive compounds of clove (*Syzygium aromaticum*) and thyme (*Tymus vulgaris*) extracts. *Journal of Food and Dairy Sciences* 11, (9): 265–269.

Fernandes, E. S., Passos, G. F., Medeiros, R., et al. 2007. Anti-inflammatory effects of compounds alpha-humulene and (−)-trans-caryophyllene isolated from the essential oil of *Cordia verbenacea*. *European Journal of Pharmacology* 569, (3): 228–236.

Filho, G. A., Cesar, J. O., and J. V. Ramos. 2013. Itabuna CEPLAC 2013. http://www.ceplac.gov.br/radar.htm.

Fischer, I. U., and H. J. Dengler. 1990. Sensitive high-performance liquid chromatographic assay for the determination of eugenol in body fluids. *Journal of Chromatography B: Biomedical Sciences and Applications*, 525: 369–377.

Francomano, F., Caruso, A., Barbarossa, A., et al. 2019. β-Caryophyllene: a sesquiterpene with countless biological properties. *Applied Sciences* 9, (24): 5420.

García-Mediavilla, V., Crespo, I., Collado, P. S., et al. 2007. The anti-inflammatory flavones quercetin and kaempferol cause inhibition of inducible nitric oxide synthase, cyclooxygenase-2 and reactive C-protein, and down-regulation of the nuclear factor kappa B pathway in Chang Liver cells. *European Journal of Pharmacology* 557, (2–3): 221–229.

Gaspar, E. M., Res, T., Gaspar, E. M., et al. 2018. Volatile composition and antioxidant properties of clove products. *Biomedical* 5, (4): 1–7.

Ghai, R., Nagarajan, K., and N. Gupta. 2014. Isolation and characterization of a novel chemical compound from *Eugenia Caryophyllus* flower bud extract. *International Journal of Pharmacy and Pharmaceutical Sciences* 6, (7): 531–536.

Gonzalez-Rivera, J., Duce, C., Campanella, B., et al. 2021. In situ microwave assisted extraction of clove buds to isolate essential oil, polyphenols, and lignocellulosic compounds. *Industrial Crops and Products* 161, 113203.

González-Rivera, J., Duce, C., Falconieri, D., et al. 2016. Coaxial microwave assisted hydrodistillation of essential oils from five different herbs (lavender, rosemary, sage, fennel seeds and clove buds): chemical composition and thermal analysis. *Innovative Food Science & Emerging Technologies* 33, 308–318.

Gopalakrishnan, N., Narayanan, C.S., and A.G. Mathew. 1988. Chemical composition of Indian clove bud, stem and leaf oils. *Indian Perfumers* 32, 229–235.

Gopalakrishnan, N., Shanti, P. P. V., and C. S. Narayanan. 1990. Composition of clove (*Syzygium aromaticum*) bud oil extracted using carbon dioxide. *Journal of the Science of Food and Agriculture* 50, (1): 111–117.

Grosso, C., Coelho, J. P., Pessoa, F. L. P., et al. 2010. Mathematical modelling of supercritical CO_2 extraction of volatile oils from aromatic plants. *Chemical Engineering Science* 65, (11): 3579–3590.

Guan, W., Li, S., Yan, R., et al. 2007. Comparison of essential oils of clove buds extracted with supercritical carbon dioxide and other three traditional extraction methods. *Food Chemistry* 101, (4): 1558–1564.

Gülçin, İ., Elmastaş, M., and H. Y. Aboul-Enein. 2012. Antioxidant activity of clove oil–A powerful antioxidant source. *Arabian Journal of Chemistry* 5, (4): 489–499.

Gupta, A., Duhan, J., Tewari, S., et al. 2013. Comparative evaluation of antimicrobial efficacy of *Syzygium aromaticum*, *Ocimum sanctum* and *Cinnamomum zeylanicum* plant extracts against *Enterococcus faecalis*: a preliminary study. *International Endodontic Journal* 46, (8): 775–783.

Gupta, A., Koolwal, N., Dobhal, M. P., et al. 2014. Biological importance of phytochemical constituents isolated from genus *Eugenia*. *Journal of the Indian Chemical Society* 91, (8): 1539–1553.

Han, X., and T. L. Parker. 2017. Anti-inflammatory activity of clove (*Eugenia caryophyllata*) essential oil in human dermal fibroblasts. *Pharmaceutical Biology* 55, (1): 1619–1622.

Haqqyana, H., Tania, V. F. W., Suyadi, A. M., et al. 2020. Kinetic study in the extraction of essential oil from clove (*Syzygium aromaticum*) stem using microwave hydrodistillation. *Moroccan Journal of Chemistry* 8, (1): 8–11.

Hatami, T., Meireles, M. A. A., and G. Zahedi. 2010. Mathematical modeling and genetic algorithm optimization of clove oil extraction with supercritical carbon dioxide. *The Journal of Supercritical Fluids* 51, (3): 331–338.

Hu, F. B., and W. C. Willett. 2002. Optimal diets for prevention of coronary heart disease. *JAMA* 288, (20): 2569–2578.

Hussain, S., Rahman, R., Mushtaq, A., et al. 2017. Clove: a review of a precious species with multiple uses. *International Journal of Chemical and Biochemical Sciences* 11, 129–133.

Hussein, G., Miyashiro, H., Nakamura, N., et al. 2000. Inhibitory effects of Sudanese medicinal plant extracts on hepatitis C virus (HCV) protease. *Phytotherapy Research: An International Journal Devoted to Pharmacological and Toxicological Evaluation of Natural Product Derivatives* 14, (7): 510–516.

Huston, C. K., and H. Ji. 1991. Optimization of the analytical supercritical fluid extraction of cloves via an on-column interface to an ion trap GC/MS system. *Journal of Agricultural and Food Chemistry* 39, (7): 1229–1233.

Imran, M., Aslam Gondal, T., Atif, M., et al. 2020. Apigenin as an anticancer agent. *Phytotherapy Research* 34, (8): 1812–1828.

Issac, A., Gopakumar, G., Kuttan, R., et al. 2015. Safety and anti-ulcerogenic activity of a novel polyphenol-rich extract of clove buds (*Syzygium aromaticum* L). *Food & Function* 6, (3): 842–852.

Ivanovic, J., Zizovic, I., Ristic, M., et al. 2011. The analysis of simultaneous clove/oregano and clove/thyme supercritical extraction. *The Journal of Supercritical Fluids* 55, (3): 983–991.

Janes, S. E., Price, C. S., and D. Thomas. 2005. Essential oil poisoning: n-acetylcysteine for eugenol-induced hepatic failure and analysis of a national database. *European Journal of Pediatrics* 164, (8): 520–522.

Jeyaratnam, N., Nour, A. H., Kanthasamy, R., et al. 2016. Essential oil from *Cinnamomum cassia* bark through hydrodistillation and advanced microwave assisted hydrodistillation. *Industrial Crops and Products* 92, 57–66.

Jimoh, S. O., Arowolo, L. A., and K. A. Alabi. 2017. Phytochemical screening and antimicrobial evaluation of *Syzygium aromaticum* extract and essential oil. *International Journal of Current Microbiology and Applied Sciences* 6, (7): 4557–4567.

Jnawali, H. N., Lee, E., Jeong, K. W., et al. 2014. Anti-inflammatory activity of rhamnetin and a model of its binding to c-Jun NH_2-terminal kinase 1 and p38 MAPK. *Journal of Natural Products* 77, (2): 258–263.

Joshi, T., Sharma, P., Mathpal, S., et al. 2020. In silico screening of natural compounds against COVID-19 by targeting Mpro and ACE2 using molecular docking. *European Review for Medical and Pharmacological Sciences* 24, (8): 4529–4536.

Kamatou, G. P., Vermaak, I., and A. M. Viljoen. 2012. Eugenol—from the remote Maluku Islands to the international market place: a review of a remarkable and versatile molecule. *Molecules* 17, (6): 6953–6981.

Kanyinda, J. N. M. 2020. Coronavirus (COVID-19): a protocol for prevention and treatment (Covalyse®). *European Journal of Medical and Health Sciences* 2, 1–4.

Kapadiya, S. M., Parikh, J., and M. A. Desai. 2018. A greener approach towards isolating clove oil from buds of *Syzygium aromaticum* using microwave radiation. *Industrial Crops and Products* 112, 626–632.

Kasai, H., Shirao, M., and M. Ikegami-Kawai. 2016. Analysis of volatile compounds of clove (*Syzygium aromaticum*) buds as influenced by growth phase and investigation of antioxidant activity of clove extracts. *Flavour and Fragrance Journal* 31, (2): 178–184.

Khalil, A. A., ur Rahman, U., Khan, M. R., et al. 2017. Essential oil eugenol: sources, extraction techniques and nutraceutical perspectives. *RSC Advances* 7, (52): 32669–32681.

Kim, J. F., Gaffney, P. R., Valtcheva, I. B., et al. 2016. Organic solvent nanofiltration (OSN): a new technology platform for liquid-phase oligonucleotide synthesis (LPOS). *Organic Process Research & Development* 20, (8): 1439–1452.

Kraus, M. 2015. Huiles essentielles: un marché mondial en croissance. *Jardins de France*, 636, 3–5.

Kubatka, P., Uramova, S., Kello, M., et al. 2017. Antineoplastic effects of clove buds (*Syzygium aromaticum* L.) in the model of breast carcinoma. *Journal of Cellular and Molecular Medicine* 21, (11): 2837–2851.

Kumar, P. S., Febriyanti, R. M., Sofyan, F. F., et al. 2014. Anticancer potential of *Syzygium aromaticum* L. in MCF-7 human breast cancer cell lines. *Pharmacognosy Research* 6, (4): 350.

Kurokawa, M., Hozumi, T., Basnet, P., et al. 1998. Purification and Characterization of Eugeniin as an Anti-herpesvirus Compound from *Geum japonicum* and *Syzygium aromaticum*. *Journal of Pharmacology and Experimental Therapeutics* 284, (2): 728–735.

Kusworo, T. D., Widayat, W., and D. P. Utomo. 2020. Fabrication and characterization of nano hybrid cellulose acetate-nanoTiO2/crosslinked polyvinyl alcohol coated membrane for crude clove oil purification. *Periodica Polytechnica Chemical Engineering* 64, (3): 304–319.

Lesgards, J. F., Baldovini, N., Vidal, N., and S. Pietri. 2014. Anticancer activities of essential oils constituents and synergy with conventional therapies: a review. *Phytotherapy Research* 28, (10): 1423–1446.

Li, H. B., Cheng, K. W., Wong, C. C., et al. 2007. Evaluation of antioxidant capacity and total phenolic content of different fractions of selected microalgae. *Food Chemistry* 102, (3): 771–776.

Ling, L. T., Radhakrishnan, A. K., Subramaniam, T., et al. 2010. Assessment of antioxidant capacity and cytotoxicity of selected Malaysian plants. *Molecules* 15, (4): 2139–2151.

Liu, H., Schmitz, J. C., Wei, J., et al. 2014. Clove extract inhibits tumor growth and promotes cell cycle arrest and apoptosis. *Oncology Research Featuring Preclinical and Clinical Cancer Therapeutics* 21, (5): 247–259.

Liu, J., Mahmood, M. S., Abbas, R. Z., et al. 2021. Therapeutic appraisal of ethanolic and aqueous extracts of clove (*Syzygium aromaticum*) and garlic (*Allium sativum*) as antimicrobial agent. *Pakistan Journal of Agricultural Sciences* 58, (1): 245–251.

Magalhães, C. B., Riva, D. R., DePaula, L. J., et al. 2010. *In vivo* anti-inflammatory action of eugenol on lipopolysaccharide-induced lung injury. *Journal of Applied Physiology* 108, (4): 845–851.

Manaharan, T., Chakravarthi, S., Radhakrishnan, A. K., et al. 2014. *In vivo* toxicity evaluation of a standardized extract of *Syzygium aqueum* leaf. *Toxicology Reports* 1, 718–725.

Marchese, A., Barbieri, R., Coppo, E., et al. 2017. Antimicrobial activity of eugenol and essential oils containing eugenol: a mechanistic viewpoint. *Critical Reviews in Microbiology* 43, (6): 668–689.

Martínez, J., Rosa, P. T., and M. A. A. Meireles. 2007. Extraction of clove and vetiver oils with supercritical carbon dioxide: modeling and simulation. *The Open Chemical Engineering Journal* 1, (1): 1–7.

Matan, N. 2012. Antimicrobial activity of edible film incorporated with essential oils to preserve dried fish (*Decapterus maruadsi*). *International Food Research Journal* 19, (4): 1733–1738.

Mbaveng, A. T., Kuete, V., Mapunya, B. M., et al. 2011. Evaluation of four Cameroonian medicinal plants for anticancer, antigonorrheal and antireverse transcriptase activities. *Environmental Toxicology and Pharmacology* 32, (2): 162–167.

Menaker, A., Kravets, M., Koel, M., et al. 2004. Identification and characterization of supercritical fluid extracts from herbs. *Comptes Rendus Chimie* 7, (6–7): 629–633.

Milind, P., and K. Deepa. 2011. Clove: a champion spice. *International Journal of Research in Ayurveda and Pharmacy* 2, (1): 47–54.

Ming, D. S., Hillhouse, B. J., Guns, E. S., et al. 2005. Bioactive compounds from *Rhodiola rosea* (crassulaceae). *Phytotherapy Research: An International Journal Devoted to Pharmacological and Toxicological Evaluation of Natural Product Derivatives* 19, (9): 740–743.

Mishra, R.P., and K. Sharma. 2014. Antimicrobial activity of *Syzygium aromaticum* L. (clove). *International Research Journal of Biological Science* 3, 22–25.

Mittal, M., Gupta, N., Parashar, P., et al. 2014. Phytochemical evaluation and pharmacological activity of *Syzygium aromaticum*: a comprehensive review. *International Journal of Pharmacy and Pharmaceutical Sciences* 6, (8): 67–72.

Mohamed, S. G., and A. M. Badri. 2017. Antimicrobial activity of *Syzygium aromaticum* and *Citrus aurantifolia* essential oils against some microbes in Khartoum, Sudan. *EC Microbiology* 12, 253–259.

Mohammed, K. A. K., Abdulkadhim, H. M., and S. I. Noori. 2016. Chemical composition and anti-bacterial effects of clove (*Syzygium aromaticum*) flowers. *International Journal of Current Microbiology and Applied Sciences* 5, (2): 483–489.

Mohanty, S., and I. E. Cock. 2010. Bioactivity of *Syzygium jambos* methanolic extracts: antibacterial activity and toxicity. *Pharmacognosy Research* 2, (1): 4.

Mollika, S., Islam, N., N., Parvin, et al. 2014. Evaluation of analgesic, anti-inflammatory and CNS activities of the methanolic extract of *Syzygium samarangense* leave. *Global Journal of Pharmacology* 8, (1): 39–s46.

Moyler, D. A. 1986. *Developments in Food Flavours*. Eds. G. G. Birch and M. G. Lindley, 119–129. London: Elsevier Applied Science.

Mytle, N., Anderson, G. L., Doyle, M. P., et al. 2006. Antimicrobial activity of clove (*Syzygium aromaticum*) oil in inhibiting *Listeria monocytogenes* on chicken frankfurters. *Food Control* 17, (2): 102–107.

Nagababu, E., and N. Lakshmaiah. 1992. Inhibitory effect of eugenol on non-enzymatic lipid peroxidation in rat liver mitochondria. *Biochemical Pharmacology* 43, (11): 2393–2400.

Nam, H., and M. M. Kim. 2013. Eugenol with antioxidant activity inhibits MMP-9 related to metastasis in human fibrosarcoma cells. *Food and Chemical Toxicology* 55, 106–112.

Nam, P. N., Lien, P. T. K., Hoa, T. T., et al. 2017. Microwave assisted soxhlet extraction of essential oil from vietnamese star anise fruits (*Illicium verum* Hook. f.) and their chemical composition. *Emirates Journal of Food and Agriculture*, 29 (2): 131–137.

Nassan, M. A., Mohamed, E. H., Abdelhafez, S., et al. 2015. Effect of clove and cinnamon extracts on experimental model of acute hematogenous pyelonephritis in albino rats: immunopathological and antimicrobial study. *International Journal of Immunopathology and Pharmacology* 28, (1): 60–68.

Nassar, M. I. 2006. Flavonoid triglycosides from the seeds of *Syzygium aromaticum*. *Carbohydrate Research* 341, 160–163.

Nasution, I. K., Susilo, B., and W. A. Nugroho. 2013. Uji kinerja alat pemurni minyak atsiri daun cengkeh (clove leaf oil) berbasis membran kitosan-selulosa. *Jurnal Keteknikan Pertanian Tropis dan Biosistem* 2, (1): 9–14.

Nejad, S. M., Özgüneş, H., and N. Başaran 2017. Pharmacological and toxicological properties of eugenol. *Turkish Journal of Pharmaceutical Sciences* 14, (2): 201.

Nikoui, V., Ostadhadi, S., Bakhtiarian, A., et al. 2017. The anti-inflammatory and antipyretic effects of clove oil in healthy dogs after surgery. *PharmaNutrition* 5, (2): 52–57.

Nirmala, M. J., Durai, L., Gopakumar, V., et al. 2019. Anticancer and antibacterial effects of a clove bud essential oil-based nanoscale emulsion system. *International Journal of Nanomedicine* 14, 6439.

Novo Belchor, M., Hessel Gaeta, H., Fabri Bittencourt Rodrigues, C., et al. 2017. Evaluation of rhamnetin as an inhibitor of the pharmacological effect of secretory phospholipase A2. *Molecules*, 22(9): 1441.

Nurdjannah, N., and N. Bermawie. 2012. Cloves. In *Handbook of Herbs and Spices*, Abington, Cambridge: Woodhead Publishing, pp. 197–215.

Ocana-Fuentes, A., Arranz-Gutierrez, E., Senorans, F. J., et al. 2010. Supercritical fluid extraction of oregano (*Origanum vulgare*) essentials oils: anti-inflammatory properties based on cytokine response on THP-1 macrophages. *Food and Chemical Toxicology* 48, (6): 1568–1575.

Ohigashi, H., and K. Koshimizu. 1976. Chavicol, as a larva-growth inhibitor, from *Viburnum japonicum* Spreng. *Agricultural and Biological Chemistry* 40, (11): 2283–2287.

Oliveira, R. A., Oliveira, F. F., and C. K. Sacramento. 2007. Essential oils: prospects for agribusiness spices in Bahia. *Bahia Agriculture* 8, (1): 46–48.

Oliveira, R. A. D., Reis, T. V., Sacramento, C. K. D., et al. 2009. Volatile chemical constituents of rich spices in eugenol. *Revista Brasileira de Farmacognosia* 19, (3): 771–775.

Oszagyan, M., Simandi, B., Sawinsky, J., et al. 1994. Supercritical fluid extraction of essential oils from mixtures of medicinal plants. In *Proceedings of the Third Symposium on Supercritical Fluids*, ed. M. Perrut, and G. Brunner, 453–458. Strasbourg: ISASF.

Öztürk, A., and H. Özbek. 2005. The anti-inflammatory activity of Eugenia caryophyllata essential oil: an animal model of anti-inflammatory activity. *European Journal of Internal Medicine* 2, (4), 159–163.

Pandey, P., Singhal, D., Khan, F. et al. 2020. An in silico screening on *Piper nigrum, Syzygium aromaticum* and *Zingiber officinale* roscoe derived compounds against SARS-COV-2: a drug repurposing approach. *Biointerface Research in Applied Chemistry* 11, (4): 11122–11134.

Peev, G., Penchev, P., Peshev, D. et al. 2011. Solvent extraction of rosmarinic acid from lemon balm and concentration of extracts by nanofiltration: effect of plant pre-treatment by supercritical carbon dioxide. *Chemical Engineering Research and Design* 89, (11): 2236–2243.

Périno-Issartier, S., Abert-Vian, M., and F. Chemat. 2011. Solvent free microwave-assisted extraction of antioxidants from sea buckthorn (*Hippophae rhamnoides*) food by-products. *Food and Bioprocess Technology* 4, (6): 1020–1028.

Pino, J. A., Marbot, R., Agüero, J. et al. 2001. Essential oil from buds and leaves of clove (*Syzygium aromaticum* (L.) Merr. et Perry) grown in Cuba. *Journal of Essential Oil Research* 13, (4): 278–279.

Pramod, K., Ansari, S. H., and J. Ali. 2010. Eugenol: a natural compound with versatile pharmacological actions. *Natural Product Communications* 5, (12): 1934578X1000501236.

Prashar, A., Locke, I. C., and C. S. Evans. (2006). Cytotoxicity of clove (*Syzygium aromaticum*) oil and its major components to human skin cells. *Cell Proliferation* 39, (4): 241–248.

Pulikottil, S. J., and S. Nath. 2015. Potential of clove of *Syzygium aromaticum* in development of a therapeutic agent for periodontal disease: a review. *South African Dental Journal* 70, (3): 108–115.

Rahman, M. F., Haykal, M. N., Siagian, N. A., et al. 2018. Synthesis and proapoptotic activity on cervical cancer cell of ester eugenol 1-(3-methoxy-4-hydroxy) phenyl-2-propylmethanoate. In *IOP Conference Series: Materials Science and Engineering*, 299, 1: 012071.

Ramos-Nino, M. E., Clifford, M. N., Adams, M. R. 1996. Quantitative structure activity relationship for the effect of benzoic acids, cinnamic acids and benzaldehydes on *Listeria monocytogenes*. *Journal of Applied Bacteriology* 80, (3): 303–310.

Rasheed, A., Laekeman, G., Totte, J., et al 1984. Eugenol and prostaglandin biosynthesis. *The New England Journal of Medicine* 310, (1): 50–51.

Rassem, H. H., Nour, A. H., and R. M. Yunus. 2016. Techniques for extraction of essential oils from plants: a review. *Australian Journal of Basic and Applied Sciences* 10, (16): 117–127.

Rathinam, P., and P. Viswanathan. 2018. Anti-virulence potential of eugenol-rich fraction of *Syzygium aromaticum* against multidrug resistant uropathogens isolated from catheterized patients. *Avicenna Journal of Phytomedicine* 8, (5): 416.

Ratri, P. J., Ayurini, M., Khumaini, K., et al. 2020. Clove oil extraction by steam distillation and utilization of clove buds waste as potential candidate for eco-friendly packaging. *Jurnal Bahan Alam Terbarukan* 9, (1): 47–54.

Reddy, L., Odhav, B., and K. D. Bhoola. 2003. Natural products for cancer prevention: a global perspective. *Pharmacology & Therapeutics* 99, (1): 1–13.

Rege, S. A., and S. A. Momin. 2018. Synergistic antioxidant activity of clove oleoresin with capsicum oleoresin and kalonji seeds extract in sunflower oil. *International Journal of Nutritional Disorders & Therapy* 2, (1): 002–006.

Rehman, M., AlAjmi, M. F., and A. Hussain. 2020. Natural compounds as inhibitors of SARS-CoV-2 main protease (3CLPRO): a molecular docking and simulation approach to combat COVID-19. *Current Pharmaceutical Design* 27, (33): 3577–3589.

Reverchon, E. (1992). Fractional separation of SCF extracts from marjoram leaves: mass transfer and optimization. *The Journal of Supercritical Fluids* 5, (4): 256–261.

Reverchon, E., Porta, G. D., and F. Senatore. 1995. Supercritical CO_2 extraction and fractionation of lavender essential oil and waxes. *Journal of Agricultural and Food Chemistry* 43, (6): 1654–1658.

Reverchon, E., and F. Senatore. 1994. Supercritical carbon dioxide extraction of chamomile essential oil and its analysis by gas chromatography-mass spectrometry. *Journal of Agricultural and Food Chemistry* 42, (1): 154–158.

Rho, H. S., Ghimeray, A. K., Yoo, D. S., et al. 2011. Kaempferol and kaempferol rhamnosides with depigmenting and anti-inflammatory properties. *Molecules* 16, (4): 3338–3344.

Riyanto, H., Sastrohamidjojo, and E. Fariyatun. 2016. Synthesis of methyl eugenol from crude cloves leaf oil using acid and based chemicals reactions. *IOSR Journal of Applied Chemistry* 9, (10): 105–112.

Rusmana, D., Elisabeth, M., Widowati, W., et al. 2015. Inhibition of inflammatory agent production by ethanol extract and eugenol of *Syzygium aromaticum* (L.) flower bud (clove) in LPS-stimulated Raw 264.7 cells. *Research Journal of Medicinal Plant* 9, (6): 264–274.

Saeed, M., Khan, M. S., Alagawany, M., et al. 2021. Clove (*Syzygium aromaticum*) and its phytochemicals in ruminant feed: an updated review. *Rendiconti Lincei. Scienze Fisiche e Naturali* 32: 273–285.

Sahraoui, N., and C. Boutekedjiret. 2015. Innovative process of essential oil extraction: steam distillation assisted by microwave. In *Progress in Clean Energy*. Eds. I. Dincer, C.O. Colpan, O. Kizilkan and M.A. Ezan, 1: 831–841. Cham: Springer.

Sallie, R., Tredger, J. M., and R. William. 1991. Drugs and the liver. *Biopharmaceutics and Drug Disposition* 12, 251–259.

Sánchez-Tena, S., Reyes-Zurita, F. J., and S. Díaz-Moralli. 2013. Maslinic acid-enriched diet decreases intestinal tumorigenesis in Apc Min/+ mice through transcriptomic and metabolomic reprogramming. *PLoS One* 8, (3): e59392.

Santos, A., Chierice, G., Alexander, K., et al. 2009. Characterization of the raw essential oil eugenol extracted from *Syzygium aromaticum* L. *Journal of Thermal Analysis and Calorimetry* 96, (3): 821–825.

Sarrami, N., Pemberton, M. N., Thornhill, M. H., et al. 2002. Adverse reactions associated with the use of eugenol in dentistry. *British Dental Journal* 193, (5): 257–259.

Scalbert, A., Manach, C., Morand, C., et al. 2005. Dietary polyphenols and the prevention of diseases. *Critical Reviews in Food Science and Nutrition* 45, (4): 287–306.

Sebaaly, C., Jraij, A., Fessi, H., et al. 2015. Preparation and characterization of clove essential oil-loaded liposomes. *Food Chemistry*, 178: 52–62.

Sofia, P. K., Prasad, R., Vijay, V. K., et al. 2007. Evaluation of antibacterial activity of Indian spices against common foodborne pathogens. *International Journal of Food Science & Technology* 42, (8): 910–915.

Su, H., Yang, M., Wan, C., et al. 2020. Renal histopathological analysis of 26 postmortem findings of patients with COVID-19 in China. *Kidney International* 98, (1): 219–227.

Sultana, K., Jayathilakan, K., and M. C. Pandey. 2017. Evaluation of antioxidant activity, radical scavenging, and reducing power of clove oil and clove oleoresin in comparison with natural and synthetic antioxidants in chevon (*Capra aegagrus hircus*) and chicken meat. *Defence Life Science Journal* 3, (1): 51.

Tampieri, M. P., Galuppi, R., Macchioni, F., et al. 2005. The inhibition of *Candida albicans* by selected essential oils and their major components. *Mycopathologia* 159, (3): 339–345.

Tanaka, T., Orii, Y., Nonaka, G., et al. 1993. Tannins and related compounds. CXXIII. Chromone, acetophenone and phenyl propanoid glycosides and their galloyl and/or hexahydroxy phenoyl esters from leaves of *Syzygium aromaticum* Merr and Perry. *Chemical Pharmaceutical Bulletin* 28, 685–687.

Tanko, Y., Mohammed, A., Okasha, M. A., et al. 2008. Anti-nociceptive and anti-inflammatory activities of ethanol extract of *Syzygium aromaticum* flower bud in wistar rats and mice. *African Journal of Traditional, Complementary and Alternative Medicines* 5, (2): 209–212.

Tejasari, M., Respati, T., Trusda, S. A. D., et al. 2020. Comparison of flavonoid from clove leaf oil cytotoxic activities with doxorubicin and cisplatin on liver cancer cell culture. *Journal of Physics: Conference Series*, 1469, (1): 012018.

Tekin, K., Akalın, M. K., and M. G. Şeker. 2015. Ultrasound bath-assisted extraction of essential oils from clove using central composite design. *Industrial Crops and Products* 77, 954–960.

Tragoolpua, Y., and A. Jatisatienr. 2007. Anti-herpes simplex virus activities of *Eugenia caryophyllus* (Spreng) Bullock & SG Harrison and essential oil, eugenol. *Phytotherapy Research: An International Journal Devoted to Pharmacological and Toxicological Evaluation of Natural Product Derivatives* 21, (12): 1153–1158.

Trongtokit, Y., Rongsriyam, Y., Komalamisra, N., et al. 2005. Comparative repellency of 38 essential oils against mosquito bites. *Phytotherapy Research: An International Journal Devoted to Pharmacological and Toxicological Evaluation of Natural Product Derivatives* 19, (4): 303–309.

Uddin, M. A., Shahinuzzaman, M., Rana, M. S., et al. 2017. Study of chemical composition and medicinal properties of volatile oil from clove buds (*Eugenia caryophyllus*). *International Journal of Pharmaceutical Sciences and Research* 8, (2): 895.

Flavor and Extract Manufacturers' Association (FEMA), Scientific Literature Review of Eugenol and Related Substances in Flavor Usage, Vol. 1. Accession No. PB-283 501, National Technical Information Service, US Department of Commerce, Washington DC, 1978.

Usman, H., and J. C. Osuji. 2007. Phytochemical and *in vitro* antimicrobial assay of the leaf extract of *Newbouldia laevis*. *African Journal of Traditional, Complementary and Alternative Medicines* 4, (4): 476–480.

Vasconcellos, M. C., Bezerra, D. P., Fonseca, A. M., et al. 2011. The *in-vitro* and *in-vivo* inhibitory activity of biflorin in melanoma. *Melanoma Research* 21, (2): 106–114.

Vijayasteltar, L., Nair, G. G., Maliakel, B., et al. 2016. Safety assessment of a standardized polyphenolic extract of clove buds: subchronic toxicity and mutagenicity studies. *Toxicology Reports* 3, 439–449.

Wael, S., Watuguly, T. W., Arini, I., et al. 2018. Potential of *Syzygium aromaticum* (clove) leaf extract on immune proliferation response in Balb/c mice infected with *Salmonella typhimurium*. *Case Reports in Clinical Medicine* 7, (12): 613.

Wang, C. C., Ho, C. T., Lee, S. C., et al. 2016. Isolation of eugenyl β-primeveroside from *Camellia sasanqua* and its anticancer activity in PC3 prostate cancer cells. *Journal of Food and Drug Analysis* 24, (1): 105–111.

Wei, M. C., Lin, P. H., Hong, S. J., et al. 2016. Development of a green alternative procedure for the simultaneous separation and quantification of clove oil and its major bioactive constituents. *ACS Sustainable Chemistry & Engineering* 4, (12): 6491–6499.

Xin, W., Huang, C., Zhang, X., et al. 2014. Methyl salicylate lactoside inhibits inflammatory response of fibroblast-like synoviocytes and joint destruction in collagen-induced arthritis in mice. *British Journal of Pharmacology* 171, (14): 3526–3538.

Xiong, G., Wang, P., Yang, J., et al. 2018. Extraction of clove essential oil by microcapsule aqueous two-phase system. *Journal of Essential Oil Bearing Plants* 21, (6): 1487–1492.

Xu, J. G., Liu, T., Hu, Q. P., et al. 2016. Chemical composition, antibacterial properties and mechanism of action of essential oil from clove buds against *Staphylococcus aureus*. *Molecules* 21, (9): 1194.

Yadav, A. S., and D. Bhatnagar. 2007. Free radical scavenging activity, metal chelation and antioxidant power of some of the Indian spices. *Biofactors* 31, (3–4): 219–227.

Yang, Y. Y., Lee, M. J., Lee, H. S., et al. 2011. Screening of antioxidative, anti-platelet aggregation and anti-thrombotic effects of clove extracts. *Journal of Physiology & Pathology in Korean Medicine* 25, (3): 471–481.

Yassin, M. T., Al-Askar, A. A., Mostafa, A. A. F., et al. 2020. Bioactivity of *Syzygium aromaticum* (L.) Merr. & LM Perry extracts as potential antimicrobial and anticancer agents. *Journal of King Saud University-Science* 32, (8): 3273–3278.

Yazdani, F., Mafi, M., Farhadi, F., et al. 2005. Supercritical CO_2 extraction of essential oil from clove bud: effect of operation conditions on the selective isolation of eugenol and eugenyl acetate. *Zeitschrift für Naturforschung B* 60, (11): 1197–1201.

Yogalakshmi, B., Viswanathan, P., and C. V. Anuradha. 2010. Investigation of antioxidant, anti-inflammatory and DNA-protective properties of eugenol in thioacetamide-induced liver injury in rats. *Toxicology* 268, (3): 204–212.

Zeković, Z., Lepojeviíc, Ž., and D. Vujić. 2000. Supercritical extraction of thyme (*Thymus vulgaris* L.). *Chromatographia* 51, (3–4): 175–179.

Zengin, H., and A. H. Baysal. 2015. Antioxidant and antimicrobial activities of thyme and clove essential oils and application in minced beef. *Journal of Food Processing and Preservation* 39, (6): 1261–1271.

Zhang, F. M., Tai, Z. G., Cai, L., et al. 2011. Flavonoids from Gypsophila elegans and their antioxidant activities [J]. *Journal of Yunnan University (Natural Sciences Edition)*, 1.

CHAPTER 18

Fenugreek Oleoresins

Chemistry and Properties

Nighat Raza and Muhammad Shahbaz

MNS-University of Agriculture

Mujahid Farid

University of Gujrat

Adeel Hakim

MNS-University of Agriculture

CONTENTS

DOI: 10.1201/9781003186205-18

18.1 INTRODUCTION

Legume plants are cheap source of high-quality foods which provide several functional and nutritional benefits. An example of such legume plants is Fenugreek. Fenugreek is a leguminous herb which belongs to Fabaceae family. It is grown in all over the world, especially in the North African and Asian countries (Ghosh et al., 2015). China, Turkey, India, Australia, Canada, southern Europe and Africa are the major countries where Fenugreek is cultivated on large scale (Ahmad et al., 2016; Moyer et al., 2003). Despite the bitter taste of fenugreek, it has been in use since 500 BC.

Fenugreek (*Trigonella foenum – graecum* L.) has different names in local languages of different areas in the world as shown in Table 18.1. It is acknowledged as an effective herb, and is being in use as a traditional medicine. The seeds of fenugreek are good source of protein as well as lipids, amino acid, biogenic medicines and lipids. These seeds are also a good source of carotene, flavonoids, saponins, choline, essential oils containing trigonelline and other functional elements (Murlidhar, and Goswami, 2012; Srinivasan, 2006). It is also found in studies that fenugreek seeds are abundant in nicotinic acid, vitamins C, A and B₁, as well as noteworthy proportion of P, Fe, Ca, Mn and Zn are present in it (Moradi, and Moradi, 2013). Both leaves and seeds of fenugreek are utilized in different dishes and food preparation, such as cheese flavoring in Switzerland, stews in Iran, roasted seeds as coffee substitute in Africa, bitter rum and syrup in Germany, curries, mixed seed powder for baking flat bread in Egypt and in dyes. Young seedlings are also utilized as vegetable (Moradi and Moradi, 2013).

TABLE 18.1 Local Names of Fenugreek

Urdu	Methi
Arabic	Hulba
Italian	Fieno Greco
Farsi	Sambelil
German	Bockshorklee, Bockshornsamen (seed)
Chinese	K'u-Tou, Hu-lu-ba,Hu-lu-pa
Spanish	Fenogreco, Alholva
French	Trigonelle, Fenugrec

Source: Snehlata and Payal (2012).

The plant of fenugreek and its seeds are diuretic, suppurative and aperient. It is found helpful for some diseases like chronic cough, dropsy, spleen and liver enlargement. Fenugreek leaves are also found to be beneficial for both external and internal burns and swelling as well as in unani (the hair falling off) (Ghosh et al., 2015; Prajapati et al., 2003). Fenugreek supports in the increase in milk flow of mother as well as comfort during child birth. The Egyptian tourists use it as tea (hilba) to eradicate stomach problems. The use of this plant is also suggested in rheumatism, in dyspepsia with loss in appetite and in diarrhea of puerperal women (Ghosh et al., 2015; Prajapati et al., 2003). Women in Egypt still use Fenugreek for menstrual pain. Fenugreek is also known to be an ecofriendly plant as it fixes nitrogen in atmospheric (PietrzAk, 2011).

18.2 BOTANICAL CHARACTERISTICS

Scientific name of Fenugreek is *Trigonella foenum-graceum* L. It is a yearly diploid plant which belongs to the family Leguminosae. Complete botanical description is depicted in Table 18.2. This specie has a feebly split core stem which grows to the height of 1–2 ft (30–60 cm) and a lengthy taproot. The leaves of fenugreek have three-lobed inversely ovate leaflets with egg-shaped stipules, petite leafstalks and jagged boundaries (Bieńkowski et al., 2016).

Fenugreek is a flowery plant. The shape of fenugreek flowers is like a boat having upturn petals and brief wings. Its color varies from light purple and yellow, to white or cream. Flowers appear in pairs or individually in the nodes of leaf (Bieńkowski et al., 2016). The odor of this plant is spicy which after touching persists on the hands. There are two verities that are present, one is cultivated and other is wild. Low Mediterranean temperatures are most suitable for the growth of fenugreek. The maturity of this plant is attained in around four months. Midsummer is generally known to be the season of flowering for this herb (Snehlata, andPayal, 2012). Flowers blooms during the month of June and July, whereas August and September are the months in which seeds attain maturity (Bieńkowski et al., 2016).

Pods of Fenugreek plant is of horned-shape having length of maximum 11 cm. These pods are narrow, curved or straight in shape, having an abruptly sharp tip. 10 to 20 cuboid seeds are present in each pod, which is separated by a crest into two uneven parts. Brown-green seeds of fenugreek are very hard but lobulated as well. Seed morphology has

TABLE 18.2   Botanical
Classification of Fenugreek

Kingdom	Plantae
Division	Magnoliophyta
Class	Magnoliopsida
Order	Fabales
Family	Fabaceae
Genus	Trigonella
Species	*foenum-graecum*

Source: Acharya et al., 2006; Ghosh
et al., 2015; Snehlata,and
Payal, 2012.

TABLE 18.3   Morphology of Fenugreek Seed

Odor	Spicy
Taste	Bitter
Colour	Yellowish brown or light brown
Appearance	Rhomboidal solid seeds. Hard, pebble-like. 3 to 5 mm long, 2 mm thick.
Bulk Density	1165.25 -1240.36 kg m^{-3} (at moisture 8.9-20.1%)
Weight	14-15g (1000 seeds)

Source: Altuntaş et al., 2005; Bieńkowski et al., 2016; Ghosh et al., 2015; Snehlata,and
Payal, 2012; Żuk-Gołaszewska,and Wierzbowska, 2017

been given in detail in Table 18.3. They can hold their germination capability for two years (Żuk-Gołaszewska, and Wierzbowska, 2017).

18.3 COMPOUNDS PRESENT IN FENUGREEK

18.3.1 Plant Chemistry

Alkaloids, fibers, mucilage and steroidal saponins are the main constitutes (50%) of fenugreek seed (Bahmani et al., 2016). Oil, carbohydrates, protein, flavonoids and aromatic compounds are the other components. (Table 18.5)

18.3.2 Alkaloids

The major alkaloid present in fenugreek is Trigonelline which has been extracted up to 36%. Other alkaloids present in the seed are carpaine choline and gentanin (Bahmani et al., 2016).

18.3.3 Steroidal Saponins

The most abundant steroidal saponins in seed are yamogenin and diosgenin (0.1% to 2.2%). Gitogenin, tigogenin, smilagenin, sarsapogenin and yuccagenin are other sapogenins present in seed. Fenugreekine is a sapogenin peptide ester which is also present in fenugreek seed (Bahmani et al., 2016).

TABLE 18.4 Fat, Protein and Carbohydrate Content in Fenugreek Seeds and Leaves

Plant Parts	Fat %	Protein %	Carbohydrate %	References
Seed	7.5	9.5	42.3	(Mandal,and DebMandal, 2016)
Seed	5–10	20–30	45–60	(Mehrafarin et al., 2010)
Seed	4	28.55	62.48	(Sulieman, Ahmed, et al., 2008)
Leaf	0.9–1	4.4	6.6	(Murlidhar,andGoswami, 2012; Snehlata, and Payal, 2012)
Seed	6–7	23–26	58	(Lu et al., 2008)
Seed	6.53	20–30	–	(Sheikhlar, 2013)

18.3.4 Oils

Unsaturated fatty acids are present in the fenugreek seed oil (6% to 10%), which are odorless and golden yellow in color. This oil can be easily dissolved in sulfur, ether, petroleum ether and benzene. Antimicrobial potential of fenugreek oil is also proven (Bahmani et al., 2016).

18.3.5 Mucilage

Endosperm of the seed contain mucilage composites that after hydrolysis produce galactose and mannose. The presence of mucilage in fenugreek seeds exhibits laxative property. The water-holding potential of fenugreek in contradiction of sodium alginate is due to the presence of mucilage. Moreover, the suspending and emulsifying effect of mucilage is acceptable (Bahmani et al., 2016). Xylene and galactomannan are also present in fenugreek and it is found to be neutral.

18.3.6 Protein Compounds

Protein content in this herb is comparatively high, which ranges from 22% to 25%. The protein is high in glutamic acid, arginine, and many essential amino acids are abundantly present like lysine, histidine, glycine and tryptophan, but low in valin, threonine, methionine and other sulfur-containing amino acids (Mirzaei, and Venkatesh, 2012). Essential and nonessential amino acids concentration is shown in Table 18.5.

18.3.7 Flavonoids

Orientin, glycoside, isoorientin, quercetin, vitexin and epigenin are the main flavonoids which are present in this plant (Mirzaei, and Venkatesh, 2012).

18.3.8 Aromatic and Other Compounds

The aromatic compounds present in fenugreek seed are hexanol, n-alkenes and sesquiterpenes. It is found that there are proteinase preventing components present in fenugreek seed. Literature reveals that vitamins like B_1, nicotinic acid, D, C and A, as well as minerals like Ca, Fe and P are also present in fenugreek (Bahmani et al., 2016).

18.3.9 Carbohydrates

Almost 8% of fenugreek seed is consist of carbohydrates (Bahmani et al., 2016).

TABLE 18.5   Amino Acid Composition Of
Fenugreek Seed

Amino Acids	(g kg-1 of protein)
Glutamic acid (Glu)	160.50
Aspartic acid (Asp)	102.00
Arginine (Arg)	91.00
Leucine (Leu)	62.60
Lysine (Lys)	57.70
Glycine (Gly)	47.50
Serine (Ser)	47.10
Isoleucine (Ile)	41.00
Proline (Pro)	39.40
Valine (Val)	38.20
Phenylalanine (Phe)	37.80
Alanine (Ala)	36.90
Threonine (Thr)	33.00
Tyrosine (Tyr)	29.60
Cysteine (Cys)	22.00
Histidine (His)	21.50
Methionine (Met)	13.00

Source: Mahfouz et al., 2012

18.4 TRADITIONAL USES OF FENUGREEK

Mankind is using Fenugreek from 2500 years ago. Some scientist compares it with qui-nine, since it is very useful in dropping fever. Smoothing effect of seed makes fenugreek a valuable source to resist gastric abscesses. The seeds support in restoring a dulled taste sense and also freshen bad breath. Oil which is extracted from seeds is also found to be useful as an emollient and softener of skin (Snehlata, andPayal, 2012). In the Balkans and Middle East, this plant is used as traditional therapy for stomach pain which is caused by the gastroenteritis or diarrhea and menstrual cycle. This remedy is also used in easing labour pains (Snehlata, andPayal, 2012). Similarly, Old herbalists of China used this herb for the treatment of male reproductive disorder and kidney complica-tions. Fenugreek seeds can be added to chutneys, pickles and other similar products, as a preservative (Snehlata, andPayal, 2012). Fenugreek has diaphoretic effect as it helps detox the body and bring on sweat. Some scientist also claim that it has beneficial effect on blood cleansing. Fenugreek also has an important role in removal of trapped pro-teins, toxic wastes and dead cells from the body and to transport nutrients to the cells, which results in good lymphatic cleansing activity. Fenugreek helps to clear congestion which keeps mucus conditions of the body (the lungs). It also acts as a mucus solvent and throat cleanser which smoothens coughing. It is also proven that fenugreek has ability to relieve bronchial complaints, colds, asthma, influenza, catarrh, sinusitis, constipa-tion, pleurisy, sore throat, pneumonia, laryngitis, emphysema and hay fever tuberculosis (Wani, andKumar, 2018). The strong smell of fenugreek can also be smelt on our skin and in under-arm sweat.

18.5 FENUGREEK OIL

Fenugreek see id also a good source of oil. Essential oils extracted from fenugreek have shown exceptional antifungal, antioxidant and antibacterial activities in the studies, have natural agents, which revealed its ability as a natural preservative agent (Mandal, andDeb-Mandal, 2016). Promising antimicrobial potential against *Escherichia coli*, *Staphylococcus aureus* and *Salmonella typhi* have been shown by the aqueous extract and seed oil of fenugreek. Aqueous extract of fenugreek is obtained by boiling its seeds in water (Verma et al., 2015). Essential oils, natural extractives and oleoresins of fenugreek are approved as GRAS (generally recognized as safe) (Hassan, A. M. et al., 2006). If the typical pungent smell of fenugreek oil is reduced, it can be used as an edible oil because physicochemical properties of fenugreek seed like ester value (190.25), acid value (4.75 mg KOH/g), free fatty acids content (2.38 mg Oleic acid/100 g), refractive index (1.464), and saponification value (195 mg KOH/g) are ideal to be consumed (Sulieman, Ahmed, et al., 2008). Oil of fenugreek is added in syrups (i.e., artificial maple syrup emulsifier) and canned food as flavouring agent. It was also found that fixed and volatile oils are also present in fenugreek seeds but in small quantity (Wani, andKumar, 2018).

18.6 OIL EXTRACTION METHOD

18.6.1 Extraction Process (Soxhlet Extraction)

18.6.1.1 Procurement of Fenugreek Seed

Akbari et al. (2019) extracted fenugreek oil with the help of Soxhlet apparatus. The seeds were procured and cleaning was done. After that drying was done in an oven at 50°C for 24 h. These dried seeds were crushed with the help of a grinder with ultra-centrifugal which was consisting of ring strainer. The moisture content of the seed was determined which was found to be 5.51 ±0.14%. This seed powder was packed in sealed vessel before extraction (Akbari et al., 2019).

18.6.1.2 Analytical Reagents and Chemicals

2,2-Diphenylpicrylhydrazyl (DPPH), Methanol with 99% purity, sodium carbonate, *n*-hexane with 99% purity, gallic acid (GA) and Folin Ciocateu reagent were used in the process (Akbari et al., 2019).

18.6.1.3 Extraction

In Soxhlet extractor, 600 mL *n*-hexane and 100 g of powdered fenugreek seed were taken and extraction was done at 65–70°C for 3 hours. After 3 hours, filtration of oil and solvent mixture was done with the help of What man filter paper No 1. The solvent was evaporated using rotatory evaporator at 40°C, and extracted oil was shifted to a circular bottle. At the end, for further analysis, obtained oil was kept at 40°C to avoid degradation of the components. Oil yield can be determined by using following equation (Akbari et al., 2019).

$$\text{Extration yield}\left(\frac{v}{w}\%\right) = \frac{\text{Volume of extracted oil}}{\text{Sample weight}} \times 100$$

Process 2

This process was adopted by Munshi et al. (2020). Fenugreek seeds of HSHM 57 variety were collected. These seeds were sifted to eliminate the extraneous materials. Cleaned seeds were wrapped in an airtight plastic container and kept at room temperature.

18.6.1.4 Preparation of FGSO (Fenugreek Seed Oil)

Oven drying of stored seeds were done for 1 day at 105±1°C (Munshi et al., 2020). Dried seeds were grounded to powder form using a lab-scale grinder and then sifted over an 80-mesh sieve. Oil extraction was done from this powder by using different solvents like petroleum ether, ethanol, acetone and hexane having boiling points of 30–60°C, 78.5°C, 56°C and 68°C respectively, in vintage Soxhlet apparatus. Then the oil sample was held in the oven at 45°C for 4 hours to obtain a solvent-free oil and then stored at room temperature. The oil obtained from this process is of dark brownish to golden yellow color (Munshi et al., 2020). Around 500 g fenugreek seed powder was used for fat removal and this extracted oil was kept at refrigerated temperature for further studies.

18.6.2 Extraction by Hydro Distillation

Plants essential oils extraction was achieved by hydro distillation in a Clevenger type device. A flask of 1 L of water was taken and dry seeds of about 200 g were immersed in it for 2 hrs. Essential oils were obtained in small bottles. Same Clevenger-type device (1928) can be used for hydro distillation of fenugreek seeds (Mehani, and Segni, 2012).

This method includes boiling of 200 g of dried seed with 1 L of water of for two hours in a flask. Then the distillation process is done with a recycling cohobage. The yield of essential oil which is obtained from fresh plant substantial (Mehani, and Segni, 2012), is find out by following formula:

$$RHEAa = \frac{HE\ mass}{Mass\ dry\ plant\ material}$$

18.6.3 Extraction of Fenugreek Seed Oil Using Subcritical Butane

This method of oil extraction was used by (Gu, L.-B. et al., 2017).

18.6.3.1 Materials

For oil extraction, fenugreek seeds were bought from a pharmacy, located at Zhengzhou, China. Fenugreek samples were grinded into powder form with the help of a Wiley Mill (Thomas Scientific, Philadelphia, PA, USA) and passed through diverse sized sieves. This seed powder was dried in drying oven at 80°C for 1 day and then kept at refrigerated temperature. Butane, other chemicals and solvents were acquired from a local chemical store (Gu, L.-B. et al., 2017).

18.6.3.2 Oil Extraction

Subcritical Butane extraction was executed using the kit procured from Henan Subcritical Biological Technology Co., Ltd., Anyang, China. For this purpose, seed powder of about

50 g was taken in the extractor. To avoid oxidation of oil during extraction, atmospheric oxygen was removed from extractor with the help of vacuum sealing. Butane was added in the form of subcritical liquid to the extractor over a metering pump. A controlling unit automatically controls the temperature according to its setting. In the end, when lipo-soluble extract reaches the separator, and evaporation of solvent occurs, the extracted oil is obtained. Quantity of oil can be found out with the help of a weighing balance (Gu, L.-B. et al., 2017).

Accelerated Solvent Extraction is another method to extract oil. This was accomplished in an Accelerated Solvent Extractor. Fenugreek seed powder (5 g) was mixed with diato-mite (15 g) and then placed in a 33 mL extraction vessel. The extractions were programmed for 3 cycles with petroleum ether solvent was added and first 5 minutes heating was done. After that a pressure of 1500 Psi at 100°C temperature is given for 30 min of extraction (5 s rinsing, 60% rinse volume,). Through a stream of N_2, the solvent was evaporated. Weighing of oil was done before storing at 4°C in a refrigerator.

The oil yield was measured with the help of following equation:

$$\text{The oil yield (wt\%)} = f_0 - f_1$$

where f_0 is the fat contents of raw materials (wt %) before extraction and f_1 are the fat contents of raw materials (wt %) after extraction. this method is with accordance to the American Oil Chemists' Society (AOCS) official method (2009) Ba 3–38 which is used to find the fat content of raw material (Gu, L.-B. et al., 2017).

18.6.3.3 Single-Factor Experiments

It is shown in the earlier studies that the most important effect on the characteristics and yield of oil among all the types studied is temperature (Gu, L. B. et al., 2017). Hence, this impact of the temperature was studied first, rather than other factors that could have influ-ence on the yield of oil. The goal of this was to choose the utmost fit temperature for the Subcritical Butane extraction of fenugreek oil from seed. In every trial, temperature was varying from 10–50°C, but particle size was upheld at 0.3 mm, the liquid/solid ratio was 30:1 and extraction time was 30 min. Other imperative factor that can affects the process of extraction is the time given for extraction. To check the effect of extraction time on yield of fenugreek seed oil, other factors were constant i.e., 40°C temperature, 30:1 liquid/solid ratio and 0.3mm particle size. Similarly, to understand the impact of fenugreek seed oil yield by the liquid/solid ratio, different ratios were used i.e., 40:1, 30:1, 20:1, 10:1, and 5:1. The remaining factors were particle extraction time 30 min, extraction temperature 40°C and size 0.3 mm. to check the effect on extraction efficiency by particles size, the ratio of liquid/solid were kept 30:1, 30 minutes' extraction time were given at40°C temperature (Gu, L.-B. et al., 2017).

18.7 OLEORESIN

Oleoresins normally comprises of the resins and fixed oils which deliver the taste and pungency to the spice and represents the odor and flavor principles of it. With the help of solvent extraction, we can obtain the oleoresins of fenugreek. There are many solvents which are available for this determination. The real composition of extracted oleoresin depends on the solvent used. Hence, when oleoresins are extracted using dissimilar solvents, a notable small variation in flavor, aroma and taste can be felt. This notable change can also be experienced from one sample to another even using the identical solvent due to a possible minor difference in parameters of extraction, like extraction temperature, degree of mixing of the solid, tie of extraction and others. To minimize this variation and more unvarying quality of oleoresin from each batch, novel and up to dated methods can be used than conservative approaches. Normally, oleoresin is isolated from extraction solvent by evaporation of the solvent without or with temperature, after solvent extraction. Generally, steroidal sapogenins (gitogenin and diosgenin obtained by hydrolysis), saponins, galactomannan resins, pigments resins which provides taste, glycosides and essential oils which provide odor are included in oleoresin.

18.8 FATTY ACID PROFILING OF FENUGREEK OIL

The oil concentration of fenugreek seed ranges between 7.8% to 8.4%, having golden-yellow colour. The oil has bitter taste and unpleasant odor (Sulieman, Ali, et al., 2008). A study was done on fenugreek oil's fatty acid composition from different regions and it was revealed that the fraction of linolenic and linoleic acid varies according to the condition and place of farming of plant (Sulieman, Ali, et al., 2008).

Several constituents of lipid have been assessed with the help of TLC-densitometry which showed that 85 percent of the neutral lipids consist of triacylglycerols, while diacylglycerols, free fatty acids and monoacylglycerols are 5.5%, 3.2% and 2.1%, respectively. Phosphotidylcholine dominates the polar fraction with 18.5%, which is followed by phosphotidylethanolamine (6%) and then phosphotidylinositol (1.5%) (Chatterjee et al., 2010). Sulieman et al. (2008) also found similar results in their study. The major free fatty acids valuation (quantitative and qualitative) was recognized by GC/MS, which revealed that linoleic acid was leading with 36% of the total fatty acids, tailed by linolenic acid, oleic acid and palmitic acid, with percentages of 18%, 13% and 9%, respectively. These results also match with the already done research (Chatterjee et al., 2010).

It is known that minor lipid classes possess significant physiological functions in animals and plants, due to this, there has been an enhanced attention by the researches to these lipids in recent years (Chatterjee et al., 2010). Examples of two such minor lipid components are N-acylethanolamines and oleamides. N-acylethanolamines have been recognized as fatty acid amides having physiological part in nervous system of mammals and as phospholipid elements in dried seeds. The other minor constituent is oleamide which has also been found in some plants recently (Wu et al., 2007). These types of lipids are yet to be found in fenugreek, if present. A study was done in which fenugreek seed oil which was extracted by different solvents, was undergone to gas chromatograph to analyze different constituents. This study exhibited that main content of fatty acid present in the oil are oleic acid (omega-9 fatty acid), *cis*-11,14,17-Eicosatrienoic acid (omega-3 fatty acid) and Linoleic acid (omega-6 fatty acid). The other fatty acids which are present in comparatively low quantity (<20%) are stearic acid, palmitic acid, behenic acid and arachidic acid. Collectively, the trans fatty acid, polyunsaturated fatty acids, monounsaturated fatty acids and saturated fatty acid content in solvent extracted oil (by hexane) was 0.00%, 71.30%, 12.95% and 15.75% respectively. Fatty acids profile of fenugreek obtained from different solvents are presented in the following graph (Munshi et al., 2020).

18.9 ANTIOXIDANT ACTIVITY

Extracted oils from plants can be used as multi-purpose additive like anti-microbial, anti-fungal and flavoring agents in cosmetics creams, drinks, foods and other products. These are not only used for above mentioned purpose but also can be utilized as antioxidant agents in different products (El-Baroty et al., 2010; Mehani, andSegni, 2012; Sarikurkcu et al., 2008). Fenugreek is among those plants that are well-known for their therapeutic properties and are in use as an herbal remedy and food source since the ancient time. The potential antioxidant and other phytochemical properties of fenugreek seed extracts have been reported in different studies (Baba et al., 2018; Mukthamba, andSrinivasan, 2017).

In a research, the oil of fenugreek seed was obtained with help of *n*-hexane by using soxhlet extraction technique. The FTIR and GC-MS examination of this oil exposed that it is good source of linoleic acid (essential omega-6 fatty acids). Linoleic acid is known to be extremely helpful for inhibition of inflammation, cancer and coronary heart diseases. The other chief components of this oil are pinene and palmitic acid, which are known to have natural antioxidant properties as it is beneficial in lowering free radicals. Current research also revealed that DPPH assay is less suitable as compared to ABTS radical scavenging assay. Hence, based on this and previous studies results, it is proposed that seed oil of fenugreek is good in contradiction of many ailments asthma, cancer, urinary infections, sexual disorder and inflammation (Akbari et al., 2019).

Oxidative stress can be induced by Acrylamide, which is a harmful element. As it was known that *Trigonella foenum-graecum* (fenugreek) possess antioxidant properties, an *in-vivo* study was carried out to explore whether seed oil of fenugreek has protecting effect against acrylamide toxicity or not. 30 male lab rats were arbitrarily divided into 4 groups. Normal saline was given to the control group. Acrylamide (20 mg/kg) was given to the second group, orally. Same quantity of Acrylamide was given to remaining groups but with supplementation of different proportions of fenugreek seed oil. It was observed that intoxication of Acrylamide amplified serum levels of AST, LDH, ALT, γ-GT, APL, cholesterol, urea, uric acid, 8-oxo-2′-deoxyguanosine, creatinine, interleukin 1 beta, tumor necrosis factor α and interleukin 6, significantly. Additionally, it impaired the concentrations and activities of the antioxidant biomarkers whereas, brain, hepatic and renal lipid peroxidation were enhanced. This rat study also revealed that supplementation of fenugreek seed oil improved the antioxidant biomarker activities and concentrations in the brain, hepatic and renal tissues, controlled the altered serum parameters and prohibited lipid peroxidation of rats suffering from acrylamide-intoxication. Hence, it is showed in this study that fenugreek seed oil protects from acrylamide-induced toxicity due to its potent antioxidant potential and free radical scavenging (Hamden et al., 2017).

18.10 RELIEVING BREAST ENGORGEMENT

The study shows that the results adopted to treat breast engorgement, particularly Fenugreek seed oil, was effective and resulting in a rapid recovery time. Furthermore, the study suggests that Fenugreek seed may be a more effective therapy of engorged breast due to its unique characteristics(Hassan, H. et al., 2020).

There would be a significant improvement in breast condition following intervention for all groups, independent of the measure used; however, the development was improved and took less time in the Fenugreek group than in the Cabbage group (p.05). Both cold Cabbage leaves and Fenugreek seed poultice were helpful in the treatment of breast inflammation. But at the other hand, Fenugreek seed was more effective at reducing breast engorgement in a shorter time period than cold cabbage leaves (Hassan, H. et al., 2020).

18.11 STEROIDS

This plant contains medicinal alkaloids, steroid chemicals, and sapogenins, and it has been used in traditional medicine for a variety of purposes (Salehi Surmaghi, 2008). This herb has been utilised to help with childbirth, digestion, and metabolism as a general tonic. Fenugreek's most significant metabolite, trigonelline, is useful in treating diabetes and lowering blood cholesterol levels.

Trigonelline is a plant hormone that is used to treat cancer (especially liver and cervical cancer) as well as migraines. The impact of trigonelline on mice revealed that it had sedative properties. This metabolite is produced by niacin, a vitamin found in foods and medical supplements that is commonly used to lower blood lipid and sugar levels (Smith, 2003).

Another significant chemical found in the seeds of this plant is diaszhenin, which is utilised to make medical steroids such as contraceptive tablets. Many research on the medicinal benefits of his plant and the identification of chemical components have been conducted. The most important biological effects and recognized chemicals associated with fenugreek seed are discussed, as well as its medicinal uses(Salehi Surmaghi, 2008).

18.12 CYTOTOXIC ACTIVITY FENUGREEK OF SEED OIL

The findings of a study showed that fenugreek seed oil modified cell morphology and reduced cell viability significantly, in a dose-proportional manner. Among cell lines, HEp-2 cells showed the greatest decrease in cell viability, followed by MCF-7 WISH and Vero cells in MTT and NRU trials. Cell viability at 1000μg/ml was 67% in MCF-7 cells, 55% in HEp-2 cells, 86% of Vero cells and 75% in WISH cells. The current study presents early screening results for fenugreek seed oil, which indicates that it has a high level of cytotoxicity against cancer cells (Al-Oqail et al., 2013). Fenugreek seeds have been found to protect against breast and colon cancers in recent studied (Amin et al., 2005; Raju, andBird, 2006). In conclusion, the results of this study show that malignant cells exposed to fenugreek seed oil have a lower cell viability (Al-Oqail et al., 2013).

The reduction in % cell viability after 24 hours of treatment in the current investigation revealed that fenugreek seed oil had significant cytotoxic effects on several kinds of malignant cells. This information is intriguing since it implies that the extract is more harmful to cancer cells than to healthy ones (Das et al., 2010).

18.13 ANTIMICROBIAL ACTIVITY

one mould, *Aspergillus niger*, two gramme negative bacteria, *Salmonella typhimurium* and *Escherichia coli*, and one gramme positive bacterium, *Staphylococcus aureus* were examined. The microorganisms used in the research were made from the University of Gezira's Food Microbiology Lab (Sulieman, Ahmed, et al., 2008).

Fenugreek oil exhibits high antibacterial action against the studied pathogens, notably *Escherichia coli*, according to the microbiological study (among bacteria). Fenugreek oil, on the other hand, was shown to have the most inhibitory impact against the fungus *Aspergillus Niger*. However, only the concentrated oil had an inhibiting impact on the organisms tested. As a result, it is strongly suggested that fenugreek seed oil be used in the food sector to extend food shelf life, as well as in the pharmaceutical and chemical industries (Sulieman, Ahmed, et al., 2008).

18.14 ANTIBACTERIAL ACTIVITY

Fenugreek oil having wide range as antiseptic property against bacteria that cause food poisoning, food decomposition, and also to those bacteria which relates to human food-borne illness. The zone diameter of inhibition (ZDI) is the parameter to determine the antibacterial activity of fenugreek seed oil (100%), it has been recorded as 15, 20, 10 mm for *Salmonella typhimurium*, *Escherichia coli* and *Staphylococcus aureus* respectively (Sulieman, Ahmed, et al., 2008). The essential oil of fenugreek exhibits constraint against *Pseudomonas aeruginosa* and *S. aureus* and the constraint against bacteria was found to be concentration dependent; the activity is noticed at lowest 12.5% (ZDI 10 and 12 mm for *P. aeruginosa* and *S. aureus*, respectively) and at highest 100% (ZDI 22 and 24 mm for *P. aeruginosa* and *S. aureus*, respectively) (Wagh et al., 2007). At 75% dilution of fenugreek essential oil, these five bacterial isolates *E. coli*, *P. aeruginosa*, *S. aureus*, *Klebsiella* and *Proteus pneumoniae* were found sensitive, based upon the ZDI 13, 12.33, 11.67, 10.5 and 9.3 mm, respectively, in accordance to the isolates (Mehani, andSegni, 2012). ZDI was determined by (Dubey et al., 2010).

All samples from essential oil of the plant fenugreek have exhibited captivating biological activity of the five bacterial strains and one fungal strain. Many studies have been assembled for the antimicrobial effectiveness of this essential oil against the microorganisms. According to the sensitivity of microbial species against the essential oil.

It has been discovered that the sensitivity of different species to the essential oil of the plant *Trigonella foenum greacum* varies depending on the concentration of the oil. All of these findings are simply the beginning of the hunt for a physiologically active natural source of material. Additional tests are required, and they must be able to corroborate the highlighted performance.

it would be interesting also to further phytochemical and biological investigations on these plants purification of the extracts obtained in order to separate the molecules responsible for the antibacterial actions, which will increase the medicinal arsenal of herbal plants Finally, we advise people to use medicinal plants responsibly, as incorrect use will almost certainly result in side effects (Mehani, andSegni, 2012).

18.15 ANTIFUNGAL ACTIVITY

The antibacterial properties of fenugreek oil and seed, which can be employed as a preservative in food or in the medical field, are well established. The growth of *Aspergillus niger*, which can produce black mould on fruits, was totally suppressed by fenugreek seed oil (Sulieman, Ahmed, et al., 2008).

18.16 FENUGREEK OIL AS A GROWTH PROMOTOR IN BROILER CHICKEN

The effect of fenugreek oil on certain blood constituents in broiler chicks revealed that adding fenugreek oil to the chicks' meals raised serum total protein and albumin levels. FEO can be employed as an effective alternative natural growth promoter in broiler diets, according to the findings of this study (Hamid, 2018).

18.17 DIABETES TREATMENT

In comparison to the diabetic group, fenugreek oil dramatically improved glucose intolerance, insulin sensitivity and blood glucose levels. After diabetic rats were given fenugreek oil, damage to the pancreatic islets and -cells was found. Furthermore, diabetic rats had decreased catalase, superoxide dismutase, glutathione and glutathione peroxidase content in the kidney, all of which were recovered to near-normal levels by the oil of fenugreek administration. In diabetic rats treated with fenugreek seed oil, elevated levels of lipid urea, creatinine, peroxidation and albumin were considerably reduced. Diabetic rats given fenugreek oil had almost normal pancreatic and kidney architecture restored. Finally, this research demonstrates the effectiveness of fenugreek oil in the treatment of diabetes, haematological disorders, and renal toxicity, which can be related to its immunomodulatory and insulin-stimulating properties, as well as its antioxidant capacity (Hamden et al., 2010).

In diabetic rats, fenugreek TG reduced -amylase activity in the small intestine by 36 percent when compared to untreated diabetic mice. Furthermore, fenugreek TG enhanced insulin sensitivity, resulting in a 43 percent reduction in blood glucose levels. Furthermore, the administration of fenugreek TG to mice having diabetes improved the glycogen rate in the musculature and liver. Furthermore, fenugreek TG (triglyceride) treatment reduced the activity of angiotensin converting enzyme in the plasma and kidney by 29 and 33 percent, respectively. Remarkably, fenugreek TG decreased the activity of lipase by 33% in the small intestine, resulting in lipid profile modulation. Furthermore, a histology investigation revealed that fenugreek TG protected hepatic renal function. Finally, these findings showed that fenugreek TG administration to mice having diabetes can make it a viable contender for industrial use as a pharmacologic mediator for hyperglycemia treatment (Hamden et al., 2017).

Diabetic rats had higher levels of renal function markers in their blood, such as blood urea nitrogen (BUN), alkaline phosphatase (ALP) and serum creatinine (Scr), which were considerably reduced by the use of fenugreek and bitter gourd oil. Furthermore, treatment with fenugreek and bitter gourd oils reduced the levels of thiobarbituric reactive compounds (TBARS) and malonaldehyde (MDA) and catalase (CAT) in the diabetic mice kidneys. The protective effect of these oils was also demonstrated by histological investigation. According to the findings, vegetable oils are useful in lowering hyperglycemia, dyslipidemia, and kidney impairment caused by diabetes side effects. As a result, they may have therapeutic efficacy in reducing diabetes side effects and may be used in conjunction with an oil diet to treat diabetes. As a result, our findings suggest that oils are an effective antidiabetic medication that can help regulate diabetes-related abnormalities like hyperglycemia, dyslipidemia, and kidney damage in STZ-induced type 2 diabetes rats. Our findings also support the idea that the use of these oils in the treatment of diabetes mellitus could have synergistic effects (Parveen et al., 2019).

18.18 WOUND HEALING ACTIVITY

Many plant products, mainly extracted oils are used as wounds healers for many centuries. According to many researches, some natural extracts, phytochemical constituents and several herbal formulations of herbal plants can be used in the treatment of wounds. Fenugreek is among those therapeutic plants which are conventionally used in traditional medicine (Moalla Rekik et al., 2016). To better understand the wound curative effect, and to comprehend the mechanism on curing wounds, the evaluation of phytochemical composition was done. Accordingly, utilization of the oil of fenugreek seed and the wound healing reference drug enhances the contraction of the skin borders to a fast recovery and accelerate the wounds healing process. The superlative curative actions are accredited to their antioxidant, antimicrobial and physicochemical possessions (Moalla Rekik et al., 2016).

18.19 Histologic Examination. To examine the epithelial tissue organization, the rebuilding of epidermal layer that covers the scar surface treated by the fenugreek oil was inspected by the hematoxylin-eosin. The higher Fibroconnective tissue renewal by fenugreek seed oil was noticed. When the microscopic inspection of the wound place treated by this oil was done, it showed a well-organized and complete epidermic regeneration. It was also observed that epithelial layer generated by the fenugreek oil was thicker as compared to the layer generated by wound healing cream "CICAFLORA" (Moalla Rekik et al., 2016).

There is a significant quantity of polyunsaturated fatty acids in fenugreek seed oil which is comprised of linolenic acid, oleic acid and linoleic acid. The predecessor of arachidonic acid is linoleic acid which has an imperative part in the inflammatory conditions including leukotrienes, prostaglandins and thromboxane's (Fetterman Jr, andZdanowicz, 2009). These increase the inflammatory process as well as act as mediators to inflammatory. Hence, the intensification in the renovation of the extracellular matrix, the local neovascularization, fibroblastic cell differentiation and migration, which increase the speed of wounds healing (Velnar et al., 2009). It is also informed in studies that fatty acids have the potential to upsurge hydration of skin as well as helpful conditions for speedy wound healing on skin and lessen trans epidermal loss of water (Miller, andMaibach, 2009).

18.20 EFFECTIVENESS ON LIVER TISSUES AND OVARIAN

An increase in interest regarding understanding the organic effect of therapeutic plants have been observed. An in vivo study on mice was done to examine the possessions of fenugreek seed oil administered on the ovarian and liver activity to check histopathological effect. In this study, orally administration with different amounts of fenugreek oil was done on Swiss female mice (albino) for ten days. The results were found to be dependent on the type of tissue and dosage of fenugreek seed oil. 0.15- and 0.1-ml administration of with fenugreek oil on mouse improved the quality and total sum of cumulus-oocyte complexes. It was observed that seed oil of fenugreek stimulated the oocytes, which were obtained from lab rats to grow in meiosis, at all quantities. The examination (Histopathological) of the ovaries obtained from rats administered with 0.05 ml of fenugreek oil and untreated rats displayed no histopathological changes.

Though, the ovaries collected by the rats which were treated with 0.15 or 0.1 ml of fenugreek seed oil exhibited development in some tissues. This was the initial research that proposed such noteworthy inspiring properties of oil of the fenugreek seed on the ovarian activity in rats (Hassan, A. M. et al., 2006).

18.21 AROMATIC COMPONENTS FOUND IN FENUGREEK OIL

The smell which comes from seeds of fenugreek is due to the volatile oils which are present in them. the oil of fenugreek comprises of many aromatic compounds like camphor, neryl acetate, b-pinene, 2,5-dimethylpyrazine, b-caryophyllene, geranial, a-selinene, 6-methyl 5-hepten-2-one, 3-octen-2-one, a-terpineol, gterpinene, a-pinene and a-campholenal. The figure 18.1 is showing the structural formula of these aromatic compound. (Hamden et al., 2011).

18.22 CONCLUSION

According to different studies, fenugreek oleoresin shows nutraceuticals and different health beneficial properties, also act as antimicrobial and antifungal factor. Studies showed the effectiveness of this oil as an antimicrobial. Additionally, fenugreek oil also contains an ample amount of antioxidants and the results of *in-vivo* studies elaborates effective results. One of the most dramatically improved results shown fenugreek oil are antidiabetic and insulin sensitivity in diabetes. Overall, based on the results of different findings it could be proposed that fenugreek oleoresin could be used efficiently for many infections

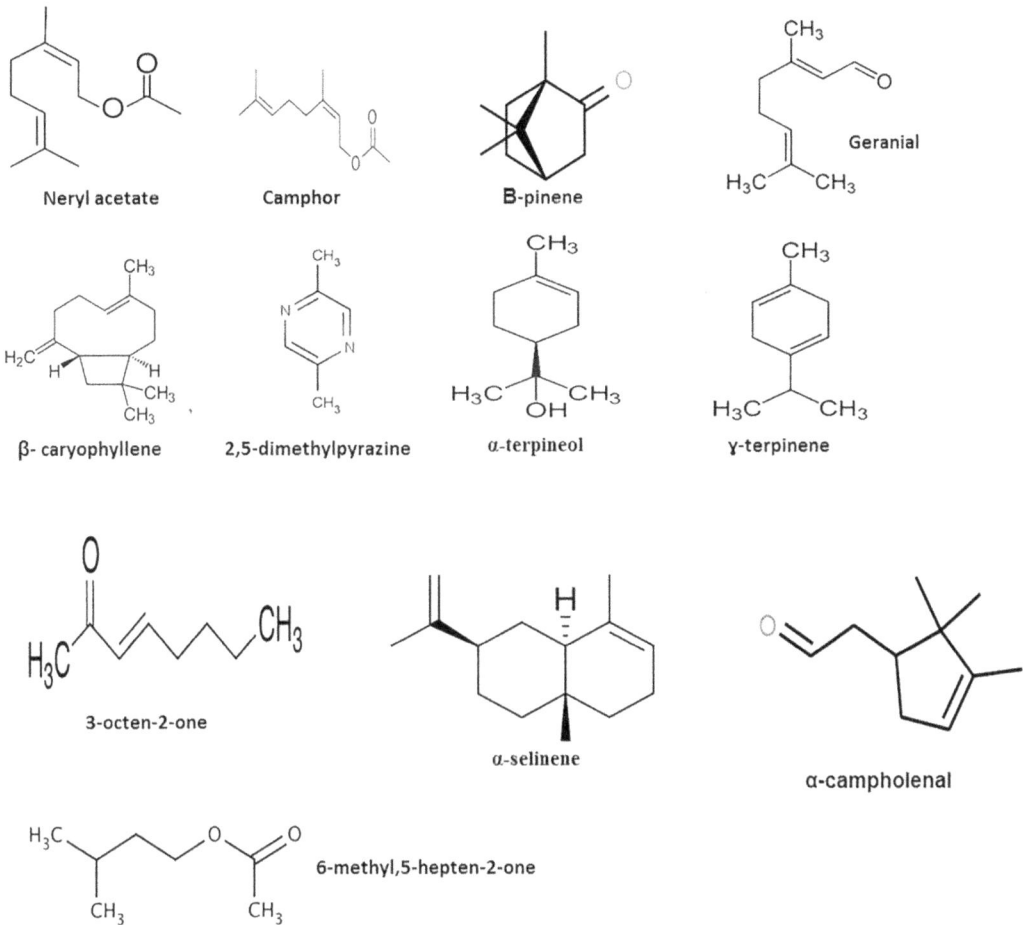

FIGURE 18.1   Aromatic components found in fenugreek oil.

such as inflammation of various body organs, cancer, asthma, sexual illness and urinary infections.

REFERENCES

Acharya, S., Thomas, J., and Basu, S. 2006. Fenugreek: An "old world" crop for the "new world". Biodiversity 7(3–4): 27–30.

Ahmad, A., Alghamdi, S. S., Mahmood, K., and Afzal, M. 2016. Fenugreek a multipurpose crop: Potentialities and improvements. *Saudi Journal of Biological Sciences* 23(2): 300–310.

Akbari, S., Abdurahman, N. H., Yunus, R. M., Alara, O. R., and Abayomi, O. O. 2019. Extraction, characterization and antioxidant activity of fenugreek (*Trigonella-foenum graecum*) seed oil. *Materials Science for Energy Technologies* 2(2): 349–355.

Al-Oqail, M. M., Farshori, N. N., Al-Sheddi, E. S., Musarrat, J., Al-Khedhairy, A. A., and Siddiqui, M. A. 2013. In vitro cytotoxic activity of seed oil of fenugreek against various cancer cell lines. *Asian Pacific Journal of Cancer Prevention* 14(3): 1829–1832.

Altuntaş, E., Özgöz, E., and Taşer, Ö. F. 2005. Some physical properties of fenugreek (Trigonella foenum-graceum L.) seeds. Journal of Food Engineering 71(1): 37–43.

Amin, A., Alkaabi, A., Al-Falasi, S., and Daoud, S. A. 2005. Chemopreventive activities of *Trigonella foenum graecum* (fenugreek) against breast cancer. *Cell Biology International* 29(8): 687–694.

Baba, W. N., Tabasum, Q., Muzzaffar, S., Masoodi, F. A., Wani, I., Ganie, S. A., and Bhat, M. M. 2018. Some nutraceutical properties of fenugreek seeds and shoots (*Trigonella foenum-graecum* L.) from the high Himalayan region. *Food Bioscience* 23: 31–37.

Bahmani, M., Shirzad, H., Mirhosseini, M., Mesripour, A., and Rafieian-Kopaei, M. 2016. A review on ethnobotanical and therapeutic uses of fenugreek (*Trigonella foenum-graceum* L). *Journal of Evidence-Based Complementary & Alternative Medicine* 21(1): 53–62.

Bieńkowski, T., Krystyna, Ż.-G., Kurowski, T., and Gołaszewski, J. 2016. Agrotechnical indicators for *Trigonella foenum-gracum* L. production in the environmental conditions of northeastern Europe. Turkish Journal of Field Crops 21(1): 16–28.

Chatterjee, S., Variyar, P. S., and Sharma, A. 2010. Bioactive lipid constituents of fenugreek. *Food Chemistry* 119(1): 349–353.

Das, A., Banik, N. L., and Ray, S. K. 2010. Flavonoids activated caspases for apoptosis in human glioblastoma T98G and U87MG cells but not in human normal astrocytes. *Cancer: Interdisciplinary International Journal of the American Cancer Society* 116(1): 164–176.

Dubey, R., Dubey, K., Janapati, Y. K., Sridhar, C., and Jayaveera, K. 2010. Comparative anti microbial studies of aqueous, methanolic and saponins extract of seeds of *Trigonella foenum-graecum* on human vaginal pathogens causing UTI infection. *Der Pharma Chemica* 2(5): 84–88.

El-Baroty, G. S., Abd El-Baky, H., Farag, R. S., and Saleh, M. A. 2010. Characterization of antioxidant and antimicrobial compounds of cinnamon and ginger essential oils. *African Journal of Biochemistry Research* 4(6): 167–174.

Farage M. A., Miller, K. W., and Maibach, H. I. 2009. Degenerative changes in aging skin. *Textbook of Aging Skin* 19: 25.

Fetterman Jr, J. W., and Zdanowicz, M. M. 2009. Therapeutic potential of n-3 polyunsaturated fatty acids in disease. *American Journal of Health-System Pharmacy* 66(13): 1169–1179.

Ghosh, B., Chandra, I., and Chatterjee, S. (2015). Fenugreek (*Trigonella foenum-graecum* L.) and its necessity. *Fire Journal Engineering Technology* 1(1): 66–67.

Gu, L.-B., Liu, X.-N., Liu, H.-M., Pang, H.-L., and Qin, G.-Y. 2017. Extraction of fenugreek (*Trigonella foenum-graecum* L.) seed oil using subcritical butane: Characterization and process optimization. *Molecules* 22(2): 228.

Gu, L. B., Pang, H. L., Lu, K. K., Liu, H. M., Wang, X. D., and Qin, G. Y. 2017. Process optimization and characterization of fragrant oil from red pepper (*Capsicum annuum* L.) seed extracted by subcritical butane extraction. *Journal of the Science of Food and Agriculture* 97(6): 1894–1903.

Hamden, K., Keskes, H., Belhaj, S., Mnafgui, K., and Allouche, N. 2011. Inhibitory potential of omega-3 fatty and fenugreek essential oil on key enzymes of carbohydrate-digestion and hypertension in diabetes rats. *Lipids in Health and Disease* 10(1): 1–10.

Hamden, K., Keskes, H., Elgomdi, O., Feki, A., and Alouche, N. 2017. Modulatory effect of an isolated triglyceride from fenugreek seed oil on of α-amylase, lipase and ACE activities, liver-kidney functions and metabolic disorders of diabetic rats. *Journal of Oleo Science* 66(-6): 633–645.

Hamden, K., Masmoudi, H., Carreau, S., and Elfeki, A. 2010. Immunomodulatory, β-cell, and neuroprotective actions of fenugreek oil from alloxan-induced diabetes. *Immunopharmacology and Immunotoxicology* 32(3): 437–445.

Hamid, H. H. A. 2018. Effect of feeding of adding fenugreek oil on the performance and blood serum profile of broiler chicks. *International Journal Current Microbiology Applied Science* 8(10): 1147–1155.

Hassan, A. M., Khalil, W. K., and Ahmed, K. A. 2006. Genetic and histopathology studies on mice: Effect of fenugreek oil on the efficiency of ovarian and liver tissues. *African Journal of Biotechnology* 5(5): 477–483.

Hassan, H., Gamel, W., Hassanine, S., and Sheha, E. 2020. Fenugreek seed poultice versus cold cabbage leaves compresses for relieving breast engorgement: An interventional comparative study. *Journal of Nursing Education and Practice* 10(5): 82–99.

Lu, F., Shen, L., Qin, Y., Gao, L., Li, H., and Dai, Y. 2008. Clinical observation on *Trigonella foenum-graecum* L. total saponins in combination with sulfonylureas in the treatment of type 2 diabetes mellitus. *Chinese Journal of Integrative Medicine* 14(1): 56–60.

Mahfouz, S., Elaby, S., and Hassouna, H. 2012. Effects of some legumes on hypercholesterolemia in rats. *Journal of American Science* 8(12): 1453–1460.

Mandal, S., and DebMandal, M. 2016. *Fenugreek (Trigonella foenum-graecum L.) Oils Essential Oils in Food Preservation, Flavor and Safety* (pp. 421–429). Elsevier.

Mehani, M., and Segni, L. 2012. Antimicrobial effect of essential oil of plant *Trigonella focnum greacum* on some bacteria pathogens. *International Science Index, Bioengineering and Life Science* 7(12): 358–360.

Mehrafarin, A., Ghaderi, A., Rezazadeh, S., Naghdi, B. H., Nourmohammadi, G., and Zand, E. 2010. Bioengineering of important secondary metabolites and metabolic pathways in fenugreek (*Trigonella foenum-graecum* L.). *Journal of Medicinal Plants* 9(35): 1–18.

Mirzaei, F., and Venkatesh, H. K. 2012. Efficacy of phyto medicines as supplement in feeding practices on ruminant's performance: A review. *Global Journal of Research on Medicinal Plants & Indigenous Medicine* 1(9): 391.

Moalla Rekik, D., Ben Khedir, S., Ksouda Moalla, K., Kammoun, N. G., Rebai, T., and Sahnoun, Z. 2016. Evaluation of wound healing properties of grape seed, sesame, and fenugreek oils. *Evidence-Based Complementary and Alternative Medicine* 2016. https://doi.org/10.1155/2016/7965689.

Moradi, N., and Moradi, K. 2013. Physiological and pharmaceutical effects of fenugreek (*Trigonella foenum-graecum* L.) as a multipurpose and valuable medicinal plant. *Global Journal of Medicinal Plant Research* 1(2): 199–206.

Moyer, J., Acharya, S., Mir, Z., and Doram, R. 2003. Weed management in irrigated fenugreek grown for forage in rotation with other annual crops. *Canadian Journal of Plant Science* 83(1): 181–188.

Mukthamba, P., and Srinivasan, K. 2017. Dietary fenugreek (*Trigonella foenum-graecum*) seeds and garlic (*Allium sativum*) alleviates oxidative stress in experimental myocardial infarction. *Food Science and Human Wellness* 6(2): 77–87.

Munshi, M., Arya, P., and Kumar, P. 2020. Physico-chemical analysis and fatty acid profiling of fenugreek (*Trigonella foenum graecum*) seed oil using different solvents. *Journal of Oleo Science* 69(11): 1349–1358.

Murlidhar, M., and Goswami, T. 2012. A review on the functional properties, nutritional content, medicinal utilization and potential application of fenugreek. *Journal of Food Processing and Technology* 3(9).

Parveen, K., Siddiqui, W. A., Arif, J. M., Kuddus, M., Shahid, S. M. A., and Adnan Kausar, M. 2019. Evaluation of vegetables and fish oils for the attenuation of diabetes complications. *Cellular and Molecular Biology* 65(7): 38–45.

PietrzAk, S. 2011. Estimation of nitrogen fixed symbiotically by legume plants. *Woda Środowisko Obszary Wiejskie* 11(35): 197–207.

Prajapati, N. D., Purohit, S., Sharma, A. K., and Kumar, T. 2003. *A Handbook of Medicinal Plants: A Complete Source Book* (pp. 554–554).

Raju, J., and Bird, R. 2006. Alleviation of hepatic steatosis accompanied by modulation of plasma and liver TNF-α levels by *Trigonella foenum graecum* (fenugreek) seeds in Zucker obese (fa/fa) rats. *International Journal of Obesity,* 30(8): 1298–1307.

Salehi Surmaghi, M. 2008. *Medicinal Plants and Herbal Therapy* (pp. 253–240). Tehran University Publication, Vol. 1.

Sarikurkcu, C., Tepe, B., Daferera, D., Polissiou, M., and Harmandar, M. 2008. Studies on the antioxidant activity of the essential oil and methanol extract of *Marrubium globosum* subsp. globosum (lamiaceae) by three different chemical assays. *Bioresource Technology* 99(10): 4239–4246.

Sheikhlar, A. 2013. *Trigonella foenum-graecum* L. (fenugreek) as a medicinal herb in animals growth and health. *Science International* 1(6): 194–198.

Smith, M. 2003. Therapeutic applications of fenugreek. *Alternative Medicine Review* 8(1): 20–27.

Snehlata, H. S., and Payal, D. R. 2012. Fenugreek (*Trigonella foenum-graecum* L.): An overview. *International Journal of Current Pharmaceutical Review and Research* 2(4): 169–187.

Srinivasan, K. 2006. Fenugreek (*Trigonella foenum-graecum*): A review of health beneficial physiological effects. *Food Reviews International* 22(2): 203–224.

Sulieman, A. M. E., Ahmed, H. E., and Abdelrahim, A. M. 2008a. The chemical composition of fenugreek (*Trigonella foenum graceum* L) and the antimicrobial properties of its seed oil. *Gezira Journal of Engineering and Applied Sciences* 3(2): 52–71.

Sulieman, A. M. E., Ali, A. O., and Hemavathy, J. 2008b. Lipid content and fatty acid composition of fenugreek (*Trigonella foenum-graecum* L.) seeds grown in Sudan. *International Journal of Food Science & Technology* 43(2): 380–382.

Velnar, T., Bailey, T., and Smrkolj, V. 2009. The wound healing process: An overview of the cellular and molecular mechanisms. *Journal of International Medical Research* 37(5): 1528–1542.

Verma, S., Yadav, S., and Singh, A. 2015. In vitro antibacterial activity and phytochemical analysis of *Mangifera indica* L flower. Extracts against pathogenic microorganisms. *Journal of Pharmacology & Clinical Toxicology* 3(3): 1053.

Wagh, P., Rai, M., Deshmukh, S., and Durate, M. C. T. 2007. Bio-activity of oils of *Trigonella foenum-graecum* and *Pongamia pinnata*. *African Journal of Biotechnology* 6(13): 1592–1596.

Wani, S. A., and Kumar, P. 2018. Fenugreek: A review on its nutraceutical properties and utilization in various food products. *Journal of the Saudi Society of Agricultural Sciences* 17(2): 97–106.

Wu, T.-T., Charles, A. L., and Huang, T.-C. 2007. Determination of the contents of the main biochemical compounds of Adlay (*Coxi lachrymal-jobi*). *Food Chemistry* 104(4): 1509–1515.

Żuk-Gołaszewska, K., and Wierzbowska, J. 2017. Fenugreek: Productivity, nutritional value and uses. *Journal of Elementology* 22(3): 1067–1080.

CHAPTER 19

Characterisation and Pharmacological Properties of Celery Oleoresin

Ruchi Sharma

Shoolini University of Biotechnology and Management Sciences

Tanu Malik

Lovely Professional University

Shailja Kumari and Somesh Sharma

Shoolini University of Biotechnology and Management Sciences

CONTENTS

DOI: 10.1201/9781003186205-19

19.1 INTRODUCTION

Celery, (*Apium graveolens* L.), is a vegetable in the Apiaceae or Umbelliferae family (Turner et al., 2020). It comes from the Mediterranean region of Southern Europe, as well as Egypt and Sweden's marshlands (Cosentino et al., 2020). Breeding started in the 19th century in Italy (Quiros, 1993). In 2017, the United States produced 79,404 tonnes of celery (AgMRC, 2019), whereas the European Union produced 335,990 tonnes (Eurostat, 2019). Celery is known by a variety of names in several languages: "Tukhme karafs" in Urdu, "Karafs" in Persian, "Ajmod" in Hindi, "Apio" in Spanish, "Sellerie" in German, and "Alkarafs" in Arabic, and the fruits are commonly referred to as "celery seeds." Apium gets its name from the Latin word "apis," which means "bee," because its little white blossoms are attractive to bees. The species name "graveolens" means "heavily scented" (Khalil et al., 2015). The word "celery" comes from the Latin word "celer" meaning "swift" and is considered a fast-acting therapeutic. It consists of three taxonomic variants that have been cultivated: celeriac (var. rapaeeum), celery (var. dulce), and smallage (var. secalinum) (Domblides et al., 2008). Celery grows best in mild, humid conditions, and the ideal temperature range for this plant is around 15°C–22°C. Growth is generally slow at low temperatures (Khalil et al., 2015). Celery necessitates a high level of humidity but not a high temperature. As a result, its best product is found in temperate locations with cool weather. Celery is a biennial plant that grows to a height of 100 cm and has a thick, firm stalk with a strong scent (Lim, 2015). Its leaves are 5–50 mm long, triangular, diamond, or spear-shaped, and have saw-teeth or lobe-shaped margins. Each umbrella contains between four and twelve branches. This plant's fruit is oval, with a width of 1.5–2 mm. It has no wings, is brown, and has black lines (Sowbhagya, 2014). The stem of celery is tall and woody, tapering into leaves. Its leaves and stalks are edible and are consumed as vegetables, depending on geography and cultivar, while its seeds are used for spicing and medicinal uses (Helaly et al., 2014). The leaves and stalks are primarily served raw in salads or cooked in soups. Celery contains the amino acid tryptophan, vitamins, dietary fibre, and minerals, all of which are beneficial to one's health (Consentino et al., 2020). Celery also includes chemicals, including sedanolide, phthalide, and 3-n-butylphthalide, which help glutathione-S-transferase (GST) function better in the liver and small intestinal mucosa (Duhamel and Vandenkoornhuyse, 2013).

19.2 BOTANICAL CLASSIFICATION

Kingdom	Plantae
Genus	*Apium*
Subclass	Rosidae
Sub-kingdom	Tracheobionta
Family	Apiaceae
Division	Magnoliopsida
Species	*Apium graveolens* Linn
Superdivision	Spermatophyta
Order	Apiales

19.3 CHEMICAL COMPOSITION

Celery has a high calorie value because of its fat content. It's also recognised for being high in vitamin C and other nutrients. Proteins, volatile oil, crude fibres, moisture, ash, starch, carbohydrates, and fixed oil are all found in its seed (Khalil et al., 2015). Fatty acids, linolenic acid, stearic acid, petroselenic acid, oleic acid, palmitic acid, and linoleic acid are present in the fixed oil (Zhou et al., 2009). This plant includes a lot of minerals, such as calcium, magnesium, and potassium, as well as a lot of sodium. A cup of chopped celery leaves contains around 100 mg of salt. Salience, sesquiterpenes, limonene, and a distinctive scent make up the essential oil. Potassium, folic acid, sodium, fibres, magnesium, chlorophyll, and silica are all abundant in it (Khalil et al., 2015; Kooti and Daraei, 2017).

19.4 PHYTOCHEMICAL COMPOUNDS

The constituents of *A. graveolens* seed extract contain carbohydrates, glycosides, flavonoids, steroids, and alkaloids in the methanolic extract. Leaves, seeds, and stems of celery contain fatty acids, (2.5%–3.5%) volatile oils (1%–3%), and sesquiterpene alcohols. The derived compounds are β-pinene, limonene (60%), selenine (10%–15%), cymene, camphene, limonene, α-pinene, sedanenolide, α-thuyene, γ-terpinene, p-cymene, β-phellendrene, sabinene, myristic, terpinolene, linoleic, 3-n-butyl phthalide, palmitoleic, petroselinic, oleic, palmitic, myristicic, stearic acid, myristoleic, α-eudesmol, β-eudesmol, and santalol (Talwari and Ghuman, 2014). Celery tuber has been reported to contain 5-methoxypsoralen and methoxsalen (8-methoxypsoralen). Seeds of celery contain 2%–3% essential oil and 15%–17% fixed oil (Kooti et al., 2015). The oil contains mostly selinene (10%), limonene (60%), frocoumarin, and its glycosides. In addition to vitamins A and C, the celery seeds contain flavonoid apigenin as the main component. In celery, a total of 16 seed extract combinations have been found, accounting for 98.7% of the total extract, the primary components of which are D-limonene and myrcene.

19.5 PHARMACOLOGICAL ACTIVITIES

Celery has many pharmacological activities as listed below.

19.5.1 Hepatoprotective Activity

A substantial action against liver damage caused by paracetamol and carbon tetra chloride has been reported using the methanolic extract of *A. graveolens* seed. When compared to silymarin, *A. graveolens* extract reduced the rise in different hepatotoxicity markers, such as aspartate transaminase, alkaline phosphatase, alanine transaminase, and albumin. Paracetamol-induced structural alterations in liver tissues were also reversed in histopathological examinations (Ahmed et al., 2002). The hepatoprotective properties of *A. graveolens* methanolic extracts were comparable to those of the standard medication silymarin (Gauri et al., 2015).

19.5.2 Hypocholesterolemic Activity

The lipid profile of rats fed a high-fat diet was investigated using a hydroalcoholic extract of celery. Celery significantly reduced triglycerides, low-density lipoprotein, and cholesterol in the treatment group as compared to the control group (Tsi and Tan, 2000). The presence of polar molecules, with amino acid/sugar moiety in the extract, as well as the effect on bile acid production, is suggested to be the mechanism of hypocholesterolemic activity (Kooti et al., 2014).

19.5.3 Antidiabetic Activity

The diabetic rat was used to assess the antidiabetic activity of the celery seed aqueous extract. It was discovered that administering the extract intraperitoneally alters the lipid profile (Roghani et al., 2007). The antidiabetic efficacy of *n*-butanol extract from celery seeds against male rats caused by streptozotocin in enhancing lipid peroxidation and antioxidant status was investigated in a study utilising *n*-butanol extract from celery seeds. These investigations showed that *n*-butanol extract (60 mg/kg body weight) or insulin treatment as a conventional medicine can control antioxidant enzyme activity, stimulate weight gain, reduce stress problems associated with diabetes mellitus, and maintain normal blood glucose levels (Al-Kurdy, 2016).

19.5.4 Antimicrobial Activity

A. graveolens volatile oil contains antifungal, antibacterial, and antiviral effects. Many bacteria, including *Salmonella typhi*, *Pseudomonas solanacearum*, *Staphylococcus aureus*, *Streptococcus pyogenes*, *Shigella dysenteriae*, *Staphylococcus albus*, and *Streptococcus faecalis* display antimicrobial activity. This plant has little activity against the pathogens *Pseudomonas aeruginosa* and *Escherichia coli* (Atta and Alkofahi, 1998). Antibacterial activity of *A. graveolens* against *E. coli* has been reported. The ethanolic extracts have more activity than the aqueous and hexane extracts (Naema et al., 2010). *Bacillus cereus*, *Citrobacter freundii*, *E. coli*, *Enterococcus faecalis*, *Enterobacter aerogenes*, *Proteus vulgaris*, *Salmonella typhimurium*, *Hafnia alvei*, *Listeria monocytogenes*, and *S. aureus* were all found to have antimicrobial activity in an ethanol extract of celery leaves and roots. Furthermore, the celery leaf ethanol extract was more efficient and effective than the celery root ethanol extract. The antibacterial activity of ethanol extracts from celery leaves and roots was stronger at higher dosages. *C. freundii* and *P. vulgaris* bacteria can be inhibited by celery extract (Sipailiene et al., 2003).

19.5.5 Antioxidant Activity

A. graveolens include a lot of phenolic compounds, which are powerful antioxidants (Jung et al., 2011). The antioxidant activity of leaves was studied (by scavenging 1,1diphenyl 2 picrylhydrazyl [DPPH] radical activity) and shown to be a powerful natural antioxidant by suppressing the oxidative process (Nagella et al., 2012). Antioxidant activity may be attributed to the constituents, including derivatives of methoxy-phenyl chromenone and L-tryptophan (Momin and Nair, 2002). Inorganic and organic extracts of celery were evaluated in another experiment, and both extracts showed excellent activity for OH and DPPH radicals. *In vivo* tests with CCl4-induced toxicity revealed strong protective effects (Popović et al., 2006).

19.5.6 Anticancer Activity

The most important bioactive component in celery oil is phthalide, which has a favourable effect on health by protecting against cholesterol, cancer, and high blood pressure (El-Beltagi et al., 2020). The most active phthalide molecule is sedanolide, which helps cancer patients decrease tumours. The active ingredients in this plant's seed oil are 3-*n*-butyl phthalide and sedanolide, which have a strong ability to induce GST, a detoxifying enzyme found in target tumour tissues (Zheng et al., 1993).

19.5.7 Anti-Infertility Activity

In rats, celery extracts were found to protect them from testicular toxicity caused by sodium valproate. The findings were backed up by histological analysis. Apigenin, a significant ingredient of the extract, could be accountable for the action (Hamza and Amin, 2007). Its protective effects against chemically induced rat testis injury were also investigated. Celery has been reported to help with testicular healing and sexual function (Kooti et al., 2014).

19.6 CELERY OLEORESINS

Oleoresins (ORs) are flavouring compounds that are extracted using a solvent from powdered spices. They have a delightful fragrance and pungency, which enhances the taste. Essential oils (EOs) can be extracted by steam distillation and can be found in varying concentrations in all spices. Because of the microbiological benefits, stability in flavour and pungency, and ease of storage and transit, ORs are preferred. Plants produce EOs as secondary metabolites, which are complex, volatile, and hydrophobic molecules (Swamy et al., 2016). It has been well documented that they have antibacterial activity against food pathogens. ORs, on the other hand, are viscous blends of EOs and resins derived from spices using organic solvents (Arshad et al., 2018). ORs can be found in liquid form when solvents such as propylene glycol are added, which makes them easier to utilise in food preparations (Bertuso et al., 2021). According to the European Food Safety Authority (EFSA), 2004, celery OR were made by extracting celery seed with extraction solvents (in compliance with Council Directive 88/344/EEC) and then evaporating the solvent. The resulting liquid form of celery seed is the most concentrated liquid form available, with 11% volatile oil and resin. Solvent extraction of the dried ripe seed of *A. graveolens* L. yields a dark green, slightly viscous, nonhomogeneous liquid with a celery-like aroma and flavour. It can be decolorised by removing some of the chlorophyll. It is soluble in most fixed oils and partially soluble in alcohol (with oily separation). The celery OR is made up of essential oil, organically soluble resins, and other compounds found in the spice. Celery seed OR is made by extracting crushed dry celery seeds using acceptable volatile solvents such as food grade hexane ethanol, ethyl acetate, or ethylene dichloride, then filtration and desolventiszation under vacuum. According to the International Organization for Standardization (ISO), as well as importing country requirements with their specified maximum permitted limits for recognised solvents, the organic solvent shall be recovered fully from the OR. OR are often referred to as "liquid celery seed," because they are easier to work with when making tinctures and extracts (Meyerhof, 1997). The OR from celery seeds should be a green liquid that flows freely and has a volatile concentration of at least 9 mL/100 g. These should smell like lemons and have a sweet herbal tone. The OR should be made using the necessary organic solvents, and then the solvent should be removed according to the importing country's requirements (Malhotra, 2006).

19.6.1 Extraction Techniques
19.6.1.1 Steam Distillation
The volatile oil is extracted from coarsely crushed celery powder/flakes by steam distillation. The powder/flakes are crushed to 30 mesh and extracted in percolators with solvent after the volatile oil has been removed. The extraction procedure is done five to six times, with one-hour contact time with the powder. To remove the solvent, the extract is collected in a miscella and treated with distillation. A high vacuum is used to eliminate the solvent residue at the end of the distillation. The resin is mixed with the volatile oil in varying proportions to form the OR. OR isolated from aged seeds may have an off-flavour due to oxidation (Sowbhagya, 2014).

19.6.1.2 Solvent Extraction
ORs can alternatively be made by extracting celery powder with a solvent (acetone or hexane) rather than steam distilling it and then removing the solvent. During the last stages of distillation when a high vacuum is applied, the finer scent of low boiling compounds may be lost to reduce solvent residues to traces in OR synthesised this way (Sowbhagya, 2014).

19.6.2 Applications of Celery Oleoresins
ORs are viscous blends of EOs and resins obtained from spices using organic solvents. Celery ORs can be found in a wide variety of processed sauces, meals, snacks, shellfish, sausages, vegetable preparations, and alcoholic and non-alcoholic beverages. Celery OR is one of the most valuable flavouring compounds because it gives food products a warm, fragrant, and appealing flavour. *A. graveolens* OR was found to be effective in reducing the growth of food pathogens, such as *L. monocytogenes* and *B. cereus*, using food-derived ORs (Bertuso et al., 2021). Nagar et al. (2020) investigated the antibiofilm and

anti-quorum-sensing activities of celery OR with *Chromobacterium violaceum* (a biosensor strain) and the pathogen *P. aeruginosa* PA01 to see whether it may be used as anti-infective agent and food preservative. Celery OR had MICs of 10% and 25% v/v against *P. aeruginosa* PAO1 and *C. violaceum* CV12472. At doses of ORs ranging from 1.56% to 50% v/v, violacein inhibition and biofilm formation were investigated. At 12.5% v/v, the celery OR showed a strong quorum sensing modulatory influence on *P. aeruginosa* PAO1 swimming, swarming, and twitching motility. Eicosadiene, benzene, methanol, and methyl ester were the primary phytoconstituents found in celery OR as determined by GC–MS, which were previously unknown. The data imply that celery possesses quantum sensing and biofilm inhibitory capabilities against Gram-negative bacteria, and that it could be used as a food intervention tool.

19.7 TOXICITY AND SAFETY

Celery, especially in Europe, is a prominent source of pollen-related food allergies (Ballmer-Weber et al., 2000). In Switzerland and France, on the basis of patient's history, over 30%–40% of individuals with food allergies were found to be sensitised to celery root, and over 30% of severe anaphylactic reactions to food are believed to be triggered by celery. Local oropharyngeal reactions, as well as various more severe forms, such as life-threatening systemic anaphylaxis, are all symptoms of celery allergy (EFSA, 2004). Flavoprotein (Api g 5), profilin (Api g 4), Api g 2 (nonspecific lipid transfer protein-LTP 1), and PR10 (Api g 1) are the most common allergens. Api g 2 and Api g 4 are potentially dangerous allergens for allergic people since they can cause anaphylactic reactions (Kooti et al., 2014). *Sclerotinia sclerotiorum* fungus, which causes dermatitis in sensitive people, has also been found on the plant. Some people are allergic to cress, which can result in anaphylaxis. Because it has a uterine-stimulating effect, it should be avoided during pregnancy (Tyagi et al., 2013). The intake of celery leaf oil is 0.001 mg/person/day, while the intake of celery OR is 1.14 mg/person/day, according to published statistics on exposure estimation. The average exposure estimation for celery seed oil, which is one of the most diffusive smells and penetrating flavours, is 0.75 mg/person/day (EFSA, 2004).

19.8 CONCLUSION AND FUTURE PROSPECTS

Celery has been grown all over the world for thousands of years and has been utilised for food flavouring, essential oil applications, and traditional medicine. Celery is mostly made up of fatty acids and flavonoids. Plant chemical composition is affected by a variety of elements, including soil type, weather, irrigation, pruning, and other horticultural methods. Celery is used in a wide range of industrial applications, including food, pharmaceuticals, and manufacturing. The presence of unsaturated fatty acids in celery OR, such as oleic acid and linoleic acid (60%–70%), causes rancidity in the OR during storage. It's time to figure out how to keep the OR stable for longer periods of time. The presence of monounsaturated fatty acids, particularly linoleic acid, can offer us with health benefits. However, more study is required on maximising yield of oil and OR using different extraction methods, especially in the developing world, where celery leaf and seed harvesting and post-harvesting processes are very comparable to the least effective traditional methods.

Numerous *in vitro* and *in vivo* investigations have demonstrated that celery seeds contain anticancer, antidiabetic, antihypertensive, antihyperlipidemic, antioxidant, antibacterial, and anti-inflammatory properties. Though celery seeds are said to offer a variety of therapeutic characteristics, randomised clinical trials are required to validate their use in the treatment of a variety of infections and chronic illnesses. Furthermore, *in vivo* and *in vitro* studies can be used to investigate the role of celery seeds in the treatment of liver illnesses, urinary tract infections, gout, and arthritis for the greatest benefit to mankind.

REFERENCES

AgMRC. 2019. Data from: Celery. https://www.agmrc.org/commoditiesproducts/vegetables/celery. Accessed on October 14, 2021.

Ahmed, B., Alam, T., Varshney, M., and Khan, S. A. 2002. Hepatoprotective activity of two plants belonging to the Apiaceae and the Euphorbiaceae family. *Journal of Ethnopharmacology* 79(3):313–316.

Al-Kurdy, M. J. J. 2016. Effects of hydroalcoholic extract of celery (Apium graveolens) seed on blood and biochemical parameters of adult male rats. *Kufa Journal for Veterinary Medical Sciences* 7(1):89–95.

Arshad, H., Ali, T. M., Abbas, T., and Hasnain, A. 2018. Effect of microencapsulation on antimicrobial and antioxidant activity of nutmeg oleoresin using mixtures of gum Arabic, Osa, and native sorghum starch. *Starch–Stärke* 70:1700320.

Atta, A. H., and Alkofahi, A. 1998. Anti-nociceptive and anti-inflammatory effects of some Jordanian medicinal plant extracts. *Journal of Ethnopharmacology* 60(2):117–124.

Ballmer-Weber, B. K., Vieths, S., Lüttkopf, D., Heuschmann, P., and Wüthrich, B. 2000. Celery allergy confirmed by double-blind, placebo-controlled food challenge: a clinical study in 32 subjects with a history of adverse reactions to celery root. *Journal of Allergy and Clinical Immunology* 106(2):373–378.

Bertuso, P. D. C., Mayer, D. M. D., and Nitschke, M. 2021. Combining celery oleoresin, limonene and rhamnolipid as new strategy to control endospore-forming *Bacillus cereus*. *Foods* 10(2):455.

Consentino, B. B., Virga, G., La Placa, G. G., Sabatino, L., Rouphael, Y., Ntatsi, G., ... and De Pasquale, C. 2020. Celery (Apium graveolens L.) performances as subjected to different sources of protein hydrolysates. *Plants* 9(12):1633.

Domblides, A., Domblides, H., and Kharchenko, V. 2008, November. Discrimination between celery cultivars with the use of RAPD markers. *Proceedings of the Latvian Academy of Sciences* 62(6):219–222.

Duhamel, M., and Vandenkoornhuyse, P. 2013. Sustainable agriculture: possible trajectories from mutualistic symbiosis and plant neodomestication. *Trends in Plant Science* 18(11):597–600.

El-Beltagi, H. S., Dhawi, F., and El-Ansary, A. E. 2020. Chemical compositions and biological activities of the essential oils from gamma irradiated celery (*Apium graveolens* L.) seeds. *Notulae Botanicae Horti Agrobotanici Cluj-Napoca* (4):2114–2133.

European Food Safety Authority (EFSA). 2004. Opinion of the Scientific Panel on Dietetic products, nutrition and allergies [NDA] to a notification from EFFA on celery leaf oil, celery seed oil and celery oleoresin pursuant to Article 6 paragraph 11 of Directive 2000/13/EC. *EFSA Journal* 2(12):155.

Eurostat. 2019. Data from: Crop production in EU standard humidity. Eurostat. http://appsso.eurostat.ec.europa.eu/nui/show.do? Accessed on October 14, 2021.

Gauri, M., Ali, S. J., and Khan, M. S. 2015. A Review of *Apium graveolens* (Karafs) with special reference to Unani medicine. *International Archives of Integrated Medicine* 2(1):131–136.

Hamza, A. A., and Amin, A. 2007. *Apium graveolens* modulates sodium valproate-induced reproductive toxicity in rats. *Journal of Experimental Zoology Part A: Ecological Genetics and Physiology* 307(4):199–206.

Helaly, A. A. D., El-Refy, A., Mady, E., Mosa, K. A., and Craker, L. 2014. Morphological and molecular analysis of three celery accessions. *Journal of Medicinally Active Plants* 2(3):27–32.

Jung, W. S., Chung, I. M., Kim, S. H., Kim, M. Y., Ahmad, A., and Praveen, N. 2011. In vitro antioxidant activity, total phenolics and flavonoids from celery (*Apium graveolens*) leaves. *Journal of Medicinal Plants Research* 5(32):7022–7030.

Khalil, A., Nawaz, H., Ghania, J. B., Rehman, R., and Nadeem, F. 2015. Value added products, chemical constituents and medicinal uses of celery (*Apium graveolens L.*)–a review. International Journal of Chemical and Biochemical Sciences 8:40–48.

Kooti, W, Ali-Akbari, S., Asadi-Samani, M., Ghadery, H., and Ashtary-Larky, D. 2015. A review on medicinal plant of Apium graveolens. *Advanced Herbal Medicine* 1(1):48–59.

Kooti, W., and Daraei, N. 2017. A review of the antioxidant activity of celery (*Apium graveolens* L). *Journal of Evidence-Based Complementary & Alternative Medicine* 22(4):1029–1034.

Kooti, W., Ghasemiboroon, M., Asadi-Samani, M., Ahangarpoor, A., Noori Ahmad Abadi, M., Afrisham, R., and Dashti, N. 2014. The effects of hydro-alcoholic extract of celery on lipid profile of rats fed a high fat diet. *Advances in Environmental Biology* 8(9): 325–330.

Lim, T. K. 2015. Colocasia esculenta. In Edible Medicinal *and* Non-Medicinal Plants. Springer, Dordrecht, 454–492.

Malhotra, S. K. 2006. Celery. In *Handbook of Herbs and Spices*. Woodhead Publishing, Cambridge, 317–336.

Meyerhof, W. 1997. *Food Chemicals Codex*. Committee of Food Chemicals Codex, Food and Nutrition Board, Institute of Medicine, National Academy of Sciences. National Academy Press, Washington, DC.

Momin, R. A., and Nair, M. G. 2002. Antioxidant, cyclooxygenase and topoisomerase inhibitory compounds from Apium graveolens Linn. seeds. *Phytomedicine* 9(4): 312–318.

Naema, N. F., Dawood, B., and Hassan, S. 2010. Iraqi medicinal plants for their spasmolytic and antibacterial activities. *Journal of Basrah Researches Sciences* 36(6).

Nagar, N., Aswathanarayan, J. B., and Vittal, R. R. 2020. Anti-quorum sensing and biofilm inhibitory activity of *Apium graveolens* L. oleoresin. *Journal of Food Science and Technology* 57(7): 2414–2422.

Nagella, P., Ahmad, A., Kim, S. J., and Chung, I. M. 2012. Chemical composition, antioxidant activity and larvicidal effects of essential oil from leaves of Apium graveolens. *Immunopharmacology and immunotoxicology* 34(2): 205–209.

Popović, M., Kaurinović, B., Trivić, S., Mimica-Dukić, N., and Bursać, M. 2006. Effect of celery (*Apium graveolens*) extracts on some biochemical parameters of oxidative stress in mice treated with carbon tetrachloride. *Phytotherapy Research* 20(7):531–537.

Quiros, C. F. 1993. Celery *Apium graveolens* L. In: *Genetic Improvement of Vegetable Crops*, G. Kallo, and B. O. Bergh, (ed.) Pergamon Press, Oxford, 523–534.

Roghani, M., Baluchnejadmojarad, T., Amin, A., and Amirtouri, R. 2007. The effect of administration of *Apium graveolens* aqueous extract on the serum levels of glucose and lipids of diabetic rats. *Iranian Journal of Endocrinology and Metabolism* 9(2):177–181.

Sipailiene, A., Venskutonis, P. R., Sarkinas, A., and Cypiene, V. 2003. Composition and antimicrobial activity of celery (*Apium graveolens*) leaf and root extracts obtained with liquid carbon dioxide. In *III WOCMAP Congress on Medicinal and Aromatic Plants-Volume 3: Perspectives in Natural Product Chemistry*, 71–77.

Sowbhagya, H. B. 2014. Chemistry, technology, and nutraceutical functions of celery (*Apium graveolens L.*): an overview. *Critical Reviews in Food Science and Nutrition* 54(3):389–398.

Swamy, M. K., Akhtar, M. S., and Sinniah, U. R. 2016. Antimicrobial properties of plant essential oils against human pathogens and their mode of action: an updated review. *Evidence-Based Complementary and Alternative Medicine* 1–21.

Talwari, G., and Ghuman, B. S. 2014. Optimization of microwave assisted process for extraction of celery seed essential oil. *Journal of Agricultural Engineering* 51(2):9–18.

Tsi, D., and Tan, B. K. 2000. The mechanism underlying the hypocholesterolaemic activity of aqueous celery extract, its butanol and aqueous fractions in genetically hypercholesterolaemic RICO rats. *Life Sciences* 66(8):755–767.

Turner, L., Lignou, S., Gawthrop, F., and Wagstaff, C. 2020. Investigating the factors that influence the aroma profile of *Apium graveolens*: a review. *Food Chemistry* 128673:1–13

Tyagi, S., Dhruv, M., Ishita, M., Gupta, A. K., Usman, M. R. M., Nimbiwal, B., and Maheshwar, R. K. 2013. Medical benefits of *Apium graveolens* (celery herb). *Journal of Drug Discovery and Therapeutics* 1(5):36–38.

Zheng, G. Q., Kenney, P. M., Zhang, J., and Lam, L. K. 1993. Chemoprevention of benzo [a] pyrene-induced forestomach cancer in mice by natural phthalides from celery seed oil. *Nutrition and Cancer* 19(1):77–86.

Zhou, Y., Taylor, B., Smith, T. J., Liu, Z. P., Clench, M., Davies, N. W., and Rainsford, K. D. 2009. A novel compound from celery seed with a bactericidal effect against Helicobacter pylori. *Journal of pharmacy and pharmacology* 61(8):1067–1077.

CHAPTER 20

Paprika Oleoresins

Chemistry and Properties

Tejasvi Bhatia and Barkha

Lovely Professional University

Garima Bhardwaj

Sant Longowal Institute of Engineering and Technology

Ajay Sharma

Chandigarh University

Vivek Pandey

VET Centre for Nanoscience

CONTENTS

DOI: 10.1201/9781003186205-20

20.1   INTRODUCTION

Capsicum, popularly known as sweet pepper or bell pepper or Shimla Mirch, is one of the highly remunerative vegetable crops. Pepper (*Capsicum annum* L.) belongs to the family Solanaceae and genus *Capsicum*. It is a vegetable and is consumed as both dehydrated and fresh spices (Bosland et al., 2012). Capsicum is categorized under the non-traditional group of vegetables (Kalloo and Pandey, 2002). Red-colored varieties of pepper (Figure 20.1) are well known as natural colorants owing to the presence of carotenoid pigments, particularly capsanthin and capsorubin (Goodwin, 2012). Powder of spicy red pepper is mainly used for aesthetic or physical purposes, and to enhance the product's aroma, color, and taste (Gordon et al., 1983). Moreover, the main interest of food technologists in carotenoids is because of their nutritional value (Govindarajan, 1986a). Another reason of interest is that they also have some pharmacological characteristics (Giovannucci, 2002).

The name paprika is mainly used by international spice traders for non-pungent red capsicum powder (Figure 20.1). The word "paprika" is Hungarian and originates from the Greek word "pepper" and the Latin word "piper," both referring to pepper. Spice paprika (bell pepper and chili) is the second-largest spice commodity globally (after black pepper) in terms of both its trade value and production volume (Lakner et al., 2018). Recently, a higher demand for oleoresins and other SMs for the improvement in taste and trade qualities of food-based products has been noted, and among various oleoresins, special interest is paid to paprika oleoresins (Govindarajan, 1986b).

The principal constituent responsible for the pungency of paprika is an alkaloid, capsaicin, followed by homodihydrocapsaicin, dihydrocapsaicin, homocapsaicin, and nordihydrocapsaicin (Davis et al., 2007). The capsaicin percentage in pungent paprika varies between 0.1% and 1% w/w (Barbero et al., 2006). Pertaining to the rich source of representative phyto compounds, pungent paprika has a prominent place in the current pharmaceutical and food industries (De Marino et al., 2008). Paprika oleoresin is an oil-soluble natural extract mainly isolated from the fruits of *Capsicum annuum* L. or *Capsicum frutescens* L. (Indian red chilies). It is highly sensitive to heat, light, and air without any antioxidant. It is known for its coloring properties pertaining to the presence of a variety of carotenoid pigments. Major coloring pigments present in the paprika oleoresin are trans capsanthin, capsorubin, beta cryptoxanthin, capsanthin 5, 6-epoxide, beta carotene,

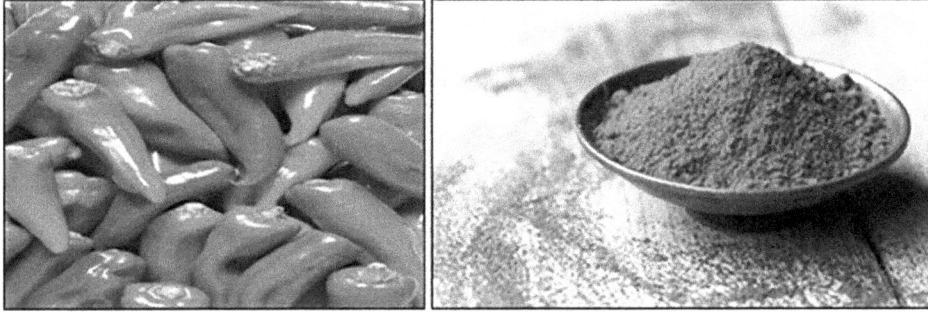

FIGURE 20.1   Red pepper and grounded paprika.

antheraxanthin, zeaxanthin, violaxanthin, and other carotenoids such as asneoxanthin and lutein.

20.2 DISTRIBUTION, PRODUCTION, AND ECONOMIC IMPORTANCE

Capsicum is cultivated around all the parts of the world, specifically in the temperate areas of European countries, South and Central America, and the subtropical and tropical regions of the Asian continent, primarily China and India (Kumar et al., 2016). The *Capsicum* genus consists of about 31 species, out of which 5 (*C. annum*, *Capsicum baccatum*, *C. frutescens*, *Capsicum chinense*, and *Capsicum pubescens*) are utilized as fresh vegetables and for the production of spices (Moscone et al., 2006). Paprika is native to the Republic of Macedonia, but it is usually distributed all over the world. The cultivation of several varieties depends on their different quality factors like taste from the very mild to the very hot. There is also a lot of variation among different species with respect to the shape and size of fruits.

Capsicum is a cool season or temperate crop and is very suited under protected cultivation as well (Figure 20.2). The yellow or red color development in fruits also occurs under low temperatures. Therefore, they can be grown in the summer season on hills and in the winter season on plains. Seed germinates best around 20°C–25°C, but the optimum temperature for the best growth is 18°C–25°C. The average daily temperature of 20°C–25°C is optimum for fruit setting in capsicum. The fruits of bell pepper are prone to sunscald at higher temperatures and very bright sunshine. Pepper requires well-drained loamy soil enriched with organic matter and the optimum sowing season is from September to February. Raising a nursery before transplanting is important in pepper. The required seed rate for normal varieties is around 1.25 kg/ha, and for hybrid varieties, it is 200 g/ha. Seed treatment with Carbendazim (@ 2 g/kg of seed) should be done prior to sowing in lines across the bed at a distance of 2.5 cm. Seeds are then covered with topsoil and paddy straw. The main field is plowed to a fine tilth prior to the transplanting of old seedlings (40–45 days) at a spacing of 30 cm. Irrigation should be provided at 10-day intervals or weekly. Application of farmyard manure (FYM) (@ 25 t/ha) and NPK (@ 40:60:30 kg/ha) as basal and 40 kg N/ha should be done on 30, 60, and 90 days after planting. Hoeing and weeding have to be carried out once and the plants are earthed up after 30 days of transplanting.

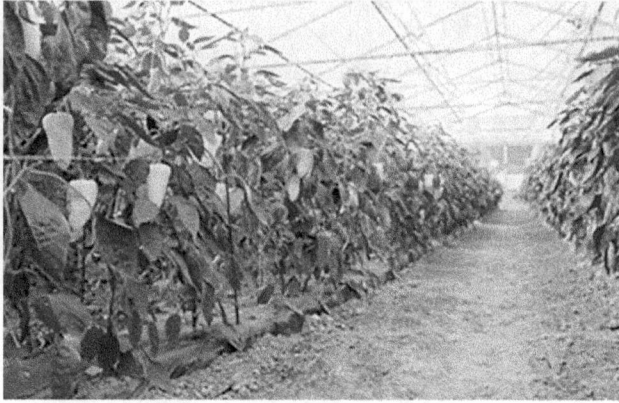

FIGURE 20.2   Bell peppers under protected cultivation.

Clipping and root pruning are two important practices in pepper cultivation that promote root development. Harvesting is done at maturity and the average yield produced is approximately 15 tons/ha in around 150–160 days. It takes around 60–70 days for the fruits to turn dark maroon from green. If the picking is done too early, farmers will not get much profit as a result of lower color development. Fruits should only be picked when they have turned dark maroon and begin to wrinkle. Dry fruits facilitate proper picking and the drying process is quickened too (<7 days) (Hilton, 1999).

After picking or harvesting, fruits should be washed properly if dirty and de-stalked (removal of petiole and seed) and split to facilitate further drying. If orange- or red-colored pods fall on the ground from the plant, they too can be split, dried, and sold as lower-grade paprika. It is recommended not to use jute bags for picking or storage as the jute fibers may lower the quality. Polythene bags should be prepared. Paprika should be stored under dry and cool conditions and should be sold out as soon as possible. Care must be taken to protect the stored produce from rodents. Prolonged storage also deteriorates the color, which ultimately decreases the crop value.

Drying of paprika can be done in different ways, i.e., sun drying, air drying, and forced drying. Sun drying is a more practical, cheaper, and efficient way of drying pods during long spells of dry weather. The harvested pods are generally laid out in a single layer over a plastic sheet spread on the open ground. The pods should be twisted once a day and left in the sun till the moisture content lowers to 20%. Air drying relies mainly on the atmospheric temperature where harvested produce is put on drying racks in the shade and the natural flow of air does the drying. Forced drying is another technique that is the most efficient and reliable means of drying paprika, regardless of weather conditions. Buildings can be converted into dryers, and heat is forced into these dryers. Tobacco dryers can also be used in paprika drying. The temperature of the dryer must not exceed 50° as the oil in the pods is adversely affected at temperatures higher than this. Grading and proper packaging of products are also important. For this purpose, superior quality fruits are graded and cleaned with a dry, soft, and clean cloth to eradicate moisture and any chemical residue present. In the case of capsicum, good-quality fruits with 2–3 lobes weighing ≤150 g are graded as B-grade fruits, whereas fruits with 3–4 lobes weighing ≥150 g are marked as A grade. Fruits that are uniform (in color, size, shape, and maturity) and free from any defects (such as bruises, decay, spots, and pesticide residues) should only be used for further packaging, whereas fruits with any defect (such as sunscald, diseased, any insect or mechanical damage) should be discarded. Generally, three grades are available for paprika based on color and external appearance:

- A grade: Dark red/maroon pods that are free from blemishes.
- B grade: Dark red/maroon pods with up to 20% blemishes.
- C grade: Paler red or orange pods with over 20% blemishes.

White pods and those that are highly blemished or diseased and do not have commercial value. Local agronomists can also be consulted for proper grading specifications.

Although open field cultivation and production of paprika can be done successfully, nowadays protected cultivation in greenhouses or poly-houses is becoming more popular. This is mainly because of several advantages of protected cultivation over conventional cultivation, such as

- enhanced productivity resulting in better yield;
- providing suitable environment for the better growth of crop plants;
- protecting from rainfall, wind, high temperatures, etc.;
- reducing the risk of injury because of insect pests and diseases, thus help to improve the yield as well as the quality of fruits;
- facilitating year-round production along with 2–3 times yield enhancement as compared to open cultivation.

Under protected cultivation, the crop period of green, as well as colored paprika, is around 7–10 months and the yield produced is about 80–100 tons/ha. Also, among various capsicum cultivars, selecting and growing hybrids in greenhouses is useful to have a constant and steady fruit and flower setting comparatively for an elongated period of 8–10 months.

20.2.1 Global Market of Paprika Oleoresin

Paprika oleoresin comprises a flavoring compound of pungent taste called capsaicin in high concentrations. High-revenue opportunity awaits for paprika oleoresin on a global level as its demand is elevating daily in pharmaceutical, cosmetic, and food industries. The need for natural flavoring colors is rising, thus pushing the revenue of paprika across the globe.

The global paprika oleoresin market is divided based on the region, application, and sales channels. The direct and indirect sales segments are placed under the sales channel of paprika oleoresin. The indirect sales are governed and categorized into wholesale, retailer, and trader. North America, Latin America, Asia Pacific and the Middle East, Africa, and Europe are the major countries placed under the area segment of paprika oleoresin.

The popularity of food and beverages has proven to be a prominent driving factor for increasing the paprika oleoresin market on a global level. Spicy food in India has also found its place in high value owing to changing lifestyles and a rise in income because of strong economic growth. Modern consumers are equipped with the knowledge of dietary and health benefits of paprika over the traditional spices that result in increasing the demand for spice in the upcoming period. Health benefits associated with paprika have made it globally popular and provided numerous growth opportunities in the market over the forecast period. The presence of carotenoids, capsaicinoids (CAPS), phenols, vitamins, and flavonoids in paprika has various pharmacological properties. Meat products, spicy culinary, cheese, cheese food coatings, and popcorn oil use paprika as a natural coloring agent. The fruit of capsicum generally comprises coloring pigments, resins, protein, pungent compounds, low volumes of volatile oil, cellulose, mineral elements, and pentosans, whereas seeds mainly contain fixed (non-volatile) oil. Triglycerides, dominantly linoleic acid and unsaturated fatty acids, constitute the fixed oil of seeds. The paprika extract has carotenoid pigments and fruit oil.

Paprika powder was originally used in the kitchen only, but now paprika powder finds a huge market as it is being utilized in the food-processing industries, chiefly snack food, sauces, and meat-processing segments. In addition to being used as a colorant, it is also utilized for flavoring and garnishing of cheese, salads, meat dishes, eggs, seafood, etc. Because of this, the commercial significance of paprika both as a vegetable and as a spice along with large-scale cultivation in tropical and subtropical areas of the world is increasing (Kannan et al., 2009). The high market value of paprika is mainly attributed to the substantial demand from the urban consumers (Kumar et al., 2018). Capsicum is rich in minerals, vitamins C and A. Sweet peppers are a good source of vitamin C. It contains about double the amount of vitamin C by weight as compared to citrus fruits. Vitamin C acts as a natural antioxidant that inhibits the growth of various reactive species in the body and help in preventing certain types of cancers (Denzongpa and Sharma, 2013). Dehydrated pepper powder is also utilized as the poultry feed to enhance the pigmentation of eggs and as a prophylactic antimicrobial agent against some microbes (Vicente et al. 2007; Lokaewmanee et al. 2013). Nowadays, constituents of paprika oleoresins are widely used in the cosmetic and pharmaceutical industries. CAPS are found to be quite effective as an analgesic, anti-cancerous, anti-inflammatory, antioxidant, and anti-obesity compound. Capsaicin also finds its uses as an analgesic in a few nasal sprays, topical ointments as well as against dermal patches to ease pain, in concentrations ranging from 0.025% to 0.25%. It can provide provisional relief from minor pains and aches in muscles and joints related to arthritis, sprains, and backache. In addition, CAPS also have beneficial effects on the gastrointestinal and cardiovascular systems.

20.3 EXTRACTION TECHNIQUES

Paprika oleoresin is a semi-viscous liquid, deep red in color, obtained from dried red paprika. Its deep red color is due to the presence of a variety of carotenoid pigments. It is an oil-soluble natural extract. *Capsicum* spp. contains numerous valuable phytoconstituents, which include polyphenols (0.5% of dry weight), carbohydrates (up to 85% of the dry weight), and minor but important bioactive secondary metabolites (SMs), such as carotenoids, CAPS, and vitamins (Arimboor et al., 2015). Mainly, there are two different methods used for the extraction of paprika oleoresins:

1. Solvent extraction

2. Carbon dioxide supercritical extraction

20.3.1 Pre-Treatments for Extraction

Dehydrated pepper is first given pre-treatment with chemicals such as sodium and potassium hydroxide, potassium carbonate, potassium bisulfate, ascorbic acid, and ethyl and methyl ester emulsions, and then oleoresins are extracted as this will enhance the quality. When treated with citric acid solutions and ethyl oleate, it was observed that both green pepper and red pepper showed a reduction in drying time and more mass transfer resistance was experienced (Doymaz and Ismail, 2013; Doymaz and Kocayigit, 2012). The pre-treatment of red pepper with $Na_2S_2O_3$, NaCl, and $CaCl_2$ before drying at 70°C resulted in enhancing its color, firmness, and quality (Vega-Gálvez et al., 2008). Pre-treatment with 5% of K_2CO_3 and 2% of ethyl oleate was found effective when drying at 50°C as it resulted in the best yield and color quality of capsicum. Researchers observed that the red color is better preserved during pre-treatments (Doymaz and Pala, 2002). Osmotic dehydration is another alternative for drying fruits. The fruits are put into the concentrated solution of solutes that have a semi-permeable membrane, and this process results in partial water removal from peppers. The moisture level was brought down at 30%–70%. Sodium chloride also acts as a driving force, as it results in quick drying when placed in an osmotic solution because of its property of synergistic effect that occurs between sodium chloride and sucrose (Ade-Omowaye et al., 2002).

It is advisable to harvest the pepper at its maturity stage as it provides more remunerative profits and also the color quality is enhanced as the fruits have turned red completely (Krajayklang et al., 2000). There is an increase in techniques for increasing the shelf life of the product, for example, freezing, refrigerating, and other atmospheric modifications, etc. Even though many preserving techniques have come to light, drying nevertheless is the most desirable one as it has given great results in reducing the level of biochemical, physical, microbiological, and chemical degradation of food and its products. This enriches the shelf life and the food can be stored for a longer period.

20.3.2 Solvent Extraction

The paprika oleoresins are obtained by solvent extraction of dried, powdered spice of red paprika fruits. During this solvent extraction, a compatible solvent system with the characteristic lipophilic/hydrophilic properties is used. The most frequently used solvents for the extraction of paprika oleoresin are trichloroethylene, hexane, ethylacetate, methylene chloride, methanol, acetone, and ethanol. The solvent selection and optimization of extraction conditions is a necessary step as it directly influences the quality and stability of the

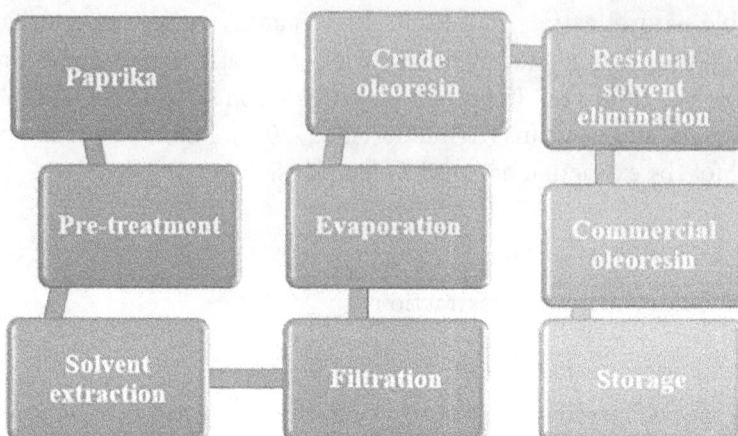

FIGURE 20.3   General outline of solvent extraction of paprika oleoresins.

final product (Mínguez-Mosquera et al., 2008). A simple solvent extraction procedure is described in Figure 20.3.

A variety of organic ingredients, including fats, oils, lipids, and proteins, can be obtained from different biological materials by this process. First, the biological material is macerated in the chosen organic solvent and then after specific time period material is filtered and finally the extract is concentrated under reduced pressure using a rotary evaporator (El Asbahani et al., 2015).

The bioactive ingredients present in paprika fruits may vary in their chemical composition from cultivar to cultivar. The process of solvent extraction of paprika oleoresin (Figure 20.4) is as follows:

- Fresh paprika fruits are first sliced and then dried using a convection oven drier at about 60°C to produce dried fruits with only about 10% water content.

- Any volatile non-aqueous solvent, more commonly hexane or ethanol, is added and permitted to precisely wet the plant material. A micellar structure is formed as the oleoresin passes into the solution along with the solvent.

- After a brief period, these micelles are removed and the existing solvent is swapped with the fresh ones to further continue the isolation process.

- The solvent is consequently removed from the crude extract by evaporation at the lowest probable temperature in order to avoid the loss of volatile aromatic constituents. This whole process is carried out in two stages, where, in the first stage, approximately 95% of the solvent is removed in a standard film evaporator, and later in the second stage, this concentrated micelle passes through partial vacuum, which removes the residue of the solvent and ultimately concentrates the micelle into an oleoresin.

- The remaining solvent, which remains with the main mass of the extracted paprika powder, is then removed by using a very high vacuum.

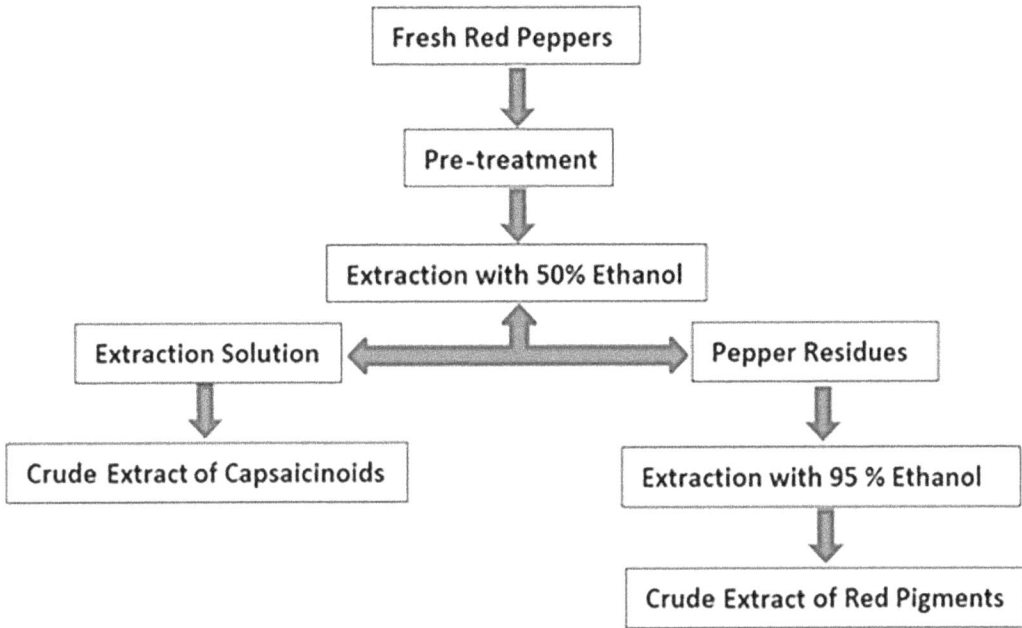

FIGURE 20.4   Solvent extraction procedure.

The total yield of oleoresin obtained depends on the solvent used and generally ranges between 11.5% and 16.5% (Govindarajan and Salzer, 1986). The pungency of extracted oleoresin mainly depends on the pungency of the original fruit. Paprika oleoresin has very little to no pungency and is mostly utilized for its coloring and flavoring potential, whereas capsicum oleoresin is mainly used as a source of higher pungency.

20.3.3 Carbon Dioxide Supercritical Extraction

In the late 19th century, extraction with supercritical fluids came to light. Carbon dioxide (CO_2) supercritical extraction for oleoresin extraction is generally used in the laboratory for research purposes and is not used for the commercial production of paprika oleoresins. This supercritical fluid extraction (SFE) is a separation technology that utilizes any supercritical fluid solvent for extraction. These are the fluids that exist at a state between the gas and liquid phases owing to their temperature and pressure, which is beyond their critical point.

The most commonly used supercritical fluid for this process is CO_2 with other choices including ethanol. At a critical pressure of 7.39 MPa and a critical temperature of 31.35°C, CO_2 starts expanding to fill its container like a gas but with a density like that of a liquid. Therefore, it is a suitable solvent for the isolation of a variety of bioactive ingredients from different biological materials, mainly because of its lower cost and non-toxic, non-flammable, and inert nature. It has a decent extraction potential to dissolve the compounds with a higher molecular weight, regardless of their nature, whether polar or non-polar. A typical scheme of commonly installed SFE plant is illustrated in Figure 20.5.

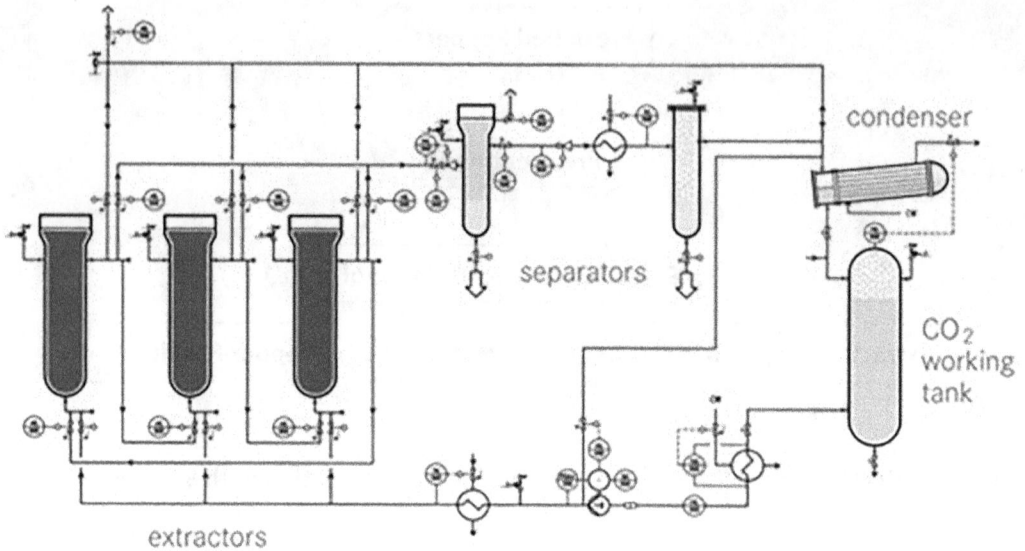

FIGURE 20.5 A typical scheme of supercritical fluid extraction plant.

The traditional extraction procedures with organic solvents were prone to isomerization and degradation, so a more efficient approach of extraction by supercritical fluid found its place in the modern world. It has reduced the thermal stress by lowering the extraction temperature conditions to 40°C. Also, compared to the traditional extraction process using Soxhlet apparatus, SFE uses supercritical fluid, thus eliminating the use of organic solvents. This manages the problems of storage and disposal of these organic solvents as well as reduces related environmental concerns.

Researchers reported continuous and discontinuous CO_2 supercritical extraction. The continuous extraction using SCF-CO_2 was done at different pressures and volumes. The range of pressure varied from 2000 to 7000 psi. Acetone and ethanol at 1% (w/w) proportion to SCF-CO_2 were taken as co-solvents. It was observed that as the pressure increased, the pigment concentration also increased. The results displayed the oleoresin recovered was 10% of the initial weight of paprika.

Discontinuous extraction was performed at two stages: the first stage with low pressure and the second stage at high pressure, and then the combination of high and low pressure ranging from 2000 to 7000 psi. The first-stage extraction displayed more lipid content extraction from paprika and a very low pigment concentration. These extractions of oleoresins were named as β-carotene-rich oils. The latter stage displayed more carotenoid pigments than lipids. The high concentrations of red pigment were obtained at high pressures (Jaren-Galan et al., 1999). The extraction curve is obtained by measuring the oleoresin yield every 30 minutes and the whole process is carried up to 10 hours. The curve plotted against oleoresin yield and extraction time displayed initial oil solubility increase, then plateau phase, and later maximum yield in the final stage (Tepić et al., 2008).

In the SFE process, the diffusion coefficients of waxes and lipids in supercritical fluids are much higher as compared to in any other liquid solvent, therefore extraction can occur more rapidly. Also, there is an additional benefit of supercritical fluids that they have no surface tension and their viscosity is much lower than liquids, which facilitates these supercritical fluids to be able to penetrate smaller pores that are normally impermeable to liquid. CO_2 extraction is usually done with a two-step separation of extracts into an essential oil and a pungent oleoresin fraction. The extract is semisolid, pasty, and viscous in nature, therefore difficult to obtain from the separation containers (Catchpole et al., 2003). The paprika extracts obtained by this process range from orange to light red to intense dark red depending on the processing conditions. This extract has many advantages over-extract, which is conventionally obtained using organic solvents, as these extracts never contain any toxic residues and solvent traces. In this process, one can also change the content of CAPS and carotenoids by varying the extraction conditions (Perva-Uzunalić et al., 2004). The key disadvantage of this process as compared to the traditional methods is the high capital necessities related to the setup for high-pressure operation. However, results have revealed the economic practicability of this method to isolate the bioactive constituents from capsicum (Fernández-Ronco et al., 2013).

20.4 CHARACTERIZATION

C. annuum L. has been characterized for its composition and carotenoid pigments. Researchers performed an experiment where they studied the best cultivator of paprika. MA1 cultivator displayed high carotenoid content in high-performance liquid chromatography (HPLC) followed by DN5 and RN2. The liquid extracts were analyzed using HPLC, and then the pigment identification was done by thin-layer chromatography and co-chromatography (Hornero-Méndez et al., 2002).

In another experiment, the carotenoid content in oleoresins of paprika and tomato was quantified using UV-visible spectroscopy. Thermal degradation experiments were also done in the same way to check their degradation rate. Acetone was used to measure the absorbance and a peak at 454 nm was obtained for paprika oleoresin and at 470 nm in tomato oleoresin. These two closely similar oleoresins can be differentiated using this technique (Abbeddou et al., 2013).

Oleoresin is widely used for its color and pungency. The color is analyzed using digital cameras and a high-vision computer system. The characterization of oleoresin and the active compound capsaicin has been done using Fourier transform infrared spectroscopy (FTIR). First, in the experiment, solvent extraction by using hexane was carried out, and then attenuated total reflectance (ATR)-FTIR at a range of 4000–450 cm^{-1} and a resolution 1 cm^{-1} was utilized. Findings showed the peaks at 3350 cm^{-1} contributing to OH/NH, 2900 cm^{-1} referring to the CH group, and 1050 for the COC group for capsaicin. Vibrational peaks because of amines were also observed in the range of 1600–1630 cm^{-1} and C–N vibrations at 1300 cm^{-1}. Oleoresin showed peaks at 1378, 1627, and 1650 cm^{-1}. Some common peaks in both oleoresin and capsaicin, such as 2857, 1517, and 1036 cm^{-1}, showed that capsaicin is present in oleoresins (Riquelme et al., 2017) (Figure 20.6). Not only for its active compound, but many fat-soluble vitamins are found in paprika oleoresin and that is also quantified by various procedures. Fat-soluble vitamins like vitamin A, D, E, and K, A acetate, E acetate, and vitamin esters were quantified in oleoresins.

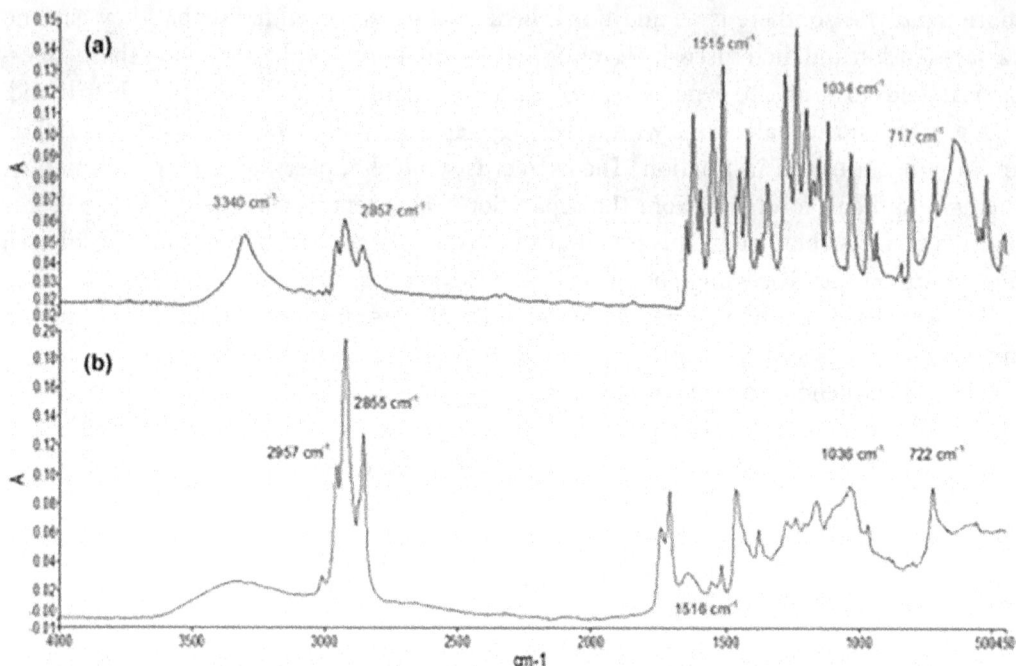

FIGURE 20.6 ATR-FTIR spectra of (a) capsaicin and (b) oleoresin (Riquelme et al., 2017).

Reverse-phase elution HPLC was used for the analysis combined with spectrophoto-metric detection by UV-visible spectroscopy. Initially, the extraction was done by using ethyl acetate. The extracts were run in HPLC having methanol/water (98:2 v/v) as mobile phase. Chromatograms were observed, and it was found that vitamins were recovered from almost 94% to 101% in range. Variations in the range of recovery of vitamins were also observed by increasing the storage of paprika up to one year. Many colored substances inherited in paprika can overlap with vitamins and can affect their deter-mination. A suitable mobile phase should be selected in HPLC for the elution. Many lipophilic samples are successfully analyzed by non-aqueous reversed-phase chroma-tography (NARP). Researchers utilized this method also to analyze paprika. Vitamins A and D were successfully quantified, but the chromatograms suggested that a stronger organic mobile phase can result in increasing the efficiency. Semi-aqueous methanol/ water resulted in no elution of vitamin D, whereas the mobile phase having methanol/ ethyl acetate gave complete elution of paprika components. Still, it was observed that the elution speed is affected by the concentration of ethyl acetate and the relation was found to be directly proportional. Another method of gradient elution was then applied, which resulted in giving vitamin elution and strong retention of the components. The chromatogram of gradient elution of paprika components is shown in Figure 20.7 (Vinas et al., 1992). Researchers also characterized oleoresin in paprika by examining micro-encapsulates that contained it. Various instrumentation techniques, such as focused ion beam coupled with scanning electron microscopy (FIB-SEM), confocal laser scanning microscopy (CLSM), X-ray photoelectron spectroscopy (XPS), and X-ray dispersion

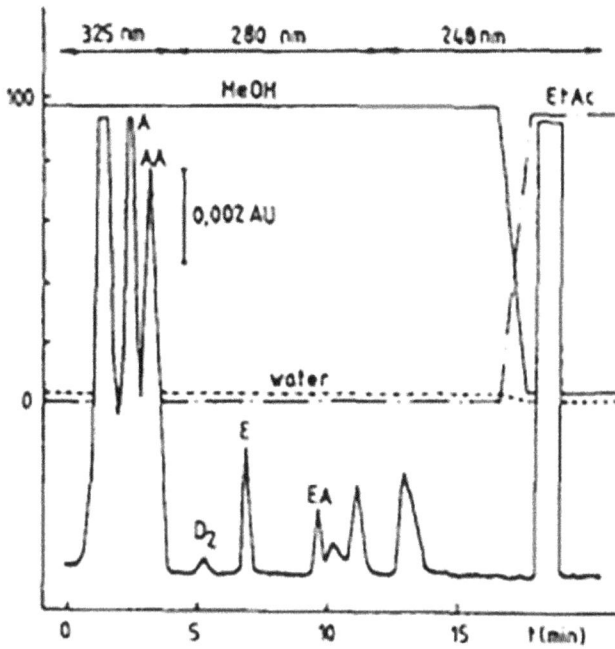

FIGURE 20.7   Chromatogram of paprika with gradient elution program (Vinas et al., 1992).

spectroscopy (EDX), were used to determine the oleoresin present in microcapsules, their morphology, and chemical constituents.

CLSM uses fluorescence to localize and visualize the compounds and is a non-destructive technique. The FIB-SEM allowed the characterization of microparticles, and linear mapping of oxygen, carbon, and nitrogen was performed by EDX that uses a focuses beam to perform the analysis (Porras-Saavedra et al., 2018).

Nuclear magnetic resonance (NMR) spectroscopy is a powerful technique used for the detection of adulteration of spices. Paprika oleoresin is a widely utilized spice all around the world. Its authenticity to its origin and adulteration of its food products can be checked by using NMR spectroscopy.

NMR analysis for 62 Asian red pepper samples comprised 9 samples from Vietnam, 17 from China, and 36 from Korea. Additional powdered red pepper samples from Korean markets were analyzed. Blind samples were analyzed with other samples to see whether they are correctly classified based on their geographical origin, as Korean samples are often more expensive than the rest.

The difference in metabolite content in samples was observed based on their origin by using NMR spectroscopy. Signals for metabolites like α-, and β-glucose, linoleic acid, unsaturated fatty acid, histidine, uridine, alanine, tyrosine, sucrose, phenylalanine, tryptophan, adenosine, and kaempferol, were obtained and quantified. Both 1H-NMR and 13C-NMR are used to determine and quantify paprika oleoresin (Pacholczyk-Sienicka et al., 2021).

Globalization and complex food chain supply have also increased food fraud all around the globe. Many food adulterants and illegal chemicals are added in various spices, and paprika is not immune to these adulterants. These additions directly affect the health of the consumer

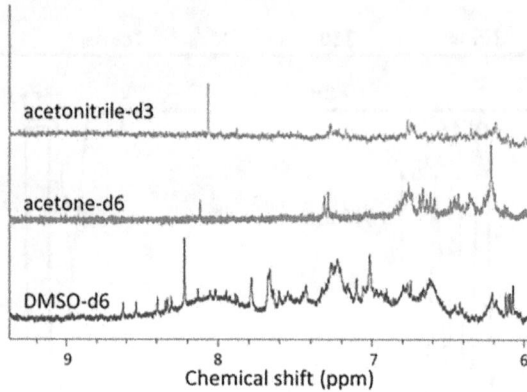

FIGURE 20.8   ¹H-NMR of paprika powder by different solvents (Hu et al., 2017).

and result in the cost of food and degrade its quality. One such illegal dye is Sudan I, which is found to be carcinogenic but is added in spices to induce freshness. Researchers determined the presence of Sudan I in paprika by using solid-state (SS) and NMR. In solid-state Sudan I was extracted by using DMSO-d6 as a solvent solution, while acetonitrile, acetone, and DMSO-d6 were utilized in NMR. The results concluded that the LOD (lowest limit of detection) is 6.7 and 208.6 mg/kg and the LOQ (lowest limit of quantification) is 22.5 and 313.7 mg/kg for NMR and SSNMR, respectively (Figure 20.8) (Hu et al., 2017).

Co-crystallization of paprika oleoresin was done to make a natural dye and to provide its applications in the food industry. The stability in the color of the free oleoresin and co-crystallized product was seen at different temperatures and light conditions. The morphology of the co-crystallized product was examined using optical microscopy. It uses a halogen light source and a polarized light filter and was seen at a magnification of 40× and 100×. The images were captured with the help of a digital camera. The morphological details reveal the orange-colored, polygonal, and irregular shapes arranged in clusters. The results of the study also concluded that there is a significant loss of color in free oleoresins compared to its co-crystallized product. This means that the co-crystallized product is less susceptible to thermal color degradations and is more stable (Figure 20.9) (Federzoni et al., 2019).

20.5 PHYSICAL PROPERTIES

Capsicum oleoresin is a viscous liquid with a clear red to dark red color and having a characteristic odor and flavor. It is partially soluble in alcohol and completely soluble in fixed oils. Oleoresin is typically the alcoholic extract of dried fruit. It is dark red and has a pungent smell. It contains capsaicin, dihydrocapsaicin, and nor-dihydrocapsaicin (Johnson, 2007). Its further properties are described in Table 20.1 (Johnson, 2007).

20.6 CHEMICAL COMPOSITION

The major constituents of paprika oleoresins are CAPS, carotenoids, flavonoids, and some volatile compounds. The chemical structures of main CAPS and carotenoids present in *C. annum* L. is shown in Table 20.2.

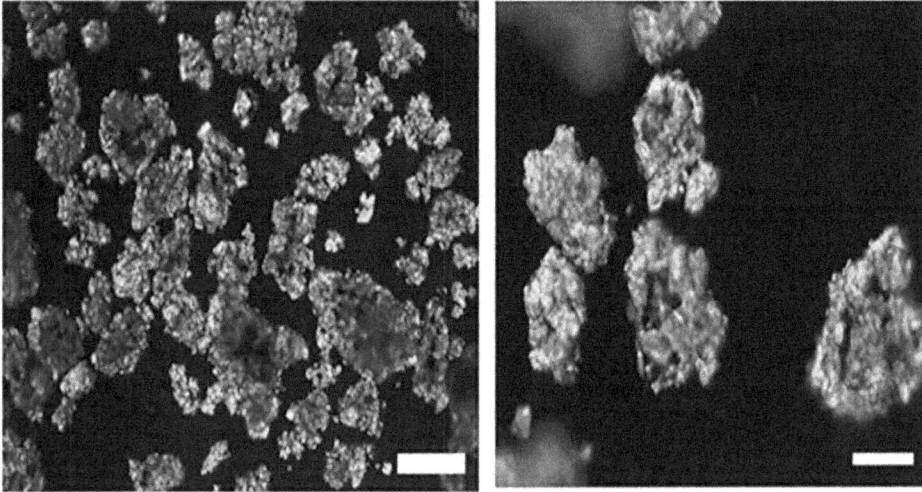

FIGURE 20.9   Images acquired from optical microscopy of the co-crystallized paprika at 40×/scale 500 μm and at 100×/scale 200 μm, respectively (Federzoni et al., 2019).

TABLE 20.1   Properties of Paprika Oleoresin

Property	Value
Form	Dark red viscous fluid, dark red-colored paste
Odor	Spicy odor
Taste	Pungent
Molecular weight	305.4 g/mole
Solubility	Fully soluble in benzene, ketone, ether, alcohol, and paraffin oils and dispersible in water
Specific gravity	1.0073–1.073 at 25°C
Melting point	≤60°C
Boiling point	≥180°C
Flash point	215°F

20.6.1 Capsaicinoids

One of the important characteristics of bell pepper is its pungent smell, which is because of the chemical group of alkaloids known as CAPS. CAPS have a vanillyl group bonded with an amide and an alkyl chain. CAPS contain mainly capsaicin ($C_{18}H_{27}NO_3$, trans-8-methyl-N-vanillyl-6-nonenamide) followed by dihydrocapsaicin and other minor derivatives, such as homocapsaicin, nordihydrocapsaicin, homodihydrocapsaicin, and various others. Different types of chilis have different contents of CAPS as it generally depends on the place where the plant was grown, temperature and intensity, fruitage, and fruit position on the plant. CAPS are very stable in oleoresins, and even during high temperature and long storage, they don't display breakdown in their composition (Berke et al., 2001). CAPS molecular structure is resistant to ionizing radiations but can decompose up to 50% exposed to 80°C or above temperature conditions. This degradation is attributed to the production of vanillyl group with acyl chain produced by cleavage of C–N bond and

TABLE 20.2   Chemical Structures of Main Capsaicinoids and Carotenoids Present in *Capsicum annum* L.

Category	Chemical Name	Structure
Capsaicinoids (CAPS)	Capsaicin	
	Dihydro-capsaicin	
	Nordihydro-capsaicin	
	Nor-capsaicin	
	Homo-capsaicin	
Carotenoids	β-Carotene	
	β-Crypto-xanthin	
	Viola-xanthin	
	Zeaxanthin	
	Anthera-xanthin	
	Cucurbita-xanthin A	
	Capsanthin	

(Continued)

TABLE 20.2 (*Continued*) Chemical Structures of Main Capsaicinoids and Carotenoids Present in *Capsicum annum* L.

Category	Chemical Name	Structure
	Capsorubin	
	Capsanthin 5,6-epoxide	

this vanillyl group is majorly attributed to the bioactivity of CAPS. These show solubility in low to medium polarity solvents like methanol, alcohol, and acetonitrile (Antonio et al., 2018).

20.6.2 Carotenoids

The red pepper is extensively utilized because of its characteristic color that makes it an attraction for the food industry. The characteristic intense red color is because of the presence of carotenoids, which are synthesized during ripening. These are a set of 750 tetraterpenoid compounds occurring in plants. They produce different colors ranging from yellow, orange to red and are known for their chromogenic functions. The structural composition of carotenoids shows eight isoprene units condensing to form C40 terpenoid compound. Every mature pepper contains carotenoid pigments as nine conjugated double-bond structures placed in the centerpolyene chain and are differentiated into two families as Red and Yellow. Red comprises capsorubin, capsanthin, and capsanthin-5,6-epoxide, and yellow comprises violaxanthin, zeaxanthin, cucurbitaxanthin A, antheraxanthin, βcryptoxanthin, and β-carotene. Combined capsanthin (30%–60%) and isomer capsorubin (6%–8%) display the majority of total carotenoids in pepper (Mínguez-Mosquera et al., 2008). Another classification placed carotenoids into two categories, namely carotenes and xanthophylls, based on their chemical structures. Cyclized and liner hydrocarbons are the characteristics of carotenes, whereas carotenes having oxygenated functional groups like –OH, $R_2C=O$, $O-CH_3$, C=O, and epoxy groups are placed under xanthophylls (Antonio et al., 2018).

Paprika oleoresin shows a color shift from green, symbolizing unripe fruit, to red, which symbolizes ripe fruit. The disappearance of chlorophyll leads to the red color in pepper followed by the process of *de novo* biosynthesis of carotenoids embarking on the ripe fruit. *De novo* biosynthesis results in esterifying xanthophylls with fatty acids, and this xanthophyll esterification is characteristic of the ripening index of the fruit. Carotenoids display a range of biological actions and applications as their consumption shows a reduced risk of cancer, enhancement of the immune system, and antioxidant production in humans (Mínguez-Mosquera et al., 2008).

20.6.3 Flavonoids

A total of 7000 secondary plant metabolites are placed under this class of compounds. These are only synthesized in plants, and because of this, they have found various bioactive applications majorly as antioxidants in mammals that are unable to synthesize them. Anti-inflammatory properties, reduction in hypertension, and arthritis are some of their other applications. The food, clothing, cosmetic, and pharmaceutical industry widely utilize flavonoids for different purposes. They protect plants again UV light and microbes and help in the growth regulation process. Pepper contains conjugated flavonoids as O-glycosides and C-glycosides derivatives. Approximately 41% of flavonoid content in pepper is present in hydrolyzed form (Antonio et al., 2018).

20.6.4 Volatile Compounds

Capsicum attracts its consumers due to its aroma, which is generally attributed to the presence of volatile compounds in it. Almost 2000 substances are found consisting of hydrocarbons, terpenes, alcohols, ketones, acids, aldehydes, phenols, esters, and lactones as volatile substances present in pepper. Some of the compound identified by the researchers are acetic acid, a-pinene, a-terpinol, acopaene, a-humulene, acalocorene, butyrate, b-caryophllene, byperene, 2-butyl acetate, b-cubebene, dimethyl sulfide, decanoic acid, dimethyl amine, hexyl n-valerate, hexanal, hexane, hexyl isobutanoate, ethyl ester propanoic acid, ethanol, ethyl 3-methylpentanoate, germacrene D, g-cadinene, isopentanoate, 3-methylpentanoate, pentyl 4-methyl-2-pentanoate, 6-methyl-4-heptenyl 2-methylpropanoate, linalool, limonene, etc. (Antonio et al., 2018).

20.7 BIOLOGICAL ACTIVITIES

20.7.1 Antifungal Properties

C. annum L. species show antifungal activity because of capsaicin. The amount of capsaicin present in the species is directly proportional to the antifungal activity. Inhibition to fungi, such as *Aspergillus flavus, Aspergillus niger,* and *Rhizopus* species, has been displayed (Riquelme and Matiacevich, 2017). Researchers also examined oleoresins as antispastic agents against fungal species *Leptographium procerum* and *Sphaeropsis sapinea* and results concluded that they exhibit moderate antifungal activity (Singh and Chittenden, 2008).

20.7.2 Antimicrobial Properties

Paprika oleoresin displays significant antimicrobial activity against bacteria, such as *Pseudomonas aeruginosa, Escherichia coli, Proteus mirabilis,* and *Staphylococcus aureus* (Adamu et al., 2005). Recently studies were done by the researchers to see whether oleoresin is an anti-bacterial product and its anti-bacterial activity was examined against Gram-positive (*Staphylococcus epidermis* and *S. aureus*) and Gram-negative bacteria (*Pseudomonas aeruginosa, E. coli*). *In vitro* disc diffusion method was used to check the resistance pattern against both bacteria by using two different varieties, i.e., curly red chili oleoresin and big red chili oleoresin. It was found that curly red chili oleoresin is a more effective anti-bacterial agent as compared to the other owing to more capsaicin content present in it. The results also displayed that Gram-positive bacteria displayed more inhibition and were more sensitive to oleoresin (Nurjanah et al., 2014).

20.7.3 Antiviral Properties

Chemical-rich capsicum has widely been studied as an antiviral agent. The chemical constituent cis-capsaicin is also known as civamide and is a migraine pain-relieving agent as also a potent agent against herpes simplex virus (HSV), as it disrupts the viral cycle (Khan et al., 2014). Researchers examined the antiviral activity of capsicum species on L20B, VERO, herpes 1, and poliovirus 1 cell lines. Methanolic, ethanolic, and acetate extracts were prepared of capsicum species and were tested against cell lines to see the inhibition of the virus. It was found that no extract displayed antiviral property against poliovirus but were effective antiviral agents in other cell lines. It was also seen that acetate extracts displayed high cytotoxicity, whereas methanolic and ethanolic extracts were non-toxic (KoffiAffoué et al., 2015).

20.7.4 Antioxidant Properties

C. annum L. comprises a variety of antioxidants at its mature red-colored stage as CAPS, ascorbic acid, lycopene, esthoxyquin, and p-coumaryl alcohol (Khan et al., 2014). Studies performed on human leucocytes declare that H_2O_2-induced DNA damage and 4-hydroxy-2-nonenal-induced damage are inhibited by various methanolic extracts from *C. annum* L. (Park et al., 2012). Phenolic groups and flavonoids contribute to the antioxidant nature of oleoresins. Oleoresins often display redox properties as they act as reducing agents like hydrogen ion donors, oxygen ions, deactivators, and metal chelators (Riquelme and Matiacevich, 2017).

20.7.5 Anti-Inflammatory Properties

Major constituents of red pepper, such as phenols and flavonoids, display anti-inflammatory property and CAPS and their compounds act as pain-reducing agents as reported by the literature (Khan et al., 2014). It has been reported that the pain of rheumatoid arthritis, noxious chemical hyperalgesia, and inflammatory heat can be reduced in their respective effects with the oral ingestion of capsaicin (Fraenkel et al., 2004). Various species, owing to their phenolic content, ascorbic acid, and CAPS, display anti-inflammatory nature. Capsaicin is the major constituent of capsicum that results in this property. *In vivo* anti-inflammatory studies in mice were conducted, where it was seen that capsaicin results in inhibiting the production of pro-inflammatory agents like PGE2 nitric oxide by the inactivation of nuclear transcription factor-kappa in murine peritoneal macrophages (Spiller et al., 2008).

20.7.6 Anticancer Properties

The major constituent of chili, capsaicin, associated with pungency, has been found efficient against both *in vitro* and *in vivo* growth of cancer cells (Mori et al., 2006). These compounds are extensively studied for their antitumor activity. HCT 116, LoVo, SW480, and Colo 205 cell lines were studied, and it was reported that capsaicin displays an anticancer effect on human colorectal cancer. Capsaicin exhibits increased apoptosis, mitochondrial dysfunction, and arrests cell cycle into G2/M phase in cell lines of SKBR-3, MCF-7, T47D, MDA-MB231, and BT-474 when studied for anticancer activity against human breast cancer. Human myeloid leukemia was also studied on HL-60, U937, and THP-1 cell lines, where capsaicin multiplies the apoptotic effects by activating the calcium-CaMKII-Sp1 pathway. Pancreatic cancer studies on PANC-1 cell line to see the capsaicin anticancer activity were also done, which showed that it arrests the growth of the tumor by inducing cell cycle arrest in G0/G1 phase (Parvez, 2017).

20.7.7 Antidiabetic Properties

Capsicum carotenoids are also known for their hypoglycemic potential as some studies showed that lipophilic carotenoid fractions of various varieties show selective inhibitory activity against α-amylase. Capsicum fruits are rich in zeaxanthin, which is used as a diet by diabetic patients as it displayed its potential as an antidiabetic agent by reducing complications and displaying antidiabetic nephritic activity. According to a study performed on a rat model having diet-streptozotocin (STZ)-induced type 2 diabetes, zeaxanthin helped in normalizing the body weight and lower the blood glucose level. It is also connected that because of antioxidant activity and modulation of lipid metabolism, capsicum also shows antidiabetic activities (Mohd Hassan et al., 2019).

20.8 SAFETY, TOXICITY, AND FUTURE SCOPE

Capsicum has been known for its health-enhancing effects and benefits ranging from acting as natural painkillers, reducing sinuses, increasing the production of digestive juices, mouth-watering resulting in a reduction of acids causing a cavity, and releasing antioxidants that help in the protection of the body. Although there are many health benefits, there are many reports of toxicity of capsaicin and carotenoids linking them with various diseases and cancers.

Capsaicin elevation can cause various reactions resulting in heat, pain, burning sensations, erythema, and stinging. Damage to the eyes, the nervous system, and the mucous membrane has also been reported by this compound. The whole response to this compound is specific from person to person, as in some it causes intense burning while in others it causes mild discomfort only. When taken in high doses, capsaicin can irritate the esophagus and stomach resulting in anal burning. Dermatitis has been experienced when excessive contact with capsaicin happened with the skin. Some studies reported the mutagenic activity of capsaicin and dihydrocapsaicin in V79 cells (Palevitch and Craker, 1996).

Researchers showed that β-carotene did not get converted into retinol as a result of high alcohol intake. This produces a high risk of lung cancer in people because of the high dose of β-carotene supplemented. Around 20–30 mg/day of β-carotene can increase the risk of cancer in heavy chain smokers.

It was also observed that niacin health benefits were suppressed because of the high intake of vitamins and selenium with β-carotene, which further induce cholesterol levels. Osteoporotic fracture risk was also found because of carotenoid dietary intake that increases the risk of hip fracture in men and women (Adadi et al., 2018)

Measurement of capsaicin acute and sub-chronic toxicity in various animal species has been measured. In mice, depending on the mode of administration, the LD50 values for CAPS in the range from 0.56 (intravenous) to 520 (dermal) mg/kg body weight were studied, and death was reported owing to respiratory paralysis. Human LD50 value by oral administration in an average person will be obtained after drinking tobacco sauces up to 1.5 quarts. The toxicity of food additive CAPS is found to be negligible in humans as no report of death because of CAPS-induced respiratory failure has been reported (Berke and Shieh, 2001).

Based on paprika extract, a toxicity study was performed in F344/DuCrj rats (Kanki et al., 2003). The paprika extract was obtained from Spanish paprika fruit with the help of extracting solvent hexane. Carotenoid content was found to be 7.5%. Rats (ten, both sexes) that were fully fed with a powdered diet were taken for the experiment. Dose levels at 0%, 0.62%, 1.25%, 2.5%, and 5% in males and females were taken in a period from 5 to 13 weeks of age. No death or remarkable histopathological changes were observed, but total serum cholesterol increased by increasing the dose showing the dose-dependency with serum chemistry.

20.9 CONCLUSION

Paprika oleoresin is extensively utilized in the modern world as a spice and natural coloring agent in the food industry, cosmetic industry, and pharmaceuticals. The characteristic pungency and red color of oleoresin contribute to its CAPS and carotenoid content. Capsaicin, dihydrocapsaicin, nordihydrocapsaicin, and homocapsaicin are the major CAPS present in pepper, whereas carotene, cryptoxanthin, zeaxanthin, lutein, capsanthin and cryptocapsin, etc. make the carotenoid content of pepper. It is also rich in flavonoids, volatile compounds, and many vitamins like vitamins A, C, D, E, and K. Oleoresin has been utilized in various fields for different applications by showing properties like antimicrobial, antiviral, anti-cancerous, antidiabetic, anti-inflammatory, antidiabetic, anti-obesity, and antioxidants. The chemical content of paprika oleoresin is characterized by various instrumentation techniques like UV-visible spectroscopy, ATR-FTIR, NMR, high-performance thin-layer chromatography (HP-TLC), thin-layer chromatography (TLC), column chromatography, mass spectroscopy, etc. to check the authenticity and quality of it. The uses of paprika oleoresin are augmenting in the modern world as it provides a safe alternative to synthetic color dyes and shows various health benefits. It is enriched in both macronutrients and micronutrients that make it a suitable candidate to be utilized in modern world diet, where nutrient deficiency is prominent among all age groups. Safe, non-toxic, and nutrient-rich paprika oleoresin is a great choice and upcoming food, cosmetic, and health supplement in the modern world.

REFERENCES

Abbeddou, S., Petrakis, C., Pérez-Gálvez, A. et al. 2013. Effect of simulated thermo-degradation on the carotenoids, tocopherols and antioxidant properties of tomato and paprika oleoresins. *Journal of the American Oil Chemists Society* 90: 1697–1703.

Adadi, P., Barakova, N. V., and Krivoshapkina, E. F. 2018. Selected methods of extracting carotenoids, characterization, and health concerns: a review. *Journal of Agricultural and Food Chemistry* 66: 5925–5947.

Adamu, H. M., Abayeh, O. J., Agho, M. O. et al. 2005. An ethnobotanical survey of Bauchi state herbal plants and their antimicrobial activity. *Journal of Ethnopharmacology* 99: 1–4.

Ade-Omowaye, B. I. O., Rastogi, N. K., Angersbach, A. et al. 2002. Osmotic dehydration of bell peppers: influence of high intensity electric field pulses and elevated temperature treatment. *Journal of Food Engineering* 54: 35–43.

Antonio, A. S., Wiedemann, L. S. M., and Junior, V. V. 2018. The genus Capsicum: a phytochemical review of bioactive secondary metabolites. *RSC Advances* 8: 25767–25784.

Arimboor, R., Natarajan, R. B., Menon, K. R. et al. 2015. Red pepper (*Capsicum annuum*) carotenoids as a source of natural food colors: analysis and stability—a review. *Journal of Food Science and Technology* 52: 1258–1271.

Barbero, G. F., Palma, M., and Barroso, C. G. 2006. Determination of capsaicinoids in peppers by microwave-assisted extraction–high-performance liquid chromatography with fluorescence detection. *Analytica Chimica Acta* 578: 227–233.

Berke, T. G. and S. C. Shieh. 2001. Capsicum, chilies, paprika, bird's eye chili. In *Handbook of Herbs and Spices*, ed. K. V. Peter, Chapter 8, Volume 1, 111–121. CRC Publishing Ltd, Washington.

Bosland, P. W., Votava, E. J., and Votava, E. M. 2012. *Peppers: Vegetable and Spice Capsicums* (Vol. 22). CABI, UK

Catchpole, O. J., Grey, J. B., Perry, N. B. et al. 2003. Extraction of chili, black pepper, and ginger with near-critical CO_2, propane, and dimethyl ether: analysis of the extracts by quantitative nuclear magnetic resonance. *Journal of Agricultural and Food Chemistry* 51: 4853–4860.

Davis, C. B., Markey, C. E., Busch, M. A., et al. 2007. Determination of capsaicinoids in habanero peppers by chemometric analysis of UV spectral data. *Journal of Agricultural and Food Chemistry* 55: 5925–5933.

De Marino, S., Iorizzi, M. and Zollo, F. 2008. Antioxidant activity and biological properties of phytochemicals in vegetables and spices (Capsicum, Laurus, Foeniculum). *Electronic Journal on Environmental, Agricultural and Food Chemistry (EJEAFChe)* 7(10): 3174–3177.

Dengzongpa, D. R. and Sharma, L. 2013. *Organic Practices of Capsicum Cultivation*. Krishi Vigyan Kendra, Gyaba, West Sikkim.

Doymaz, I., and Ismail, O. 2013. Modeling of rehydration kinetics of green bell peppers. *Journal of Food Processing and Preservation* 37: 907–913.

Doymaz, İ., and Kocayigit, F. 2012. Effect of pre-treatments on drying, rehydration, and color characteristics of red pepper ('Charliston' variety). *Food Science and Biotechnology* 21: 1013–1022.

Doymaz, I., and Pala, M. 2002. Hot-air drying characteristics of red pepper. *Journal of Food Engineering* 55: 331–335.

El Asbahani, A., Miladi, K., Badri, W., et al. 2015. Essential oils: from extraction to encapsulation. *International Journal of Pharmaceutics* 483: 220–243.

Federzoni, V., Alvim, I. D., Fadini, A. L., et al. 2019. Co-crystallization of paprika oleoresin and storage stability study. *Food Science and Technology* 39: 182–189.

Fernández-Ronco, M. P., Gracia, I., de Lucas, A., et al. 2013. Extraction of *Capsicum annuum* oleoresin by maceration and ultrasound-assisted extraction: influence of parameters and process modeling. *Journal of Food Process Engineering* 36: 343–352.

Fraenkel, L., Bogardus, S. T., Concato, J., et al. 2004. Treatment options in knee osteoarthritis: the patient's perspective. *Archives of Internal Medicine* 164: 1299–1304.

Giovannucci, E. 2002. A review of epidemiologic studies of tomatoes, lycopene, and prostate cancer. *Experimental Biology and Medicine* 227: 852–859.

Goodwin, T. 2012. *The Biochemistry of the Carotenoids: Volume I Plants*. Springer Science & Business Media.

Gordon, H. T., Bauernfeind, J. C., and Furia, T. E. 1983. Carotenoids as food colorants. *CRC Critical Reviews in Food Science and Nutrition* 18: 59–97.

Govindarajan, V. S. 1986a. Capsicum - Production, technology, chemistry and quality. Part II. World production and trade. *CRC Critical Reviews in Food Science and Nutrition* 23(3): 207–287.

Govindarajan, V. S. 1986b. Capsicum - Production, technology, chemistry and quality. Part III. Chemistry of the color, aroma and pungency. *CRC Critical Reviews in Food Science and Nutrition* 24(3): 245–533.

Govindarajan, V. S., and Salzer, U. J. 1986. Capsicum—production, technology, chemistry, and quality—Part II. Processed products, standards, world production and trade. *Critical Reviews in Food Science & Nutrition* 23: 207–288.

Hilton, M. D. 1999. Small-scale liquid fermentations. *Manual of Industrial Microbiology and Biotechnology* 49–60.

Hornero-Méndez, D., Costa-García, J., and Mínguez-Mosquera, M. I. 2002. Characterization of carotenoid high-producing *Capsicum annuum* cultivars selected for paprika production. *Journal of Agricultural and Food Chemistry* 50: 5711–5716.

Hu, Y., Wang, S., Wang, S., and Lu, X. 2017. Application of nuclear magnetic resonance spectroscopy in food adulteration determination: the example of Sudan dye I in paprika powder. *Scientific Reports* 7: 1–9.

Jaren-Galan, M., Nienaber, U., and Schwartz, S. J. 1999. Paprika (*Capsicum annuum*) oleoresin extraction with supercritical carbon dioxide. *Journal of Agricultural and Food Chemistry* 47: 3558–3564.

Johnson Jr, W. 2007. Final report on the safety assessment of *Capsicum annuum* extract, *Capsicum annuum* fruit extract, *Capsicum annuum* resin, *Capsicum annuum* fruit powder, *Capsicum frutescens* fruit, *Capsicum frutescens* fruit extract, *Capsicum frutescens* resin, and capsaicin. *International Journal of Toxicology*, 26 Suppl 1: 3–106.

Kalloo, G., and Pandey, A. K. 2002. Commendable progress in research. *The Hindu Survey of India*, 159–163.

Kanki, K., Nishikawa, A., Furukawa, F., Kitamura, Y., et al. 2003. A 13-week subchronic toxicity study of paprika color in F344 rats. *Food and Chemical Toxicology* 41: 1337–1343.

Kannan, K., Jawaharlal, M., and Prabhu, M. 2009. Effect of plant growth regulators on paprika review. *Agricultural Reviews* 30: 229–232

Khan, F. A., Mahmood, T., Ali, M., Saeed, A., et al. 2014. Pharmacological importance of an ethnobotanical plant: *Capsicum annuum* L. *Natural Product Research* 28: 1267–1274.

KoffiAffoué, C., Adjogoua, E. V., Yao, K., et al. 2015. Cytotoxic and antiviral activity of methanolic, ethanolic and acetate extracts of six varieties of Capsicum. *International Journal of Current Microbiology and Applied Sciences* 4: 76–88.

Krajayklang, M., Klieber, A., and Dry, P. R. 2000. Colour at harvest and post-harvest behaviour influence paprika and chilli spice quality. *Postharvest Biology and Technology* 20: 269–278.

Kumar, P., Chauhan, R. C., and Grover, R. K. 2016. Economic analysis of capsicum cultivation under polyhouse and open field conditions in Haryana. *International Journal of Farm Sciences* 6: 96–100.

Kumar, S., Patel, N. Saravaiya, S. 2018. Analysis of bell pepper (Capsicum annuum) cultivation in response to fertigation and training systems under protected environment. *Indian Journal of Agricultural Sciences* 88. 1077–1082.

Lakner, Z., Szabó, E., Szűcs, V., et al. 2018. Network and vulnerability analysis of international spice trade. *Food Control* 83: 141–146.

Lokaewmanee, K., Yamauchi, K., and Okuda, N. 2013. Effects of dietary red pepper on egg yolk colour and histological intestinal morphology in laying hens. *Journal of Animal Physiology and Animal Nutrition* 97: 986–995.

Mínguez-Mosquera, M. I., Pérez-Gálvez, A., and Hornero-Méndez, D. 2008. Color quality in red pepper (*Capsicum annuum*, L.) and derived products. In: *Color Quality of Fresh and Processed Foods*, eds. C. A. Culver and R. E. Wrolstad, 311–327, American Chemical Society.

Mohd Hassan, N., Yusof, N. A., Yahaya, A. F., et al. 2019. Carotenoids of capsicum fruits: Pigment profile and health-promoting functional attributes. *Antioxidants* 8(10): 469. https://doi.org/10.3390/antiox8100469.

Mori, A., Lehmann, S., O'Kelly, J., et al. 2006. Capsaicin, a component of red peppers, inhibits the growth of androgen-independent, p53 mutant prostate cancer cells. *Cancer Research* 66: 3222–3229.

Moscone, E. A., Scaldaferro, M. A., Grabiele, M., et al. 2006. The evolution of chili peppers (Capsicum-Solanaceae): a cytogenetic perspective. In *VI International Solanaceae Conference: Genomics Meets Biodiversity* 745: 137–170.

Nurjanah, S., Sudaryanto, Z., Widyasanti, A., et al. 2014. Antibacterial activity of *Capsicum annuum* L. oleoresin. In *XXIX International Horticultural Congress on Horticulture: Sustaining Lives, Livelihoods and Landscapes (IHC2014): V World* 1125: 189–194.

Pacholczyk-Sienicka, B., Ciepielowski, G., and Albrecht, Ł. 2021. The application of NMR spectroscopy and chemometrics in authentication of spices. *Molecules* 26(2): 382. https://doi.org/10.3390/molecules26020382.

Palevitch, D., and Craker, L. E. 1996. Nutritional and medical importance of red pepper (*Capsicum* spp.). *Journal of Herbs, Spices & Medicinal Plants* 3: 55–83.

Park, J. H., Jeon, G. I., Kim, J. M., et al. 2012. Antioxidant activity and antiproliferative action of methanol extracts of 4 different colored bell peppers (*Capsicum annuum* L.). *Food Science and Biotechnology* 21: 543–550.

Parvez, G. M. 2017. Current advances in pharmacological activity and toxic effects of various *Capsicum* species. *International Journal of Pharmaceutical Sciences and Research* 8: 1900–1912.

Perva-Uzunalić, A., Škerget, M., Weinreich, B., et al. 2004. Extraction of chilli pepper (var. Byedige) with supercritical CO_2: effect of pressure and temperature on capsaicinoid and colour extraction efficiency. *Food Chemistry* 87: 51–58.

Porras-Saavedra, J., Alamilla-Beltrán, L., Lartundo-Rojas, L., et al. 2018. Chemical components distribution and morphology of microcapsules of paprika oleoresin by microscopy and spectroscopy. *Food Hydrocolloids* 81: 6–14.

Riquelme, N., and Matiacevich, S. 2017. Characterization and evaluation of some properties of oleoresin from *Capsicum annuum* var. cacho de cabra. cacho de cabra. *CyTA Journal of Food*, 15(3): 344–351.

Singh, T., and Chittenden, C. 2008. In-vitro antifungal activity of chilli extracts in combination with *Lactobacillus casei* against common sapstain fungi. *International Biodeterioration & Biodegradation* 62: 364–367.

Spiller, F., Alves, M. K., Vieira, S. M., et al. 2008. Anti-inflammatory effects of red pepper (*Capsicum baccatum*) on carrageenan-and antigen-induced inflammation. *Journal of Pharmacy and Pharmacology* 60: 473–478.

Tepić, A. N., Dimić, G. R., Vujičić, B. L., et al. 2008. Quality of commercial ground paprika and its oleoresins. *Acta Periodica Technologica* 39: 77–83.

Vega-Gálvez, A. L. M. S., Lemus-Mondaca, R., et al. 2008. Effect of air drying temperature on the quality of rehydrated dried red bell pepper (var. Lamuyo). *Journal of Food Engineering* 85: 42–50.

Vinas, P., Campillo, N., García, I. L., and Córdoba, M. H. 1992. Liquid chromatographic determination of fat-soluble vitamins in paprika and paprika oleoresin. *Food Chemistry* 45: 349–355.

Vicente, J. L., Lopez, C., Avila, E., Morales, E., et al. 2007. Effect of dietary natural capsaicin on experimental *Salmonella enteritidis* infection and yolk pigmentation in laying hens. *International Journal of Poultry Science* 6: 393–396.

Index

Note: **Bold** page numbers refer to tables; *italic* page numbers refer to figures.

For Product Safety Concerns and Information please contact our EU
representative GPSR@taylorandfrancis.com
Taylor & Francis Verlag GmbH, Kaufingerstraße 24, 80331 München, Germany

www.ingramcontent.com/pod-product-compliance
Lightning Source LLC
Chambersburg PA
CBHW080133220326
41598CB00032B/5052

9 781032 030029